Kath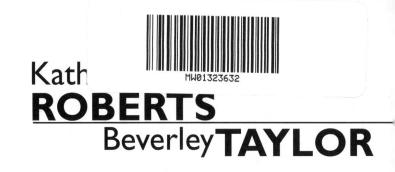
ROBERTS
Beverley **TAYLOR**

Nursing Research Processes
An Australian Perspective
second edition

THOMSON

Australia · Canada · Mexico · Singapore · Spain · United Kingdom · United States

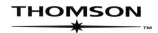

102 Dodds Street
Southbank Victoria 3006

Email highereducation@thomsonlearning.com.au
Website http://www.thomsonlearning.com.au

First published in 1998
This second edition published in 2002
10 9 8 7 6 5 4 3 2
05 04 03 02

Copyright © 2002 Nelson Australia Pty Limited.

COPYRIGHT
Apart from fair dealing for the purposes of study, research, criticism or review, or as permitted under Part VB of the Copyright Act, no part of this book may be reproduced by any process without permission. Copyright owners may take legal action against a person who infringes on their copyright through unauthorised copying. Enquiries should be directed to the publisher.

National Library of Australia
Cataloguing-in-Publication data

Roberts, Kathryn L. (Kathryn Louise), 1943–.
   Nursing research processes: an Australian perspective.

   2nd ed.
   Bibliography.
   Includes index.
   Tertiary students.
   ISBN 0 17 010402 8.

   1. Nursing – Research – Australia. 2. Nurses – Research – Australia. 3. Research – Australia – Management. I. Taylor, Beverley J. (Beverley Joan), 1951–. II. Title.

610.73072094

Editor: Robyn Whiteley
Project editors: Jo Tayler and David Parnham
Publishing editor: Glen Sheldon
Text designer: John Canty
Cover designer: Jo Groud
Cover illustrator: Rosanna Vecchio
Indexer: Fay Donlevy
Typeset in Bembo in 11.5/13 pt by Susan Lawrence
Production controller: Sally Chick
Printed in Singapore by Markono

This title is published under the imprint of Thomson.
Nelson Australia Pty Limited ACN 058 280 149 (incorporated in Victoria) trading as Nelson Thomson Learning.

Foreword

I was very pleased to have had the opportunity to write the foreword for the first edition of this book; I am even more pleased to have been invited to introduce this second edition.

The evaluation of nursing activity and the generation of knowledge for nursing practice is now of central importance in any health system that has embraced the concept of evidence-based practice. Evidence-based nursing focuses on the need for nurses to use those interventions that are supported by the most up-to-date evidence or knowledge available. The evidence-based approach acknowledges the difficulties faced by busy practitioners in keeping up to date with an ever-growing literature in health care and emphasises the importance of providing them with condensed information gathered through the systematic review of the international literature on a given topic.

Despite nursing's relatively recent interest in research, there is a growing amount of evidence on which to base practice. The recent establishment of nursing in the universities has generated research training, which has contributed significantly to the development of nursing as an academic discipline and is beginning to make a contribution to an evidence base for practice. The first edition of this book played an important part in the development of research-mindedness and research activity in Australian nursing. Drawing on feedback from readers, the authors have made substantial revisions to strengthen the content and I congratulate them on their continuing work on dispelling the myths that surround research through writing in a way that is accessible and enjoyable.

Alan Pearson

This book is dedicated:

by Kathryn Roberts, to Ron Roberts, for his mentorship, editorship and, most of all, his love;

by Bev Taylor, to the memory of David Ariaratnam, a Bachelor of Nursing (Honours) student, who drowned tragically at Byron Bay on 12 February 1997 – for all he would have loved to have known about nursing research;

and by both of us, to all of the nurses in Australia who have undertaken research for the purpose of advancing the knowledge base of our discipline.

Contents

Foreword	*iii*
Preface	*xii*
Acknowledgements	*xiii*

Section 1: Preparing and planning for research

Chapter 1: Research and nursing — 1
by Kathryn Roberts and Beverley Taylor

Chapter objectives	1
Introduction	2
Nurses 'doing' research	2
History of nursing research and influences on it	3
The current scene	6
Knowledge and research	7
Types of nursing research	12
Summary	21
Main points	21
Review questions	23
Discussion questions	24
References	24

Chapter 2: The research question — 28
by Kathryn Roberts

Chapter objectives	28
Introduction	29
Finding nursing research problems: sources and strategies	29
Criteria for selecting problems	33
Stating the problem/question/purpose of the study	37
The process	38
Stating an hypothesis and identifying variables	39
Summary	40
Main points	41
Review questions	41
Discussion questions	43
References	43

Chapter 3: Reviewing the literature — 45
by Kathryn Roberts

Chapter objectives	45
Introduction	46
Why review the literature?	46
Identifying relevant literature	47
Possible resources	49

The mechanics of searching	53
Selecting literature	58
Acquiring your own collection of information	59
Reading and documenting the information	61
Critiquing individual reports	63
Putting it together	71
Summary	72
Main points	72
Review questions	73
Discussion questions	74
References	75

Chapter 4: Research and its relationship to theory — 76
by Kathryn Roberts

Chapter objectives	76
Introduction	77
Theory – what is it?	77
Historical usage of theoretical frameworks in nursing research	79
Use of nursing and health theories and models in nursing research	79
How to use a conceptual framework in a research study	87
Developing theory from research	88
Summary	88
Main points	88
Review questions	89
Discussion questions	91
References	91

Chapter 5: Ethics in nursing research — 95
by Kathryn Roberts

Chapter objectives	95
Introduction	96
Historical examples of unethical research conduct	96
Codes of ethics and research ethics guidelines	98
Protecting the rights of human participants	99
Ethical aspects of research in special cases	112
Human Research Ethics Committees	115
Research ethics in the practice of nursing	118
Scientific misconduct	118
Reading a research report: ethical considerations	120
Summary	120
Main points	121
Review questions	121
Discussion questions	123
References	123

Chapter 6: Obtaining approval and support for your project 126
by Kathryn Roberts and Beverley Taylor
    Chapter objectives 126
    Introduction 127
    The research proposal 127
    Funding 166
    Obtaining informal approvals 166
    Summary 167
    Main points 168
    Review questions 169
    Discussion questions 170
    References 170

Section 2: Designing and doing research
Chapter 7: Quantitative research methodology **175**
by Kathryn Roberts
    Chapter objectives 175
    Introduction 176
    Major types of research designs 176
    Validity in scientific research 179
    Types of experimental designs 183
    Summary 194
    Main points 194
    Review questions 195
    Discussion questions 197
    References 197

Chapter 8: Quantitative methods 199
by Kathryn Roberts
    Chapter objectives 199
    Introduction 200
    Choosing a setting 200
    Defining the population 201
    Sampling 202
    Quantitative methods of obtaining data 207
    Summary 234
    Main points 234
    Review questions 236
    Discussion questions 237
    References 237

Chapter 9: Quantitative data collection and management 241
by Kathryn Roberts
    Chapter objectives 241
    Introduction 242
    Preparing for data collection and management 242

The process of data collection	249
Management of data and products of analysis	254
Pilot study	258
Summary	260
Main points	261
Review questions	262
Discussion questions	263
References	263

Chapter 10: Quantitative data analysis — 265
by Kathryn Roberts

Chapter objectives	265
Introduction	266
Quantitative data analysis	266
Scales	267
Descriptive statistics	268
Introduction to probability and inferential statistics	277
Want to learn more about statistics?	288
Summary	288
Main points	288
Review questions	289
Discussion questions	290
References	290

Chapter 11: Interpreting quantitative findings — 292
by Kathryn Roberts

Chapter objectives	292
Introduction	293
Preparation	293
Interpreting descriptive findings	293
Relationship findings	294
Summary	300
Main points	300
Review questions	301
Discussion questions	303
References	303

Chapter 12: Qualitative interpretive methodologies — 304
by Beverley Taylor

Chapter objectives	304
Introduction	305
Research as a means of generating knowledge	305
Defining epistemology and ontology	306
Some common qualitative theoretical assumptions	307
Differences between quantitative and qualitative research	308

Postmodern influences on contemporary epistemology and
  ontology   309
Differences between interpretive and critical qualitative methodologies 310
Postmodern alternatives for qualitative methodologies   311
Grounded theory   313
Phenomenology   319
Ethnography   324
Historical research   328
Summary   332
Main points   332
Review questions   333
Discussion questions   335
References   335

Chapter 13: Qualitative critical methodologies 340
by Beverley Taylor

Chapter objectives   340
Introduction   340
Common qualitative critical theoretical assumptions   342
Critical methodologies compared with poststructuralism   343
Poststructuralism compared with postmodern thought   344
Defining critical terms   345
Action research   347
Feminisms   352
Critical ethnography   359
Nursing research discourse reflecting postmodern influences   362
The co-author's postscript to postmodernism   366
Summary   367
Main points   367
Review questions   368
Discussion questions   370
References   370

Chapter 14: Qualitative methods 374
by Beverley Taylor

Chapter objectives   374
Introduction   375
Choosing congruent methods   375
Research contexts and participants   376
Rigour in qualitative research   377
Methods that may be used in qualitative research   382
Summary   398
Main points   399
Review questions   401
Discussion questions   402
References   403

Chapter 15: Qualitative data collection and management — 406
by Beverley Taylor

Chapter objectives	406
Introduction	407
Forms of qualitative data	407
The usefulness of qualitative data	408
Strategies for collecting the data	412
Use of computers in qualitative data collection and management	416
Summary	418
Main points	418
Review questions	420
Discussion questions	421
References	422

Chapter 16: Qualitative data analysis — 423
by Beverley Taylor

Chapter objectives	423
Introduction	424
Approaches to analysing qualitative data	424
Other methods of text analysis	434
Computer systems that manage qualitative data	438
Examples of completed qualitative analyses	440
Adjust analytic methods with a rationale	442
The analysis of images as qualitative data	443
Summary	443
Main points	444
Review questions	445
Discussion questions	447
References	447

Chapter 17: Interpreting qualitative findings — 449
by Beverley Taylor

Chapter objectives	449
Introduction	450
Differentiation between analysis and interpretation	450
Qualitative research findings as relative interpretations	452
Qualitative findings in relation to methodological approaches	454
Qualitative interpretive and critical categories of interpretive processes	455
Processes for synthesising qualitative interpretive and critical results	457
Summary	464
Main points	465
Review questions	467
Discussion questions	468
References	468

Section 3: Disseminating and applying research

Chapter 18: Disseminating the findings   470
by Kathryn Roberts and Beverley Taylor

Chapter objectives	470
Introduction	471
The research report	471
The written report	473
Presenting a report at professional meetings	501
Writing for a wider audience	505
Summary	508
Main points	508
Review questions	509
Discussion questions	511
References	511

Chapter 19: Using nursing research   513
by Kathryn Roberts

Chapter objectives	513
Introduction	514
Applying nursing research to practice	514
Summary	524
Main points	525
Review questions	526
Discussion questions	527
References	527
Glossary	*530*
Answers to review questions	*540*
Index	*541*

Preface

When the first edition of this book was published in 1998, students were at last able to access a research text written by Australian nurse-researchers. The success of the first edition reflects the warm reception of the Australian nursing context and content. In this, the second edition, we have continued the use of Australian nursing research examples, updating them where possible to portray the current research scene.

Another feature of the first edition that was well received was the equal space devoted to quantitative and qualitative research approaches, which reflected the coming of age of qualitative research in nursing in this country. In this edition, the content falls into three sections – preparation and planning, design and execution and, finally, dissemination and application of both qualitative and quantitative research. We feel that this arrangement makes access more convenient.

Our decision to make the text user-friendly, by using a more informal voice than had traditionally been used in such texts, was a resounding success and is continued in this edition of the book. We have also taken note of feedback from users and have incorporated main points and student exercises (through review questions and discussion questions) as well as a larger number of examples and much more content on postmodernism.

Although this book was written initially for undergraduate nurses, other people have found it useful also, for example nurses in clinical practice, and honours and postgraduate students.

We hope that the second edition will also be well received.

Kathryn Roberts
Bev Taylor

Acknowledgements

The authors would like to acknowledge the contribution of their respective universities, Northern Territory University and the Southern Cross University, towards the making and revision of this book.

The authors and publisher would like gratefully to credit or acknowledge permission to reproduce text material:

Allen, D.G. 1995, p. 458, 'Hermeneutics: philosophical traditions and nursing practice research', *Nursing Science Quarterly*, vol. 8, no. 4, 174–182. Reprinted by permission of Sage Publications; Bailey, S. 1998, p. 31, 'An exploration of critical care nurses' and doctors' attitudes towards psychiatric patients', *Australian Journal of Advanced Nursing*, vol. 15, no. 3, 8–14, ANF; Black, A. & Childs, G. 1994, p. 29, 'Staff attachment and loss in a long-term baby ward', *Contemporary Nurse*, vol. 4, no. 4, 153–161; Borbasi, S. 1996, p. 323, 'Living the experience of being nursed', *International Journal of Nursing Practice*, vol. 2, 222–8, Blackwell Science; Brink, P. & Wood, M. 1994, pp. 29, 41, *Basic Steps in Planning Research*, London: Jones & Bartlett, Sudbury, MA, 2, http://www.jbpub.com. Reprinted by permission; Burns, S. & Grove, N. 1993, pp. 323–4, 379, *The Practice of Nursing Research: Conduct, Critique and Utilisation*, Philadelphia: W.B. Saunders Company, 71, 64; Cheek, J. 2000, pp. 345, 437, 438, *Postmodern and Poststructural Approaches to Nursing Research*, 124, 51, 52, © 2000 by Sage Publications, Inc., California. Reprinted by permission of Sage Publications; Chenoweth, L. & Kilstoff, K. 1998, pp. 350, 351, 'Facilitating positive changes in community dementia management through participatory action research', *International Journal of Nursing Practice*, vol. 4, 175–88, Blackwell Science; Chinn, P. & Kramer, M. 1993, p. 11, *Theory and Nursing: A Systematic Approach*, St Louis: Mosby Year Book; Emden, C. 1998, pp. 435, 436, 'Conducting a narrative analysis', *Collegian*, vol. 5, no. 3, 34–9, RCNA; Emden, C. & Sandelowski, M. 1998, pp. 381, 382, 'The good, the bad and the relative: conceptions of goodness in qualitative research: part one', *International Journal of Nursing Practice*, vol. 4, no. 4, 206–12; Erickson, H., Tomlin, M. & Swain, M. 1983, p. 8, *Modeling and Remodeling: A Theory and Paradigm for Nursing*, Englewood Cliffs, NJ: Prentice-Hall, 29; Fahy, K. 1997, pp. 363, 364, 'Postmodern feminist emancipatory research: is it an oxymoron?', *Nursing Inquiry*, vol. 4, 27–33, Blackwell Science; Fawcett, J. 1989, p. 10, *Analysis and Evaluation of Conceptual Models of Nursing*, 2nd edn, Philadelphia: F.A. Davis, 5; Fiveash, B. 1998, pp. 326, 327, 'The experience of nursing home life', *International Journal of Nursing Practice*, vol. 4, 166–74, Blackwell Science; Glass, N. 1998, pp. 355, 356, 'The contested work place: reactions to hospital based RNs doing degrees', *Collegian*, vol. 5, no. 1, 24–31, RCNA; Glass, N. & Davis, K. 1998, pp. 353, 364, 365, 366, 'An emancipatory impulse: a feminist postmodern integrated turning point in nursing research', *Advances in Nursing Science*, vol. 21, no. 1, 43–52, University of Connecticut; Glass, N. 2000, pp. 352, 353, 354, 'Speaking feminisms and nursing', in J. Greenwood (ed.), *Nursing Theory in Australia: Development and Application*, Frenchs Forest: Pearson Education Australia, pp. 357, 360, 362, 363, 368, 369; Gray, G. & Pratt, R. (eds) 1991, pp. 17–18, *Towards a Discipline of Nursing*, Melbourne: Churchill Livingstone, 7; Hicks, C. 1996, p. 518, *Undertaking Midwifery Research*, Edinburgh: Churchill Livingstone, vii, by permission of the publisher; Jackson, D. & Raftos, M. 1997, pp. 357, 358, 'In uncharted waters: confronting the culture of silence in a residential care institution', *International Journal of Nursing Practice*, vol. 3, 34–9, Blackwell Science; Johnstone, M.-J. 1999, p. 330, 'Reflective topical autobiography: an underutilised interpretive research method in nursing', *Collegian*, vol. 6, no. 1, 24–9, RCNA; Jones, C. & Chapman, Y. 2000, pp. 321, 322, 'The lived experience of seven people treated with autologous bone marrow/peripheral blood stem cell transplant', *International Journal of Nursing Practice*, vol. 6, 153–9, Blackwell Science; Josipovic, P. 2000, p. 327,

'Recommendations for culturally sensitive nursing care', *International Journal of Nursing Practice*, vol. 6, 146–152, Blackwell Science; Keatinge, D. et al. 2000, p. 349, 'The manifestation and nursing management of agitation in institutionalised residents with dementia', *International Journal of Nursing Practice*, vol. 6, 16–25, Blackwell Science; Kellett, U. 1998, p. 323, 'Meaning-making for family carers in nursing homes', *International Journal of Nursing Practice*, vol. 4, 113–19, Blackwell Science; Koch, T., Kralik, D. & Kelly, S. 2000, p. 350, 'We just don't talk about it: men living with urinary incontinence and multiple sclerosis', *International Journal of Nursing Practice*, vol. 6, 253–60, Blackwell Science; Leininger, M. 1970, p. 324, *Nursing and Anthropology: Two Worlds to Blend*, New York: John Wiley & Sons, 48–9; Leininger, M. 1985, p. 324, *Qualitative Research Methods in Nursing*, New York: Grune & Stratton, 35, 238; Lincoln, Y.S. 1995, p. 381, 'The making of a constructivist – a remembrance of transformations past', in E.G. Guba (ed.), *The Paradigm Dialogue*, Newbury Park: Sage Publications; Logan, P. 1999, p. 278, 'Venepuncture versus heel prick for the collection of the newborn screening test', *Australian Journal of Advanced Nursing*, vol. 17, no. 1, 30–6, ANF; Lumby, J. 1991, p. 7, 'Threads of an emerging discipline', in *Towards a Discipline of Nursing*, G. Gray & R. Pratt (eds), 478, by permission of the publisher Harcourt Australia; Lumby, J. 1997, p. 356, 'Liver transplantation: the death/life paradox', *International Journal of Nursing Practice*, vol. 3, 231–8, Blackwell Science; Lyneham, J. 2000, p. 31, 'Violence in New South Wales Emergency Departments', *Australian Journal of Advanced Nursing*, vol. 18, no. 2, 8–17, ANF; McTaggart, R. 1991, p. 347, 'Principles for participatory action research', *Adult Education Quarterly*, vol. 41, no. 3, 168–87. Reprinted by permission of Sage Publications; Moody, L. 1990, p. 7, *Advancing Nursing Science through Nursing Research*, vol. 2, 20, by Sage Publications, Inc., California. Reprinted by permission of Sage Publications; Pearson, A. et al. 1997, pp. 516, 521, Evidence-based nursing: an examination of nursing within the international evidence based health care practice movement. Discussion Paper No. 1, Royal College of Nursing Australia, 3, 1; Powers, P. 1996, p. 437, 'Discourse analysis as a methodology for nursing inquiry', *Nursing Inquiry*, vol. 3, 207–17, Blackwell Science; Robertson, J. 1994, pp. 37–8, 'Intermittent intravenous therapy: a comparison of two flushing solutions', *Contemporary Nurse*, vol. 3, no. 4, 174–9; Rosenau, P. 1992, pp. 309, 310, 312, 341, 344, 345, 406, 458, 459, *Post-Modernism and the Social Sciences: Insights, Inroads and Intrusions*, New Jersey: Princeton University Press, 15, 42, 63, 78, 96, 31, 57, 80, 137, 15, 3, 14, 13, 85, 96, 120; Rossiter, J. & Yam, B. 1998, p. 327, 'Promoting the nursing profession: the perceptions of non-English-speaking background high school students in Sydney, Australia', *International Journal of Nursing Practice*, vol. 4, 213–19, Blackwell Science; Russell, R.L. 1990, p. 331, *From Nightingale to Now: Nurse Education in Australia*, Sydney: Harcourt, back cover of book, by permission of Harcourt Australia; Santamaria, N. 2000, p. 37, 'The relationship between nurses' personality and stress levels reported when caring for interpersonally difficult patients', *Australian Journal of Advanced Nursing*, vol. 18, no. 2, 20–6, ANF; St John, W. 1999, pp. 316, 317, 'Beyond the sick role: situating community health nursing practice', *Collegian*, vol. 6, no. 1, 30–5, RCNA; Speedy, S. 1987, p. 353, 'Feminism and the professionalization of nursing', *Australian Journal of Advanced Nursing*, vol. 4, no. 2, 20–8, ANF; Street, A. 1995, p. 220, *Nursing Replay: Researching Nursing Culture Together*, Melbourne: Churchill Livingstone, 105; Walter, R., Davis, K. & Glass, N. 1999, pp. 354, 355, 'Discovery of self: exploring, interconnecting and integrating self (concept) and nursing', *Collegian*, vol. 6, no. 2, 12–15, RCNA; Wellard, S. & Palaster, L. 1996, pp. 359, 360, 361, 'An evaluation of two methods of pre-cannulation skin disinfection', *Australian Journal of Advanced Nursing*, vol. 14, no. 1, 132–6, ANF; Yuginovich, T. 2000, pp. 328, 329, 'More than time and place: using historical comparative research as a tool for nursing', *International Journal of Nursing Practice*, vol. 6, 70–5, Blackwell Science; Zeitz, K. 1999, pp. 322–3, 'Nurses as patients: the voyage of discovery', *International Journal of Nursing Practice*, vol. 5, 64–71, Blackwell Science.

Every attempt has been made to trace and acknowledge copyright holders. Where the attempt has been unsuccessful, the publisher welcomes information that would redress the situation.

Research and nursing

chapter objectives

The material presented in this chapter will assist you to:

- describe the ways that nurses can carry out research
- understand the historical evolution of nursing research
- understand what knowledge is and how it is produced
- distinguish between the various types of research paradigms
- use computers in nursing.

Introduction

Research is 'a careful search or inquiry, a course of critical investigation' (Sykes 1976). Have you ever asked why people do research when it takes so much skill, time, money and patience? Nurses want to find answers to questions so that they will stand up to scrutiny by their peers. Nursing research is a systematic process of investigating phenomena of interest, the general purpose of which is to add to the body of knowledge about the practice of nursing and about health in humans. For example, nurses may wish to study what factors are important in the promotion of health and the prevention of illness. They may also want to find the best solution to a practice problem. Or they may be curious about some phenomenon such as dying.

Is nursing a research-based profession? Not yet. Although the tendency for nurses to conduct research and heed research findings is increasing, there is still insufficient research. There is also a time lag between development and implementation of research. Further, theory derived from research is not immediately applied to the everyday work, concerns and issues of clinical nursing practice.

We need more clinical research in nursing so that we can show that we have based our care on the best available practice. This means using research evidence to support our clinical decision-making. We can also use research findings to demonstrate that clients have improved health as a result of nursing care and that nursing therefore makes a valuable contribution to the health of our society. We must do this if we want to preserve our professional status and guard against encroachment on our practice by other occupational groups.

In this chapter, we shall discuss how nurses can participate in nursing research, give a brief account of the history of nursing research, address the nature of knowledge in general and nursing knowledge in particular, describe paradigmatic approaches to nursing research and introduce the topic of computers in nursing research.

Nurses 'doing' research

Nurses can participate in nursing research in various ways. At an independent level, a nurse may conduct the whole project alone. This takes a considerable amount of training, preferably to the doctoral level. At an interdependent level, a nurse may participate in a research project in collaboration with other researchers. Interdependence implies that the nurse makes a contribution to the conceptualisation, implementation, evaluation and dissemination of the project. At a dependent level of participation, a nurse may be a data collector for another researcher's project, but does not make a significant contribution to the conceptual part of the project.

Nursing research provides many opportunities to collaborate with nurses in the discipline of nursing and with people from other disciplines who are interested in nursing and health. Because nursing involves the areas of person, nursing, environment and health, there is a great deal of scope for collaboration in projects that have a specific focus or that cover a range of domains. It may be possible to set up collaborative projects in which nurses undertake research with other nurses, with other health care researchers, or with people from other disciplines.

Nurses in practice, administrative and teaching settings have opportunities to collaborate with other nurses on research projects. For example, a group of clinicians working within the same ward or unit may have a specific practice question they wish to pursue. Also, they may like to work with nurses across various wards or units in the same health care facility, or to collaborate on a larger project that may require more research participants and the expertise of multiple researchers. Nurses working in practice, administration and teaching may choose to collaborate on research projects that are informative for them in their various nursing roles.

Nurses can also collaborate with researchers from other health care disciplines. Health care requires the expertise of many workers qualified in different fields of practice, such as doctors, physiotherapists, speech therapists, nutritionists, occupational therapists and so on. The complexity of human problems when body dysfunction is present means that the overall needs of patients are often best met by multi-disciplinary teams in hospitals and community organisations. Many research questions that can directly benefit patient care can be raised within multi-disciplinary teams. In these cases, nurses may choose to work with other health care workers on research projects, but they must guard their interests and resist the efforts of others to take over or downplay their contributions.

A great deal of expertise may be available to nurse researchers who are open to working with specialists from disciplines other than nursing and health-related disciplines. Researchers with a background in human sciences, such as sociology, psychology and education, may be invaluable sources of assistance and support for anyone undertaking nursing research. For example, a researcher skilled and experienced in reflective practice and critical perspectives for change may facilitate collaborative research projects with nurses in their work settings.

Research collaboration is possible between nurses and other nurse researchers, other health care researchers, and researchers from other disciplines. It may take time, energy, opportunities and organisational skills before projects get under way, but the rewards can be many for nursing and for the other people with whom the nurses collaborate.

History of nursing research and influences on it

Florence Nightingale, who documented the factors that affected the morbidity and mortality of soldiers wounded in the Crimean war, has been hailed as the first nurse-researcher. After the time of Nightingale, the centre of nursing research activity changed to the United States, where the history of nursing research has been further described by Moody (1990) and Abdellah and Levine (1994). Australia is following the American trends, but 20 years later. The main reason for this is not that Australian nurses are backward in comparison with American nurses, but that it took 20 years longer for us to initiate the major prerequisite for the development of nursing research, which was the entry of basic nursing education into the tertiary education system.

During the first half of the twentieth century, nursing went through a phase in which service was paramount. There was almost no clinical nursing research during this period, the emphasis being on the improvement of nursing through better management. This reflected an industrial trend towards efficiency through the development of such strategies as the assembly line.

In Australia, an academic period of nursing began in the 1950s, and is still with us in the 2000s. Post-basic nursing education was the first area to enter that phase. Nurses began to do post-basic tertiary diplomas in education and administration at colleges of advanced education when these courses became available from the New South Wales College of Nursing and the Royal College of Nursing, Australia in Melbourne, Perth, and Brisbane. Nurses took these courses to acquire credentials for advancement in the teaching and administration of nursing. Then nurses began to do undergraduate degrees in those disciplines, but there was little research involved in these courses. By the early 1980s, many nurses anticipated that nursing would move into the tertiary education sector, and decided to emulate what they saw happening in other disciplines by preparing themselves with postgraduate degrees. Because postgraduate nursing degrees did not as yet exist in this country, they acquired degrees in education, management, and behavioural sciences. The research produced by these nurses accounted for the bulk of research activity at that time.

Because these nurses had to do degrees in disciplines other than nursing, their research resulted in the development of non-nursing knowledge rather than nursing knowledge. Their research was on such topics as the education, administration, psychology, sociology and anthropology of nurses. This might at first sound like a heretical statement. But, if you think about it, the knowledge of nursing education that has been built up through research is knowledge about education, not about the practice of nursing. Similarly, knowledge about the psychology or sociology of nurses is knowledge about psychology or sociology, not about nursing practice. That is not to say, of course, that the knowledge of concern to nurses should be limited to nursing practice knowledge.

The move of basic nursing education into the tertiary education sector was an important influence on the development of nursing research in this country, but it was an indirect influence, as it did not result directly in an increased production of nursing research. It did, however, create a demand for nurses with postgraduate education who could teach the courses, and it built up a pool of educated nurses who would later enter postgraduate courses and do research.

The demand for basic tertiary education courses for nurses began when nurses in higher professional positions began to study for advanced educational qualifications and to examine their own education programs. They began to realise that they were the only health profession that was not educated in the tertiary education system to degree level and questioned why this was so.

A period of professional lobbying ensued under the auspices of professional organisations that banded together, despite their previous differences, to achieve the goal of tertiary education for nurses. Many reports recommending a transfer of nursing education to the tertiary sector were additional fodder for arguments (Russell 1990).

This lobbying was resisted fairly strongly by both the Commonwealth government and the tertiary education system, ostensibly because nursing did not need a college education and the quality of care would suffer if nurse training started turning out theoretical rather than practical nurses. However, a major factor contributing to the resistance was undoubtedly fear about the cost of the transfer. Nursing education had come out of the states' health budgets while tertiary education was funded under the Commonwealth budget, so a transfer meant that costs would be shifted from the states to the Commonwealth. Nevertheless, by 1978, six pilot basic nursing education programs had been established across Australia. These were at Cumberland College of Health Sciences in Sydney, Riverina College of Advanced Education in Wagga Wagga, Lincoln Institute of Health Sciences and Preston Institute of Technology in Melbourne, Sturt College of Advanced Education in Adelaide, and Western Australian Institute of Technology in Perth (Russell 1990). These courses were at the undergraduate diploma level and did not normally feature research, which was not seen as core business of the colleges.

The Dawkins reforms in the tertiary education sector, implemented in the late 1980s, resulted in the merger of colleges of advanced education and universities. As a result, the basic nursing entry to professional practice became a baccalaureate degree, with nursing research units being incorporated into the courses.

After the basic degree courses had been established, postgraduate courses in nursing began to develop and to a large extent they have replaced courses in nursing education and administration as the area of choice for nurses' study. The PhD is still the main doctoral degree completed by nurses (Roberts 1996b) but, whereas in the 1980s it was possible to do a PhD only in a non-nursing discipline, by the 1990s it was possible to do a PhD in clinical nursing. By the mid-1990s the transition to university education for nurses was almost complete, with a hierarchy of courses in the discipline of nursing being available.

The establishment of nursing as a university discipline has also had the effect of increasing the production of nursing research. This has happened not only as a consequence of more nurses doing postgraduate research degrees, but also because of an increasing recognition that there is a lack of nursing research.

During this academic phase of nursing, other influences on nursing research were operating. Those nurses who were doing advanced degrees were looking for an outlet to publish the papers they had written during the course of their studies. The Royal Australian Nursing Federation saw an opportunity and, in 1983, launched the *Australian Journal of Advanced Nursing* to cater for a higher level of scholarly discourse than had been available in other nursing journals. It published articles on nursing research, but there was also a focus on nursing education (McConnell & Paech 1993; Roberts 1995). This is not surprising when it is considered that most nurse-researchers were nurse-academics who were working for graduate degrees that generated research in nursing education.

Professional nursing organisations have also had some influence on nursing research. The Royal College of Nursing, Australia has fostered nursing research through the development of a Research Society, a national database of nurse-researchers, nursing research workshops, research grants and continuing education initiatives on evidence-based practice. The Australian Nursing Federation (1997) developed a set of national standards that gives a framework for nursing research. These evolved from a draft set of standards developed by the Western Australian Research Network (1994). The Australian Nursing Council Inc. has promoted research through the incorporation of a competency statement about nursing research in the ANCI competencies for beginning nursing practice (ANCI 2000). It has also included research in the Code of Ethics (ANCI 1993).

The nursing profession in Australia has entered a clinical phase of nursing. Basic nursing education focuses on clinical nursing, but higher qualifications are also being undertaken primarily in clinical nursing, with a range of advanced courses at the graduate diploma and master's degree level. Research degrees are focusing on clinical practice. The nurse-practitioner movement to expand the scope of nursing practice is being established. There is discussion about licensure for advanced practice.

The current scene

The level of the nursing research culture in Australia is still embryonic, one reason being that nurses do not do enough research. Wright, Brown and Sloman (1996) reported that only 40 per cent of their sample of New South Wales nurses had participated in a research project, and only 30 per cent had conducted nursing research.

Some reasons for this lack of research activity are attributable to the culture of nursing itself: nurses see research activity as something beyond normal practice; the hierarchy in health care agencies does not encourage it; and the system of promotion does not reward it adequately. The dissemination of research beyond conferences demands a capability in scholarly writing, but the culture of nursing has been predominantly a culture that transmits knowledge in oral rather than written forms (Parker, Gardner & Wiltshire 1992), and many nurses are uncomfortable with scholarly writing.

Another reason for a lack of nursing research is that until recently the nursing profession had not produced many qualified nurse-researchers, because nursing education has only recently entered the universities, the traditional training ground for researchers in all disciplines. We have not yet had time to build up the tradition of research groups that is common in other disciplines. It also needs to be recognised that the first nurse-academics in the unified national system of universities had to make a discipline shift in order to focus on nursing research.

Other reasons concern the nature of nurses. Nurses want to do things promptly and effectively, with a minimum of fuss and to the best of their abilities. Being busy people already, they may argue that they do not have the time or energy to go home from work and catch up on the latest research by subscribing to and reading nursing journals. Nurses are also practical people. While it may be interesting to pontificate on theoretical issues in nursing, they need to get the work done. The research they are most likely to do will be that which works on a practical level and is likely to produce a better way of doing what they already do.

There is still a lack of published research. Only a few years ago, Lumby (1991, p. 478) stated that 'Australian nurses are in their infancy in nursing research publications, with only one journal in which to publish'. However, in the 1990s various other nursing journals were started, all featuring research. These include *Collegian, Contemporary Nurse, International Journal of Nursing Practice, Nursing Inquiry,* and *The Australian Journal of Holistic Nursing.* The change in focus of nurse-academia from education to nursing has resulted in an increase in the publication of clinical nursing research and a decrease in nursing education research (Roberts 1996b).

Knowledge and research

What is knowledge?

Knowledge is knowing or familiarity gained through the senses (Sykes 1976), primarily sight and hearing. For us to believe something, it must be both true and verifiable: it must agree with observed facts and be consistent with the general body of established knowledge. Knowledge is more than true belief; it must be able to be justified – we must be able to explain why what we believe is true (Maddox 1993).

What is nursing knowledge?

Moody has defined scientific knowledge as knowledge 'generated from systematic study, through qualitative or quantitative modes of inquiry; this knowledge is commonly accepted by its community of scholars' (Moody 1990, p. 20). This definition acknowledges that nursing knowledge has been developed through research and inquiry, not only in the traditional 'hard' quantitative scientific approach, but also in the 'soft' qualitative research approach. The need for balance in the ways of knowing has been applied at a practical level in this book, as we have tried to integrate and ensure equality of representation of both the quantitative and qualitative research approaches.

The question of what constitutes nursing knowledge subsumes other questions such as: 'What is nursing?'; 'Is nursing knowledge unique?'; 'Who can contribute to nursing knowledge?'; 'What kinds of knowledge can various people contribute?'; and 'What produces nursing knowledge?' In this section, brief answers will be offered to each of these secondary questions, before attempting to answer the primary question: 'What constitutes nursing knowledge?' In addition, we will ask: 'How is nursing knowledge transmitted?'

What is nursing?

Nursing scholars have given various answers to the question: 'What is nursing?' Here are some of their answers.

Nursing:

- [puts] us in the best possible condition for Nature to restore or to preserve health – to prevent or to cure disease or injury (Seymer 1955, pp. 334–5).
- requires the application of scientific knowledge and nursing skills and affords the opportunities for constructive work in the care and relief of patients and their families (Frederick & Northam 1938, p. 3).
- [is] a significant, therapeutic, interpersonal process (Peplau 1952, p. 16).
- [involves] assisting the individual (sick or well) in the performance of those activities contributing to health, or its recovery (or to a peaceful death) that he would perform unaided if he had the necessary strength, will, or knowledge (Henderson 1955, p. 4).
- involves the concept of self-care, putting the responsibility back into the hands of the person receiving care, with the nurse giving assistance only as it was required (Orem 1959; Kinlein 1977).
- is a service to individuals and to families; therefore, to society. It is based upon an art and science which mould the attitudes, intellectual competencies, and technical skills of the individual nurse into the desire and ability to help people, sick or well, cope with their health needs, and may be carried out under general or specific medical direction (Abdellah et al. 1960, p. 24).
- acknowledges the supportive role of the nurse (Orlando 1961; Rogers 1961; Wiedenbach 1964).
- [is] a process of action, reaction, interaction, and transaction (King 1971, p. 22).
- [is a matter of] promoting man's adaptation in his physiological needs, his self-concept, his role function and his interdependence relations during health and illness (Roy 1976).
- involves the unique therapeutic value of the nurse-patient relationship in nursing encounters (Paterson & Zderad 1976; Watson 1981, 1985; Chinn & Jacobs 1983; Benner 1984; Leininger 1985, 1995; Parse, Coyne & Smith 1985; Dunlop 1986, 1988; Parker 1988; Pearson 1989; Kretlow 1989–90; Lawler 1991; Lumby 1991; McMahon & Pearson 1991; Carper 1992; Taylor 1992).
- is what happens between nurses and patients in contexts of care (Taylor 1994, 2001).

Even though there is no agreement on what nursing is, Erickson, Tomlin and Swain (1983, p. 29) found common features in what nurses say collectively. They concluded that the mission of nursing is to:

> assist persons with their responses to health and illness states; with their self-care practices in relation to their health [with their coping and adapting]; to achieve a state of [optimum] wellness by way of an interpersonal process.

Is nursing knowledge unique?

Is there something about nursing that gives it a brand of knowledge that it can claim as its own? In other words, can nursing claim to be a discipline? Disciplinary status is assigned to those areas of inquiry that can demonstrate that their knowledge constitutes something unique, different from other areas of knowledge interests.

Donaldson and Crowley (1978, p. 113) define a discipline as a 'unique perspective, a distinct way of viewing all phenomena, which ultimately defines the limits and nature of its inquiry'. Opinions differ as to whether nursing is a discipline or whether it relies on borrowed knowledge that is applied from other disciplines, such as physics, chemistry, history, philosophy, psychology, sociology, and so on.

Nursing might more correctly be described as a 'practice discipline', because it is concerned with the development of professional knowledge and skills. This label of 'practice discipline' has been central in the debates about whether nursing has a body of knowledge that is unique to its concerns, whether the core of nursing is the human experiences of patients and nurses, and whether nursing can claim that knowledge arises out of the work of its practitioners.

The scholars who claim that nursing is a practice discipline argue essentially that nursing is careful people-oriented work, of a health-related nature, which is informed by practice knowledge (Smyth 1986; Visintainer 1986; Pearson 1988; Tillett, 1994). In contrast, the opposing argument uses the label of 'practice discipline' to argue the reverse – that the practice theory of nursing is borrowed from other disciplines and comprises mainly scientific and moral knowledge (Beckstrand 1978a, 1978b, 1980). It also argues that, of itself, nursing has nothing or little to offer as unique understandings to itself, or to other established disciplines.

We would argue that, while nursing knowledge of clients and health incorporates a wide spectrum of knowledge derived from other disciplines, it is in the application of that knowledge to nursing practice that it becomes a part of nursing knowledge. For example, nurses study about how social status, culture, educational level, and perception impact on the client's health status.

The relationship of research-based theory and practice

Views differ as to whether a theory–practice gap exists, and if it does, how wide it is. Beckstrand (1978a, 1978b) Donaldson and Crowley (1978) and Gortner (1983) have argued previously that the concerns of practice and theory are separate; that nursing is an applied science; that nurses with the mandate to research nursing should not be involved in nursing practice; and that practice informs practitioners, but not the disciplinary content of nursing. In other words, they do not think that clinicians have anything to offer the knowledge base of the practice discipline.

However, those views have been countered. It has been argued that theory and practice can be mutually synergistic (Pearson 1988). Carper (1992) acknowledged that nursing is known in a variety of ways, therefore practice knowledge is valid. Nurses who are practitioners can be theorisers of their own work (Smyth 1986). The practice of nursing can inform the discipline of nursing by virtue of its nature and location as the central business of nursing (Tilden & Tilden 1985; Visintainer 1986). Moccia (1986) offered a compromise between the opposing views about theory and practice by suggesting that both perspectives can create a dialogue to reconcile their apparent contradictions.

What is the metaparadigm of nursing?

The unique perspective of each discipline is judged by its metaparadigm. The metaparadigm of a discipline comprises the fundamental ideas on which its knowledge is founded. Fawcett (1989, p. 5) explained that:

> The metaparadigm of each paradigm of each discipline ... is the first level of distinction between disciplines. It is not unusual, however, to find that more than one discipline is interested in the same or similar concepts.

There is consensus in the nursing literature on the metaparadigm of nursing. In relation to nursing's metaparadigm, Kemp (1983, p. 610) wrote that:

> ... there is general agreement that the domain of nursing is person, environment, health, and nursing. By specifying the domain of nursing, research and practice should reflect common goals of providing nurses with knowledge within these four conceptual dimensions.

This means that knowledge that can be claimed to be unique to nursing is concerned directly with any or all of the four domains that represent the scope of nursing. Given that the domains are broad, this means that there are many interpretations of what constitutes nursing knowledge, by whom, how, and for what purposes.

Who can contribute to nursing knowledge?

This is a tricky question, because the answers may be judged by various people to be either too exclusive or too inclusive. Essentially, the debates run in either direction, with some people arguing for 'the middle road'.

People who take an exclusive position say that nurses should be the researchers of nursing. Their justification of this position is that nurses know nursing best and therefore they are the best able to generate important nursing research questions and areas of interest. Furthermore, they can most effectively access and work with other nurses, health workers, and clients in nursing and health care settings. The rationale might also include statements that nurses are best able to analyse and interpret effectively what they observe, gather and compile, given that they have inside knowledge of the culture of nursing.

People who argue for inclusiveness say that any person who has something worthwhile to offer can contribute to nursing knowledge. This means that sociologists, psychologists, educationists, or anyone for that matter, can contribute to nursing, as they have done already (Street 1990, 1991, 1992, 1995; Brown & Seddon 1996a, 1996b).

People who make 'middle road' arguments confirm their position by asking the questions: 'Who has contributed to nursing knowledge?'; 'Why?'; 'How?'; 'Has this person made an important contribution?'; 'In what way has this knowledge contributed to nursing?' In other words these people are not interested in who has contributed, but they look at the value of the contributions to nursing knowledge and practice.

In this book, we have tended to take the middle road, presenting any knowledge that has contributed to nursing in any or all of its domain concepts (person, environment, health, and nursing), regardless of the work role or disciplinary bias of its author.

What kinds of knowledge can various people contribute?

Scholars in nursing have acknowledged various ways of knowing. This means that all kinds of knowledge are seen as being worthy contributors to the practice discipline of nursing. Carper (1992) suggested four fundamental patterns of knowing in nursing: empirics, the science of nursing; aesthetics, the art of nursing; the component of personal knowledge in nursing; and ethics, the moral component. She acknowledged the contribution of all the patterns of knowing in increasing nurses' awareness of the diversity and complexity of nursing knowledge. She emphasised that all forms of knowing have their place, and that none is mutually exclusive.

Chinn and Kramer (1993) agree with Carper and emphasise the effects of 'patterns gone wild'. They warn that:

> Empirics removed from the context of the whole of knowing produces control and manipulation ... Ethics removed from the context of the whole of knowing produces rigid doctrine and insensitivity to the rights of others ... Personal knowing removed from the context of the whole of knowing produces isolation and self distortion ... Aesthetics removed from the context of the whole of knowing produces prejudice, bigotry and lack of appreciation for meaning.

How is nursing knowledge transmitted?

Nursing knowledge is transmitted primarily through scholarship in the discipline. There are four types of scholarship in nursing: theoretical, clinical, teaching and research (Roberts 1996b). These have been derived from Boyer's (1990) typology of integrative scholarship, which relates to theoretical scholarship; scholarship of application, which is clinical scholarship in nursing; scholarship of discovery, which is research scholarship; and teaching scholarship. Teaching, theoretical, and clinical scholarship are not research scholarship in the sense of research as it has been defined above. They do, however, have a reciprocal relationship with research scholarship. They raise questions that are answered by research, and research in turn helps to build up that body of knowledge and, in turn, scholarship.

What is the proper focus of nursing research?

One of the problems in delineating areas of concern for nurse-researchers is the awesome breadth of knowledge that nurses must concern themselves with in their care for the client. Becoming a nurse involves time studying about many things that impinge on the health of people, such as sociology, psychology, anatomy, physiology, microbiology, and anthropology. And those are only the underpinnings for the study of clinical nursing and health. It is no wonder that nursing research has had so many different directions. One rule of thumb that may help you to decide on the boundaries of nursing research is that nursing research is research that concerns those areas over which nurses have control of the decision-making in their practice. For example, if in your practice you can specify the way that you give intravenous medications, then a research question concerning whether those medications should be given 'bolus dose' or 'over time' might be an appropriate question to investigate.

As early as 1978, authors in the nursing literature were summarising a dialogue with the conclusion that three general themes for nursing research activity had emerged: principles and laws that govern life processes, well-being and optimum functioning of human beings, sick or well; patterning of human behaviour in interaction with the environment in critical life situations; and processes by which positive changes in health status are effected (Donaldson & Crowley 1978). Simply put, nursing research is research about people attaining, maintaining and regaining health. This includes the practice of nursing people through the various stages of illness. It is through the research on people and the practice of nursing that knowledge is built.

Nursing research must therefore be directed primarily to the improvement of the quality of client care. Nursing professionalism and morale spin-offs should be secondary outcomes (Neyle & West 1991). While education research and nursing systems research will continue to be of interest to nurse-academics and nurse-administrators, they are now becoming minor rather than major areas of nursing research focus in Australia (Roberts 1996b).

Types of nursing research

Nursing research, like all research, can be either basic or applied. Basic research develops fundamental knowledge and tests theory. Studies of clients' health states, their ability to care for themselves, and their perceptions of phenomena pertaining to health and illness are cases in point. An example is the study of parental attitudes to immunisation (Roden 1992). Applied research concerns the application of knowledge to specific situations. It addresses problems, such as the best way to practise nursing. A study comparing two types of neonatal cord care (Barclay et al. 1994) is an example of applied research.

Overview of nursing research paradigms

A paradigm is a broad view or perspective of something. Some people may even say that a paradigm is a 'world view', so you can see that it is a comprehensive approach to a particular area of interest. The paradigm of a profession not only concerns the content of the professional knowledge, but also the processes by which that knowledge is produced.

Various approaches to doing research can be classified paradigmatically. For example, researchers may speak of quantitative or qualitative research, or they may refer to certain paradigms across all the possible kinds of knowledge that can be generated through research. A paradigmatic view provides overall, overarching categories, in which can be placed certain kinds of research and ways of knowledge generation and verification.

A student who is new to research will find that there is a lot of detail to be learnt about the various research approaches. This can be very confusing for researchers who are trying to get an overview of the possibilities and problems confronting them. With this in mind, we have organised this book into distinct chapters that give information on quantitative and qualitative research. We have also introduced the concept of two forms of qualitative inquiry, to sort out the differences in qualitative research methodologies. In Chapter 12 we have also described how the qualitative research methodologies differ from one another and from quantitative research.

The three major categories of research we have used to structure this book generate and verify empirico-analytical (quantitative), interpretive (mostly qualitative), and critical (mostly qualitative) forms of knowledge. In addition, nurses use the ideas of postmodernism in their research, but as this approach resists categorisation it will be dealt with outside the confines of a paradigm. These distinctions will be described in Chapters 12 and 13, but a brief introduction to them will be given here.

Science and empirico-analytical (quantitative) research

Traditional science has had a strong influence on nursing research. Science is:

> a collection of propositions, ranging from reports of observations to the most abstract theories accounting for these observations ... the end product of research, the careful statement in approved technical terms of something that has been empirically determined to be so, and perhaps also of a tentative explanation of why it is so (McMullin 1987, p. 3).

Science can also be thought of more broadly as being all the things that a scientist does that affect the scientific outcome in any way. This can include any influences on the scientist, whether or not the scientist is conscious of them (McMullin 1987). This definition incorporates the first definition. It allows scholars and philosophers to suggest that there is no such thing as a totally objective approach to science; that scientists impose their own values and beliefs upon their research.

Empirico-analytical research is interested in observation and analysis by the scientific method. The scientific method is basically a set of rules for how to do research that can be considered to be rigorous, in the sense that it can be shown to test something over and over again and be consistently accurate (reliability).

It also shows that it is testing what it actually intends to test (validity) rather than other things that are there unnoticed (extraneous variables). To achieve this, the scientific method demands that research be as free as possible from the distorting influences of people, such as their ideas, intentions and emotions (subjectivity). In other words, research needs to show that due consideration has been given to achieving objectivity. It is a process that is common to all disciplines that produce scientific knowledge. The scientific method has traditionally been regarded as the best way to build knowledge. It comprises both induction, a theory-building approach, and deduction, a theory-testing approach.

Another requirement of the scientific method is that the only research questions that can be legitimately asked are those that can be structured in ways that can be observed and analysed (by empirico-analytical means) and measured by numbers, percentages and statistics (quantified). This is why research using the scientific method is also referred to as empirico-analytical and/or quantitative research.

Empirico-analytical and/or quantitative researchers want to reduce things of interest to their most focused and smallest parts (reductionism) in order to study them. They do this because of an underlying assumption that there are cause and effect links between certain objects and subjects (variables). It is assumed that these cause and effect relationships have a far greater chance of being discovered if the variables in a study are carefully controlled and manipulated. Researchers take a great deal of care to design their projects to ensure that they are observing and analysing the effects of what they intend to study so that they can demonstrate to 'the scientific community' that the results are statistically significant. This means that they try to confirm or dispute the degree of certainty they can place in cause and effect relationships through mathematical explanations.

Nursing has been identified as a science because it uses primarily the empirical method for its research inquiry. Nurses adopted the empirical scientific method because they believed that it was the best way of developing nursing knowledge and of promoting the acceptance of nursing as a valid discipline. The classification of nursing as a science allies nursing to empirical science, especially when decisions about research funding and research ethics are concerned.

The quantitative research process

The steps of the scientific quantitative research process are as follows (Moody 1990, p. 89):

- identifying the problem or phenomenon of interest
- explicating the linkage of the research question or problem to a theoretical framework
- formulating testable research questions or hypotheses
- designing the study
- refining the research questions/hypotheses and how the data will be collected
- specifying the sample/participants to be studied

- planning for data management
- collecting data
- analysing data
- interpreting the findings
- identifying conclusions
- making recommendations
- disseminating findings.

This book will follow this sequence of the nursing research process. However, this is an iterative process – that is, one moves back and forth between the steps rather than completing one phase entirely before going on to the next.

The quantitative research process attempts to find out scientific knowledge by the measurement of elements. This may be at four levels: description, in which elements of a phenomenon are counted; correlation, in which relationships of two or more elements are investigated; explanation, in which one element explains another; and prediction, in which the activity of one element can be predicted from that of another. The quantitative research process uses an empirical method in which data are collected by means of our senses, primarily sight.

The quantitative research process may involve an inductive process in which a lot of data are collected and described. For example, if you wanted to find out the average of some characteristic of people, you could go out and measure many people and calculate the mean. However, you would then have to test your findings to see if they hold up generally. You would do this by measuring a lot more people of varying kinds and seeing if most of the measurements fell near the average. Many quantitative designs involve testing relationships between phenomena, usually by proposing an hypothesis or statement about the relationship between the variables. Then data are gathered, findings analysed, and conclusions drawn about the findings.

Qualitative research

In this book we make a distinction between qualitative interpretive and critical research, noting that the principal difference is that interpretive forms are concerned mainly with creating meaning, while critical forms focus on causing socio-political change. Postmodern influences on research can be considered as extending combinations of qualitative interpretive and critical research, taking a highly eclectic view of knowledge generation and validation methods and processes.

Qualitative interpretive research

Qualitative research is interested in questions that involve human consciousness and subjectivity, and value humans and their experiences in the research process. Qualitative research involves finding out about the changing (relative) nature of knowledge, which is seen to be special and centred in the people, place, time and conditions in which it finds itself (unique and context-dependent). Qualitative research uses thinking that starts from the specific instance and moves to the general pattern of combined instances (inductive), so it grows from the ground up to make larger statements about the nature of the thing being investigated.

Rather than starting with a statement (hypothesis), qualitative research begins a project with a statement of the area of interest, such as: 'This research will explore the nature and effects of nurse–patient relationships in intensive care units'. The measures for ensuring validity in qualitative research involve asking the participants to confirm that the interpretations represent faithfully and clearly what the experience was/is like for them. Reliability is often not an issue in qualitative research, as it is based on the idea that knowledge is relative and is dependent on all of the features of the people, place, time and other circumstances (context) of the setting. People are valued as sources of information and their expressions of their personal awareness (subjectivity) are valued as being integral to the meaning that comes out of the research. Rather than saying that something can be claimed as being statistically significant, qualitative research makes no claims to generate knowledge that can be confirmed as certain (absolute).

Interpretive research aims mainly to generate meaning. It tries to explain and describe, in order to make sense of things of interest.

Qualitative critical research

All the statements made for qualitative interpretive research apply to critical research, but there is a difference between the two in terms of their intention to bring about social and political change. Qualitative critical research aims overtly to bring about change in the status quo. By working collaboratively with participants as co-researchers to address research problems systematically, qualitative researchers try to find answers and use them to bring about change. These differences will be discussed further in Chapters 12 and 13. The major difference between interpretive and critical qualitative research is in the main intention of what they hope to achieve through the research process. Essentially, interpretive research is about making meaning while critical research is about causing change.

Postmodern influences on research

The postmodern era has provided an eclectic extension to what we are naming in this book as qualitative interpretive and critical research. It is not possible to claim postmodernism as a third research paradigm in this book, as postmodern thinking questions many of the taken-for-granted assumptions about knowledge generation and validation in research, and resists taking on the authority of a 'grand narrative'. Instead, we can discuss postmodern influences on research methods and processes. Postmodernism seeks to 'turn on their heads' cherished notions of the importance of author, text, subject, history, time, theory, truth, representation and politics (Rosenau 1992). Taken altogether, postmodernism requires researchers to redefine their basic assumptions, intentions and roles and to make adjustments to their present ways of viewing and doing research. These influences will be discussed further in Chapters 12 and 13.

The qualitative research process

As was pointed out earlier, there are similarities in the processes for quantitative and qualitative research. All projects need a well-planned beginning; a careful middle section when the data are collected, analysed, and interpreted; and a thoroughly executed end stage in which the results are written up and disseminated. However, there are also differences between quantitative and qualitative research processes.

Qualitative research tends to define the word 'process' differently from the accepted dictionary usage, which is synonymous with a set of steps or methods. Qualitative research defines process as the 'how' of research, especially in relation to how the people in the research relate to one another. Therefore, there are some common features of research processes that identify qualitative research projects as being different from quantitative research projects. These include features of language, and also the degree of participant involvement in, and the sense of group ownership of, the research.

The differences lie in the use of language, the degree of involvement and collaboration of the research participants, and the 'ownership' of the project. Quantitative researchers tend to refer to the people they have accessed in the research as 'subjects'. By objective means, subjects are exposed to carefully prepared methods and instruments such as surveys, questionnaires, clinical trials and so on.

In contrast, qualitative researchers tend to refer to the people they have accessed in the research as 'participants'. By means that value the participants' subjectivity, researchers claim to 'work with' participants when doing qualitative research projects.

There are variations in the degree of participant involvement in qualitative research. For example, critical forms of qualitative research pay far more attention to ensuring a high degree of research participant involvement and collaboration. This is evidenced by the tendency of many of the researchers who use critical methodologies to refer to participants as co-researchers. Critical researchers also try to minimise the effects of power differences between the researcher and the participants/co-researchers. Friendships that last throughout the life of the project and beyond may even develop between the people involved in the research.

In qualitative critical methodologies such as feminist and action research approaches, and those reflecting postmodern influences, there is a tendency for participants/co-researchers to have an influential voice in the overall conduct of the project. This means that the project may run according to the wishes and directions of the group, and that they develop a strong sense of joint ownership of the project. This sense of ownership may be reflected in the acknowledgement in the research report of all the people involved in its direction. Ownership may also manifest in the publication of jointly authored journal articles and the presentation of jointly prepared papers at professional conferences.

Shifting paradigms

There has been a recent shift of focus towards qualitative research in nursing. However, most nursing research in Australia is still within the quantitative paradigm (Roberts 1996b), although authors such as Gray and Pratt (1991, p. 7) have argued that 'the debate has shifted from the quantitative versus qualitative research methods, to that of exploring and promoting the relative strengths of particular qualitative research approaches'. It has been suggested that in nursing, the qualitative and quantitative paradigms will converge in time and that nurses will develop their own unique strategies (Tinkle & Beaton 1983).

Although postmodernism resists being represented as a paradigm, it should be noted that it has an important effect on the present trends in shifting paradigms. Postmodern thinking allows nurses to create highly imaginative research strategies to replace the rigid rules and methods that have been reflected in modernist (taken simply to mean here, quantitative and qualitative) research projects. Affirmative postmodern influences encourage researchers to move from their reliance on the 'scientific method' to be guided by their feelings, personal experience, empathy, emotion, intuition, subjective judgement, imagination, creativity and play (Rosenau 1992). The inclusion of these subjective elements constitutes a major departure from the rules of the 'scientific method' reflected in quantitative research, and constitutes an extension of qualitative researchers' ideas about the role of relative and personal knowledge in their projects.

Using computers in nursing research

Computers have become so much an indispensable tool of the researcher that we are going to talk about them in the first chapter. Even if you, as a student, are not required to understand computers in order to carry out a research project, you will need to understand something about them if you are going to read research reports competently.

Researchers use computers in almost every phase of the research process. They use them as terminals to conduct a search of the literature and to download full text articles, to record data, and to analyse both qualitative and quantitative data; as word processors to write the research documents and to compile bibliographies and lists of references. They even use them to design the posters by which they present the findings.

Computers have taken the hard labour out of some parts of the research process. For example, improved access to databases has simplified the identification of relevant literature. However, the use of computers has also complicated other parts of the research process, such as data analysis, as more sophisticated data analysis techniques have become the norm.

Structure of a computer

If you are under 30 years of age, you may feel you can safely skip this section.

Computers are composed of innumerable components grouped into half a dozen structures: the keyboard, forgetful memory (RAM), never forgetful memory (hard disk or CD-ROM), portable memory (floppy disk), and the central processor (which takes messages from all the above and displays the result on the screen or printer or sends it to another computer linked by phone line). By the time this chapter appears in a book, computers will be operating 10 times faster and hold 10 times as much information as the machine on which this chapter is being composed. And they will cost less!

What is important is how these components affect the user. The program you need to do your word processing or analyse your data will be either on your network or on the hard disk of your machine, or you may have to install it from a floppy disk or CD-ROM onto your hard disk. When you want to use the program, your central processor will grab parts of the program from the hard disk, stick bits of it into RAM, and 'run' the program. The more RAM you have, the bigger can be the pieces the central processor uses at any one time and the faster it will operate – up to a point. It will take the information you have keyed in initially (or stored in earlier sessions) and process it according to your instructions. As a prudent user, you will then ask the central processor to make a backup copy on a floppy disk or tape, or your allocated memory area on the network. Next week, when the computer crashes because your cat chewed the power cord, you will not have to repeat the tedious process of rekeying in all your information.

Types of computers

There are two kinds of computers: those that are hooked up to a network and those that are self-sufficient. It makes no difference whether your computer is Apple, IBM or IBM compatible: the value of what emerges from the machine depends totally on the integrity of the whole analytical process. If you are operating from a network, the choice of 'applications' (programs) available to you is probably so vast that your problem will be trying to pick the appropriate one or to find a simple version. If you are operating from your own personal computer your problem will be to choose 'software' (programs) that meets your needs and your wallet.

For the purpose of a typical nursing research project, the basic entry level computer these days will more than suffice. These machines have enough capacity to drive a respectable word processor and a sufficiently powerful statistical analysis program or qualitative software analysis program. To give examples without necessarily endorsing a particular product we could suggest that most basic word processor programs, such as Microsoft Word and ClarisWorks, and spreadsheet programs, such as Excel, Lotus123, or ClarisWorks, easily handle the basics of what will be discussed in this book. And such programs are usually supplied with the machine! Your word processor should be able to produce a neat research proposal or report, and also have the ability to integrate graphics.

For quantitative data analysis, 'StatView' or a network version of Statistical Package of the Social Sciences (SPSS) will do anything and everything, all at once, but the interpretation is still up to the user. Here, you need the capability to draw up tables and graphs; fit regression lines; work out means, standard deviations, probabilities and Pearson correlation co-efficients and so forth, but do not worry – all will be revealed in later chapters of the book!

For qualitative data analysis, software packages such as NUD*IST or N-Vivo or Ethnograph can be purchased that take all of the hard 'cut and paste' work out of the analysis. NUD★IST was developed in Australia and is very popular here. An example of a study that used NUD★IST is by Siebold, Miller and Hall (1999). They used the package to analyse pre- and post-birth interviews. Other studies using NUD★IST as the data analysis software package analysed patient satisfaction with nursing care (O'Connell, Young & Twigg 1999) and Darwin women's attitudes to using condoms for safe sex (Roberts & Cahill 1997; Roberts 1999).

In addition, voice-recognition programs are now beginning to be used to assist with audiotape transcription processes. This involves using the voice-recognition program to enter the data into the computer. The researcher listens to the audiotape recording and repeats it into the computer speaker, whereupon the program converts it into text. However, this technology is still not well enough developed to make this a smooth process. Like any other program, learning the commands, which in this case can be voice-activated as well as keyboard or mouse-activated, represents quite a lot of work. An evaluation of three different voice-recognition software programs showed that the IBM Via-Voice had a lower mean error rate than the Dragon Systems Naturally Speaking program (Devine, Gaehde & Curtis 2000).

As we have seen, computers can now be used to assist with any part of the research process. However, you need to remember that no computer program substitutes for the thinking process.

Backing up

This section is not about reversing direction. It is about creating peace of mind by making duplicates of every computer file that you create. Every chapter ever written about the basics of handling documents on computer stresses the importance of backing up. This is undoubtedly because such chapters are written by people who have had some experience in the game. They have all lost data. To summarise – you can never have too many backups. In the process of your research program, ask yourself: 'How much data can I afford to lose?' Think about the possibility of fire, power failure, hard disk failure, losing your briefcase with the only backup copy inside or even theft. (Someone stole a $5000 laptop from a car in Jabiru last year. No problem, the computer was insured for $5000. But it held the only copy of two years' work on its hard disk. What was its value? $50 000?). Remember Murphy's (Sod's) Law: 'If anything can go wrong, it will.' And here's a corollary: 'It will go wrong at the worst possible time' – for example, the night before your assignment or thesis is due.

If what you are working on is not worth a dollar for the floppy disk (re-usable almost indefinitely) or the two minutes it takes to copy it, then forget it. But even a document as simple as this chapter has been saved to disk every 10 minutes during composition and was copied to floppy disk and copied to the hard disk on another computer, all as a matter of course. You have been warned. Make an extra copy and store it in an independent place. One of us emails her working files to herself from work to home or vice versa at the end of the day – they are then secure, offsite and easily retrievable; and the process is quick and inexpensive.

Computer etiquette

It is important when using a computer to be considerate of other researchers. One way that you can do this is to abide by the rules concerning access to your institution's machines. You should familiarise yourself with your institution's policies on the use of its computers.

Researchers often belong to a list such as 'NURSRES' whose members discuss research issues. When communicating by email, be courteous. If you belong to a list, familiarise yourself with the 'netiquette'. Most lists post out sets of guidelines to new people to help them fit in. Your fellow list members are unlikely to tolerate behaviour such as 'flaming' (destructive personal criticism). Failure to abide by the norms of behaviour on a list can lead to expulsion from the list by its owner or moderator.

Legal aspects

You should be aware of some of the legal aspects of communicating by electronic means. Some types of behaviour, such as defamation, can be a civil offence. A person was sued in Australia recently for slandering a colleague by email. Remember that anything you distribute to a public email list can be treated as a publication.

It is also possible to commit a criminal offence when using email. Similar laws apply to email as apply to regular forms of communication, such as postal mail. Therefore anything that is illegal to distribute through the postal system cannot legally be distributed by email. The data-handling rules concerning confidentiality and privacy of patient information also apply if the data are stored on a computer.

Supplying others with copies of software for which they need a licence is also illegal. It is as important to observe copyright regulations with regard to software as it is with other things. However, some software is free and distributed over the World Wide Web.

Summary

In this chapter, we have described how nurses can carry out and participate in nursing research. We have outlined a brief history of nursing research in Australia, and the influences that have promoted and hindered its development. We have given a brief exposition on what knowledge is and how it is produced and how research contributes to the development of nursing knowledge. We have described the different paradigms of nursing research and discussed the differences between them. Finally, we have explained how you can use computers in nursing research. Now, you are ready to get started on the research process by asking your research question, or stating your research problem.

Main points

- Nursing is in the process of becoming a research-based profession.
- Nurses can participate in research at an independent, interdependent or dependent level and can collaborate with researchers in other disciplines.

- Nursing research began with Florence Nightingale and has passed through a service period and an academic period and is now in a clinical period.
- Nursing research is lacking because of a lack of research culture in nursing, a lack of qualified nurse-researchers and the practical nature of nurses themselves.
- Nursing scholars have given various answers to the question: 'What is nursing?', and even though there is no agreement on what nursing is, common features are that the mission of nursing is to assist persons with their responses to health and illness states and with their self-care practices in relation to their health (i.e. with their coping and adapting); and to achieve a state of (optimum) wellness by way of an interpersonal process.
- Nursing can be described as a 'practice discipline', because it is concerned with the development of professional knowledge and skills, because it has a body of knowledge that is unique to its concerns, and because that knowledge arises out of the work of its practitioners.
- The metaparadigm of a discipline comprises the fundamental ideas on which its knowledge is founded, and in nursing there is general agreement that the domain of nursing is person, environment, health, and nursing.
- A paradigmatic view provides overall, overarching categories for research approaches of knowledge generation and verification, and the three major categories of research we have used to structure this book are empirico-analytical (quantitative), interpretive qualitative, and critical qualitative forms of knowledge, plus some postmodern ideas that lie outside the confines of a paradigm.
- Postmodern influences on research can be considered as extending combinations of qualitative interpretive and critical research, taking a highly eclectic view of knowledge generation and validation methods and processes.
- Qualitative interpretive research aims to generate meaning by explaining and describing areas of human interest.
- Qualitative critical research aims overtly to bring about change in the status quo by working collaboratively with participants as co-researchers to address research problems systematically.
- Postmodernism is NOT a paradigm, because postmodern thinking questions many taken-for-granted assumptions about knowledge generation and validation in research, and resists taking on the authority of a 'grand narrative'.
- Qualitative research defines process as the 'how' of research, especially in relation to how people in the research relate to one another. Therefore, some common features are the importance of language, and the high degree of participant involvement in, and the sense of group ownership of, the research.
- Affirmative postmodern thinking allows nurses to create highly imaginary research strategies to replace the rigid rules and methods that have been reflected in modernist (taken simply to mean here, quantitative and qualitative) research projects, and to move away from their reliance on the 'scientific method' to be

guided by their feelings, personal experience, empathy, emotion, intuition, subjective judgement, imagination, creativity and play.
- Computers are now an indispensable tool in nursing research.
- It is important to keep backups.
- Users musts conform to 'netiquette' and legal constraints.

Review Questions

1 Florence Nightingale's most important contribution to research in health was:
   a development of nursing theory in Notes on Nursing
   b compilation of statistics on soldiers' morbidity and mortality
   c study of the best ways to acquire provisions
   d experimenting with wound care techniques

2 The predominant influence on the development of Australian nursing research was:
   a development of postgraduate study in universities
   b conducting research in undergraduate degrees
   c research in sociology, education and psychology
   d professional organisations

3 The embryonic level of nursing research culture in Australia could be attributed to:
   a nurses' attitude to nursing research
   b the oral culture in nursing
   c lack of encouragement by the system
   d all of the above

4 Nursing can be described as a 'practice discipline' because:
   a it is concerned with the development of professional knowledge and skills
   b it has a body of knowledge that is unique to its concerns
   c nursing knowledge arises out of the work of its practitioners
   d all of the above

5 The general agreement that the domain areas of nursing are person, environment, health, and nursing, is nursing's:
   a metaparadigm
   b paradigm
   c methodology
   d philosophy

6 Basic research:
   a develops fundamental knowledge
   b concerns the application of knowledge
   c tests the best way to address nursing problems
   (d) takes in all of the above

7 An example of a research paradigm is:
   a qualitative research
   b experimental research
   (c) grounded theory
   d descriptive research

8 Empirico-analytical research is:
   a applied to critical research
   b interpretive
   c unconcerned with numerical analysis
   (d) deductive

9 Qualitative research:
   a is concerned with measurement
   b claims to generate absolute knowledge
   (c) values people as sources of information
   d establishes validity through hypotheses

10 Qualitative and quantitative research differ in their:
   (a) need for a well-planned beginning
   b need for care in data collection
   c use of language
   d requirement for dissemination

Discussion Questions

1 Is nursing a research-based profession? Discuss.
2 What forms the knowledge base of nursing?
3 Compare and contrast the types of knowledge as described by Carper.
4 Should the focus of nursing research be the nurse, the client or the practice?
5 What is the difference between quantitative and qualitative research?

References

Abdellah, F., Beland, I., Martin, A. & Matheney, R. 1960, *Patient-Centered Approaches to Nursing*, Macmillan, New York.
Abdellah, F. & Levine, E. 1994, *Preparing Nursing Research for the 21st Century*, Springer, New York.
Australian Nursing Council, Inc. 1993, *Code of Ethics for Nurses in Australia*, ANCI, Canberra.

Australian Nursing Council, Inc. 2000, *National Competencies for the Registered and Enrolled Nurse*, ANCI, Canberra.

Australian Nursing Federation 1997, *Standards for Research for the Nursing Profession*, ANF, Melbourne.

Barclay, L., Harrington, A., Conroy, R., Royal, R. & LaForgia, J. 1994, 'A comparative study of neonates' umbilical cord management', *Australian Journal of Advanced Nursing*, vol. 11, no. 3, 34–40.

Beckstrand, J. 1978a, 'The need for a practice theory as indicated by the knowledge used in the conduct of practice', *Research in Nursing and Health*, vol. 1, 175–9.

Beckstrand, J. 1978b, 'The notion of a practice theory and the relationship of scientific and ethical knowledge to practice', *Research in Nursing and Health*, vol. 1, no. 3, 131–6.

Beckstrand, J. 1980, 'A critique of several conceptions of practice theory in nursing', *Research in Nursing and Health*, vol. 3, no. 2, 869–79.

Benner, P. 1984, *From Novice to Expert: Uncovering the Knowledge Embedded in Clinical Practice*, Addison-Wesley, Menlo Park, California.

Boyer, E. L. 1990, *Scholarship Reconsidered: Priorities of the Professoriate*, Carnegie Foundation for the Advancement of Teaching, Princeton, New Jersey.

Brown, C. & Seddon, J. 1996a, 'Nurses, doctors and the body of the patient: medical dominance revisited', *Nursing Inquiry*, vol. 3, 30–5.

Brown, C. & Seddon, J. 1996b, 'The social body and the mechanical body: can they coexist in nurse education?', *Journal of Advanced Nursing*, vol. 23, 651–6.

Carper, B. 1992, 'Fundamental patterns of knowing in nursing', in *Perspectives on Nursing Theory*, 2nd edn, ed. L. Nicholl, J B Lippincott Co., Philadelphia.

Chinn, P. L. & Jacobs, M. K. 1983, *The Emergence of Nursing Theory*, C.V. Mosby Co., St Louis.

Chinn, P. L. & Kramer, M. 1993, *Theory and Nursing: A Systematic Approach*, Mosby Year Book, St Louis.

Devine, E., Gaehde, S. & Curtis, A. 2000, 'Comparative evaluation of three continuous speech recognition software packages in the generation of medical reports', *Journal of the American Medical Informatics Association*, vol. 7, no. 5, 462–8.

Donaldson, S. & Crowley, D. 1978, 'The discipline of nursing', *Nursing Outlook*, vol. 26, no. 2, 113–20.

Dunlop, M. 1986, 'Is a science of caring possible?', *Journal of Advanced Nursing*, vol. 11, 661–70.

Dunlop, M. 1988, *Science and Caring: Are They Compatible? Shaping Nursing Theory and Practice: the Australian Context*, La Trobe University, Lincoln School of Health Sciences: Department of Nursing, Melbourne.

Erickson, H., Tomlin, M. & Swain, M. 1983, *Modeling and Remodeling: A Theory and Paradigm for Nursing*, Prentice-Hall, Englewood Cliffs, New Jersey.

Fawcett, J. 1989, *Analysis and Evaluation of Conceptual Models of Nursing*, 2nd edn, F. A. Davis, Philadelphia.

Frederick, H. & Northam, E. 1938, *A Textbook of Nursing Practice*, Macmillan, New York.

Gortner, S. 1983, 'Knowledge in a practice discipline: philosophy and pragmatics', Keynote Address American Academy of Nursing Meeting, American Academy of Nursing, Minneapolis, Minnesota.

Gray, G. & Pratt, R. 1991, 'Prologue' in *Towards a Discipline of Nursing*, eds G. Gray & R. Pratt, Churchill Livingstone, Melbourne.

Henderson, V. 1955, *Textbook of Principles and Practice of Nursing*, Macmillan, New York.

Kemp, V. A. 1983, 'Themes in Theory Development' in *The Nursing Profession: A Time to Speak*, ed. N. L. Chaska, McGraw-Hill, New York.

King, I. M. 1971, *Toward a Theory for Nursing: General Concepts of Human Behavior*, John Wiley & Sons, New York.

Kinlein, M. L. 1977, *Independent Nursing Practice with Clients*, Lippincott, Philadelphia.

Kretlow, F. 1989–90, 'A phenomenological view of illness', *Australian Journal of Advanced Nursing*, vol. 7, no. 2, 8–10.

Lawler, J. 1991, *Behind the Screens: Nursing, Somology, and the Problem of the Body*, Churchill Livingstone, Melbourne.

Leininger, M. 1985, *Qualitative Research Methods in Nursing*, Grune & Stratton, New York.

Leininger, M. 1995, *Transcultural Nursing: Concepts, Theories, Research and Practices*, 2nd edn, McGraw-Hill/Greyden Press, Columbus.

Lumby, J. 1991, 'Threads of an emerging discipline', in *Towards a Discipline of Nursing*, eds G. Gray & R. Pratt, Churchill Livingstone, Melbourne.

Maddox, H. 1993, *Theory of Knowledge*, Freshet Press, Castlemaine, Australia.

McConnell, E. & Paech, M. 1993, 'Trends in scholarly nursing literature', *Australian Journal of Advanced Nursing*, vol. 11, no. 2, 28–32.

McMahon, R. & Pearson, A. (eds) 1991, *Nursing as Therapy*, Chapman and Hall, London.

McMullin, E. 1987, 'Alternative approaches to the philosophy of science', in *Scientific Knowledge: Basic Issues in the Philosophy of Science*, ed. J. Kourany, Wadsworth Publishing Co., Belmont, California.

Moccia, P. (ed.) 1986, *Theory Development and Nursing Practice: A Synopsis of a Study of the Theory–Practise Dialectic*, National League for Nursing, New York.

Moody, L. 1990, *Advancing Nursing Science through Nursing Research*, vol. 2, Sage Publications, Newbury Park, California.

Neyle, D. & West, S. 1991, 'In support of a scientific basis', in *Towards a Discipline of Nursing*, eds G. Gray & R. Pratt, Churchill Livingstone, Melbourne.

O'Connell, B., Young, J. & Twigg, D. 1999, 'Patient satisfaction with nursing care: a measurement conundrum', *International Journal of Nursing Practice*, vol. 5, no. 2, 72–7.

Orem, D. 1959, *Guides for Developing Curricula for the Education of Practical Nurses*, Government Printing Office, Washington DC.

Orlando, I. J. 1961, *The Dynamic Nurse–Patient Relationship*, Putnam, New York.

Parker, J., Gardner, G. & Wiltshire, J. 1992, 'Handover: the collective narrative of nursing practice', *Australian Journal of Advanced Nursing*, vol. 9, no. 3, 31–7.

Parker, J. M. 1988, Theoretical perspectives in nursing: from microphysics to hermeneutics, paper presented at the Third Nursing Research Forum, Lincoln School of Health Sciences, La Trobe University, Melbourne.

Parse, R., Coyne, B. & Smith, M. 1985, *Nursing Research: Qualitative Methods*, Brady Communications, Bowie, Maryland.

Paterson, J. & Zderad, L. 1976, *Humanistic Nursing*, John Wiley & Sons, New York.

Pearson, A. 1988, *Primary Nursing – Nursing in the Oxford and Burford Nursing Development Units*, Croom Helm, London.

Pearson, A. 1989, Translating rhetoric into practice: theory in action, paper presented at the National Nursing Theory Conference, Adelaide, S.A.

Peplau, H. E. 1952, *Interpersonal Relations in Nursing*, Putnam, New York.

Roberts, K. 1995, 'Early Australian nursing scholarship: the first decade of the AJAN: Part 2: Scholarship', *Australian Electronic Journal of Nursing Education*, vol. 1, no.1.

Roberts, K. 1996a, 'A profile of nurse-academics in Australian universities', *Collegian*, vol. 3, no. 3, 4–9.

Roberts, K. 1996b, 'A snapshot of Australian nursing scholarship 1993–94', *Collegian*, vol. 3, no. 1, 4–10.

Roberts, K. 1999, 'Attitudes to condom use in a group of Darwin women', *Australian Journal of Rural Health*, vol. 7, 166–71.

Roberts, K. & Cahill, S. 1997, 'Condom use in Aboriginal women', *Australian Journal of Rural Health*, vol. 5, 43–7.
Roden, J. 1992, 'Child immunisation levels in Sydney's Western Metropolitan Region: parental attitudes and nurses' roles', *Australian Journal of Advanced Nursing*, vol. 9, no. 3, 18–24.
Rogers, M. 1961, *Educational Revolution in Nursing*, Macmillan, New York.
Rosenau, P. 1992, *Post-Modernism and the Social Sciences: Insights, Inroads and Intrusions*, Princeton University Press, New Jersey.
Roy, C. 1976, *Introduction to Nursing: An Adaptation Model*, Prentice-Hall, Englewood Cliffs, New Jersey.
Russell, R. L. 1990, *From Nightingale to Now: Nurse Education in Australia*, Harcourt Brace Jovanovich, Sydney.
Seymer, L. (ed.) 1955, *Selected Writings of Florence Nightingale*, Macmillan, New York.
Siebold, C., Miller, M. & Hall, J. 1999, 'Midwives and women in partnership: the ideal and the real', *Australian Journal of Advanced Nursing*, vol. 17, no. 2, 21–7.
Smyth, J. 1986, The reflective practitioner in nurse education, paper presented at the Conference Proceedings of the Second National Nursing Education Seminar, *Visions into Practice*, Adelaide, S.A.
Street, A. 1990, *Nursing Practice: High Hard Ground Messy Swamps and the Pathways In Between*, Deakin University Press, Geelong, Victoria.
Street, A. 1991, *From Image to Action: Reflection in Nursing Practice*, Deakin University Press, Geelong, Victoria.
Street, A. 1992, *Inside Nursing: a Critical Ethnography of Clinical Nursing Practice*, State University of New York Press, New York.
Street, A. 1995, *Nursing Replay: Researching Nursing Culture Together*, Churchill Livingstone, Melbourne.
Sykes, J. (ed.) 1976, *Concise Oxford English Dictionary*, University Press, Oxford.
Taylor, B. 1992, 'From helper to human: a reconceptualisation of the nurse as person', *Journal of Advanced Nursing*, vol. 17, 1042–9.
Taylor, B. 1994, *Being Human: Ordinariness in Nursing*, Churchill Livingstone, Melbourne.
Taylor, B. 2001, *Being Human: Ordinariness in Nursing* (adapted and reprinted), Southern Cross University Press, Lismore, N.S.W.
Tilden, V. & Tilden, S. 1985, 'The participant philosophy in nursing science', *Image: Journal of Nursing Scholarship*, vol. 17, no. 3, 88–90.
Tillett, L. 1994, 'Nola J Pender: the Health promotion model', *Nursing Theorists and Their Work*, C.V. Mosby Co., St Louis.
Tinkle, M. & Beaton, J. 1983, 'Toward a new view of science: implications for nursing research', *Advances in Nursing Science*, vol. 5, no. 2, 27–36.
Visintainer, M. A. 1986, 'The nature of knowledge and theory in nursing', *Image: Journal of Nursing Scholarship*, vol. 18, no. 2, 32–8.
Watson, J. 1981, 'Nursing's scientific quest', *Nursing Outlook*, vol. 29, no. 7, 413–16.
Watson, J. 1985, *Nursing: Human Science and Human Care. A Theory of Nursing*, Appleton-Century-Crofts, Norwalk, Connecticut.
Western Australian Research Network 1994, 'Planning and conducting research' in *Handbook of Clinical Nursing Research*, J. Robertson (ed.), Churchill Livingstone, Melbourne.
Wiedenbach, E. 1964, *Clinical Nursing: A Helping Art*, Springer Publishing Co., New York.
Wright, A., Brown, P. & Sloman, R. 1996, 'Nurses' perceptions of the value of nursing research for practice', *Australian Journal of Advanced Nursing*, vol. 13, no. 4, 15–18.

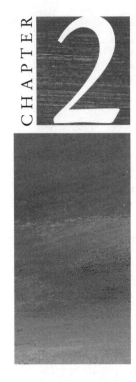

CHAPTER 2
The research question

chapter objectives The material presented in this chapter will assist you to:

- identify which persons can help you with finding research problems
- understand the usefulness of literature in finding research problems
- state the criteria for selecting research problems
- state a research problem and ask a specific research question
- refine the question, formulate an hypothesis and identify variables.

Introduction

Every research project begins with a research question that asks about the answer to a problem and therefore guides the study. A clearly stated research question is essential for smooth progress through the project. A research question should be 'an explicit query about a problem or issue that can be challenged, examined, and analysed and that will yield useful new information' (Brink & Wood 1994, p. 2).

Research problems and research questions are different, although the terms are sometimes used interchangeably. Generally, the research problem will be stated as a sentence, while the research question will be more specific and stated as a question. For example, in a study on staff attachment and loss in a long-term baby ward, the research problem was 'the effects of caring for long stay sick infants on the professional caregivers themselves' (Black & Childs 1994). The research questions were: 'Does attachment or bonding occur? If so, how does it form and what are its implications? Can and should staff be better prepared for dealing with this unique kind of emotional workplace stressor? Does providing the best care in itself put the staff member at risk?' In this chapter, we will refer mainly to research problems.

Beginners who are about to start a research project expect that it will be easy to find a problem to research. They are surprised to discover that finding the right research problem can be one of the most difficult parts of the research process. The difficulty lies partly in the boundless number of potential research problems in a field as broad and under-researched as nursing. But it is also not easy to recognise suitable research topics if you are not familiar with the research process and with previous research in the area. In older, established university disciplines, research groups with specific research themes have been developed and the chief researcher has a list of potential problems from which students may choose. In nursing, this tradition has not yet developed because the leaders have not had time to get to that point. Therefore, there is less direction available for aspiring researchers. However, there is acknowledgement of the interests and experience of students such as mature registered nurses, which results in collaborative efforts to ensure that topics arise from the clinical field.

Despite the difficulty in choosing a problem, a good research project clearly rests on the quality of the problem. In this chapter, you will learn some sources of research problems, their criteria and how to state them. Then you will learn how to restate your problem as one or more hypotheses, and to identify the variables.

Finding nursing research problems: sources and strategies

People

Your own interests are a source of research problems. You need to identify your interests and formulate a problem that reflects them, a problem for which you really want to find the answer. You will be familiar with the territory and the terminology and thus be able to judge the relevance and significance of the problem.

Critical observation of other nurses' practice will lead to problem formation. Just analysing the conversation in the tearoom may lead to ideas for research topics. In practising nursing, one often asks whether a particular approach is the best way to carry out a nursing intervention. Why are procedures done a certain way? Are they based on scientific findings or on tradition or opinion? For example, how many minutes is the optimum time for handwashing before an aseptic procedure? Is the use of clean paper towels sufficient, or is it necessary to use sterile towels? You can also ask what factors encourage or discourage specific client outcomes, such as post-operative pain, and think about how you might measure the outcomes. You can listen to what your clients say or do not say during nursing interactions.

Your own nursing experience is a source of research problems. You can examine your own practice for observations or questions that you have asked. Look at what is happening and ask how it ought to be different. You can also ask questions about the nature and effects of phenomena and relationships in nursing. Ideas for research topics that come to you in the course of your experience are often more relevant and interesting to you than those that are remote. You may find that you have more enthusiasm for researching a problem that could have some impact on your own practice or practice setting. What has frustrated you at work? As an example, the difficulties that nurses encountered with handover practices led to an action study of ways to improve them (McKenna & Walsh 1997). Client problems can also be a source of ideas. For example, a client focus group of women with multiple sclerosis who suffered from incontinence met during a research project and decided to take action (Koch & Kelly 1999).

Your lecturer or supervisor may be a source of research problems. If you are doing an individual research project, you may find that your supervisor has a list of problems that you can tap into. In any case, your supervisor should be able to help you find a problem and to discuss the implications of selecting that problem. Your supervisor will also help you to refine your general ideas into a more specific focus.

Your colleagues may be able to help you find a problem. Brainstorming with your friends and colleagues about problems they have encountered may help to clarify your ideas. Tuning into conversations on the Internet will also be a source of ideas. You can talk to colleagues at work, at professional meetings and at conferences, particularly research conferences. Listening to speakers at conferences, particularly if they are nursing leaders, can give you a feeling for the issues of the moment. The informal part of the conferences is fertile ground for the generation of new questions. Ideas and issues emanating from these situations can become research problems.

When you have identified an area of interest, talking to the expert clinicians in the field can lead you to research problems that they have identified. Such problems will probably be topical, relevant, and worthwhile.

The research literature

The professional literature is a rich source of problems. Once you have examined your experience and identified your area of interest, have a look at the relevant research periodicals. Reading a study will often suggest ideas about how it could have been improved, and thus lead to ideas for further research. For example, Barclay and colleagues found that the separation of the umbilical cord in neonates was faster in those not treated with antiseptics. Examination of the methodology and results revealed that the study had not used a randomising procedure. Furthermore, the very small percentage of babies who did contract infections had not had their cords swabbed for microbiology after the infection (Barclay et al. 1994). The presence of these infections, even though they were not cord infections, weakened the findings slightly. Reading this study could stimulate a researcher to replicate it using randomisation and swabbing the cords of any babies who contracted infection.

Similarly, although there has been an increasing interest in research into death and dying, a review of the literature shows that there has been little focus on qualitative approaches to the phenomenon, or on death from a child's perspective. Semmens and Peric found that the literature tended to treat children's and adults' views of death as though they were identical, so they were curious to see if children's experiences were different (Semmens & Peric 1995–6). They used a qualitative approach to explore children's experiences of a parent's chronic illness and death. In this way, they were able to go beyond the published accounts of death, to explore something new and important in understanding how children's reactions may be different from those of adults.

Another source of inspiration can be the recommendations at the end of a research report. For example, at the end of a study exploring violence towards nurses in New South Wales emergency departments, Lyneham (2000) stated:

> Further research is required to examine the issues of non-reporting, security and precipitating factors so that there can be a concerted effort to find real solutions and protect emergency nurses from harm.

This recommendation could lead the reader to plan a similar study that incorporates these recommendations in its design.

Sometimes, in reading through the literature, you will see certain research themes emerging. For example, two articles on gender bias in cardiac conditions (Hildon 1994; Broom 1995) appeared in the literature in late 1994 and early 1995. The emergence of these articles may have been in response to the criticism that research into heart disease was male-dominated. A researcher looking for a topic could explore such an emerging theme if it were suitable in other respects.

The literature may also reveal a gap that needs to be filled. For example, Bailey stated that 'there exists a scarcity of published research on the issues relevant to the care of psychiatric patients within an acute care stetting' and that 'only one study is currently to be found in the literature directly pertaining to the attitudes of critical care nurses and doctors towards patients who have attempted suicide' (Bailey 1998). She then proceeded to carry out a study on the attitudes of critical care doctors and nurses towards psychiatric patients. Similarly, O'Brien and Spry (1995) found that the literature relating to career structures did little to describe the expanding role of the Clinical Nurse Consultant from the practitioner's point of view. Accordingly, they set up an action research project to track the role transitions of these nurses from ward-based experts to facility-oriented resource people.

There may also be variations in findings that lead to the design of a study to settle the argument. For example, there were inconsistencies in the findings on the use of cabbage leaves in breast engorgement that led the author and colleagues to carry out a study comparing cabbage leaves and cold compresses and another comparing chilled and room-temperature cabbage leaves (Roberts 1995a; Roberts, Reiter & Schuster 1995). The inconsistent findings of these studies led to a further study (comparing cabbage leaf extract with a placebo) and the development of an instrument to measure breast engorgement objectively.

The literature can also provide examples of studies that you may wish to replicate. Replication is repeating a study using the same methodology. Replications is generally considered to be desirable in order to verify existing findings and increase their validity by carrying out identical research with a variety of subjects in different settings. However, there are few studies published that replicate others so we have a large number of small, unrelated studies with a limited generalisability of results (Nieswiadomy 1993). There is a need for more research that builds upon earlier research and addresses its limitations. Be aware, however, that originality is a requirement for research projects in many higher degrees. It is also important to realise that in some cases replication may not be seen as necessary or advisable. This is especially true if you are taking a qualitative approach, which assumes that people are unique in their respective contexts and that absolute replication is not possible. In such cases, the research would still need to be original, but not necessarily based on the research method used previously.

Professional trends

Major events that affect the profession can also be a source of research topics. By reading those columns of journals that deal with professional issues, you can get advance warning of these trends and use them to help you select a topic. One such event was the introduction of diagnosis related groups in Australia in the 1990s in order to contain costs. This event was a watershed for nursing research as it stimulated the use of a variety of managed care systems and highlighted the need for outcome measures that would show the costs of the nursing component of care (Abdellah & Levine 1994). Another issue was the impact of unqualified carers on client care, which also generated research studies. There will be many issues for the third millennium, for example the impact of the introduction of the role of the nurse-practitioner or advanced practice nurse. A good place to find issues is in editorial columns of journals.

Identified research priorities

Research priorities that have been identified already are a useful source of problems. A prioritisation of clinical research problems was carried out for oncology nurses by Chang and Daly (1996) and for rural nurses by Bell, Daly and Chang (1997). The latter study found that community care in relation to reducing length of stay in hospitals, allocation of time for health promotion and illness prevention, professional isolation, and delivery of updates and counselling skills education were all seen as research priorities by rural nurses. You could also set your own priorities by looking at the status quo and asking what are the most important things to change, or asking your colleagues what they see as priorities.

Nursing or health theories are another source of research problems. There is a great need for more testing of the large number of nursing theories. Theories postulate that there are certain relationships between concepts and these can be tested out using research techniques. The theory may predict a certain outcome and it is necessary to test the theory to see if it is applicable in practice. Very few nursing research projects operate at the level of testing theory (Moody et al. 1988; Roberts 1995b) but some use the theory as a framework for organising the research. For example, a study of the effect of boomerang pillows on respiratory capacity used Levine's conservation principles as a conceptual framework (Roberts, Brittin & deClifford 1995). The role of theories as conceptual frameworks for nursing research will be explored further in Chapter 4.

There are many sources of research problems, if you remain open to the possibilities inherent in your work and look for them in your reading and discussion with colleagues. It is very important to get the right problem in terms of relevance, significance and feasibility. Spending time in the beginning can pay dividends by preventing the waste of time and energy involved in the selection of a problem that is unsatisfactory.

Criteria for selecting problems
The researcher

You, the researcher, must have the appropriate experience and skills to address the research problem. Frequently, research experience is related to qualifications. Beginning skills can be learned in undergraduate programs, although many undergraduate programs are now focusing on the preparation of research consumers rather than researchers. Advanced research skills are learned in research degrees, specifically honours, research masters' and doctoral degrees. You must also understand some of the assumptions that underlie the use of certain methodologies, for example, grounded theory.

An inexperienced researcher should select a problem that can use a simple design, instruments and analytical process. It is better to carry out a simple project well than do poorly in a complex one. Complicated designs requiring sophisticated measurement techniques and complex data analyses are best left to more experienced researchers. If physical equipment is involved, you need to consider whether you have the technical expertise to run it.

You must have adequate knowledge of the general area you are preparing to research if you are to research it effectively. It is easier to research in an area with which you are familiar since you will already know the terminology and major ideas. For example, a midwife would find it easier to do research in midwifery from a theoretical base of midwifery knowledge. Familiarity with relevant theories and concepts will assist you to plan research that is linked to theory. Knowledge of previous research in the area will also help you to select an appropriate problem to research.

Interest in the problem is also a criterion. You should research in an area that you are interested in and choose a problem for which you want to find the answer. This will help you to maintain enthusiasm for the project during the difficult periods. You will probably produce a better result if you are interested in what you are doing. The interest factor is more important in a longer project than in a shorter one since it is more difficult to sustain interest over a longer period.

The problem

The problem selected should fall within the general area of nursing if it is to be considered nursing research. The debate about what constitutes nursing research is continuing; for example, where the boundaries lie between nursing and medical research, and research in behavioural science. A rule of thumb is that if nurses have control over the decision-making in that area of practice, it is a suitable subject for nursing research. Research about client health is also valid for nursing. A good question to ask yourself is 'How is this relevant to nursing?' The answer should show a link to nursing's major domain concepts of person, health, environment, and nursing.

The importance of the research problem is also a criterion (Barnard 1986). For a beginning researcher, it need not be a problem that solves all of the important questions in nursing. Nevertheless, it should be a question that is worth answering. Nursing journals are paying increasing attention to significance for nursing, particularly in the areas of clinical application. For example, the journal *Clinical Nursing Research* requires the author to address the question of clinical significance of the research. Since you are going to put a lot of time and effort into your study, you should select a topic that will produce findings of benefit to some person or group – the client, the nurse, the health care agency, the community, or society. Will the answer to your research question have the potential to lead to improvements in client health, community health or nursing practice? Will it lead to changes in protocols or policies in your institution? Will the study lead to the development of knowledge? Perhaps it will test a theoretical proposition or explore a new area of knowledge.

You should also consider feasibility, or whether the research can actually be carried out. By their very nature, some problems are difficult or impossible to research. For quantitative research, you need to choose variables that can be measured using the current technology. For example, it would be impossible to assess neonates' attitudes to neonatal intensive care units. For qualitative research, the question needs to be stated broadly enough to permit a full explanation of the phenomenon to be measured. It should also be aligned to the theoretical assumptions of how knowledge is produced through research. Taylor was interested in exploring the meaning of ordinariness, so she used some ideas from phenomenology (Taylor 1994). For example 'being-in-the-world' means the claim that people are aware of the answers to larger life questions by virtue of living in their bodies every day. Using this concept, she set up a phenomenological research approach that would give her the widest possible means of gathering in whatever insights she could from nurses and patients so that they could tell her what the ordinariness of being human in nursing meant to them.

Legitimacy is also a criterion. Just because a study can be carried out does not mean it should be. A research problem should not reflect a moral position. Areas such as religious beliefs, politics, or ethics are frequently value-laden. For example, 'Should nurses assist with euthanasia?' is not a suitable research topic because it is trying to answer a moral question. Moral questions should be answered by ethical debate rather than by research. This does not mean that value-laden, subjective areas cannot be researched, however. It is a matter of eliminating the 'should' aspect of the question. Questions such as the above can be rephrased to something like 'What is the lived experience of nurses assisting with euthanasia?' or 'What are the attitudes to death of nurses who have assisted with euthanasia compared with those who have not?'

Research questions which show that the researcher is biased and trying to prove a point are also unsuitable. For example, a research question such as 'Why are the graduates from University X incompetent?' indicates bias on the part of the researcher and is not a suitable research question. These questions can frequently be rephrased in a different way, for example: 'What perception of their own competence is held by graduates of University X?'

Ethical standards are also a criterion. You should not proceed with any research project that involves harming or deceiving the subjects, coercing the subjects to participate, or exposing them to risks out of proportion to the benefits of the research. Any research project must comply with the ethical guidelines of the NHMRC and the relevant human research ethics committee(s) or else it will not be approved. You can find further information about the ethics of research in Chapter 5.

Resources

You need to be sure that you have sufficient time to carry out the project. A research project almost invariably takes longer than you expect; you need to make sure that the project itself will not consume more time than is available to complete it. You should consider the nature of the project. If you are using a collaborative process between the researcher and the participants, such as action research, it will take longer than, say, a questionnaire. You should also consider the nature of the problem you are studying. For example, a study of client progress through a lengthy treatment would not be feasible if you only have one semester to carry out the project. You should also consider the time you can spend working on the project. You will need to balance the time necessary for the project with your other work and personal commitments. Finally, you should consider if data would have to be collected at a particular time of year or month and how that fits your schedule.

Money is also a consideration. Be sure that you can afford the project. Virtually every project has some cost attached. Some universities allocate money to students for research projects and may provide equipment such as computers and software. However, they do not usually support the costs of expensive student projects. You should clarify at the outset the amount of financial support that will be provided. If the amount available from the university, your own funds and other sponsors is not sufficient, you will need to rethink the project and scale it down to a more realistic level, or choose another topic.

In deciding whether or not you can afford a project, consider its real costs, the budget available, and the cost–benefit ratio. Before making a final decision, you should make a list of all projected expenses, including an adjustment for price rises. There will probably be costs for obtaining literature, including photocopying, computer searches, books and journal subscriptions. For carrying out the project, you may need stationery and other consumables such as cartridges for the printer. You may need to pay the participants in your project. If you are doing a postal survey, postage (including return postage for questionnaires) will be a major cost. Printing questionnaires and self-addressed envelopes will also be significant costs. If you are doing field research involving interviews, audiotapes will be a significant cost. You may need to rent or purchase equipment such as tape recorders, video cameras, computers or instruments if they are not available through your institution. You may need to hire labour for data collection and management. If your project involves travel, you will have transportation, accommodation and, possibly, living costs to consider. You may also have communication costs such as telephone calls and faxes. For the data analysis stage, you may need to purchase computer software or hire specific services. For the writing-up stage, you will need more stationery and consumables. There is no such thing as free research!

In selecting a problem, you must consider the people you will need to help you undertake the project. For example, there may be gatekeepers who can give or withhold permission to enter facilities for data collection. The gaining of administrative support is one of the highest priorities when beginning nursing research in clinical settings (Fry, Mortimer & Ramsay 1994). You will need to secure permission from gatekeepers before undertaking the project, at the problem formation stage. If you are employed in a clinical facility, you may need to negotiate with the authorities for the use of the facilities, or for time off to carry out the project.

Availability of the people that you need to study for the research is an important consideration. Your being convinced of the value of your research does not mean that people will be queuing up to help you with it. Clinical research is notorious for subjects disappearing. When you get out in the field you may find that you cannot locate enough people who meet the criteria for participating in your study, particularly if they are unusual. Potential participants may be geographically difficult to access, in the case of Aboriginal people in remote areas, or they may be hard to find, for example illegal injecting drug users. Sometimes people may be involved already in other studies and will not have the time for involvement in two studies, or their participation in one study precludes their taking part in another. Even if potential participants are eligible, they may be unwilling to help, especially if there is any discomfort involved. Some people are afraid to talk to a researcher on sensitive topics such as criminal behaviour or domestic violence in case of unwanted consequences. Sometimes people just do not trust a researcher, for example elderly people may not be willing to sign a consent form because relatives have told them not to sign any documents.

There can also be procedural difficulties with accessing participants. For example, if the proposed participants are children, parental consent is required. The authorities and medical staff in the clinical facilities must agree that your study can take place. In addition, you will need to go through the appropriate channels for approval in your institution such as your supervisor, the human research ethics committee, and all of the other required committees.

Stating the problem/question/purpose of the study

It is normal for there to be a general statement of purpose or aim of the study. This is usually found near the beginning of the study and sets out concisely, in broad terms, what the study hoped to accomplish, or its goals and aims. Its purpose is to orient the reader to the study. An example of a statement of purpose is: 'The aim of this study was to investigate interpersonal stress in a group of registered nurses and to explore the possible cognitive mediating function of the personality construct of *Lifestyle* proposed by Individual Psychology (IP)' (Santamaria 2000). In another example, the purpose of a study that compared the use of normal saline and heparinised saline in flushing intravenous cannulae was 'to determine which (if either) solution was better suited to paediatric patients' (Robertson 1994). In a third study, the stated purpose was 'to investigate the incidence of restraint in nursing homes and factors that contribute to decisions to apply restraints' (Koch 1994). Another study using a historical survey method stated that its purpose was 'to examine trends in published Australian nursing literature' (McConnell & Paech 1993). Note that in all of these, the purpose of the study is stated concisely, and gives the reader a general idea of what the study hoped to accomplish.

The more specific problem or question that the study seeks to answer can be stated either as a declarative statement or a question. Stating it as a question helps you to clarify exactly what it is that you want to find out. For example,

Robertson went on to pose the research question(s) for the above study on flushing solutions for cannulae as:

> whether flushing the cannula with normal saline, rather than heparinised saline, resulted in a difference in the: reason for removal of the IV cannula, incidence of phlebitis, incidence of blocked cannulae, and number of days an indwelling, intermittent intravenous cannula remained functional (Robertson 1994).

The greater specificity of this set of questions tells the reader exactly what Robertson was measuring and foreshadows the variables that would be measured.

One way of structuring a research question is to divide it into a stem, which is the 'who, what, when, where or why' part of the question, and a topic, which is what the question is about (Brink & Wood 1994, p. 10).

Research questions can be formulated at three levels (Brink & Wood 1994). The first level is descriptive. Questions at this level are exploratory, frequently looking at new groups or trying to supply missing data. They do not try to investigate relationships among variables or demonstrate cause and effect. Usually they have a stem of 'what?' or 'who?' Qualitative research questions are usually descriptive by their very nature although relationships may be explored during the study and theory may be developed. An example of a qualitative research question is: 'What are the important characteristics which Koories identify as leading to a personal state of mental health or well-being?' (Turale 1994). In this question, 'what are' is the stem, and 'the important characteristics which Koories identify as leading to a personal state of mental health or well-being' is the topic.

The second-level question is focused on the relationship between two or more variables and the direction of the relationship, or how one varies or correlates with the other. For example, McConnell and Paech examined the relationship between date of publication and the characteristics of articles in the first eight years of the *Australian Journal of Advanced Nursing* (McConnell & Paech 1993). The stem in the question is 'what is the relationship' and the topic is 'between time published and the characteristics of articles in the first eight years of the *AJAN*'.

The third level of question is one in which the research question asks 'why', or explores cause and effect. The 'why' is frequently explained by the theory. For example, a study designed to find out whether kangaroo mother care (KMC) was superior to conventional incubator care hypothesised that babies who received KMC would have more stable temperatures than those in conventional care because prolonged contact with the mother's skin helped to stabilise them. At level 3, you can predict what will happen and provide a theory based on previous research findings to explain it (Brink & Wood 1994).

The process

The first step in formulating a research question is either to brainstorm topics or to make a list of potential topics, using the sources given earlier in this chapter. Write your ideas down on paper, the whiteboard, or the computer and play with them.

Then select what seems to you the best idea and discuss it with colleagues, your supervisor or experts in the field. Evaluate the topic in terms of the criteria given previously, then narrow it down to a feasible topic. Finally, write a statement of purpose and then state your research problem as a question or set of questions. During this process, you will be reading the literature to become an expert on the topic and this will help you with the formation of relevant research questions.

Once the research problem and its consequent question or questions have been formulated, you will need to refine them. Frequently, the initial question is too broad and beyond the limits of a feasible study, making it necessary to narrow down the problem until you have a research question that you can undertake. The narrowing-down process can relate to the topic or the setting for the research. You can narrow the topic by removing its less important parts. Alternatively, you can narrow the number of settings in which you will conduct the study, or the types of participants you include. It may be necessary to restrict the topic in several dimensions. Suppose you want to investigate the impact of managed care plans on nursing outcomes. To look at all kinds of care plans in all types of hospitals and for all types of clients would clearly be a lifetime's work, so you have to narrow down the topic to a few outcomes for one type of client in one type of hospital.

Stating an hypothesis and identifying variables

Once you have stated your problem, you need to develop an hypothesis that will give you a working basis for investigation. Although stating an hypothesis might seem difficult at first glance, it is not. Basically, an hypothesis is only a statement of what the researcher thinks is going to be the outcome of the investigation. We formulate hypotheses all the time, although we may not recognise them. For instance, we may say 'Every time I forget my umbrella, it rains'. This could be restated as a research hypothesis: 'On the days when I forget to take my umbrella, it is more likely to rain than on days when I remember to take it'.

In a research project, it is customary to formulate a formal research hypothesis that speculates about the relationship between two variables. In order to be an hypothesis, it must state a possible relationship, and it must have at least two variables that enter into the relationship.

A variable, as its name suggests, is something that varies. In the example above, there are two variables, whether I forget or remember my umbrella, and whether or not it rains. The variable that can be controlled by the researcher is called the independent variable. The variable that is not controlled by the researcher, or the variable that is hypothesised to be affected by the independent variable, is the dependent variable. It is helpful to think of the dependent variable as the outcome variable. In the example above, you could think of the weather as the dependent variable, and the remembering of the umbrella as an independent variable. However, this is not strictly correct as you are not manipulating your memory. In instances where the researcher does not control the independent variable, it is more correct to speak of research variables than of independent and dependent variables.

Let us take a nursing example. In a study comparing the effectiveness of venepuncture and heel prick in a newborn screening test, an hypothesis was not stated explicitly (Logan 1999). However, the implied hypothesis was that there would be no significant difference in the time taken to do the test and the crying behaviours of the babies. This hypothesis suggests that there will be no difference, which is appropriate when the researchers cannot really predict a direction for a difference. This is called a null hypothesis. If the researchers had evidence to suggest that one of the methods was more effective than the other, they might have stated a directional hypothesis that 'the time taken to do the heel prick will be longer than that taken to do the venepuncture'. Or vice versa. By now you will have spotted that the variables are the method of obtaining blood and the time taken. Since it is the method of obtaining blood that is varied by the researcher, that is the independent variable. Since it is the time taken to obtain the blood that is the outcome, that is the dependent variable.

Research hypotheses can be stated as directional hypotheses, meaning that the researcher is speculating about the direction that the findings will take. In order to do this, the researcher must have some grounds for stating a direction. These can consist of a theoretical prediction, previous research findings, or a logical argument.

Even when you express a directional hypothesis, it is usually converted to a null hypothesis, because, in statistical analysis, it is customary to try to demonstrate that you reject the statement that there is no difference in the groups, rather than saying that there is a difference. This will be discussed further in Chapter 10.

Each hypothesis should be able to be tested, or it is not an hypothesis. Also, each hypothesis should deal only with one relationship and one set of variables. However, a study may have more than one hypothesis being tested.

Variables are, as stated above, the parts of an hypothesis that vary. They should be defined in terms of the concept that they measure. Variables should also be stated in terms of how they are going to be measured, which is not always stated in the hypothesis itself. For example, if you were going to measure blood pressure, you should state whether you are measuring it with a sphygmomanometer, or with a direct sensor in the blood vessel.

Summary

In this chapter, we have looked at the reasons that research problems are important. We have seen that you, your colleagues, the literature and theories are sources of problems. We have examined the criteria for selecting a research problem in terms of the researcher, the problem, and resources. We have also looked at the process of framing a research question and at the different levels of question. We have addressed how to narrow down a broad topic into a manageable one. Finally, we have discussed how to formulate an hypothesis.

Main points

- A research question is 'an explicit query about a problem or issue that can be challenged, examined, and analysed and that will yield useful new information' (Brink & Wood 1994, p. 2).
- A research problem will be stated in broader terms and as a sentence, while a research question will be more specific and stated as a question.
- Difficulties in finding a research problem can be attributed to too much choice and a lack of familiarity with either the research process or previous research in the area.
- People, the research literature, professional trends and identified research priorities can be a source of research questions and problems.
- The researcher should have the requisite characteristics and an interest in the problem; the problem should be important, legitimate, and able to be researched.
- The statement of purpose or aim sets out concisely the goals and aims of the study.
- There are three levels of question: descriptive or exploratory level, relationship finding (correlational) and causal or hypothesis testing.
- The process of finding a problem is to make a list of potential topics, select what seems to you the best idea, discuss it with colleagues or experts, evaluate the topic and then narrow it down to a feasible topic.
- When the topic has been identified, you write a statement of purpose, state your research problem as a question or set of questions and refine it as necessary.
- An hypothesis is a testable statement of the expected outcome that speculates about relationship between variables. Each hypothesis deals with one relationship only, and may be directional or non-directional (null).
- A variable is something that varies: the independent variable is varied by the researcher and affects the dependent variable; the dependent or outcome variable is not controlled by the researcher and is affected by the independent variable.
- Variables should be defined in terms of the concept that they measure and be stated in terms of how they are going to be measured.

Review Questions

1. A research problem will:
    a. be stated as a sentence ✓
    b. be an explicit query
    c. state an hypothesis
    d. describe the participants

2   Which of the following people is normally a source of nursing research problems?
    a   lecturer
    b   medical staff
    c   librarians
    d   a and c

3   Which of the following is a criterion for selecting research problems?
    a   researcher's skills and experience
    b   importance of the problem
    c   degree of difficulty of project design
    d   all of the above

4   Which of the following would **not** be a legitimate research question?
    a   Does dressing technique A result in faster healing than technique B?
    b   What is the lived experience of post-traumatic stress syndrome?
    c   Should nurses carry out termination of pregnancy procedures?
    d   How do clients cope with adaptation to HIV-positive status?

5   Which of the following would be an example of a descriptive-level research question?
    a   What is the relationship between personality type and self-caring abilities?
    b   What factors do diabetic clients identify as important in achieving self-care?
    c   Do men have higher levels of access to health care than women?
    d   All of the above

6   Which of the following would be an example of a second-level research question?
    a   What is the relationship between gender and heart disease?
    b   Is dressing technique A more effective in promoting wound healing than dressing technique B?
    c   What is the incidence of immunisation in the population of city C?
    d   Which is the more efficient conductor of ECG stimuli, water or gel?

7   Which of the following is a third-level research question?
    a   Do babies who get less cuddling have higher rates of 'failure to thrive' than babies who get more cuddling?
    b   What is the experience of gay people in their contact with nurses?
    c   What is the relationship between age and attitudes to safe sex?
    d   Does gender influence the client's attitude to pain?

8   In a research question, the stem identifies the:
    a   hypothesis
    b   variables
    c   person or object being researched
    d   relationship statement

9   Which of the following is a directional hypothesis?
    a   What is the lived experience of caring for the terminally ill?
    b   There will be a higher rate of HIV in persons who do not practise safe sex than in those who do.
    c   There will be a relationship between gender and tolerance to pain.
    d   There will be no difference in self-caring abilities in males and females.

10 In the hypothesis 'There will be a higher rate of infection in clients who are treated with a gauze dressing than with an occlusive dressing', which is the dependent variable?
    a   gauze dressing
    b   clients
    c   modality of treatment
    d   rate of infection

Discussion Questions

1. Differentiate between a research problem and a question.
2. List four major sources of research problems and state why they are useful.
3. Discuss five constraints on the research topic.
4. Discuss five criteria that a research problem should meet.
5. Define 'hypothesis' and 'variable' and state the subtypes of each.

References

Abdellah, F. & Levine, E. 1994, *Preparing Nursing Research for the 21st Century*, Springer, New York.

Bailey, S. 1998, 'An exploration of critical care nurses' and doctors' attitudes towards psychiatric patients', *Australian Journal of Advanced Nursing*, vol. 15, no. 3, 8–14.

Barclay, L., Harrington, A., Conroy, R., Royal, R. & LaForgia, J. 1994, 'A comparative study of neonates' umbilical cord management', *Australian Journal of Advanced Nursing*, vol. 11, no. 3, 34–40.

Barnard, K. 1986, 'Research utilization: the researcher's responsibilities', *Maternal Child Nursing*, vol. 11, 150.

Bell, P., Daly, J. & Chang, E. 1997, 'A study of the educational and research priorities of registered nurses in rural Australia', *Journal of Advanced Nursing*, vol. 25, no. 4, 794–800.

Black, A. & Childs, G. 1994, 'Staff attachment and loss in a long term baby ward', *Contemporary Nurse*, vol. 4, no. 4, 153–61.

Brink, P. & Wood, M. 1994, *Basic Steps in Planning Research*, Jones & Bartlett, London.

Broom, D. 1995, 'Women and heart disease', *Collegian*, vol. 2, no. 1, 16–19.

Chang, E. & Daly, J. 1996, 'Clinical research priorities in oncology nursing: an Australian perspective', *International Journal of Nursing Practice*, vol. 2, no. 1, 21–8.

Fry, A., Mortimer, K. & Ramsay, L. 1994, 'Clinical research and the culture of collaboration', *Australian Journal of Advanced Nursing*, vol. 11, no. 3, 11–17.

Hildon, A. 1994, 'Gender bias in cardiology: are women missing out on PTCA?' *Australian Journal of Advanced Nursing*, vol. 12, no. 1, 6–11.

Koch, S. 1994, 'Restraining nursing home residents', *Australian Journal of Advanced Nursing*, vol. 11, no. 2, 9–14.

Koch, T. & Kelly, S. 1999, 'Identifying strategies for managing urinary incontinence with women who have multiple sclerosis', *Journal of Clinical Nursing*, vol. 8, no. 5, 550–9.

Logan, P. 1999, 'Venepuncture versus heel prick for the collection of the newborn screening test', *Australian Journal of Advanced Nursing*, vol. 17, no 1, 30–6.

Lyneham, J. 2000, 'Violence in New South Wales emergency departments', *Australian Journal of Advanced Nursing*, vol. 18, no. 2, 8–17.

McConnell, E. & Paech, M. 1993, 'Trends in scholarly nursing literature', *Australian Journal of Advanced Nursing*, vol. 11, no. 2, 28–32.

McKenna, L. & Walsh, K. 1997, 'Changing handover practice: one private hospital's experience', *International Journal of Nursing Practice*, vol. 3, no. 2, 128–32.

Moody, L., Wilson, M., Smyth, K., Schwartz, R., Tittle, M. & Van Cott, M. 1988, 'Analysis of a decade of nursing practice research: 1977–86', *Nursing Research*, vol. 37, no. 6, 374–9.

Nieswiadomy, R. 1993, *Foundations of Nursing Research*, Appleton & Lange, Norwalk, Connecticut.

O'Brien, B. & Spry, J. 1995, 'Expanding the role of the clinical nurse consultant', *Australian Journal of Advanced Nursing*, vol. 12, no. 4, 26–32.

Roberts, K. 1995a, 'A comparison of chilled cabbage leaves and chilled gelpaks in treating breast engorgement', *Journal of Human Lactation*, vol. 11, no. 1, 17–20.

Roberts, K. 1995b, 'Early Australian nursing scholarship: the first decade of the AJAN: Part 2: Scholarship', *Australian Electronic Journal of Nursing Education*, vol. 1, no. 1.

Roberts, K., Brittin, M. & deClifford, J. 1995, 'Boomerang pillows and respiratory capacity in frail elderly women', *Clinical Nursing Research*, vol. 4, no. 4, 465–71.

Roberts, K., Reiter, M. & Schuster, D. 1995, 'A comparison of chilled and room temperature cabbage leaves in treating breast engorgement', *Journal of Human Lactation*, vol. 11, no. 3, 191–4.

Robertson, J. 1994, 'Intermittent intravenous therapy: a comparison of two flushing solutions', *Contemporary Nurse*, vol. 3, no. 4, 174–9.

Santamaria, N. 2000, 'The relationship between nurses' personality and stress levels reported when caring for interpersonally difficult patients', *Australian Journal of Advanced Nursing*, vol. 18, no. 2, 20–6.

Semmens, J. & Peric, J. 1995–6, 'Children's experiences of a parent's chronic illness and death', *Australian Journal of Advanced Nursing*, vol. 13, no. 2, 30–8.

Taylor, B. J. 1994, *Being Human: Ordinariness in Nursing*, Churchill Livingstone, Melbourne.

Turale, S. 1994, 'Ballarat Koorie life experiences: learning about Koorie perceptions of mental health and illness', *Australian Journal of Mental Health Nursing*, vol. 3, no. 1, 16–28.

CHAPTER 3

Reviewing the literature

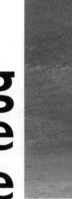

chapter objectives

In this chapter, you will learn how to review the literature that bears on the research problem by identifying, obtaining, reading and sorting it. The material in this chapter will assist you to:

- understand why you should review the literature
- locate possible sources of relevant literature
- set up an efficient system for keeping track of sources
- identify the literature that is pertinent to the project
- obtain the identified literature
- effectively read the literature that has been obtained
- extract the relevant information from the literature
- critique research reports
- set up an efficient system for dealing with references.

Introduction

The literature is the total body of writing that deals with the topic being researched. It comprises theoretical and research papers together with any other relevant material. It may include books, articles in periodicals, conference proceedings, unpublished papers and personal communications from other researchers.

The term 'review of the literature' has several meanings. In the sense of the act of reviewing the literature, it means to read, sort and analyse the work, putting it into some kind of order. It also involves critiquing individual research reports. These are the two senses of 'review of the literature' that we will deal with in this chapter. In the sense of the outcome of reviewing the literature, the phrase means that section of a paper, thesis or dissertation that presents an integrated evaluation of previous theory and research. How you go about writing a literature review will be dealt with in Chapter 6.

Beginning researchers often find the thought of dealing with the literature to be quite overwhelming, particularly when it is on a topic that has been well researched. It may seem an impossible task not only to read and understand all the literature but also to critique it and to organise it into a sensible framework. Nevertheless, it is essential to acquire, read and make sense of all relevant research on the topic. Researchers must understand the work that has gone before if they are to know how and where their study will fit into the overall work and add to that body of knowledge.

Why review the literature?

A beginning researcher may wonder why it is necessary to review the literature. It might seem more effective simply to decide what you want to research and then go and do it. However, reviewing the literature helps you develop a comprehensive understanding of the topic, making you aware of what is known and what questions need to be answered. This can help you to decide exactly what to research and how to go about it.

Familiarity with the body of literature on a topic will help you to identify how your proposed study will fit into the body of literature already available. For example, you might discover that the question you wanted to answer has been researched already using a particular theoretical framework.

Reviewing the literature can also help you to narrow down the topic for your study. In reading the literature, you may see that your topic is too broad and would entail too many areas of investigation. Knowing the literature can help you select a facet of the topic that would be beneficial to study and that can be kept within realistic bounds.

Reviewing the literature can also help you with the design of your study. By exposure to the approach used by previous researchers investigating the area, you can see whether the designs chosen are usually experimental, phenomenological or historical. For example, you would find that homelessness has usually been studied using interview and field work because the homeless are impossible to access through survey methods such as postal questionnaires.

Reviewing the literature can also help you with the details of the study's methodology. You will be able to see the specifics of the previous designs, how they related to their theoretical frameworks, how the data were collected and how they were analysed.

However, you should be aware that in some qualitative approaches, justification is given for not reviewing the literature prior to the study. In some qualitative research approaches, such as grounded theory, it is not appropriate to do more than a superficial reading of the literature in order to identify whether the topic needs to be studied. This will be discussed later in Chapter 12.

Identifying relevant literature

The first step in reviewing the literature is to identify possible sources. In today's world, in which an enormous amount of information is readily available, even the identification of information can be time-consuming. It is important to understand the process of identifying relevant literature and to use that process efficiently in order to select only that which bears directly on your topic. This approach will minimise the amount of work involved.

Preparing to search

Before heading off to the library, it is important to organise your search. Being systematic in both searching and record-keeping is the key to an efficient search. Even if you think you have a small topic that requires little organisation, it is important to get into good habits of searching and record-keeping that will become second nature to you. Not only will these habits stand you in good stead in simple projects, they will be useful for non-research projects and for larger research projects, should you progress to them.

You need to start by defining your topic in sufficient detail to enable you to find the relevant information. In previous chapters, we looked at how you select, narrow and refine your topic. By now, you should have a good idea of the key words that define your topic. It is essential to know these before starting your search so that you can use them as terms under which to look.

Beginning researchers often wonder when to search for material. For quantitative research, you will always search at the beginning of the project. If it is a longer project, say a year, you will search at the end as well in order to make sure that you have included the latest information. If it is a very long project, such as a major thesis, you will need to do a top-up search at least every six months. This is not difficult in these days of electronic media.

For qualitative research, there is a different approach to timing the review of the literature. You may choose not to review the literature before undertaking a study because it can narrow a study too early and too much, causing you to miss important observations. You may choose to review the literature as the study progresses so that you can see what others are doing, or wait until the end. The problem with the latter approach is that you may spend much time and energy finding what is already known. A middle ground is to read the literature for highlights of major findings and theories only, thus achieving an informed stance but still remaining open to possibilities.

Setting boundaries to the search

Students also find it difficult to decide how much to search and frequently underestimate the amount of time it takes to do a search. How much to search will depend on your experience, searching skills, and financial resources. You should normally spend no more than one-quarter of your time reviewing the literature. It is important to search enough to be sure that you have found all of the relevant information but do not search so much that you are in danger of sinking under the weight of information. You should not spend so much time reading that you never carry out the research project. On the other hand, if you do not spend enough time reading you may miss important information. The extent of your reading depends partly on how much information is available on your exact topic. If there is not very much, it may be necessary to read related material. If there is a lot, it may be necessary to narrow the topic. Difficulty in locating sources can also influence the amount of time available for reading.

It is best to begin at the most current references and work your way back until you cannot find any more. If the topic is new, then it may not be necessary to go back very far. For instance, the topic of AIDS was unheard of before 1980. If the topic is in and out of vogue, then beware of stopping the search prematurely as there may be more information in earlier years. As a rule of thumb, 10 years is a reasonable period to search, with those papers leading you to previously published 'classics' that should be included.

Another factor that affects the extent of your search is your reason for doing it. If you are doing a brief undergraduate project, your lecturer should not expect you to have every reference ever written on the topic, and a dozen main papers will normally be sufficient. At the other end of the spectrum, a PhD thesis will normally require an extremely thorough review of the literature. The higher up the academic ladder you climb, the more comprehensive and exacting will be your review of the literature. A world expert on a topic will be thoroughly conversant with the literature on that topic.

Financial constraints can also have a bearing on how much you search. While sources close to home are reasonably cheap to photocopy, it is expensive to acquire material on interlibrary loan. Often, universities have funds dedicated to interlibrary loan materials for students, so it is wise to check with your supervisor or lecturer about sources of money for this purpose.

Your own expertise in searching can also be an important factor. Students just beginning to learn about research will not be as skilled at uncovering sources or using other resources.

Sometimes it is necessary to narrow either the scope of the literature review or the topic reviewed. If the topic is producing too much literature, it may be too complex and you should narrow it to make it more manageable. You may be reading non-research material that does not belong in a literature review. If so, you should narrow your search to look only at actual research papers and exclude non-research material or, at most, read it for background information. It is important to identify the boundaries of your search. Sometimes a diagram or flow chart of the topic and design is helpful to identify the limits of the literature review.

Possible resources
Who can help you?
We tend to think of literature resources as paper-based or electronic but it is important to remember that there are people who can be of great assistance and who are often happy to help students. First, if it is a class project, consult your lecturer. Lecturers have almost invariably done research themselves, or they would not be assigning you a research project. Frequently they will help you to narrow down the topic or point you in the direction of some appropriate resources. However, before you consult them, make sure you have thought through the topic somewhat and can talk about it. If it is a thesis or dissertation, you should consult your supervisor frequently, as it is part of his or her job to assist you in this way.

Secondly, consult your colleagues. They may have some material on the subject. Also, if they know you are interested in a topic, they may keep their eyes open for information for you. They can also help you to talk through the topic and may give you ideas or a perspective on the topic that you had not thought of. Electronic mail allows researchers to contact colleagues easily and discuss common interests. For example, NURSRES is a list of a large number of nurses interested in research and a message to them will usually result in some useful resources or dialogue. However, be warned that a request that shows that you have not first made an attempt to find the information yourself will not usually be well received. You must first do a thorough search through the indexes (see section below headed Indexes).

The library staff will also be helpful. They know how to find information and are usually willing to help, provided you do not expect them to do all your work for you. The staff at the circulation or information desk can help you locate items that you need. Similarly, the staff familiar with the catalogue can help you find out whether an item is in the library. The interlibrary loan staff can help you to obtain items that you need from other libraries. Some libraries have specific reference librarians for particular areas of knowledge and they are familiar with the main materials in that area. The reference librarian can advise you on the type of search that will be most productive. This advice can include which databases to use, and which strategies will be most effective for searching.

Most libraries have orientation sessions on how to use the technology, especially CD-ROM or World Wide Web (WWW) databases. The librarian can also help you find items that are not in the usual databases.

Types of literature sources

There are various types of materials available. One distinction is between primary and secondary sources. Primary sources are those written by the author and have the advantage of being the author's own ideas. Secondary sources are those to which an author refers. They have the disadvantage of being filtered through the writer's own attitudes and biases, but sometimes you cannot access the source in any other way. A clue to a secondary source is a reference 'cited by …' Indeed, the Review of the Literature section of any paper is full of secondary sources.

Another distinction is between scholarly and unscholarly work, scholarly works usually being the more valuable sources for research purposes. Such works as theoretical papers, reports of research methodologies, procedures or instruments, reports of research results, review papers and books written by authorities are scholarly literature. Refereed journal articles are considered more scholarly than non-refereed articles. A refereed journal article is one that has been sent out for peer review before being accepted for publication. Sources from the lay literature, newspapers and magazines are not scholarly work. Anecdotal or impressionistic reports or opinions on how to carry out health care are not normally scholarly. You should use them for background reading only. Similarly information obtained from the World Wide Web is unlikely to be scholarly unless it is from a refereed journal that is accessible from the web.

Useful sources of literature

Books

Books are not usually in the forefront of research unless they are research books. This is primarily because of the time lag of up to five years between the time a research report project is written up, appears in a journal and is then cited in a book. However, books can be valuable sources of literature and ideas. Their bibliographies can also be a useful source of references. There are now electronic databases of books that are in print. For example, the database WorldCat lists all books in print. It is accessible through a portal called First Search, which lists many databases. These may be available at your library.

Conference proceedings

Conference papers and proceedings are also useful and can be listed as references. Sometimes there will have been a conference on exactly the topic you are researching. These documents are usually harder to access, but they can sometimes be obtained on interlibrary loan. With the growth of electronic media, this type of paper will probably become more accessible.

Reports

Reports from government and institutions are also useful sources of information. These are becoming easier to access now that many institutions are listing their reports on their web sites. For example, the Australian Bureau of Statistics has a large number of statistical reports that can be ordered for a nominal sum. Some reports can be difficult to find out about and to access but reading the bibliographies of journal articles and other reports can lead you to relevant reports, as can searching the indexes.

Theses

A thorough search of the literature will include a search for relevant theses. It is possible to find information about theses on the FirstSearch master database of databases. The specific database is 'Dissertations' and it lists theses, in some cases back as far as 1975. However, the listings are incomplete. Not all universities list their theses this way and not all theses are listed by the universities that do list them. A search by the author for Australian nursing theses listed only 25 theses, which is a gross under-representation of the number of theses that have been done. The list is of abstracts only so if you want to read beyond the abstract, you must still obtain a copy of the thesis on interlibrary loan. However, the abstracts themselves are useful to get an idea of what has been done in the field. If you need to satisfy the criterion of originality for a doctoral thesis, it can help you to rule out certain topics that have been researched already.

Journals

Professional journals are the most valuable resource for researchers. These journals have varying degrees of scope for their various audiences. The scope varies from broad interest journals such as the *Australian Journal of Advanced Nursing*, *International Journal of Nursing Practice*, and *Nursing Inquiry* to more specific specialty journals such as the *Australian and New Zealand Journal of Mental Health Nursing*, or concept-specific journals such as the *Australian Journal of Holistic Nursing*. Journals can be discipline-specific to nursing, for example *Collegian* or *Contemporary Nurse*, or they can be multi-disciplinary, like the *Australian Journal of Rural Health*. Some journals are dedicated to research, such as *Clinical Nursing Research*, *Nursing Research* and *Western Journal of Nursing Research*. Some journals have a particular methodological focus, for example *Qualitative Health Research*. Others also include theoretical scholarship and/or clinical scholarship. Frequently nursing knowledge incorporates knowledge from other disciplines, so journals of those disciplines may be a useful source of material. These disciplines may include medicine, public health, anthropology, sociology and psychology, and paramedical disciplines such as physiotherapy or occupational therapy.

Journals can be international, for example *Clinical Nursing Research*, which accepts papers from any country, or they can have a national focus, for example *Collegian*, or *Contemporary Nurse*, which deal with Australian research. State-based journals have a more restricted focus, for example *The Lamp*, which is concerned mainly with events in New South Wales. You can find resources for your topic, depending on how specific it is, in a few journals or in many.

Electronic journals, or journals published only on the Internet, are also being developed. The *Online Journal of Issues in Nursing* emanates from the United States, and the *Australian Electronic Journal of Nursing Education* comes from Australia. Electronic journals will undoubtedly proliferate. They are gradually becoming accessible through your university information technology services or library.

Articles

The bibliography or reference section of useful articles will probably contain references to other useful articles. The text of the article will be a guide to selecting articles from that bibliography to follow up.

Indexes

Each discipline usually has an index that lists the articles in most relevant journals by keyword headings. These may be cumulative indexes that do not necessarily publish abstracts, or they may be abstract indexes. Examples include Psychology Abstracts (known electronically as PsychLit), Sociological Abstracts, and ERIC (Education Resources Information Centre). There is even a dissertation index, Dissertation Abstracts International, which lists doctoral theses and has an electronic version. There are highly specific indexes such as CANCERLIT, which indexes all articles to do with cancer. The most useful one for nursing is CINAHL (Cumulative Index of Nursing and Allied Health Literature), which lists most nursing and health journals. MEDLINE, which indexes mainly medical literature but also indexes some nursing literature, can also be useful. The Health ROM indexes public health literature and has the full text of documents from organisations such as the NHMRC. You should ask the librarian to help you identify the most appropriate index, particularly if your topic is at all obscure. All of the relevant indexes can be accessed through a master index of databases such as FirstSearch. FirstSearch acts as a portal to the individual indexes and makes it easy to use more than one of them.

Indexes are usually a prime source of information because they index most journals that you will want to access and they are updated frequently. Articles are indexed by author and topic so you can find all articles by a particular author or authors. This can be useful if you know the authorities in the field. However, it is more likely that you will want to use the topic index to search for literature on a particular topic. In order to do this, you will need to use the keywords that you identified earlier. If you are having trouble finding information by using your keywords, it is useful to use the thesaurus function on the index. It will lead you to the exact keywords to use.

With the widespread use of computers, abstracting indexes are now exclusively on computer. Computer literature searches are effective because they are fast, accurate, current and comprehensive. They are flexible, since they allow searching by journal name and year of publication as well as by author and topic. You can also exclude certain types of references, for example non-research articles or those not written in English. You can also restrict the years of publication to those of interest to you.

With the arrival of Internet technology, the abstracting indexes are now accessible via the WWW. Modern libraries have switched over to this technology, with online computer terminal access to the databases. The databases can even be accessed from your home computer via your library web page if you are an authorised user.

Searching a database index is a fast, efficient process that you can do yourself. In addition, you can print out the results of your search, or even download it to your personal computer for printing or for inserting into an electronic reference manager. Furthermore, you can now download entire research articles from some databases and print them on your own printer. You can also have them emailed to you. You can learn details of how to use these specific methods by an orientation at your library.

The mechanics of searching

Essentially, the principle is that you enter the keyword or combination of keywords, and the database will list every article on that subject. For example, if you were searching for information on 'body position' and 'respiratory capacity', the search would turn up every article that had listed those two keywords. You can also search by author if you know a writer in the field. It is possible to narrow the search, for example restricting the search to items written in English, research articles, or those from certain years only. Then, you can read through the list, ignoring items that are unsuitable and marking those that you want to follow up. You can then print or download your list of marked items and go in one layer deeper, finding the abstract of each article if the index has it. Sometimes reading the abstract will rule out further searching for the article. Alternatively, you may wish to mark the reference as a key source that you must follow up. You can print each abstract separately, which gives you a very good beginning to your collection of material. You can also download the details, including abstracts, into an electronic reference manager.

Information required

For each reference you obtain, you will need sufficient information to be able to use any citation or document referencing system. The usual information required for each item is the author or authors' name(s) and initials; the year; the month, volume and issue for periodicals; and the publisher and city of publication for books. For edited books, you will need the editor's name and initials (or the editors' names and initials) as well as the name(s) and initials of the author(s) of the section and the title of the section. You may require further information if you are using a non-standard referencing system. References printed from an electronic database such as CINAHL will usually contain all of the necessary information.

Most libraries these days have an electronic reference retrieval system. However, if you are in a library that has less up-to-date technology and you need to record references yourself on cards or paper, it is important to train yourself to write down all of the required information. This will avoid your spending time later on tracking missing information. It is important to be accurate since these references will end up in your reference list, which must be correct. It is useful to add to the reference item a running record of where you have looked for it, or where you found it, and on what date. You can also record when you read it, if you are working on a longer project.

Filing your references

As your search progresses, you will build up a list of references, probably generated by a computer database and either printed as hard copy, or saved onto a computer diskette for storage electronically. You may also have references from other sources, such as conference proceedings, that were not listed electronically, and which you have had to write by hand on cards or slips of paper. You need to file all references systematically. You will need to consider how you are going to organise these references. Only some of them will end up in your bibliography, but you need to keep track of all references obtained, even the useless ones. The larger the project, the more crucial it is to do this.

To organise these references, you will need some sort of filing system, which can be simple or sophisticated, cheap or expensive. Paper-based systems are the cheapest and simplest to use, but require double handling of information. A simple, cheap system is a shoe box or plastic flip-top box with cardboard dividers and references written on pieces of paper or index cards. If you are using computer printout, separate it into individual references for filing and later assembly of relevant ones into a bibliography and put them in your filing box. Later you can assemble relevant references into a bibliography.

Much more sophisticated and efficient is the use of a word processing program on a computer. You can compile a 'library' of references which can be typed in, copied and pasted from the list of references in the electronic database, or downloaded electronically from a database. You are encouraged to use this type of system if you can because it allows you to keep a running reference system without having to write or type the details more than once.

Whatever method you use, it is usual to organise your references by author. You can use the universal 'find' facility of the word processor to find references on a particular topic in your word processor file. Once the details have been entered into your word processor, they can be cut and pasted into your reference list at the end of the word-processed report. Not only is this method more efficient, it is also more accurate because there is less opportunity to make typographical errors.

At the most complex technological end of reference management, there are computer programs such as EndNote and ProCite that allow you to keep a database of your references. You can create a 'library' of references or citations that you can insert into the word processor document of your assignment. You can keep a separate library for each topic or integrate all your references into one library. Figure 3.1 shows you an EndNote library.

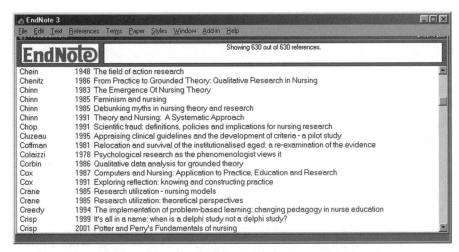

Figure 3.1 EndNote library

Figure 3.2 shows you an individual entry of one reference into EndNote.

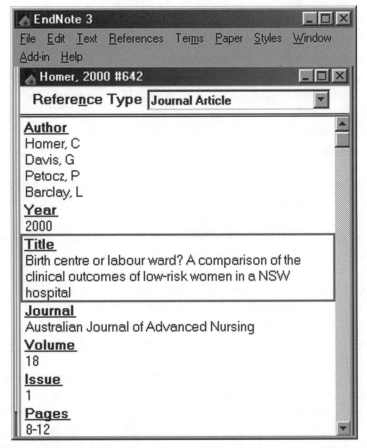

Figure 3.2 EndNote reference

This system has three major advantages. First, it is efficient, since you have to enter an item into the library only once regardless of how often you use it.

Secondly, it is flexible, since you can insert and delete references easily and change the citation format with one command. Thirdly, it is more accurate, since there is never a problem with mismatching citations in the document and the reference list(s). The more sophisticated programs have inbuilt capability to download items and abstracts from an electronic database such as CINAHL directly into your electronic library of references. This relieves you of the necessity of typing them in and eliminates transcription errors. Anyone doing a large research project would find such a program invaluable. The disadvantage is that it is relatively expensive.

There are two useful ways to organise the references: by topic or alphabetically by author. For larger projects, you may wish to have sections in your filing system in which to put items that you are obtaining on interlibrary loan or those that you find are not useful. Within these categories, you can still file items alphabetically by author. The author system is more useful since items may not always fit neatly into topics and since referencing systems are usually author-based. Electronic systems normally index by author but word-searching facilities enable you to retrieve items by topic.

Where do you find the sources?

Now that you have your list of potential references, the next problem is where to find them as easily and economically as possible. It is important to realise that you will be unlikely to find all of them. This problem is more acute now than ever before because electronic media can give you a list of everything written on a topic regardless of how accessible it is. Unless you are doing a PhD thesis it is not necessary to find everything, just the main sources.

The obvious place to start looking is in libraries. There are various types of libraries that may be useful. University libraries carry a large range of resources. Hospital libraries may carry resources that a university library does not have. Members of professional associations will have access to their associations' libraries. Some government departments have specialist libraries, for example drug and alcohol or family planning libraries. Public libraries may have useful material, depending on your topic. Electronic libraries are also starting to become available. For example, the Virginia Henderson Library is now open. It is run by Sigma Theta Tau, the nursing honour society in the United States. It was named after Virginia Henderson, one of the most prominent nurses of the twentieth century.

Libraries will have materials available in the reference section, the shelves, and the current serials section. Larger libraries may have separate journal and book areas. Some may also have closed stacks from which only the librarian can retrieve items. The National Library in Canberra operates exclusively on a closed stack basis – the reader submits an order form for each item, then the library staff locate the item and give it to the reader.

If you live in a large city, you may need to visit several libraries. This is cheaper than interlibrary loans unless your institution provides the latter service free of charge. It is helpful to identify which libraries have the journals you are looking for. The librarian will be able to assist you by looking up the information on an index of journal locations. If you locate enough items in another library to justify a trip, it is then worthwhile to visit.

A library's catalogue is the index for information. The catalogue will normally be electronic, stored on a computer that may be linked to a network of library computers. You can search through the catalogue by author, title, and subject, with variations on these themes. You select the search mode, for example key word, and then type in the information. The computer then searches its database and prints the items on the screen. Computer searching is fast and it can also give you up-to-date information about the status of the item — whether it is checked in, or in closed reserve, for instance.

Each library item is classified either alphabetically, numerically, or by a combination of letters and numbers. One popular system is the Dewey Decimal System, which uses a three-number prefix, a decimal point and a multi-number suffix. Nursing and medical items are listed at 610. The other main system is the Library of Congress system, which uses a combination of letters and numbers. Nursing items are listed at RT. Once you are familiar with either system, you will find it is easy to use.

In the library it is also useful to browse the shelves, particularly if you have identified fairly clearly what you are looking for. Sometimes you will find information in current issues of serials which often have their own section in the library. You may find some items on the re-shelving shelves. Historical research may require a search of the Archives.

There is a growing amount of information available on the information superhighway, or 'infobahn', for example reports by government agencies, or position statements from client support groups. These can be accessed on the WWW, using programs such as Netscape. Powerful search engines such as LYCOS, YAHOO and AltaVista will assist you to find information on any topic. It is possible to download documents to your own computer through these media. However, take care with information accessed from these sources because there is no guarantee as to the accuracy or quality of the information, especially for research purposes. Unlike professional, refereed journals, which are subject to a peer review process, there is no control over what is put up on the WWW.

Don't overlook informal locations such as in-house collections of materials or personal libraries of your colleagues.

If you cannot obtain an item easily by the above methods, then it may be necessary to acquire it using the interlibrary loan service of your institution. Universities and hospitals both have interlibrary loan services, with specialist librarians. The librarian consults the index of locations of books or journals on the Australian Bibliographic Network, and sends for the item. The lending library then either sends the book or a photocopied article to your institution, and your library loans you the book or sells you the photocopy. Usually the item is sent by post, but in cases of extreme urgency a journal article can be faxed or emailed. However, the interlibrary loan option is expensive and the library may pass on costs to you. It is also relatively slow if items are posted rather than faxed or emailed. It can take a month or longer if the host library is understaffed or has to recall a book from a borrower. If the item is in an overseas library, it can take even longer. It is wise to allow plenty of time to acquire items on interlibrary loan.

Libraries are now increasingly using electronic delivery services to obtain items that they do not hold themselves. Indeed, the increasing availability of journal articles from the Internet will probably eventually make that part of the interlibrary loan service obsolete.

Selecting literature

Before you start reading the literature, you need to select what is the appropriate literature to read. The aim of this exercise is to end up with the most relevant literature – and only literature that is relevant. Suppose that you are doing a search for material on a topic such as the effect of circumcision on the infant's ability to breastfeed in the immediate post-operative period. There is a huge body of literature on breastfeeding and a large amount of literature on circumcision. It would be impossible to read all of it and most of it would not directly bear on your topic, although some might be useful background reading. You would want only research articles about the relationship between circumcision and breastfeeding. You would not be interested in articles debating the advantages of circumcision unless they contained observations relevant to breastfeeding. Similarly, you would not want articles on breastfeeding that did not address circumcision. Therefore you would combine the two keywords 'circumcision' and 'breastfeeding' on the computer literature search, which would then extract only articles that dealt with both topics. Figure 3.3 shows you the interaction between the two bodies of literature. By looking only for articles dealing with both topics, you will save yourself a considerable amount of time.

When searching for literature, you can eliminate many items by reading the abstract. It is best to do this at the literature search stage to avoid wasting time and money. However, not all entries in an index have abstracts and it is then necessary to look at the article itself. If it is necessary to read the article, just skim lightly through the introduction and conclusions. By reading those, it is often possible to decide whether the article is relevant. You can also eliminate articles that are in non-research journals since you are interested only in research. When you have eliminated the irrelevant and the unobtainable, you will be left with only a small percentage of your original sources. This is normal and it shows the ability to discriminate between useful and irrelevant literature.

You should also consider whether the article is written by someone who has the authority and credibility to produce a valuable article. Other considerations about the quality of the article are the date when the study was carried out and

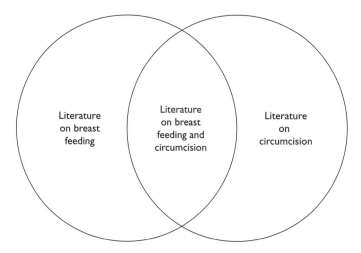

Figure 3.3 Elimination of irrelevant literature

the type of journal in which it appears. If it is a refereed journal you can be assured that the article was reviewed by at least two peers of the writer. This system of peer review entails the journal editor sending out the article to two identified reviewers who critique the article using a similar process to the critique method detailed later in this chapter. The editor then sends the critiques to the author, who revises the article. This process continues until the article either meets the standards of the editor and reviewers or the author gives up or decides to send the article to another journal. Thus, the peer review system helps to maintain a standard of excellence in research scholarship.

Acquiring your own collection of information

Having decided that the article or other material is relevant, you now have the problem of how to capture this information for your own future use. You should decide which method to use before you undertake close reading of any material. The pre-technology approach is to take notes of key ideas by hand from the article. This is time-consuming and has the disadvantage that the notes are your own interpretation of the material and thus subject to bias. Also, if you want to consult the reference later, you will have to look it up again. However, this method is relatively cheap and can be effective provided you do not need much information from the source.

The second method is to capture the article in hard copy. This can be done by photocopying it. This method is more expensive, but more flexible. Photocopying captures the entire article, conference paper or section of a book. You can take the material elsewhere to work on and to re-read as many times as you like, which you will need to do when new ideas or insights occur. Be sure that each photocopy has physically written on it information about the volume, year, issue, and so forth. The current trend is for journals to print this information at the top or bottom of the page, but not all do. You can either write it on the photocopy or photocopy your reference information onto a blank space on the article when you are photocopying it. When photocopying material, make sure that you do not infringe the copyright laws. It is against the law to copy more than 10 per cent of a book. Most libraries have near the photocopy machines signs informing you of the copyright laws.

You can also capture a hard copy of a document by downloading it from a computer source and printing it. You would be likely to do this from a WWW document or from an electronic source of a journal that has what is called 'full text' capability. More and more libraries are converting journal subscriptions to electronic form. The advantages of this are obvious. The library reduces its need for shelf space for journals, and researchers are able to have virtually instantaneous access to documents including from a home computer via the library portal if they have the appropriate authorisation and password information.

The most technologically advanced method is to store the document electronically rather than in hard copy, but please ensure that you have a backup. You can download the article directly into the computer or receive it by email if you have the authorisations from your library or you wish to pay for it. Alternatively, if you have a scanner and Optical Character Recognition (OCR) software on your computer, you can scan your photocopied article for reading and storage. The scanner scans the entire document into the computer page by page. The OCR software then creates a word processor document on your computer that you can use as you wish provided you obey the law. This technology is becoming more accessible as the price of scanners is now under $200. However, be warned that optical scanning technology is still not perfect and you may find you have to spend time correcting errors that the spellchecker finds on the transcribed copy. Advanced users of this technology are using CD-ROM burners, which are also becoming cheaper, to store large volumes of information that they can then read from the CD-ROM. The inclusion of a CD-ROM reader as standard equipment in a computer has made this practicable. This system is obviously of great benefit as the information is then very portable from home to university and so forth. Imagine travelling around Australia with your laptop writing your thesis using your collection of references on CD-ROM and your reference manager program!

By using these techniques, you should end up with a collection of all of the material relevant to your topic and be ready to process it.

You will also need to organise the copies of the literature that you have if there are more than a few papers. An expanding file is useful for this purpose, or a portable file – a box with file hangers. If there is a large amount of material or you are involved in several projects, you may want to invest in a filing cabinet. The articles can then be filed by author or by topic. If you have scanned electronic copies, you can organise them on computer in various files and perhaps even store them on a CD-ROM. The latter method will require a CD-ROM burner and appropriate software.

Reading and documenting the information

The next step is to read the relevant material. At this stage, you may need to narrow down your topic even further, or you may redirect it slightly as a result of your reading. The first stage in reading is to read all the material superficially once or twice. This will give you a feeling for the important issues in the topic and methodologies of research previously used on the topic. The next stage is to read the material critically, identifying major points. This may require several readings, but you should at this stage be reading only the most relevant material.

Reading a research report

In order to become familiar with the body of research on your topic, you will have to read research reports. It is helpful to understand the structure of a research report. They usually follow a logical standard order. The **title**, of course, comes first. Next comes the **abstract**, which summarises the study. The **introduction** will give the problem being researched, its scope and its significance. The **theoretical framework** will be identified and its relationship to the study will be discussed. The previous findings will then be summarised and specific research questions given. If it is a quantitative design, specific hypotheses and variables will be identified, either formally or informally. This section usually answers the questions 'what' and 'why'. If it is a qualitative study, hypotheses and variables will not be stated, rather the project will be introduced in exploratory terms, and the theory underlying the choice of methods may be described, because qualitative research usually outlines the basis on which knowledge of a particular kind is collected and analysed.

The **methodology** section will outline the design of the study, the subjects used and the methodology used to answer the research question, including methods of data collection and analysis. In the **results** section, the findings of the study will be given. The **discussion** section will discuss the significance of the findings and how they relate to previous findings and the theoretical framework. Conclusions and recommendations for implementing the findings will then be given. At the end of the paper, the references will be given. This section usually answers the questions 'how', 'when', where' and 'to whom'.

In reading research reports, beginning researchers often have problems with the scholarly language used, particularly research terminology and statistics. Sometimes it seems as though the writer has difficulty in communicating in plain language, particularly if using a formal style of writing. These are conventions that have grown up over the years. Unfortunately, if you want to learn to read research, you have to come to terms with the language. It is really no different from being dropped into the middle of some nursing specialty such as critical care and having to learn the jargon. If you are reading research in a clinical area that is your own specialty, you should be familiar with the clinical terminology. It is usually the research terminology that is difficult. The best way to handle this problem is to read the paper and make notes of the words you do not understand. Look these words up in your research textbook, making particular use of the glossary. Then re-read the paper. Sometimes a paper requires several readings before you will understand it, but it usually gets easier with each reading. It may help to get together a group of students and do this as a group exercise.

Documenting key ideas from the readings

Since it is impossible to work with a considerable number of whole reports, it is necessary to identify the key passages so that you can refer to them again. There are several ways of doing this. Whichever method you use, you must be able to link the source and the idea so that you can attribute the idea to its rightful source and thus avoid plagiarism.

One system is to indicate key ideas on a photocopy of the article or book chapter. This method works best where there is little material on the topic. You can indicate the key ideas with highlighters, even developing a colour scheme for coding topics. Another way is to make symbols in the margin of the paper. This system can also be adapted for use on an electronic copy of a paper, using keyboard symbols. This method is faster initially but has the disadvantage that you have to go back and use the whole document every time you want to refer to an idea.

Another way is to organise material under topic headings so that you have all of your ideas on one topic together. The keywords that you used for your literature search are a start, but you will probably need subheadings. For example, in kangaroo mother care research, one key outcome is weight gain. In reading the literature, one would have assembled information concerning the findings of various studies for weight gain. If these are filed under the heading of weight gain, it makes it easy to find all of the material on weight gain.

One way of organising key ideas is a paper-based method – you write them down on separate cards or pieces of paper with identifying headings at the top. A 12.5 by 20 cm filing card or one-third of an A4 sheet of paper is ideal for this purpose. The cards are more expensive but more robust and easier to flick through when you are looking for a particular bit of information. They can also be re-used by using the reverse side. At the top of the card, write the author and date of the source on the left hand side. This will allow you to find the passage again in the original article. Also write the keyword under which the idea fits at the top of the card on the right hand side. This will allow you to file the idea under keyword headings in a filing box. Then write the key idea on the card. This method forces you to be selective and to think about how the idea fits into the picture. Then file the card under the keyword heading in a shoe box or other file. The accumulated cards under the keyword headings will form the beginning of a draft of the paper. All you need to do is sort them into a logical sequence and start writing.

If you have access to a word processor, a much more modern and flexible way to do the above procedure is to type key ideas into the word processor rather than writing on paper, using the same principles of identifying the information. This can be done either as you read or by first taking notes manually and then typing them into the word processor. By doing the former, you avoid double work for yourself.

You can then either print out the information and file it mechanically as above, or file it electronically in the computer by creating a file for each keyword and pasting the information in there. Be sure to keep the author, date and keyword identifiers attached to each piece of information so that you can cite them when you are writing the paper. You can also cut and paste the information into various files that are the electronic equivalent of the sections of the shoebox or flip-top box.

If you have an electronic copy of the whole document, either generated by your scanner or downloaded from a database, you can adapt several of the above techniques to the electronic copy. You can use italics, symbols or bold font to emphasise key passages. You can use the colour facility of the word processor to colour-code key passages. You can copy and paste chunks of the manuscript into your various keyword files. In writing your paper, you could even copy quotations directly from the electronic version. The same principles of identifying the passages by author and date and attributing cited material to the original author also apply to this method.

Critiquing individual reports

A critique is a balanced assessment of both the positive and negative qualities of a research report, developed through a process of critical appraisal. A good critique offers constructive criticism, with suggestions as to how the researcher could have improved the research report.

People critique research reports for several reasons. One is to promote student learning. Most research training will require students to learn to critique existing research reports in order to teach them to differentiate good research from bad. Critiquing will teach students to discriminate wisely about what to include in a review of the literature. Learning to critique also helps students to interpret their own research findings in light of previous findings. Another reason for critiquing is for clinicians to evaluate research reports in terms of whether they offer a foundation for change in clinical practice, which we will discuss in Chapter 19. Still another is for researchers to scrutinise research reports for their suitability for a literature review in a research proposal or report. Finally, critiquing can be done by experienced researchers who review journal submissions to make recommendations on the publication of an article.

A good way to learn about what constitutes a critique is to look at some models. If you want to see some critiques of journal articles, try reading the critiques that frequently accompany articles in *Clinical Nursing Research* and *Western Journal of Nursing Research*. However, a journal critique may not be complete because the author may be able to raise only major points in the space available. The reader must rely on the reviewer to evaluate the research on all of the relevant criteria below and raise significant issues in the critique.

If you have to choose an article on which to practise critiquing, you will find that those in refereed journals offer less scope for critique than those in non-refereed journals. Research reports in refereed journals have already been critiqued before publication. They are therefore more likely to be high-quality reports, although the perfect report has not yet been published. Reports in non-refereed journals are more likely to offer scope for finding flaws. If you want to find out whether a journal is refereed, look at the introductory part of the journal where information about it is given, or look in the 'Instructions to Authors' section. One of these will usually say whether the journal requires manuscripts to be peer reviewed.

Critiquing quantitative research reports

The process of critiquing, assuming you have selected appropriate material, is to read through the article quickly for general meaning, then read it in detail several times, asking questions about the article and taking notes. Then you build the material in your notes into a structured, logical argument. You may choose to use the same structure as a research report, looking at the introduction, method, results and discussion in turn. Indeed, it would be wise to read the section in Chapter 18 on research reports before attempting to critique. Right now, we are not going to provide extensive examples to follow. However, you might like to use the examples provided in Chapters 6 and 18 for practice in critiquing.

When critiquing a research report, you should ask general questions about the quality of the research and the document reporting it, and specific questions about parts of the research. We will look at these in turn. In assessing the general quality of the research, we need to ask the question about whether it is significant, that is, do the findings make a difference? For example, there may be studies that give instruction about research design, but which did not get results that could impact on clinical practice. It is also important to ask whether the study is sound science: does it have a good methodology; does it have a good design? Does it have a logical progression of links between the purpose of the study, the method, the findings, and the conclusions? With regard to the quality of the writing of the report, is it well written with a smooth flow between parts? Is it clear and concise and stated in terms that the reader can understand easily?

In assessing the research report, you need to ask whether it is complete. Most journals require authors to use the IMRAD system, or Introduction, Method, Results, and Discussion. The National Standards Institute of the United States of America adopted this system as the industry standard (Day 1998). Does the report have all of these sections? Are they in a logical order? According to Day (1998), IMRAD is a logical order because it progresses from problem to solution. However, in critiquing, remember that some journals have particular formats that they require authors to follow.

Preliminaries

When you start your critique, look at the title first.

- Is it concise, yet informative?
- Does it indicate the research approach?

An example of a title that does this is: 'Birth centre or labour ward? A comparison of the clinical outcomes of low-risk women in a NSW hospital' (Homer et al. 2000). This title tells you that the study compared clinical outcomes of low-risk maternity clients in a labour ward and a birth centre. When you see a phrase such as 'the effects of' in a title, it usually means an experimental or quasi-experimental approach. Similarly, a title such as 'The lived experience of suffering' (Daly 1995) indicates a phenomenological study on what it is like to suffer.

The next area for appraisal is the abstract. Most articles these days have abstracts for the convenience of their readers.

- Does the abstract correctly and concisely describe the problem, methods, design, results, conclusions and implications?
- Does it provide a good basis for deciding whether or not the study is worth reading?

Introduction

- Does the introduction explain the purpose of the study, that is, what the study was investigating?
- Does it state the actual problem the researcher investigated or the question the researcher answered?
- Does it give a rationale for doing the study in terms of a theoretical question, unanswered previous research findings, or observations of the researchers or their colleagues?
- Does it set the study in context – does it give the background to the study in terms of some previous work that led to the study question?
- Does it set the scope of the problem, or the limits of the study?
- Does the introduction talk about the potential importance of the study – how this study would advance knowledge on this topic, what significance might it have? In other words, does it answer the question 'so what?'

Literature review

The next part of the introduction in a quantitative study will address the conceptual framework of the study and the literature review or previous findings.

- Does the study have a conceptual framework or not?
- If so, is it an appropriate framework for the study?
- Is it a nursing framework or a framework from another discipline, for example sociology?
- Has the author linked the framework to the research question? In what way?
- Are the concepts clearly defined?
- Is the literature relevant to the topic and the concepts being investigated?
- Is it directly related or is it more marginal?
- Is appropriate literature from the conceptual framework included?
- Is the review comprehensive and complete?
- Are classic and current sources included?
- Is there a majority of primary sources?

- Is the literature review just a summary of individual research publications, or is it an integrated review that includes an objective analysis of the strengths and weaknesses of the various studies?
- Does the review develop logically, producing an argument that justifies carrying out the study?
- Does the author summarise the key points of the literature review?

Hypotheses and variables
- If the study design goes beyond description, are there hypotheses? Are they stated or implicit? If stated, are they clearly stated?
- Do the hypotheses flow from the problem statement or arise from the previous findings?
- Do the hypotheses suggest a proposed relationship between two or more variables?
- Are the hypotheses stated as directional or null hypotheses?
- Are they capable of being tested?
- Are they operationally defined (stated in terms that allow the reader to see how they will be measured)?
- Do the hypotheses make it clear what variables are being tested?
- Are the dependent, independent and extraneous variables conceptualised or defined? In operational terms?

Methodology
Generally, the methodology should give enough detail to permit replication of the study. For example, if it is an experiment, the exact procedures for administering the treatment should be given. The methodology section is usually broken down into subsections according to the journal's formula. There may be variations in the organisation of this section depending on the journal. The main subsections are usually the design, participants (subjects), setting, procedures for data collection and analysis, and the instruments and materials.

- Has the author addressed all sections?

The methodology section should give the design fairly early so that the readers will know whether they are reading about a descriptive study or an experiment.

- Is the design the most appropriate one to answer the research question?
- Was the selected design likely to control threats to validity, thereby promoting internal validity?
- If it was an experimental design, was the way of testing the hypotheses valid?
- Has the author included a section about the participants?
- Has the paper stated what the target population was and how the participants were selected, that is, what the sampling procedures were?
- Does the sample appear to be representative of the target population or is it biased in some way?
- What type of sample was it and how could this impact on the findings?

- How many participants were selected, and was it enough to ensure valid findings?
- How did the researcher determine how many should be in the sample, for example was a power analysis used?
- What processes were used to recruit the participants?
- After the sample was recruited, what procedures were used to assign them to groups if warranted?
- Were there any losses of participants from the sample during the study and did this affect the findings?
- Did the author report on the ethical aspects of the study?
- Was permission gained from the appropriate human research ethics committee or committees?
- Did the participants volunteer to take part in the study?
- Was informed consent obtained?
- Were participants protected from potential physical, social, psychological and financial harm?
- Were the procedures of the study designed so as to protect the privacy, confidentiality and anonymity of the participants where appropriate?
- Did the author report on what instrument or instruments were used, including their suitability?
- Did the instrument measure accurately with sufficient sensitivity?
- How was it developed, and by whom?
- If the instrument was previously in existence, did the author report the validity and reliability?
- Did the author get permission from the owner of the copyright on the instrument?
- If the instrument was researcher-developed, was the trialling procedure reported, including acceptable validity and reliability tests?
- Who collected the data? Did the data collectors have the appropriate training on the instrument?
- Did the author report the data collection procedures in detail?
- Was a pilot study done?
- Were data processing and management procedures reported? Were they accurate?
- Were data analysis procedures reported in sufficient detail, including statistical tests? Were they adequate?

Results
- Is the results section concise and clearly presented?
- Are the graphics and tables informative and necessary?
- Do the data appear to be sufficient, valid and reliable?
- Did the author describe the participants and their relevant characteristics?
- Did the author give all of the results that were related to the research question or hypotheses?
- Were the findings consistent with the hypotheses?

- Were the findings statistically significant with levels of significance given?
- Were the findings clinically significant?

Discussion

This section should wrap up the report. It should be concise but should bring out the important aspects of the study. A poor discussion section only summarises the findings. A good discussion section discusses their meaning and significance.

- Does the discussion section discuss the contribution made by the study to the development of knowledge?
- Does it point out the strengths and weaknesses of the study and how weaknesses could be addressed in future research?
- Does it relate the findings to the conceptual framework?
- Does it compare the findings with the previous findings identified in the review of the literature?
- Does it say how the findings of this study extend the previous findings?
- Does it say whether the findings could be generalised to other people?
- Do the authors discuss any relevant implications for practice?
- Are any conclusions drawn from the findings; if so, are they appropriate?
- Are any recommendations made for further research, theoretical development or practice?
- Do the recommendations arise appropriately out of the conclusions?

References

- Are the majority of references recent?
- Are they complete and accurate?
- Are all citations listed in the references? Are all of the references cited in the study?

You may not address all of the points above in every critique because they may not all be relevant to the research being critiqued.

Critiquing qualitative research reports

In the preceding section you were given many important questions to ask to assist you in critiquing quantitative research reports, and many of these apply equally well to qualitative reports. Keeping in mind the questions raised previously, this section will emphasise some key questions to ask when critiquing a qualitative research report. The approach taken here will be to use the structure for writing qualitative research reports presented in Chapter 18 of this book, as a basis on which to raise questions for research critique.

The points for critiquing a qualitative research report will be listed and some explanation will be given as necessary. You may find that many of the points have been covered elsewhere in this book. There are close and direct connections between critiquing qualitative research and qualitative research processes (Chapter 1), the format of a qualitative proposal (Chapter 6), presenting the results in qualitative research (Chapter 17) and the elements of a qualitative research report (Chapter 18).

Title, research summary and literature review

Qualitative critiques begin with attention to preliminaries. Look again in the preceding section at what has been written about how to critique the title, the research summary or abstract, and the literature review. All of the questions apply equally well to qualitative as to quantitative research.

It is important to check that the literature review contains all of the elements of a good literature review as described in this chapter. Remember, it is probably more difficult to write a literature review than it is to critique it. Some specific questions that can be asked to assess the completeness of a literature review in a qualitative report are:

- What is the relationship between the literature review and the research area/questions that are considered to be important in the area that has been selected for study? What rationale is given for their selection?
- What do the practitioners, administrators, researchers, governments, community, media, and so on have to say about the area? To what extent are these views represented?
- What key ideas have been raised? What has been seen as problematic? Have solutions and/or actions been proposed and/or evaluated in response to perceived difficulties?
- Has the material been identified clearly as to paradigms of knowledge? Has the material challenged existing knowledge and theory, or does it serve to reinforce current conceptions?
- What research methods have been employed in these studies? Have these research methods been appropriate in terms of the research questions that have been investigated? Is there attention to ensuring that the methods are congruent with the underlying theory guiding the research approach (methodology)?
- What are the major findings associated with these studies? Do they reflect an approach that is quantitative, qualitative or a combination of both?
- What debates have there been in the area with respect to both the content of the research and the underlying theory guiding the research approach (methodological) aspects? What have been the main issues involved in these debates?
- What important issues appear to have been overlooked in the area? Are there any gaps, omissions, or 'silences' in the literature?
- What 'common threads' emerge in terms of issues, debates, research findings, and themes? How can these 'common threads' guide an evaluation of the knowledge that has been gathered to date, and how can they be employed to propose important and potentially fruitful areas for further enquiry?

Research plan, including methodology, methods and processes

The body of a qualitative report contains sections on the methodology, methods and processes. The definitions for each of these sections, as they apply specifically to qualitative research, will be given in Chapter 6. Questions follow that you need to keep in mind in order to critique a qualitative project in relation to methodology, methods and processes.

Methodology
- What theoretical assumptions about the way knowledge is generated underlie the methods?
- Have explanations been given of the basic nature and intent of the chosen methodology?
- Is there an explanation of how the methodology relates to this project?
- Are the main references to the methodological literature included?

Ethical requirements
In qualitative research, it is important to critique the ways in which the ethical rights of the participants were safeguarded throughout the project. The report should be checked carefully to see that it includes explanations regarding the ethical requirements. Some questions to ask are:

- Has ethical clearance been obtained?
- From which committees was ethical clearance obtained?
- Are there comprehensive statements about appropriate ethical considerations?
- Are there indications that informed consent, privacy and anonymity were honoured?
- Has any attention been paid to maintaining the integrity of ethical considerations and interpersonal relationships throughout the research?

Methods and processes
Some questions that may guide the critique of methods and processes are:

- Is the sequence of the research methods clearly explained?
- How were participants enlisted into the project?
- Has an explanation been provided of the reasons for the number of participants in the project?
- Are the processes used appropriate for the underlying methodological ideas of the project? That is, does the project demonstrate as appropriate a level of negotiation, collaboration and sharing of power between the researcher and participants as might be reasonably expected?
- Is there a clear account of how the data were collected?

Analysis and interpretation
Some questions that may guide you in critiquing the analysis and interpretation phase of the project are:

- Are the analysis and interpretation phases easily discernible in the report?
- Has a rationale been given for the choice of analysis methods?
- Have the steps in analysis been set out clearly?
- Has the researcher explained who did the analysis, that is, was it done by an individual or by a group?
- Are the processes described clearly as to how the individual/group went about doing the analysis?

- Are there examples of the data organised in their analysed form?
- Are excerpts provided of actual dialogue between researchers/co-researchers/participants?
- Have sub-themes/collective themes/competing discourses been described clearly?
- Has the researcher explained who made the interpretations?
- Is there a clear account of how the interpretations were made?
- Are the interpretations set out systematically and clearly?
- Is there a clear account of how the interpretations were validated?

Discussion, insights, recommendations, suggestions and conclusions

Some questions to guide the critique of this part of the research report are:

- Does the report document provide a comprehensive discussion of the findings/insights/examples of changed practice that emerged from the project?
- Does the report offer practical suggestions and/or recommendations for nurses and nursing practice?
- Are the final discussion and conclusions congruent with the overall plan, methodology, methods and processes of the research?

In summary, the questions relating to critiquing a research report's preliminaries apply equally well to qualitative as they do to quantitative research critiques. Even so, there are some differences to note in critiquing a qualitative research report. It is important to be aware of the differences and to judge the overall integrity of a qualitative project on qualitative research assumptions of what equals a good research report.

It is useful to keep a brief summary of your critique of the articles that you read. As well as the citation, you can record the problem studied, the theoretical framework, the methodology, your own evaluation of the work and how it links into your work. You may not feel that this is necessary if you only have a few articles to deal with but it is important for keeping order in a larger body of literature. Most of the information, except your evaluation, is already present in the abstract of the article. You can make handwritten evaluations. You can also type this sort of summary straight into a word processor. If you are downloading information from an electronic database you can copy the abstract, which gives you a ready-made summary of the article, written by the author. You can either copy and paste the abstract into your word processor document or you can download it into an electronic reference manager. You can also enter other comments or information into the word processor document or the space provided for notes on the entry in the reference manager.

Putting it together

The reasons for reviewing the literature were given at the beginning of the chapter. By the time you have obtained and read the information, you should have a good overview of the literature on the topic. By the time you have read it thoroughly several times and made notes, you should be starting to see patterns and to understand how various parts fit into the whole. You should be able to follow the important themes through the literature. You may even begin to see where you could shape your study further, usually by narrowing it. For example, if you used literature on kangaroo mother care of pre-term infants it becomes clear that there is a group of studies dealing with infant outcomes and another group that deals with maternal outcomes. In planning a study on kangaroo mother care, you would decide whether you were going to study maternal outcomes, infant outcomes, or both. If you decided to study maternal outcomes only, the literature on infant outcomes would become redundant and vice versa.

If you are interested in exploring literature acquisition and review techniques in more detail, there are books on the subject, such as *Health Sciences Literature Review Made Easy* by Garrard (1999).

The process of reviewing the literature may seem at first to be a chore that is difficult and complex. As you move through the process, however, you will find that the time and energy that you invest will bring rewards in terms of learning new ideas. You will also feel a sense of accomplishment when you have become thoroughly conversant with the literature on a topic. You can discuss the topic intelligently with other researchers. You are now ready to move on to writing a literature review.

Summary

In this chapter, you have learned the meaning of 'review of the literature', and the reasons for reviewing the literature. You have learned ways of identifying possible sources and how to assess the sources for relevance. You have also learned ways of organising this process. Finally, you have learned how to critique individual research reports. You are now ready to move on to considering your conceptual framework (if it is appropriate) and writing a research proposal.

Main points

- The literature is the total body of writing dealing with the topic being researched.
- In preparing to search, be systematic, define your topic, identify key words, set boundaries to the search.
- A search can be limited by availability of time and information, financial constraints and the skills of the searcher.
- Colleagues, experts, librarians and lecturers can be resources.
- Information can be found in books, reports, journal articles, conference papers, electronic indexes, email and the WWW.
- Keep good records of the details of your search using a suitable manual or electronic organising system.

- In selecting material, stick to the topic, exclude non-research material, eliminate non-obtainable material and consider the quality of the source.
- Types of reading can include reading superficially and critically.
- Research reports have a distinct structure including the preliminaries, introduction, methodology, results and discussion.
- Information can be extracted from your readings by photocopying, downloading off the Internet, or a note-taking system.
- Key points can be recorded on cards, in a word processor, or by a highlighting system on hard copy.
- References can be compiled using a manual card system, a word processing system or an electronic reference manager.

Review Questions

1 The literature includes:
   a everything ever written on the subject
   b the research findings relevant to the topic
   c anecdotal accounts of the topic
   d recommendations for specific procedures

2 A comprehensive literature review is:
   a more important to do initially in quantitative research
   b more important to do initially in qualitative research
   c equally important to do initially in both quantitative and qualitative research
   d not important as to the timing in either type of research

3 Approximately what is the maximum proportion of the time devoted to a project that should be spent reviewing the literature?
   a 5 per cent
   b 15 per cent
   c 25 per cent
   d 40 per cent

4 In making a search, it would be reasonable to search as far back as:
   a five years
   b ten years
   c 20 years
   d 40 years

5 Reasons for finding a great deal of literature on the research question might include:
   a the topic is too broad
   b anecdotal material is being included
   c the search is going too far back
   d all of the above

6. Which of the following is considered to be highest quality type of literature for research?
   a. research papers in a refereed (peer-reviewed) journal
   b. secondary sources
   c. books
   d. research reports in conference proceedings

7. The most useful abstracting index for nursing literature is:
   a. NHMRC
   b. ERIC
   c. Medline
   d. CINAHL

8. The advantage of an electronic reference management system is that it:
   a. involves less handling of references
   b. is cheap
   c. enables electronic downloading of references
   d. a and c

9. Which of the following is most characteristic of a quantitative research article?
   a. provision of excerpts of dialogue
   b. comprehensive discussion of the findings
   c. discussion of theoretical assumptions about how knowledge is generated
   d. relating the findings to a conceptual framework

10. Which of the following is most characteristic of a qualitative research article?
    a. discussion of procedures for obtaining ethics clearance
    b. description of the instrument used
    c. discussion of themes and sub-themes
    d. description of the pilot study

Discussion Questions

1. What are the different meanings of the term 'review of the literature'?
2. How would you prepare to search for literature and what boundaries would you set?
3. List five major sources of literature.
4. Discuss the advantages and disadvantages of the different methods of keeping track of or filing your references and the information extracted from them.
5. Define 'critique' and outline the process used.

References

Daly, J. 1995, 'The lived experience of suffering', in *Illuminations*, ed. R. Parse, National League for Nursing, New York.

Day, R. 1998, *How to Write and Publish a Scientific Paper*, 5th edn, Cambridge University Press, Cambridge.

Garrard, J. 1999, *Health Sciences Literature Review Made Easy: The Matrix Method*, Aspen Publishers Inc., Gaithersburg, Maryland.

Homer, C., Davis, G., Petocz, P. & Barclay, L. 2000, 'Birth centre or labour ward? A comparison of the clinical outcomes of low-risk women in a NSW hospital', *Australian Journal of Advanced Nursing*, vol. 18, no. 1, 8–12.

CHAPTER 4

Research and its relationship to theory

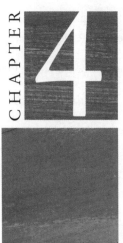

chapter objectives

The material presented in this chapter will assist you to:

- define terms related to theories and models
- understand the relationship between theory and research
- describe the ways in which major nursing and health theories have been used in research
- discuss ways in which a theoretical framework can be used in nursing and health research.

Introduction

Nursing research is linked with nursing theory in a reciprocal relationship. Research findings are 'incorporated into theory by human scientists ... to describe, explain, predict and prescribe important aspects of our lives' (Greenwood 1996). Research can lead to the revision of existing nursing theory through testing that theory. Conversely, research using qualitative methodologies such as grounded theory can lead to the development of useful theories for nursing and health. Both of those approaches can lead to the development of knowledge in the discipline of nursing.

Research into the health status of the client and the practice of nursing can lead to the development of useful theories for health and nursing. Even if a research project concerns a basic nursing procedure or phenomenon, it can lead to the development of theoretical knowledge (Brown 1964). Deriving theory from research data is an inductive approach. Many instances of data are collected and then a theory is proposed that fits the observations. This approach is associated with qualitative research designs such as grounded theory and phenomenology.

Theory can stimulate research when a researcher has ideas that are based in nursing theory. These ideas about the potential outcomes of the study form the framework of a study. The conceptual framework of a research study is like the skeleton of the body, or a frame of a building: it gives structure. This structure helps to plan the work, to know how the parts fit together, to know where to add parts on, and to provide a place to attach the other parts. All parts of the research project are linked to the theory, thus forming a coherent whole. Using theory as a conceptual framework is a deductive approach that is associated primarily with quantitative research methodology.

Research can also answer questions about theory through theory-testing. For example, a researcher might decide to test one of the propositions of an existing nursing theory against a new group of clients or in a nursing situation in which previous research on that proposition has not been carried out. Theory-testing is a deductive approach associated primarily with quantitative research design. At this stage in the development of theory-based research, very little testing of nursing theory has been carried out.

In this chapter, we will meet some definitions concerning theory, explore in more detail the links between theory and research, discuss the use of major nursing and health theories in research in nursing and health with examples, and explain specific ways in which a theoretical framework can be used in nursing and health research.

Theory – what is it?

A theory is an attempt to describe, organise or explain a phenomenon or group of phenomena of a discipline in a language appropriate to the discipline. Furthermore, models and theories organise our knowledge in an orderly, coherent way, thus providing a 'map' of the knowledge of the discipline.

Theories of nursing and health describe and explain nursing and health. They define the practice of nursing, and they deal with knowledge about health in humans. They may describe or explain the relationship between the nurse and the client. For example, Orem's Self-Care Deficit Nursing Theory states that nurses devise nursing systems to care for clients at different dependency levels (Orem 2001).

In order to understand the nature of a theory, it is necessary to understand its component parts and related terms, such as phenomenon, concept, and model. A phenomenon is something that happens and that can be perceived directly by the senses, for example, electricity. A phenomenon may be visible; for example lightning is a visible form of electricity. A phenomenon may also be invisible, for example the electricity that runs through electrical wires is not visible.

A concept is an abstract generalised idea that describes a phenomenon or a group of related phenomena, for example caring, blood pressure, or stress. Concepts range from the fairly concrete e.g. 'photograph' to the more abstract, for example 'health'. A concept may be inferred from direct measurements, for example central venous pressure may be measured directly using a manometer. A concept may also be inferred from indirect measurements such as measuring pain by means of visual analogue pain scales. A concept may also be explored through qualitative research methodologies. The major concepts in the discipline of nursing have been identified as nursing, person, environment and health. Very abstract concepts, for example 'well-being', are sometimes called constructs. Constructs such as energy fields may sometimes be identified through research.

A model is a structure that represents phenomena or concepts. A model may show the physical structure of what it represents, for example a model aeroplane. However, a model may also use language to describe what it represents, in which case it is called a theoretical or conceptual model.

Theories and models are generally considered to be at several different levels of complexity. The least complex level is a descriptive-level model, which identifies the major elements of a phenomenon by naming them. For example, Henderson's fourteen-needs model just lists the client's needs (Henderson 1966). The next level is a descriptive model that classifies its components by grouping them in meaningful categories. For example, all nursing diagnoses have been classified into eleven functional health patterns (Gordon 1982).

The next level of complexity of a model or theory is one in which the relationships between the concepts in the theory or model are shown. For example, the Neuman Systems Model shows the relationships between the core body structure and the lines of defence that surround it (Neuman 1995). The next level explains the relationships, or why the concepts are related. For example, in her Self-Care Deficit Nursing Theory, Orem explains the link between self-care, self-care demands and self-care agency (Orem 2001). The highest level is prescriptive-level theory, in which it is hypothesised that a certain intervention will result in a predictable outcome (Dickoff, James & Wiedenbach 1968). It is this level that promotes theory-testing. However, predictability may not be an issue for some research methods that emphasise induction.

Historical usage of theoretical frameworks in nursing research

Nursing research has not had a good record of using theoretical frameworks. In an early study of the use of five major nursing theories in the literature, Silva found that there was a lack of integration of models throughout the studies, little evidence of either systematic extension or replication of research based on nursing models, little validation of the models by the theorist, and lack of testing of assumptions and propositions within the models (Silva 1987). Further studies of nursing research published overseas have shown that only half of the articles in the specific nursing research and specialty journals, such as *Nursing Research* and *Heart and Lung*, used nursing theory frameworks (Brown, Tanner & Padrick 1984; Moody et al. 1988). Those using a theory or model used it as an organising framework rather than testing it (Brown, Tanner & Patrick 1984; Moody et al. 1988). For those articles that used a theoretical framework, behavioural science theories – Orem's Self-Care Deficit Nursing Theory, Rogers's Unitary Human Beings Theory and Roy's Adaptation Theory – were the frameworks most often used (Brown, Tanner & Patrick 1984; Moody et al. 1988).

In Australia, in a study of the first decade of literature in the *Australian Journal of Advanced Nursing*, it was found that about a quarter of all articles had a theoretical framework (Roberts 1995). Fewer than a third of research articles had a theoretical framework, and this proportion did not increase over the decade. Behavioural science frameworks were most common, and Orem's Self-Care Deficit Nursing Theory was the most common nursing theory used. In addition, there was a low level of application of the theory. Thirteen articles cited only the theory, a further eight demonstrated conceptual links with the theory, while twelve used the theory as an organising framework and only one article tested the theory. These findings indicate a low level of usage and application of theoretical frameworks, particularly nursing frameworks.

In a snapshot study of one recent year of Australian nurse-academics' nursing scholarship, most research articles did not use a theoretical framework (Roberts 1996). Of the few that did, the majority used a nursing framework. However, we must not blame the authors entirely. It appears that some clinical research journals do not like the use of theoretical frameworks. The author has twice had clinically focused research journals require that a theoretical framework be removed before the article was accepted for publication (Roberts 1999).

Use of nursing and health theories and models in nursing research

The latter half of the twentieth century saw the development of a considerable number of models and theories of nursing and health. However, some of these attracted more research interest than others. The most-researched theories are those that contain concepts with sufficiently precise definitions to provide a useful research framework. There are two major groups of these: grand theories that are broad in scope and middle-range theories that are more restricted in scope. The former are used in researching every part of nursing whereas the latter have been used in nursing specialty research. These theories will be described briefly below. For more information, the publication on the original theory should be consulted.

Grand theories

The grand theories most used for conceptual frameworks in studies listed in CINAHL are Orem's Self-Care Deficit Nursing Theory (Orem 2001), Levine's conservation model (Levine 1991), the Neuman Systems Model (Neuman 1995), Roy's Adaptation Model (Roy & Andrews 1991), and Rogers's Energy Fields Model (Rogers 1994).

Orem's Self-Care Deficit Nursing Theory

Orem's model, called the Self-Care Deficit Theory of Nursing, was developed initially in the 1970s but it has continued to evolve and Orem's book is now in its fifth edition (Orem 2001). The model comprises three related theories: the theory of self-care, which describes and explains self-care; the theory of self-care deficit, which describes how clients need nursing; and the theory of nursing system, which describes and explains relationships necessary for nursing to take place.

The theory of self-care proposes that people will normally act in a rational way to care for themselves and their dependants. People can therefore develop and function optimally, be healthy and achieve a sense of well-being. In doing so, they meet requirements, or self-care requisites. These are of three types: universal, or those required by everyone regardless of their age; developmental, or those required at a particular stage in the person's development; and health deviation, or those relating to the person's state of health, or health care. Care requisites may be met through self-care, care of dependants, or nursing care.

The theory of self-care deficit proposes that, at times, persons or their dependants will have a greater need for self-care than they can fulfil. This creates a self-care deficit or a need for care to be provided by an external source, such as a nurse.

The theory of nursing system links the nurse and the client by proposing that nurses act to provide nursing care for people or groups of people who are unable to meet their own or their dependants' needs for self-care. The nursing systems that the nurse and client devise can be wholly compensatory, in which the nurse performs all care for the client, partially compensatory, in which the nurse and client share the care, or supportive-educative in which the nurse supports and educates the client.

Orem's theory has been used fairly extensively in nursing research, in a broad range of topics (Eben et al. 1994). Orem has developed a complete set of assumptions and propositions, which are testable. Many doctoral theses based on her theory have been carried out and many research papers have been published that have been at some level based on her theory. Several tools have been developed to assess self-care and attitudes to self-care. These include Denyes's Self-Care Agency, Kearney and Fleischer's Exercise of Self-Care Agency, and Hanson and Bickel's Perception of Self-Care Agency (McBride 1991). In Australia, studies have been done on teaching self-care skills for headaches (Del Fante 1985), differing attitudes to self-care of hospital and community nurses (Yelland & Sellick 1988), and use of relaxation for the promotion of comfort and pain relief in clients with advanced cancer (Sloman et al. 1994). Sloman and colleagues used Orem's concept of self-care to conceptualise the study. They reasoned that patients experiencing severe cancer pain could use relaxation techniques and gain a degree of self-control. Participants were randomly assigned to three groups: one that received relaxation techniques, a group that received relaxation training and a control group that received no relaxation training. The researchers found that the patients who received relaxation training perceived that they were more relaxed. The study also found that there was a reduction in p.r.n. medication for those groups. The researchers concluded that the nurse could play a supportive-educative role in encouraging and teaching self-relaxation in cancer patients and thereby promote client self-care in accordance with Orem's theory. In England, a more recent study (Lauder 1999) explored the concept of self-neglect using Orem's theory.

Levine's Conservation Principles

Many years ago, Levine, one of the early nurse-theorists, developed her four Conservation Principles to provide a structure for teaching medical-surgical nursing (Artigue et al. 1994). The four Conservation Principles are: conservation of energy, of structural integrity, of personal integrity, and of social integrity. The Principle of Conservation of Energy refers to balancing energy output and energy input to avoid excessive fatigue. The Principle of Conservation of Structural Integrity refers to maintaining or restoring the structure of the body by prevention of physical breakdown and the promotion of healing. The Principle of Conservation of Personal Integrity refers to the maintenance or restoration of the patient's sense of identity and self-worth. Finally, the Principle of Conservation of Social Integrity refers to the patient's status as a social being who interacts with others, particularly significant others (Levine 1990).

Levine's model views the person as an holistic being, able to adapt and preserve its integrity with the external environment. If any of these principles is altered, the person's health status is changed. The nurse acts therapeutically to help the client conserve energy and maintain integrity or adapt to changes in energy or integrity. When further adaptation cannot occur, the nurse supports the individual and family while care is needed.

Levine's model is undergoing a recent resurgence. It has been used as a conceptual framework in several studies. These include client-based studies such as one on fatigue in clients with congestive cardiac failure (Schaefer & Potylycki 1993). In Australia, Levine's framework has been used in two studies of boomerang pillows (Roberts et al. 1994; Roberts, Brittin & deClifford 1995). In the study of the effect of boomerang pillows on frail elderly women, a comparison of volumes before and after 10 minutes on a boomerang pillow showed that the lung volume was significantly lower after using the boomerang pillows. It was argued that the use of these pillows may lead to less conservation of energy in these women (Roberts, Brittin & deClifford 1995).

Roy's Adaptation Model

The Roy Adaptation Model views the individual as a system that constantly adapts in response to stimuli from its external or internal environment. Stimuli can be classed as 'focal' immediate stimuli; 'contextual' contributing stimuli; or 'residual' background stimuli (Roy & Andrews 1991). Each person has a level of adaptation that can be tolerated with ordinary adaptive responses. The response can be positive if adaptation occurs in a way that contributes to the achievement of goals such as survival or growth, or ineffective if it does not. Each person has two mechanisms for responding to stimuli and controlling adaptation: the regulator or physiological mechanism, and the cognator or behavioural mechanism. Persons adapt in four modes. The physiological mode deals with physiological responses. The three psychosocial modes are the self-concept mode, which deals with psychic integrity; the role function mode, which deals with social roles; and the interdependence mode, which deals with interactions with other people.

Roy's model has been used extensively as a conceptual framework in many doctoral theses and published research studies in nursing research. The research studies have been carried out in the field of paediatric nursing, midwifery nursing, neonatal nursing, and gerontological nursing. The emphasis on babies and children is not surprising as Roy developed her model originally for paediatric nursing. Roy's model was used in experiment to determine whether the effect of caregiving relatives' level of involvement in care increased their satisfaction with nursing home care (Toye & Blackmore 1996). They found that it did not.

Neuman Systems Model

Neuman's model views the client's system as consisting of the basic structure or core, surrounded by layers of defences, rather like the layers of an onion. The basic structure is the energy resources, comprising all basic variables that compose intrinsic human factors related to survival, such as genetic and ego structures, and regulation of body temperature. The basic structure is immediately surrounded by the flexible lines of resistance, which represent the body's resources that help defend against stressors, for example the immune system. Outside the flexible lines of resistance is the normal line of defence, which is a constant stability state for the individual who has adjusted to stressors. The outermost ring is the flexible lines of defence which is another shield against stressors or environmental forces that may alter the stability of the system. Stressors are of three types. Intrapersonal stressors are forces occurring within the individual, e.g. negative emotions. Interpersonal stressors are forces that occur between one or more individuals, e.g. role expectations. Finally, extrapersonal stressors are forces occurring outside the individual, e.g. financial circumstances. The nurse acts, using prevention to intervene in the interaction of the client with stressors. Primary prevention occurs when a stressor is suspected or identified; secondary prevention occurs after symptoms from stress have occurred; and tertiary prevention occurs after the active treatment and leads back to primary prevention.

Neuman's model has also been used extensively in nursing research. Neuman (1995) reports that her model is one of the three most frequently utilised models for nursing research. It is used extensively for graduate students' research projects and has identified future study and practice impact (Louis 1995). Abstracts of many studies using the Neuman model are presented in Neuman's book. Many published clinical research studies and several doctoral theses have used the Neuman Systems Model as an organising framework. The studies have been in the areas of premature infants, high dependency nursing, pain, stress, anxiety, and health promotion. These topics reflect the emphasis in Neuman's theory on stress and prevention.

Neuman herself has identified additional topics for further research using her model. She suggests that evaluation of primary preventive health education programs for school children, availability of alternative health care delivery services for clients, development of primary prevention programs for adults in the middle years of 40 to 60, and evaluation of multi-disciplinary health promotion programs are appropriate contemporary issues for exploration and research with the Neuman model (Beckman et al. 1994). There does not as yet appear to be any published research by Australian nurse-researchers using the Neuman Systems Model.

Rogers's Theory of Unitary Human Beings

Rogers postulated that human beings are dynamic energy fields inseparable from their environmental energy fields. In Rogers's paradigm, the four major concepts are: energy fields, a universe of open systems, pattern, and pan-dimensionality (Daily et al. 1994). Rogers saw the fundamental unit of the living and the non-living as the energy field. A unitary human being is an energy field that is not limited by time and space. It is identified by its unique pattern and its characteristics cannot be predicted from knowledge of the parts. An environmental energy field is an energy field that is similar to a human energy field. Each person is a human energy field that incorporates its own specific environmental energy field. These form open systems that exchange energy with each other. Both fields are changing all the time. The pattern is seen as a wave and includes behaviours, qualities, and characteristics of the field. Rogers postulated three principles of homeodynamics: the Principle of Helicy, or the continuous variety of human and environmental field patterns; the Principle of Integrality, or the continuous mutual human–environmental field interaction and processes, and the Principle of Resonancy, or change from lower to higher frequency of the wave patterns as the person develops and becomes more complex (Daily et al. 1994).

Recent studies using Rogers's conceptual model as a base have been numerous, as have doctoral theses using Rogers's theoretical framework. Studies have concerned therapeutic touch, parental attachments, addictions, and perception of time. There does not appear to be any published research by Australian nurse-researchers using the Science of Unitary Human Beings.

Middle-range theories and models

These theories and models include Leininger's Model of Transcultural Care (Leininger 1995), King's Theory of Goal Attainment (King 1981), Benner's Model of Skill Acquisition (Benner 1984), Watson's Theory of Human Caring (Watson 1979), Johnson's Behavioral Systems Model (Johnson 1990), Newman's Health as Expanding Consciousness (Newman 1994), Mercer's Maternal Role Attainment Model (Bee, Legger & Oetting 1994), Parse's Theory of Human Becoming (Parse 1992) and Peplau's Model of Psychodynamic Nursing (Peplau 1991). There has been little research in Australia using these models.

Research using Leininger's Model of Transcultural Care as a theoretical framework has not been published widely (Alexander et al. 1994). However, in the United States many cultures have been studied as part of research into transcultural nursing and care (Alexander et al. 1994). This research has been slow to be funded because qualitative research has not been as successful in attracting funding as quantitative research. One would think that Leininger's model would be a very relevant one for studying people in such a multicultural society as Australia. However, the author could find only a few published research studies by one Australian nurse-researcher, Omeri, that used the Leininger model. These are studies of culture care of Iranian immigrants in New South Wales (Omeri 1997), and utilisation of culturally congruent strategies to enhance recruitment and retention of Australian Indigenous nursing students (Omeri 1999). In the study on Iranian immigrants, Omeri used Leininger's model to develop care that was compatible with the women's cultural beliefs.

King (1981) developed a Theory of Goal Attainment. King's model is a systems model that conceptualises the person as an open system interacting with the environment. The individual is seen as a personal system that is a part of a group. A group is an interpersonal system that is a part of a social system. These systems interact with each other. This theory has led to a small amount of nursing research. It has been used in a variety of studies overseas in which goal attainment was investigated (Ackermann et al. 1994). Areas of focus include adolescent health, women's health, cardiac rehabilitation, family health and nursing home clients.

Benner's Model of Skill Acquisition in Nursing has basically used research to uncover the knowledge embedded in clinical practice (Alexander & Keller 1994). Benner has stated that 'the lack of charting of our practices and clinical observations deprives nursing theory of the uniqueness and richness of the knowledge embedded in clinical practice' (Benner 1984, p. 2). This knowledge is central to the advancement of nursing practice and to the development of nursing science. Benner's model has been used as the theoretical framework in several research studies pertaining to specialist nursing education and clinical career ladders, including Alexander and Keller (1994).

Watson developed a model incorporating 10 carative factors that nurses should use. Watson and others have attempted to research the 10 carative factors of Watson's model (Barnhart et al. 1994), but this is difficult because of the abstract nature of the theory and the limitations of caring in the clinical setting, for example brief encounters with clients. The theory was clinically validated by researchers using qualitative methodology (Barnhart et al. 1994). There have been several studies using Watson's Theory of Caring, primarily on clients' and nurses' perceptions of caring.

Johnson's Behavioral Systems Model proposes seven behavioural subsystems that classify human behaviour, including the biological subsystem and the achievement subsystem. The model has been used in several research studies on the visually impaired, cancer sufferers, and the elderly. Furthermore, Derdiarian has developed and tested an instrument (Derdiarian 1988, 1991) and has tested the model in a research study (Derdiarian 1990).

Newman's Model of Health as Expanding Consciousness uses the concepts of movement, space, time and consciousness to depict health (Newman 1986). It has attracted a limited amount of research, perhaps because of its abstract nature. Newman herself has been developing a research methodology consistent with her theoretical paradigm (Newman 1994). Several researchers have undertaken studies about time, space and movement, particularly in the study of the elderly (Keffer et al. 1994).

In the specialist area of maternal–child health, Mercer's Theory of Maternal Role Attainment has been used in a few published studies in the maternal–child nursing area (Bee, Legger & Oetting 1994). The work of Mercer's predecessor, Rubin, was used as the theoretical rationale for a study by Barclay and Martin on episiotomy care in Australia (Barclay & Martin 1983). They argued that the theory of the attainment of the maternal role encompassed a phase of 'taking in' the stresses of labour and delivery and that the enjoyment of 'taking on' motherhood would be diminished by pain, including the pain of the episiotomy. Therefore, any midwifery interventions that could diminish the pain would enhance the 'taking on' of motherhood. In their study of treatment of the episiotomy wound, they compared the treatments of warm sitz bath, iced sitz bath and ray lamp against an untreated control group. While they found no difference in the groups with regard to healing and incidence of infection, they found that the group using an iced sitz bath perceived less pain than the other groups. They concluded that the use of iced sitz baths was more likely than the other methods to reduce pain, which was an important consideration in taking on the role of mother (Barclay & Martin 1983).

Peplau's Model of Psychodynamic Nursing identifies four phases of the nurse–client interaction and delineates such aspects of the role of the nurse as teacher and resource person (Peplau 1991). Peplau's model, developed originally in the 1950s, has been used as a conceptual framework in a limited amount of research over 30 years, mostly in psychiatric nursing (Brophy et al. 1994). The Peplau model is another that has undergone a revival in recent times, led by Forchuck in Toronto, Canada.

Parse's model was developed using Rogers's model as a foundation, along with concepts from existential-phenomenological thought (Lee, Schumacher & Twigg 1994). Parse's model is very abstract and involves the notion that health is a lived experience in which humans structure meaning multi-dimensionally, move towards greater diversity, and reach beyond the self. Parse's model has been used for a growing body of research. Studies using Parse's methodology are qualitative in approach and phenomenological in nature. Parse has developed a research methodology that is congruent with her theory and the phenomenological research tradition (Parse 1995). Research using Parse's model appears to centre on the elderly and on the lived experience of human emotions such as grieving. Parse's theory has been used in several research studies concerned with the lived experience of health, being elderly, being unemployed or homeless, grieving, and laughter. In Australia, Professor John Daly at the University of Western Sydney has done research using Parse's methodology to study the lived experience of suffering (Daly 1995).

The Health Belief Model is a model that seeks to explain factors that influence people to take preventive 'health' action. It was originally developed and extended by Becker (1974). This model hypothesised that persons would generally not seek preventive care or health screening unless they had some relevant health motivation and knowledge, saw themselves as potentially vulnerable and the condition as threatening, were convinced of the value of intervention and foresaw few difficulties in undertaking the recommended action (Becker 1974). The Health Belief Model suggested that the likelihood of taking a recommended preventive health action was promoted by the perceived threat of the disease and the perceived benefits of preventive action but was inhibited by perceived barriers to preventive action. Perceived threat was affected by perceived susceptibility to the disease and the perceived seriousness of the disease. Modifying factors such as age, sex, personality, and cues to action affected the perceived threat of the disease.

Becker and colleagues suggested that the original Health Belief Model was in need of modification in response to research findings. They developed the Preventive Health Behaviour Model. The Preventive Health Behaviour Model, despite its name, is really a model of prevention of disease. The Preventive Health Behaviour Model suggests that the likelihood of complying with individual 'health-related' behaviours could be predicted by motivation, value of illness threat reduction, and probability that the compliant behaviour will reduce the threat. These were moderated by modifying and enabling factors such as demographic variables, structural variables (for example cost), attitudes, interaction, and enabling variables such as experience.

In her 1982 book, *Health Promotion in Nursing Practice*, Pender proposed a modification of the Health Belief Model (Pender 1982). Pender proposed two phases in the model – the decision-making phase and the action phase.

The decision-making phase comprises individual perceptions and factors, and constitutes the perceived barriers and the cues to action. The benefits of preventive action are moved to the individual perceptions sector of the model. The cues to action are moved to the action phase of the model.

The Health Belief/Preventive Health Behaviour model was used as a theoretical framework for a study by Agars and McMurray evaluating the effects of three different methods of breast self-examination on nurses' personal BSE practice (Agars & McMurray 1993). The researchers used a pre-test/post-test design to follow three groups, using a BSE instruction booklet, a film and group discussion, and individual teaching. They found that each group had a significant improvement but the nurses given the film and discussion had the most improvement. The researchers found that barriers to action were more predictive of behaviour before the instruction and perceived susceptibility was more predictive after the instruction.

In her 1982 book, Pender also proposed the Health Promotion Model (Pender 1982), which represented a breakthrough in that she turned everything around. Rather than preventing disease, the person was promoting health. The model was revised in her 1987 book (Pender 1987).

The Health Promotion Model uses the concept of perceived self-efficacy. The model was developed from an extensive review of health research. The central proposal of the model is that the individual has cognitive-perceptual (thinking and sensing) factors that are modified by situational, personal and interpersonal characteristics to result in the participation in health-promoting behaviours in the presence of a cue to action (Tillet 1994). The cognitive-perceptive factors have a direct effect on the decision, whereas the modifying factors have an indirect effect through the cognitive-perceptual factors. Pender's Health Promotion Model has been used as a theoretical framework for investigating the health-promoting activities of clients in all age groups.

How to use a conceptual framework in a research study

The theoretical framework is used in all stages of the research project. The first step in using a conceptual framework is to choose a theory or model that is suited to the research question. For example, if clients from another culture are involved, transcultural nursing may be the theory of choice. If stressors are involved, then the Neuman Systems Model would be appropriate. If independence is a major concept, then the Orem Self-Care Deficit Nursing Theory would be appropriate. However, it is inappropriate to stretch a theory to fit something for which it was not intended.

It is important to examine the relationship between the question asked and the theoretical framework. You should ensure that the question is congruent with the conceptual framework and that it is phrased in the language of the theory. You then state testable hypotheses, defining variables that have been derived from the concepts of the theory. You should define the variables in the theory in a way that is consistent with the theory. If there are relationships between the variables, you should state them in terms of the theory. You can use the conceptual model to help find and interpret the literature. The concepts and variables, defined in terms of the model, can be used as key words to retrieve and organise the literature. This will help you to select appropriate literature and exclude inappropriate literature.

The methodology of the study, including data analysis, should be congruent with the model. For example, Parse's model has its own suggested method of data analysis.

You can use the model as a guide to interpreting the findings and judging their significance. In writing up the report, you can use the model to provide a structure for organising the literature review, the presentation of the results and the discussion. If used appropriately, it leads to an integration of the parts of the study.

Developing theory from research

Research can generate theory. Usually, this is done by inductive reasoning in which the researcher makes many observations of the phenomenon under investigation and then uses the data to generate theoretical insights that describe or explain the phenomenon. The researcher proceeds from a relatively theory-free base so as to observe without pre-formed judgements. For example, in her study of nurses' practice when shifting from the institutional setting to the client's home, St John used a grounded theory approach to develop a theory of nursing practice (St John 1999). Irurita (1999) also used a grounded theory method to explore the problem of patient vulnerability. General theory-producing approaches to research, usually qualitative, are: grounded theory, phenomenology, historical research, hermeneutics and critical analysis. These will be explored in greater depth in Chapters 12 and 13.

Summary

In this chapter, we have examined the relationship between research and theory, seeing that research can either be based on a theoretical framework, or can lead to the development of theory by acting as a precursor for theory. We have looked at the historical utilisation of theoretical frameworks in nursing research. We have examined some specific theories of nursing and their usage in research. Finally, we have explored the process of using a theoretical framework in a research project.

Main points
- A theory is an attempt to describe, organise or explain a phenomenon or group of phenomena of a discipline in a language appropriate to that discipline.
- Theories can organise knowledge in an orderly, coherent way, thus providing a 'map' of knowledge of nursing discipline, describe and explain nursing and

health, define the practice of nursing; and describe or explain the relationship between the nurse and the client.
- Theory can provide a conceptual framework for a study and be tested by research.
- Research can generate theory, leading to the development of useful theories for nursing and health.
- Nursing theories have minimal usage in nursing research. Of existing nursing theories, Orem's theory is most utilised.
- Grand theories that can be used include: Orem's Self-Care Deficit Nursing Theory, Levine's Conservation Model, Neuman's Systems Model, Roy's Adaptation Model, and Rogers's Energy Fields Model.
- Middle-range theories and models that can be used include: Leininger's Transcultural Care Model, King's Theory of Goal Attainment, Benner's Model of Skill Acquisition, Watson's Theory of Human Caring, Johnson's Behavioral Systems Model, Newman's Health as Expanding Consciousness Model, Mercer's Maternal Role Attainment Model, Parse's Theory of Human Becoming and Peplau's Model of Psychodynamic Nursing.
- To use a conceptual framework in a research study, choose a theory or model suited to your research question, then ensure all parts of the study are congruent with the concepts of the chosen theory and use the language of the theory. Use the model to interpret the findings of the study.

Review Questions

1. Which of the following statements is true?
    a. Research can generate theory.
    b. Theory can generate research.
    c. Practice can generate research.
    d. all of the above

2. A phenomenon:
    a. is normally invisible
    b. is composed of models
    c. can be directly perceived by the senses
    d. can have all of the above characteristics

3. The type of theory that is usually used in specialty research in nursing is:
    a. grand theory
    b. middle-range theory
    c. highly specific theory
    d. inductive theory

4 Which of the following is a grand theory?
   a Orem's Self-Care Deficit Theory of Nursing
   b Leininger's Model of Transcultural Care
   c Benner's Model of Skill Acquisition in Nursing
   d Mercer's Maternal Role Attainment Model

5 Which of the following is a middle-range theory?
   a Rogers's Theory of Unitary Human Beings
   b King's Theory of Goal Attainment
   c Neuman's Systems Model
   d Levine's Conservation Principles

6 Which of the following would be the most suitable conceptual framework for a study on heat transfer in premature infants?
   a Levine's Conservation Principles
   b Maternal Role Attainment
   c Health as Expanding Consciousness
   d Health Promotion Model

7 Which of the following would be the most suitable conceptual framework for a study on acclimatisation to the tropical climate?
   a Orem's Self-Care Deficit Theory of Nursing
   b Roy's Adaptation Model
   c Benner's Skill Acquisition Model
   d Leininger's Transcultural Nursing Model

8 Which of the following would be the most suitable as a conceptual framework for a study on stress?
   a Roy's Adaptation Model
   b Orem's Self-Care Deficit Theory of Nursing
   c Neuman's Systems Model
   d Rogers's Theory of Unitary Human Beings

9 Which of the following would be the most suitable as a conceptual framework for a study using the phenomenology methodology?
   a Parse's Human Becoming Theory
   b Orem's Self-Care Deficit Theory of Nursing
   c Roy's Adaptation Model
   d Leininger's Transcultural Nursing Model

10 Which of the following would be the most suitable conceptual framework for a research study on women's attitudes to breast self-examination?
    a Benner's Skill Acquisition Model
    b Roy's Adaptation Model
    c Parse's Human Becoming Theory
    d Orem's Self-Care Deficit Theory of Nursing

Discussion Questions

1. Define 'theory' and discuss the relationship between practice, theory and research.
2. Differentiate between 'grand' and 'middle-range' theories.
3. State which grand theory is most used in nursing research and give examples of it.
4. List five middle-range theories and give examples of their use in nursing research.
5. Discuss how nursing theories can be used in nursing research.

References

Ackermann, M., Brink, S., Clanton, J., Jones, C., Marriner-Tomey, A., Moody, S., Perlich, G., Price, D. & Prusinski, B. 1994, 'Imogene King: theory of goal attainment', in *Nursing Theorists and Their Work*, 3rd edn, ed. A. Marriner-Tomey, C. V. Mosby, St Louis.

Agars, J. & McMurray, A. 1993, 'An evaluation of comparative strategies for teaching breast self-examination', *Journal of Advanced Nursing*, vol. 18, 1595–1603.

Alexander, J., Beagle, C., Butler, P., Dougherty, D., Robards, K., Solotkin, K. & Velotta, C. 1994, 'Madeleine Leininger: cultural care theory' in *Nursing Theorists and Their Work*, 3rd edn, ed. A. Marriner-Tomey, C.V. Mosby, St Louis.

Alexander, S. & Keller, S. 1994, 'Patricia Benner: from novice to expert – excellence and power in clinical nursing practice', in *Nursing Theorists and Their Work*, 3rd edn, ed. A. Marriner-Tomey, C.V. Mosby, St Louis.

Artigue, G., Foli, K., Johnson, T., Marriner-Tomey, A., Poat, C., Poppa, L., Woeste, R. & Zoretich, S. 1994, 'Myra Estrin Levine: four conservation principles', in *Nursing Theorists and Their Work*, 3rd edn, ed. A. Marriner-Tomey, C.V. Mosby, St Louis.

Barclay, L. & Martin, N. 1983, 'A sensitive area', *Australian Journal of Advanced Nursing*, vol. 1, no. 1, 12–19.

Barnhart, D., Bennett, P., Porter, B. & Sloan, R. 1994, 'Jean Watson: philosophy and science of caring', in *Nursing Theorists and Their Work*, 3rd edn, ed. A. Marriner-Tomey, C.V. Mosby, St Louis.

Becker, M. 1974, 'The health belief model and sick role behavior', *Health Education Monographs*, vol. 2, 409.

Beckman, S., Boxley-Harges, S., Bruick-Sorge, C., Harris, S., Hermiz, M. & Steinkeler, S. 1994, in *Nursing Theorists and Their Work*, 3rd edn, ed. A. Marriner-Tomey, C.V. Mosby, St Louis.

Bee, A., Legger, D. & Oetting, S. 1994, 'Ramona T Mercer: maternal role attainment', in *Nursing Theorists and Their Work*, 3rd edn, ed. A. Marriner-Tomey, C.V. Mosby, St Louis.

Benner, P. 1984, *From Novice to Expert: Excellence and Power in Clinical Nursing Practice*, Addison-Wesley, Menlo Park, California.

Brophy, G., Carey, E., Noll, J., Rasmussen, L., Searcy, B. & Stark, N. 1994, 'Hildegard E Peplau: psychodynamic nursing', in *Nursing Theorists and Their Work*, 3rd edn, ed. A. Marriner-Tomey, C.V. Mosby, St Louis.

Brown, J., Tanner, C. & Padrick, K. 1984, 'Nursing's search for scientific knowledge', *Nursing Research*, vol. 33, no. 1, 26–32.

Brown, M. 1964, 'Research in the development of nursing theory: the importance of a theoretical framework in nursing research', *Nursing Research*, vol. 13, no. 2, 109–12.

Daily, J., Maupin, J., Murray, C., Satterly, M., Schnell, D. & Wallace, T. 1994, 'Martha E Rogers: unitary human beings', in *Nursing Theorists and Their Work*, 3rd edn, ed. A. Marriner-Tomey, C.V. Mosby, St Louis.

Daly, J. 1995, 'The lived experience of suffering', in *Illuminations*, ed. R. Parse, National League for Nursing, New York.

Del Fante, A. 1985, 'Teaching self care skills for migraine and tension headaches', *Australian Journal of Advanced Nursing*, vol. 2, no. 3, 4–8.

Derdiarian, A. 1988, 'Sensitivity of the Derdiarian Behavioral System Model instrument to age, site, and stage of cancer: a preliminary validation study', *Scholarly Inquiry for Nursing Practice*, vol. 2, no. 2, 103–21.

Derdiarian, A. 1990, 'The relationships among the subsystems of Johnson's Behavioral Systems Model', *Image: Journal of Nursing Scholarship*, vol. 22, no. 4, 219–24.

Derdiarian, A. 1991, 'Effects of using a nursing model-based assessment instrument on quality of nursing care', *Nursing Administration Quarterly*, vol. 15, no. 3, 1–16.

Dickoff, J., James, P. & Wiedenbach, E. 1968, 'Theory in a practice discipline: part 1. practice-oriented theory', *Nursing Research*, vol. 5, 415–35.

Eben, J., Gashti, N., Hayes, S., Marriner-Tomey, A., Nation, M. & Nordmeyer, S. 1994, 'Dorothea E Orem: self-care deficit theory of nursing', in *Nursing Theorists and Their Work*, 3rd edn, ed. A. Marriner-Tomey, C.V. Mosby, St Louis.

Gordon, M. 1982, *Nursing Diagnosis: Process and Application*, McGraw-Hill, St Louis.

Greenwood, J. 1996, 'Nursing research and nursing theory', in *Nursing Theory in Australia: Development and Application*, ed. J. Greenwood, Harper Educational Australia, Sydney.

Henderson, V. 1966, *The Nature of Nursing: A Definition and Its Implications for Practice, Research, and Education*, Macmillan, New York.

Irurita, V. 1999, 'The problem of patient vulnerability', *Collegian*, vol. 6, no. 1, 10–15.

Johnson, D. 1990, 'The behavioral systems model for nursing', in *Nursing Theories in Practice*, ed. M. E. Parker, NLN–PUBL 1990 #15–2350, National League for Nursing, New York.

Keffer, M., Hensley, D., Kilgore-Keever, K., Langfitt, J. & Peterson, L. 1994, 'Margaret A Newman: model of health', in *Nursing Theorists and Their Work*, 3rd edn, ed. A. Marriner-Tomey, C.V. Mosby, St Louis.

King, I. M. 1981, *A Theory for Nursing: Systems, Concepts, Process*, Delmar Publishers, Albany, New York.

Lauder, W. 1999, 'Constructions of self-neglect: a multiple case study design', *Nursing Inquiry*, vol. 6, no. 1, 48–57.

Lee, R., Schumacher, L. & Twigg, P. 1994, 'Rosemarie Rizzo Parse: man-living-health' in *Nursing Theorists and Their Work*, 3rd edn, ed. A. Marriner-Tomey, C.V. Mosby, St Louis.

Leininger, M. 1995, *Transcultural Nursing: Concepts, Theories, Research and Practices*, 2nd edn, McGraw-Hill/Greyden Press, Columbus.

Levine, M. 1990, 'Conservation and integrity … Levine's conservation model', in *Nursing Theories in Practice*, ed. M. E. Parker, NLN–PUBL 1990 #15–2350, National League for Nursing, New York.

Levine, M. 1991, 'The conservation principles: model for health', in *Levine's Conservation Model: A Framework for Nursing Practice*, eds K. Schaefer & J. Pond, F. A. Davis Co., Philadelphia.

Louis, M. 1995, 'The Neuman model in nursing research: an update', in *The Neuman Systems Model*, 3rd edn, ed. B. Neuman, Appleton & Lange, Norwalk, Connecticut.

McBride, S. 1991, 'Comparative analysis of three instruments designed to measure self-care agency', *Nursing Research*, vol. 40, no. 1, 12–16.

Moody, L., Wilson, M., Smyth, K., Schwartz, R., Tittle, M. & Van Cott, M. 1988, 'Analysis of a decade of nursing practice research: 1977–86', *Nursing Research*, vol. 37, no. 6, 374–9.

Neuman, B. 1995, *The Neuman Systems Model*, 3rd edn, ed. B. Neuman, Appleton & Lange, Norwalk, Connecticut.

Newman, M. 1986, *Health as Expanding Consciousness*, National League for Nursing, New York.

Newman, M. 1994, *Health as Expanding Consciousness*, 2nd edn, National League for Nursing, New York.

Omeri, A. 1997, 'Culture care of Iranian immigrants in New South Wales, Australia: sharing transcultural nursing knowledge', *Journal of Transcultural Nursing*, vol. 8, no. 2, 5–16.

Omeri, A. 1999, 'Using culturally congruent strategies to enhance recruitment and retention of Australian nursing students', *Journal of Transcultural Nursing*, vol. 10, no. 2, 150–5.

Orem, D. 2001, *Nursing: Concepts of Practice*, 6th edn, C.V. Mosby, St Louis.

Parse, R. 1992, 'Human becoming: Parse's theory of nursing', *Nursing Science Quarterly*, vol. 5, no. 1, 35–42.

Parse, R. 1995, 'Research with the human becoming theory', *Illuminations*, ed. R. Parse, National League for Nursing, New York.

Pender, N. 1982, *Health Promotion in Nursing Practice*, Appleton & Lange, New York.

Pender, N. 1987, *Health Promotion in Nursing Practice*, 2nd edn, Appleton & Lange, New York.

Peplau, H. 1991, *Interpersonal Relations in Nursing: a Conceptual Frame of Reference for Psychodynamic Nursing*, G Putnam's Sons, New York.

Roberts, K. 1995, 'Early Australian nursing scholarship: the first decade of the AJAN. Part 2: Scholarship', *Australian Electronic Journal of Nursing Education*, vol. 1, no. 1.

Roberts, K. 1996, 'A snapshot of Australian nursing scholarship 1993–4', *Collegian*, vol. 3, no. 1, 4–10.

Roberts, K. 1999, 'Through a looking glass', *Clinical Nursing Research*, vol. 8, no. 4, 299–301.

Roberts, K., Brittin, M. & deClifford, J. 1995, 'Boomerang pillows and respiratory capacity in frail elderly women', *Clinical Nursing Research*, vol. 4, no. 4, 465–71.

Roberts, K., Brittin, M., Cook, M. & deClifford, J. 1994, 'Boomerang pillows and respiratory capacity', *Clinical Nursing Research*, vol. 3, no. 2, 157–65.

Rogers, M. 1994, 'The science of unitary human beings: current perspectives', *Nursing Science Quarterly*, vol. 7, no. 1, 33–5.

Roy, C. & Andrews, H. 1991, *The Roy Adaptation Model: The Definitive Statement*, Appleton & Lange, Norwalk, Connecticut.

Schaefer, K. & Potylycki, M. 1993, 'Fatigue associated with congestive heart failure: use of Levine's Conservation Model', *Journal of Advanced Nursing*, vol. 18, no. 2, 260–8.

Silva, M. (ed.) 1987, *Conceptual Models of Nursing*, Annual Review of Nursing Research, Springer Publishing Co. New York.

Sloman, R., Brown, P., Aldana, E. & Chee, E. 1994, 'The use of relaxation for the promotion of comfort and pain relief in persons with advanced cancer', *Contemporary Nurse*, vol. 3, no. 1, 6–12.

St John, W. 1999, 'Beyond the sick role: situating community health nursing practice', *Collegian*, vol. 6, no. 1, 30–5.

Tillet, L. 1994, 'Nola J Pender: the health promotion model', in *Nursing Theorists and Their Work*, 3rd edn, ed. A. Marriner-Tomey, C.V. Mosby, St Louis.

Toye, C. & Blackmore, A. 1996, 'Satisfaction with nursing home care of a relative: does inviting greater input make a difference?' *Collegian*, vol. 3, no. 2, 4–6, 8–11.

Watson, J. 1979, *The Philosophy and Science of Caring*, Little, Brown & Co., Boston.

Yelland, J. & Sellick, K. 1988, 'Community health and hospital-based nurses: differing attitudes to self-care', *Australian Journal of Advanced Nursing*, vol. 5, no. 2, 3–7.

CHAPTER 5

Ethics in nursing research

chapter objectives The material presented in this chapter will assist you to:

- cite examples of unethical research
- outline the NHMRC Statement on Human Experimentation
- discuss the principle of beneficence
- discuss the principle of respect for human dignity
- discuss the principle of justice
- outline the role and function of the institutional ethics committee
- discuss issues in collaborative research
- analyse research issues in clinical practice
- recognise scientific misconduct
- evaluate the ethical aspects of a research paper.

Introduction

Ethics is concerned with moral questions and behaviour. In nursing, research is usually concerned with investigating the effects of nursing interventions on people. Therefore ethics in nursing research concerns moral questions and behaviour in nursing research. Research participants' rights must be respected throughout the research process. Ethical researchers guarantee that no harm was done to any person involved in the research process. They also guarantee the validity of the research findings so that clinicians who apply those findings to client care can have confidence in them.

Sometimes there are problems in reconciling scientific rigour with ethical research practices and there are many examples of researchers acting unethically with disastrous consequences. This chapter demonstrates the need for ethics surveillance and principles of ethical research conduct. It discusses the obligations of nurses to conform to high ideals.

Historical examples of unethical research conduct

There have been numerous instances of researchers harming participants in the name of medical research. Indeed, research history abounds with examples of disregard for ethical behaviour, whether from ignorance or indifference to the welfare of others. Many researchers have committed unethical acts in their desire to develop knowledge or their drive to accumulate research papers for their own glory. In the eighteenth century, medical researchers deliberately injected bacteria into people to see if they would cause venereal disease and typhoid fever. In the nineteenth century, doctors tested surgical operations and anaesthetics on slaves (McNeill 1993).

More has been documented about unethical research practices in the twentieth century. In the 1920s, the United States Public Health Service carried out what has become known as the Tuskegee Syphilis Study, in which researchers deliberately did not treat 400 American Negro men for syphilis even after treatment was available, simply to observe the natural outcomes of the disease. The study was carried on over 40 years and terminated only in the 1970s because of moral outrage. A public health nurse, Eunice Rivers, was involved in carrying out that study and it is partly because of her success in recruiting and retaining participants that the study continued for so long (Vessey & Gennaro 1994). The Tuskegee study had disastrous and long-reaching results because many African American believe HIV is an instrument of genocide that has been made by humans (Thomas & Quinn 1991).

The most famous unethical medical experiments were carried out in the Second World War. Doctors in the Nazi concentration camps carried out medical experiments, presumably to improve the efficiency of the camps and to advance their own careers by building up a research profile. They carried out these experiments on camp prisoners, particularly identical twins and persons they considered subhuman on racial grounds. People were subjected to transplants, high-altitude decompression and submersion in ice-water. Doctors tested the efficiency of different methods of killing and the effects of starvation (Caplan 1992). While some of these experiments concerned developing knowledge that could apply to flying or to exposure of sailors at sea, they nevertheless violated human rights. Participants were selected on racial grounds, were forced to participate, and were harmed by their participation. Most did not survive but those who did sustained permanent physical and psychological damage.

In the same era, the Japanese conducted germ warfare 'experiments' on the Chinese in mainland China using anthrax, cholera, typhoid, typhus and bubonic plague. They subjected some Chinese to prolonged exposure to X-rays, replacement of human blood with horse blood, and murder by surgical experiments. Again, their motives were to advance the war and their own careers. They may have killed 3000 people in all (McNeill 1993).

During the same war, the Australian Department of Defence subjected many Australian servicemen to high levels of exposure to mustard gas in tropical conditions. These trials were unethical not only because the government already knew that the outcome would be unfavourable but also because the servicemen were not informed of the risks and so could not give informed consent. Many received burns as a result and although the Department of Defence will not disclose information, it is believed that there has been some out-of-court settlement (McNeill 1993).

In the post-war period, the New Zealand Cancer Study at the National Women's Hospital in Auckland, described by Johnstone (1999), is a classic example of unethical research. A gynaecologist, Dr Herbert Green, had a theory that pre-cancerous changes in the cervix (carcinoma in situ) would not necessarily progress to carcinoma if untreated. In the study, which had been approved by the hospital ethics committee, he set up an experiment in which 817 women were treated and 131 women (without their knowledge) were in the untreated group. The women in the untreated group had a mortality rate of four times that of the treated group. The study was eventually stopped because of pressure from the hospital colposcopist and pathologist. At the subsequent inquiry, the judge found that the study had been unethical because the women had not given informed consent, the study design was poor, there had been inadequate scientific and ethical review, and there was a known risk that the women would die if untreated. The judge criticised the other doctors and administrators for failing to intercede on the women's behalf. The judge also found that the hospital ethics committee was inadequate because it comprised mainly medical doctors, had a limited understanding of ethical research, did not require informed consent, and did not assess the scientific merit of projects adequately. The New Zealand Medical Council found the chair of the hospital ethics committee guilty of unprofessional conduct for his failure to review the study adequately but as he was retired, he was not subjected to any further action. The Medical Council dropped the charges against the gynaecologist because he was mentally and physically unfit to face them (*Weekend Australian* 27 Oct. 1990).

Lest we think that the record is any better in recent times, in 1992 questions were asked about consent procedures used in the Tamoxifen breast cancer prevention study in the USA and about subject recruitment materials for a women's health initiative clinical trial (Vessey & Gennaro 1994). Recently, in the United Kingdom, over a period of 40 years, hospitals removed and stored, without parents' consent, the hearts of more than 10 000 children (*Sunday Age* 19 Sep. 1999, p. A20, cited in *Monash Bioethics Review* 1999). The hearts were removed during routine post-mortem examinations, for which the parents had given consent; however, the parents were unaware that the hospitals had retained the hearts for research purposes and that the babies had been buried without their hearts.

More locally, there is at present an inquiry into the practice of a Sydney mortuary in selling to researchers organs removed at autopsy.

These examples show that, at every period in recent history, researchers have exploited participants, often people at their mercy. In all of these cases, the researchers' dedication to research or to their own advancement led to disregard for the welfare of the individual participants. The ethical researcher will select means that are consistent with what the research can achieve and will ensure that no harm arises from the study.

Codes of ethics and research ethics guidelines

Several codes of ethics have been developed since the Second World War. In the course of judging those accused of the concentration camp atrocities, the Nuremburg Tribunal, in 1949, promulgated the Nuremburg Code of research ethics, which formed the basis for subsequent codes. In 1964, the World Medical Association adopted the Declaration of Helsinki, which distinguished therapeutic research, in which participants receive beneficial treatment, from non-therapeutic research, which does not benefit participants but may benefit future patients. The Declaration of Helsinki stated that researchers should exercise even greater care to protect participants from harm in non-therapeutic research than in therapeutic research and that ethics committees should require strong, independent justification for exposing a healthy volunteer to substantial risk of harm just to gain new scientific information.

In Australia, the National Health and Medical Research Council (NHMRC) developed the Statement on Human Experimentation (NHMRC 1992a) This statement was updated recently to become a more general statement applying to all research on humans, not just medical research, which was the focus of the earlier version (Spriggs 1999). The statement exemplifies the principles of ethical research and the rights of participants that are discussed in this chapter. All researchers who carry out projects involving human participants will be required by the human research ethics committee (HREC) of their institution to read this statement before carrying out the research. The statement will be available from your research management unit. This statement is currently under review. Dodds (2000) argues that the recent version still does not provide sufficient guidance for HRECs.

The national nursing associations in the United States, Canada and the United Kingdom have developed guidelines for conduct in nursing research. In Australia, the WA Teaching Hospitals Nurse Researchers Network developed a set of Standards for Nursing Research, which stated that 'nurses undertaking research will respect the basic human rights of the individual at all times' (Robertson 1992). The WA group submitted the standards to the Australian Nursing Federation, which reviewed the standards, and incorporated them into their own beginning standards (Robertson 1992). The standards, published by the ANF in 1997, are, along with the NHMRC guidelines, the national standards for ethics in nursing research. In addition, the Royal College of Nursing, Australia has stated in its document *Nursing Targets into the Twenty-first Century: A National Statement* that nursing research will be fostered by 'recognition as a legitimate, professional, ethical and socially relevant area of inquiry' (RCNA 1992).

Thus, there are several codes to guide the researcher and the research consumer. Professional nurses must be familiar with a relevant code of ethics for nursing research. Nurse-researchers will use the code to guide their action, thus ensuring ethical research. Nurses who read research for its applications to practice will be able to judge the ethical aspects of research papers. Nevertheless, it is not sufficient for you as a nurse merely to be familiar with a code of ethics. You must understand the principles behind the code of ethics. These are outlined in the following section.

Protecting the rights of human participants

Participants' rights/principles

The Belmont Report in the United States has cited three principles that underpin most research standards: beneficence, respect for human dignity, and justice (National Commission for the Protection of Human Subjects of Biomedical and Behavioral Research 1978).

Principles of beneficence and non-maleficence

Beneficence is 'doing good'. In the nursing or medical research context, this means that the researcher's aim should be to produce results that ultimately will benefit individuals or society as a whole through better treatment. In the research context, beneficence can be achieved by producing outcomes that will benefit humankind.

More crucial, however, is the principle of non-maleficence or doing no harm. In applying this principle, nurse-researchers need to consider the potential for harm to or exploitation of the participants and whether the risks of the research outweigh the benefits. It is important to apply this principle in the planning and implementation stages of the research. HRECs examine applications closely to ensure that they meet this principle.

The right not to be harmed means that human participants should not be harmed as a result of participating in a research study. Obviously, the examples of experiments cited earlier, such as the New Zealand study on cervical cancer, resulted in harm to the participants. In this context, harm means excessive harm beyond slight discomfort involved in such things as blood tests. The researcher should always respect the rights, beliefs, and autonomy of the individual participant.

The right not to be harmed includes being protected from harm through being involved in research studies of dubious scientific merit. The researcher has the ethical responsibility to the scientific nursing community to ensure the integrity of the study throughout the process, from planning to publication. Ethical aspects related to good science include the value of the study in terms of the development of knowledge in nursing or health, the use of an appropriate and valid theoretical framework and methodology for the question. The HREC is usually the arbiter of what is 'good' science. This assumes that the HREC members have the necessary expertise to decide what is good science, a value judgement that may affect whether they approve qualitative research. At present, the only scientist required to be on an Australian HREC is a medical doctor with a research background, which is almost certain to be in the positivist tradition. Thus the authority in the power structure determines the criteria for 'good' or 'valid' science. This means that qualitative projects may be viewed less favourably because the authority has been socialised into a view that experimental research is the only valid methodology.

Only persons who have the qualifications and facilities to conduct the work properly should conduct or supervise research. If researchers or supervisors fall short in knowledge or experience, they should seek the help of a consultant. This has been a problem for nursing research in Australia in its beginning phases because we have not yet developed a critical mass of qualified researchers, and many of those whom we do have received their research training in other disciplines. This has meant that they have had to make a discipline shift, teaching themselves to apply research techniques from other disciplines to nursing research.

Specific harm to research participants can include physical harm, psychological harm, emotional harm, social harm, financial harm, and exploitation. Physical harm can range from minor discomfort to permanent injury or death. The Nazi and Japanese wartime experiments resulted in death for thousands of people. The New Zealand Women's Hospital experiment was a classic example of extreme physical harm including death from cervical cancer. The experiment on the Australian troops resulted in permanent injury to participants.

Research studies can also cause psychological harm, by damage to the participant's mind from taking part in the study. A classic example of a study that caused psychological harm is the Milgram obedience experiment in which the researcher encouraged participants to administer electric shocks to other people (Milgram 1963). This experiment was carried out after the Second World War in an attempt to show that people will obey orders from superiors regardless of the results. An actor played the part of the subject of the experiment and in reality there was no electricity connected. With the encouragement of the researcher, the participants continued to escalate the amount of 'electric current' to lethal levels despite the 'subject's' agonised pleas to stop. We can only speculate on the psychological harm suffered by the real subjects of the experiments, even if they were debriefed later.

Qualitative research can also cause emotional harm, for example in the interview process when the researcher seeks intimate details of participants' lives. Emotional harm can result from invasion of privacy when a researcher obtains information that the participant would rather have kept secret or perhaps has revealed in an unguarded moment and later regrets doing so. It can be distressful for participants to recollect memories that they would prefer to avoid. Emotional harm can also result from disclosure of confidential information by the researcher, which could lead to embarrassment to the participants or worse. Unauthorised use of organs from patients has caused anguish for relatives.

Research could also cause social harm if, for example, the research interfered with the participant's kinship and family relationships, or the participant lost employment as a result of participating in the research project. For example, if people participated in a study on AIDS that led to disclosure of their condition to family and/or employers, that could cause irreparable social harm.

Financial harm could result if, say, the researcher or health agency charged the participant for investigative tests associated with the project. This is less likely in Australia where the individual does not pay directly for tests under Medicare. However, there is still financial harm in charging the government for research tests for which the researcher should pay because the taxes that people pay for Medicare will be higher. Another example of financial harm is a nurse practising independently carrying out a research project and billing the client for time used for the research. Other potential costs to the participants are the loss of their time and the hidden costs of participating such as baby-sitting or transport costs. People have a right to decide how to use their time effectively. Exploitation occurs if the researcher uses the participants' contribution for profit in any way, such as the selling of names for a mailing list, or expecting the participants to participate in ongoing research projects because they participated in the initial research project.

Tension can arise between the ethical consideration of doing no harm on the one hand and the need for scientific rigour on the other. For example, the accepted test of a new drug or treatment is a classic experiment in which one group of patients receives the new treatment and another group receives a placebo. A placebo is a treatment that looks exactly the same as the active treatment but does not contain the drug. The question then arises whether it is ethical to withhold the treatment from one group. If the treatment turns out to be beneficial, then the placebo group may be harmed by not having the treatment. The issue of fair access to experimental drugs may arise in terminal illness, as happened with AIDS in the 1990s. If, on the other hand, the treatment has unforeseen side effects, the experimental group may be harmed. There is also a question as to whether it is ethical to remove patients from established treatment to test a new drug. There is a risk of complications to the patient who is not even receiving standard treatment but receives a placebo instead.

At all costs, researchers must avoid harming participants. One way of doing this is to test out a new treatment, wherever possible, on animals or tissue cultures. This is not foolproof because, for example, some drugs may be teratogenic for certain species and not others. Testing on animals, at worst, does not consider an animal's right not to be harmed and, at best, judges that the prevention of harm to humans justifies the harm to the research animals. Most universities now have an animal ethics committee that ensures the humane use of animals for research purposes.

Researchers can also avoid harm by making provision in the research protocol to stop the study if there is reason to suspect that harm would result from continuing it. In addition, the researcher must remove individual participants from the study if there is evidence that they are suffering untoward effects. The safety of the participants must in all cases take priority over the research project. The NHMRC requires that an emergency contact number be given to all research participants so that they can contact the researcher if they are having any adverse effects. In addition, studies of new drugs or procedures should have statistical analysis built into them that ensures that the study concludes as soon as it is possible to ascertain the potential value of the drug or procedure. This allows the commencement of the new treatment for those receiving a placebo, or conventional treatment if the new drug or procedure is clearly superior, or resumption of the participants' previous treatment if that is superior. Thus, there is minimal risk for the participants.

In considering research proposals for their potential to do harm, the researcher and the HREC balance the risks to the participants with the benefits to society or the profession. The benefits should normally outweigh the risks. There are several potential benefits to the participants. There is the possibility of accessing a new nursing intervention or medical treatment that would otherwise not be available. There is also the opportunity to acquire knowledge and experience by participating in the research process. There is a possible material reward for participation. Participants may also achieve increased awareness of an experience through reliving it. Finally, participants such as the terminally ill may be comforted by the knowledge that they are helping others and advancing scientific knowledge.

If costs outweigh benefits, the researcher should not carry out the project. In an ethical trial, the advantage of the experimental treatment over the conventional treatment should not yet have been established. If an experiment has the potential to result in a valuable new treatment and if the participants know and accept that they have only a limited chance of getting the real treatment, the benefits outweigh the risks.

Principle of respect for human dignity

This principle affirms the rights of humans to determine their own actions, or the right to self-determination. It concerns the right to decide whether to participate in a research project after full disclosure about the project. Participants have the right to self-determination, full disclosure and freedom from harassment. They also have the right to refuse to participate and to withdraw from a study at any time without penalty.

Informed consent

Informed consent is the agreement of the participant to take part in the research project after having been thoroughly briefed about the project and its possible outcomes. Informed consent has two elements: information and consent. Ethical research involves full disclosure of information to the prospective participant. This will include the identity of the researcher, the purpose and nature of the study, the right to refuse to participate, the right to withdraw at any time, the responsibilities of the researcher, possible benefits of the study, possible risks or side effects, any alternative treatments, and measures to be taken to protect privacy and to ensure anonymity and confidentiality. As a researcher, you should give information to the participants in a form and language that they can understand easily. This is usually done in the form of a plain language statement, which is written so that it is comprehensible to a layperson who does not have an advanced education. Figure 5.1 shows an example of a plain language statement.

DARWIN PARENTS' ATTITUDES TO KANGAROO MOTHER CARE

A research team consisting of Professor Kay Roberts, Professor Jenny Watson and Ms Bev Turnbull, all from Northern Territory University, and Ms Christine Paynter and Mrs Beryl McEwan of the Special Care Nursery at Royal Darwin Hospital are carrying out a project to investigate Darwin parents' attitudes to the experience of kangaroo mother care (KMC). The aim of the project is to find out about the perceptions of mothers who do KMC concerning the experience and the perceptions of fathers about the experience of their partners giving KMC.

We would greatly appreciate your assistance in providing information about your own experiences. However, there is absolutely no pressure on you to participate and your care will in no way be affected by a refusal to participate. We will obtain your baby's doctor's consent for you to participate in the project.

If you agree, you will contacted by a researcher to interview you at the Special Care Nursery or another mutually convenient place.

You will be interviewed by a member of the research team and your experiences and attitudes to KMC will be discussed. The interviewer will record the interview on audiotape. The information will help us to improve the care for other parents who decide to undertake KMC.

The audiotapes will be transcribed by a confidential transcriber. All information collected will remain:

1. ANONYMOUS: Your name and address must be known to the interviewer but it will never be mentioned on the transcript of the tape or in the report of the research, and your personal details will be locked away, quite separate from the other material.
2. CONFIDENTIAL: You will not be able to be identified by anything that is written in the text of the research paper.

The same care will be taken with the names or characteristics of anyone you mention in the interview.

If you would like more information before you decide, contact Professor Kay Roberts, on 8046 6071, who will be happy to answer questions. You may also use this number at any time during the project, if you need information.

If, during the course of the project, you have any concerns about the project or the researcher, you may contact the Executive Officer of the Northern Territory University Human Research Ethics Committee, who is not connected with this project and who can pass on your concerns to appropriate officers within the University. The Executive Officer can be contacted on 8046 6070.

If you decide to participate, please fill in the consent form that is attached to this letter, and give it to a member of the research team. We will contact you soon, to arrange your participation. After the consent form is signed, you may still withdraw from the study at any time, without penalty of any kind.

Whatever your decision on this matter, thank you for devoting some time to reading this statement and considering its contents.

Figure 5.1 Example of a plain language statement

Silva and Sorrell (1984) demonstrated that research participants did not always understand procedures to which they had consented and that the amount, clarity and complexity of information affected participants' comprehension of information they had been given. Age, occupation or gender did not affect comprehension, but illness, passage of time and amount of threatening information did. It is therefore important to be vigilant in ensuring that the participant understands the nature of the study. The full disclosure of information may also be problematic in cross-cultural research such as that with Indigenous or migrant participants where problems of differences in language, cultural values and beliefs may be present. Written consent may not be feasible and arrangements must be made to record the consent in some other way, for example by audiotape recording.

Informed consent can also be a problem if, as happens in exploratory ethnographic research, the researcher cannot state the problems and research questions at the outset. The researcher should discuss difficulties openly with the participants during the study and obtain their consent. The researcher and the participants make mutual decisions concerning ethical issues throughout the study.

Informed consent can also be a problem when the participants cannot speak English. Special provisions must be made to translate the consent form and plain language statement into the participants' first language. If participants cannot read well, it may be necessary to make arrangements to have the plain language statement read out to them.

Participants must agree to participate in the project and they or, in the case of those not able to give consent, their agents, are the only ones who can make this decision. The participant must give consent without any coercion or unfair inducement. Coercion is the obtaining of research participants through their fear that harm will befall them if they do not enter the study. Examples of persons vulnerable to coercion are patients who fear inferior treatment or nursing care if they do not take part in the medical research project, or students who are afraid of failing a course if they refuse to participate in a research project for the lecturer. Some groups are especially susceptible to coercion. Patients are especially vulnerable when their clinician is also the researcher, which is at the base of the NHMRC requirement that the clinician and researcher be different people. Unfair inducement is the holding out of undue material gains for the purposes of recruiting research participants. A reasonable monetary payment that merely compensates participants for inconvenience or time spent is not unfair inducement. For example, the payment of participants at a rate equivalent to an hourly wage is a reasonable recompense for time and expenses, but offering more than this, especially to captive participants, is not ethical. An example of unfair inducement is offering prisoners a remission off their sentence if they take part in a research project. The NHMRC guidelines for ethical aspects of qualitative health research point out that the crucial issue is whether the potential participants' belief that there is some gain for taking part affects their freedom to consent (NHMRC 1995).

Participants must also be free to withdraw from the study at any time. In qualitative research, where unforeseen events may occur, the researcher should remind participants periodically of their right to withdraw. Participants must be able to withdraw without a penalty, such as discriminatory treatment from a researcher who has some power over the participants. There is a moral dilemma in the use of participants who are unconscious or otherwise unable to give their own informed consent in that they are unable to withdraw from a study themselves and must rely on their agents.

The researcher must obtain informed consent from participants before collecting data. An agent can act for either the researcher or the participant. The participant usually signs a document that is specific to that study and includes all of the relevant information. The same considerations of language and literacy apply to the consent form. An example of a consent form is seen in Figure 5.2.

CONSENT TO BE A RESEARCH PARTICIPANT
BOOMERANG PILLOWS STUDY

Professor _____, Ms _____, Ms _____ and Ms _____ are nurses undertaking a comparison of boomerang and straight pillows and the way that they affect breathing. To do the study, they need to position people on both types of pillows and compare the results using a machine to measure the breathing. If I agree to be in the study, I will have my breathing measured sitting, and at rest in bed on both types of pillows. *This study should take approximately 45 minutes of my time.* There should be no adverse effects from participating in this study. There will be no benefit to me, although the study may produce information of use to nurses in the future.

I have had the opportunity to talk to one of the researchers about the study. I may reach Professor _____ at _____ if I have any questions later. I have received a copy of this form to keep. I have the right to refuse to participate or to withdraw at any time without any jeopardy to me.

_____   _____
Participant's signature   Investigator's signature

_____   _____
Date   Date

Figure 5.2 Example of a consent form

While a written document with the participant's signature is usual practice, if the research is sensitive, for example on sexual topics, or the participant feels particularly vulnerable, for example where criminal behaviour is concerned, a formal verbal agreement may be recorded on audiotape (NHMRC 1995). The NHMRC guidelines also state that it is not always possible to obtain written consent from all observed persons.

Obtaining consent can be problematic in some situations, particularly in naturalistic observation. Consent is not necessary for observation in public places such as the street. In large institutions, where there are many people being observed, it may be impractical to obtain written consent from everyone being observed. Consent from the institution, with general information to the employees about the project, must suffice. Applying the principle of consent can also be difficult in cultures that do not possess the Western idea of individualism and where the family and community make the decisions (Davis 1990). There are also situations in which written consent is unnecessary. The return of a questionnaire implies consent since the prospective respondent is free to refuse to participate by throwing the questionnaire away. Indeed, it is better research practice to have anonymous questionnaires. A signature on a consent form attached to a questionnaire invalidates the anonymity of the respondent and diminishes the validity of the data. However, a plain language statement explaining the project is still necessary and should be sent as an attachment to the letter.

Special participants

Special participants are persons who have a diminished ability to give informed consent and are therefore at risk of exploitation. Some special participants have an impaired ability to understand information. Such persons include developmentally disabled people, confused elderly, and mentally ill persons who may or may not have the capacity to give informed consent, depending on their mental state. Persons in a dependent relationship are also special participants because they are unable to give their own consent. These include children, elderly persons who cannot give free consent, wards of state, and unconscious patients.

These groups should be treated with the same ethical standards as all others and require even greater protection because of their inability to give informed consent. Special participants should not be used as research fodder because of their vulnerability to exploitation. They should be used only for therapeutic research from which they have some hope of deriving a benefit, or in situations in which other populations are not suitable to answer the questions posed by the study (NHMRC 1999).

The principle of obtaining informed consent from special participants is that informed consent should be obtained from an agent, a person who has the intelligence or capability to give it on behalf of the other dependent person. The person giving informed consent should be in a legal capacity to the proposed participant, such as a parent or guardian. Children are considered to be below the age of legal consent, and consent should be obtained from the parents or legal guardian. Consent should also be obtained from the child where the child is of sufficient maturity and intelligence to make this feasible.

However, obtaining informed consent from such groups as the elderly is not always straightforward. Elderly people frequently have visual and hearing impairments that can make the use of written consent forms inappropriate (Madjar & Higgins 1996). The reluctance of elderly people to sign documents of any sort because of the perceived threat of loss of autonomy has been noted by Madjar and Higgins, and borne out by my own experience of collecting data with elderly women (Roberts, Brittin & deClifford 1995), where one woman refused to participate in the study because she had a policy of not signing any documents unless her son was present. Madjar and Higgins (1996) raise the issue of whether it is better to conform to the requirement to get a signature on a piece of paper or to allow such people to participate on the grounds that it is not ethical to deny them participation in the study. They believe that researchers should be allowed to use their discretion in such situations.

An interesting issue has arisen with regard to obtaining consent for the use in research studies of tissues and body parts that were obtained for clinical purposes. For example, slides may be taken for diagnostic purposes and a research project later planned in which it is intended to use those slides. Should consent be obtained? In many cases it is difficult to track down the clients to get their permission. It is possible to avoid this situation by obtaining at the time of collection of the material consent to use the slides or tissues for later research purposes. Of course, if a research project is planned before the tissues are collected, consent should be obtained. It should not just be assumed that if the tissues are there, they can be used freely for research purposes.

Deception

Sometimes a researcher seeks to deceive participants to facilitate data collection or because giving full information can lead to invalidation of the study. This is most likely to occur in methods involving participant observation (NHMRC 1995). Participants might not behave naturally if they know they are being observed, especially in cases where illicit activity is concerned. Participants might also censor information at interview if they know the real purpose of the study.

Deception can be passive, where the researcher omits to give information to participants, or active, where the researcher actually tells lies to the participants. Passive deception usually involves covert data collection or obtaining data by false pretences without actually lying. Techniques for covert data collection include observing participants who do not know they are being observed, interviewing participants who do not know that what they say will become research data, or participating in activities with a group who do not know they are participants. For example, a nurse-researcher might wish to study the conversation of nurses at tea breaks. Believing that if the nurses knew they were being observed their behaviour might change, the nurse-researcher might elect to collect data on them without their knowledge. Covert research can also take place through the study of confidential documents (NHMRC 1995). More sinister techniques involve the use of devices such as one-way mirrors or hidden video cameras and microphones.

Apologists for covert data collection justify it by saying that it is sometimes the only way to obtain valid data. However, studies may be unethical if the design involves covert observation of subjects behaving in ways that they would not wish a researcher to observe or record, or that they might later regret. It can be argued that nurses ought to be able to carry out work without unknowingly being observed by a researcher and that researchers who use covert observation fail to take into consideration the feelings of the subjects when they find out that they were observed without their knowledge. In ethnographic studies, it is sufficient to get permission from the community. Individual consent is necessary only if specific data, for example, interviews, are sought.

Active deception consists of deliberately withholding some information or giving false information about the study to secure people's participation. The researcher may resort to this when knowledge of the true purpose of the study would invalidate the findings. The Milgram obedience experiment cited earlier in this chapter is a classic case of deception. Another less harmful instance of deception occurred in England. A researcher asked nurses to evaluate the same research paper that had two false names and qualifications on them: one paper was purported to have been written by a doctor and one by a nurse; both were female (Hicks 1992). The participants thought they were critiquing the papers but the true purpose of the study was to see whether nurses ascribed greater research expertise to doctors than to nurses. There was no difference in the perceptions of the quality of the paper overall, but the participants ascribed superior research methodology and statistical analysis to the paper supposedly written by the doctor. The other classic method of active deception is the use of placebos in experiments. The researcher should inform participants that they have an equal chance of getting a placebo or the treatment.

Is it ever justifiable to deceive research participants, for example if the benefits of the research to society outweigh the risks to the individual? The NHMRC guidelines for ethics in qualitative research say that 'in nearly all cases research which is covert or deceptive is unethical and should not be undertaken' (NHMRC 1995). However, the guidelines also state that the HREC must make a decision as to whether the potential social benefits of the research outweigh the participants' right to know, with the participants' well-being taking priority. Most authorities now consider any deception to be unethical because the deliberate withholding of information violates the autonomy or right to self-determination of the participant. Deception means lying to participants either by commission or omission. If the participants find out they may never again trust that researcher or any other. Despite this, however, deception is still routinely practised in research in some disciplines, for example psychology.

Principle of justice

The principle of justice is that all participants have the right to be treated fairly and with respect and courtesy at every stage of the research process, from the design of the project to the reporting of findings. At the design stage, it is necessary to build fair selection and treatment of participants into the process. Participants should be selected on criteria related to relevance to the topic rather than availability or on inability to refuse. The Australian Army study of mustard gas calls into question whether the soldiers were truly volunteers. Once the group has been selected, each participant should have an equal chance of receiving the active treatment both for reasons of fairness and for reasons of scientific validity. The researcher should assign participants to the group randomly, not on the basis of favouritism. If the researcher is in a position of authority over participants, participants who decline to participate or who withdraw from a study should not be penalised in any way, regardless of the effect of their withdrawal on the research project. The informed consent document or another written agreement that outlines the commitment of the participant and the researcher in terms of time, procedures and benefits, should be adhered to by the researcher. The participants should be provided with access by telephone or in person to the researcher in case of problems, and the researcher should provide any necessary assistance if inadvertent side effects occur. At the end of the study, any promised benefits or reports should be provided.

Anonymity

Anonymity means the concealment or obscuring of the identity of the participants. Total anonymity occurs when even the researcher cannot identify the research participants, for example when a questionnaire is returned anonymously. Partial anonymity occurs when the researcher knows the identity of the participants but conceals it from any outsiders. If anyone beyond the team knows the identity of the participants, or can link findings to any participant, then the participants do not have anonymity. For example, while reading a book chapter detailing a research project in which I had been a participant, I saw my initials and geographical location as part of a code that documented a quotation. The passage also gave sufficient information to enable a reader to identify me. I considered that my anonymity had been breached.

The researcher should act at all times in such a manner as to protect the anonymity of the participants and should build appropriate procedures into the study design to separate the identity of the participants from the data. For example, if the design of the study requires that a written consent form is attached to the data, this is separated from the data as soon as possible and the data are entered into the computer using a code number or pseudonym. If the design of the study requires the linking of two sets of data, a list is created that records the participants' names and pseudonyms or code numbers but this is stored in a different place. An alternative to this is a code number or combination of numbers and letters such as the participant's mother's maiden initials, number of siblings and so forth. This code, which may be used according to a formula generated by the researcher but which will be unique to each participant, will be attached to all protocols. If the researcher must know the identity of the participants, as happens in qualitative research, the full name of the person should not be used in the primary data, including tape recordings. A pseudonym or code number should be used in the transcribed or processed data. With this type of data also, a list linking the code numbers or pseudonyms should be kept separately and securely.

An issue has arisen recently with respect to anonymity and research on the Internet. Some researchers have been posting questionnaires to all members of a list of subscribers to the Internet, using the facility that allows them to post one message through the central listserver to all members of the list. If respondents unwittingly use the 'reply to all' option, rather than the 'reply' option which goes back only to the individual initiating the response, the answered questionnaire goes back to all of the members of the list. This obviously destroys the anonymity of the respondents. The correct procedure is for the researcher to warn respondents to send the answered questionnaire back to the address of the researcher. This procedure keeps the data in the hands of the researcher who can then institute procedures to separate the data from the names and thus protect the anonymity of the participants.

Privacy

Privacy in the research context refers to the right of participants to decide which information they wish to disclose. Participants have a right to privacy, particularly concerning their attitudes, beliefs, behaviours, opinions, and records such as diaries and other private papers. Researchers do not have any automatic right to information by virtue of the fact that they are doing a research project and they must not invade the privacy of the participant beyond what is reasonable and what is approved by the HREC for the purposes of the study. Even then, researchers must be sensitive to the private nature of some information and guard its confidentiality. Invasion of privacy can also occur in covert data collection, which was discussed under the topic of informed consent. Watching people in non-public places for data collection when they are not aware of it is an invasion of privacy.

A special problem concerning privacy of records has arisen since epidemiological research has become popular and it has become increasingly commonplace for nurses and other health professionals to carry out research utilising records that identify the individual. Often access is sought by nurse-researchers for records of births and deaths, which are open to inspection for the purposes of research at the discretion of the appropriate state or territory registrar. In addition, records of living persons are often needed for research purposes. The principle laid down by the NHMRC is that medical records should be made available for legitimate research purposes; in practice, this means HREC-approved research projects. This principle also has legal force since several states, including New South Wales, Victoria, Queensland and South Australia, have statutes providing access to hospital medical records for research purposes (NHMRC 1985). The issue that then arises is whether the individual needs to give consent to their use. However, the task of tracking down all persons whose records one might wish to access to obtain written consent would be impossible. Even if it were possible, it might alarm some participants, as could happen if one wished to do a study on the link between previous miscarriages and probability of abortion. With regard to the use of medical records, there is a distinction between information obtained for further experimentation, and the study of records. In the former case, informed consent must be obtained for any research that adds further risk to the participants. In the case of a pure study of records, consent from the individuals is not necessary. However, it is possible to build in consent for future examination of records into an initial consent form.

Procedures can be put in place to safeguard the privacy of records. Where two types of records are linked together, once the linkage has been made, the names must be removed from the file and replaced with a code number. The list linking the names and code number or pseudonym must be kept in a secure place. It is recommended that standard measures be taken to ensure anonymity and confidentiality, as discussed in the previous sections.

Anonymity may be violated if the identity of the participants is not concealed in the reporting or publication stage. This can happen if the researcher reveals a cluster of characteristics that would identify a person, for example 'a female professor at University X' where there is only one.

Right to confidentiality

The researcher has the responsibility to keep data confidential so that individuals are not compromised. This means that you do not allow anyone access to the data unless they are authorised to have it, and you do not tell anyone information given to you in confidence.

Maintaining confidentiality includes protecting data from unauthorised access. You can prevent inadvertent unauthorised data access by storing data in a secure place such as a locked filing cabinet. This is especially important for data that are not anonymous. Researchers must refuse any requests for data access from unauthorised persons. You can also prevent identification of participants by concealing their names and identities in a report. Even geographical locations should be concealed if they are easily identified.

During the course of a research project, the participants may tell the researcher confidential information. The researcher has an obligation to respect the participants' wishes concerning the confidentiality of information as far as possible. Confidentiality is especially important for sensitive data such as that concerning sexual matters or use of illicit drugs, or while the participants' names are linked to the data. Confidentiality is broken if you disclose information to persons outside the project, either by careless gossip or by allowing unauthorised persons to access the data.

In qualitative research in which new information may arise because of its unpredictable nature, participants should periodically be reminded of their right to withhold information. Confidentiality in qualitative research can be difficult to maintain in small settings where everyone knows everyone else. However, in some qualitative projects, participants may choose to be named.

In the case of medical records, the researcher must exercise care concerning confidentiality and ensure that the information is restricted to those who need it.

Sometimes, persons in authority may pressure the researcher for access to data; for example in a study of health in an industrial setting, the participants' supervisor may ask to see data on workers. This should not be granted. The only persons in authority who can legitimately demand access to confidential research data are police who have a search warrant.

The NHMRC guidelines on ethics in qualitative research point out that researchers need to be aware that they cannot guarantee participants absolute confidentiality because they may be legally compelled to testify in court (NHMRC 1995). If, for example, a participant confessed to a crime, in some states or territories the researcher could be called to testify in court and would not be able to claim client-professional privilege.

A moral dilemma concerning confidentiality may arise if one discovers irregularities in practice during the course of a research project. This places the researcher in a difficult position – whether to break confidentiality and report irregularities to the authorities, or to keep quiet about them and condone patient abuse. Reporting to the authorities will likely jeopardise the continuation of the research, whereas keeping silent will allow the researcher to retain the trust of the participants.

Broken confidentiality destroys trust and may have consequences for the present and later research. If confidentiality is broken during the project, the researchers may be asked to leave before the project is completed, with disastrous consequences for the outcome of the research project. If participants feel that they have been betrayed, they are not likely to consent to further research by that researcher. Furthermore, they are unlikely to grant access to future researchers. The ethical dilemma is whether to give priority to the research or to patient safety. The resolution of such a dilemma is not easy. The researcher may wish to start with a discussion with the participants about the problem and try to raise their awareness of the problem and attempt to solve the problem that way. If the problem cannot be resolved 'in house', the researcher must make a decision based on the moral issue. The safety of clients must take priority over research aims. The NHMRC guidelines on ethics in qualitative research state that the researcher is not legally protected against mandatory reporting if abuse is seen during a study (NHMRC 1995).

Ethical aspects of research in special cases
Embryos and foetal tissue

Since the development of *in vitro* fertilisation (IVF), research on the human embryo or foetus has become more controversial. The embryo is the product of the union of the sperm and ova at fertilisation and before implantation. The foetus/foetal tissue is the continuation of the embryo from the time of implantation to the time of complete gestation, regardless of its status at birth. The foetal membranes, placenta, umbilical cord and amniotic fluid are considered to be part of the foetus before separation (NHMRC 1992c). There is concern about experimentation on embryos, either spare embryos left over from IVF treatment or embryos specifically created for research purposes. The central issue is whether embryos have human status and therefore should be protected from harm. To decide whether embryos have human status requires a determination of when life begins. These issues are under debate in legal, moral, religious and research areas. In recent times, several states (South Australia, Victoria and Western Australia) have enacted legislation that restricts experimentation on human embryos and that overrides guidelines of government agencies. Embryos, which are of concern in IVF, are treated differently from the foetus and foetal tissue, which are considered to exist when implantation occurs. The sperm and ova produced for IVF should be treated as belonging to the donors rather than the institution or researcher and the donors' wishes concerning the usage of these must be respected. Embryos belong to the donors or a single surviving donor. At present it is considered unethical to store frozen embryos for more than 10 years, grow them beyond the stage at which implantation would normally occur or conduct cloning experiments designed to lead to the production of multiple genetically identical humans (NHMRC 1992b). However, the law does permit stem cell research which could lead to cures for genetic diseases.

According to the NHMRC guidelines, it may be ethical to carry out experiments on the foetus *in utero* where they may promote life or health of the foetus or where the research provides the mother with information about the health or normality of the foetus, thereby giving her choices concerning the future treatment and disposition of the foetus. It is unethical to administer drugs to or carry out any procedure on the mother to find out any harmful effects on the foetus, even if abortion is anticipated. Once abortion is inevitable, some research procedures may be permissible. Consent should be obtained from the mother and where practicable the father before the research commences and permission should be obtained for use of foetal tissues, including cells, membranes, placenta, umbilical cord and amniotic fluid to be stored or propagated in tissue culture. Permission to transplant cells into a human recipient should also be specifically obtained. The decision to approach the mother for consent to such research must be made by the clinician rather than the researcher (NHMRC 1992c).

There are also issues concerning research on a separated pre-viable foetus or foetal tissue. A pre-viable foetus is one that has not reached an age of 20 weeks gestational age and that weighs 400 g or less. The foetus should have separated by natural processes or lawful means, should not be dissected while there is any obvious sign of life, and should be removed from the nearby clinical area before research is carried out. Again, there should be separation of clinical and research decision-making to avoid a conflict of interest (NHMRC 1992c).

Indigenous participants

Indigenous participants are not special participants under the previous definition; nevertheless their situation requires special consideration. The history of relationships between Indigenous people and non-Indigenous researchers has produced a suspicion of the motives of non-Indigenous researchers. Research involving Aboriginal and Torres Strait Islander communities must take account of sensitive ethical issues, particularly with regard to culture. The Special Purposes Committee of the NHMRC convened a national conference in 1986 in Alice Springs from which it emerged that a high priority was ethics in relation to Aboriginal and Torres Strait Islander health. A national workshop of ethics in Indigenous health was then held in New South Wales in 1987, attended by 30 Indigenous representatives from all around Australia. From this workshop, a set of advisory notes, later converted to comprehensive guidelines, was developed. At the time of the workshop, the Medical Research Ethics Committee believed that the issue of Aboriginal and

Torres Strait Islander communities deserved special consideration because it had an obvious level of poor health that past research had failed to address. It cited reasons for this failure as a priority of interest in scientific research or research interests of white Australians and an insensitivity among researchers to the 'values, needs and customs' of Aboriginal and Torres Strait Islander peoples. Specific concerns were: lack of understanding of cultural values concerning gender issues, inappropriate treatment of organs post-mortem, inappropriate requests for and handling of blood and other biological specimens, and publication of inappropriate pictures, such as of dead people (NHMRC 1992c). Prior to the guidelines, the lack of appreciation of ethical issues in research on Aboriginal and Torres Strait Islanders had led to deficient practices including approval being sought from individuals instead of from the appropriate community authority, lower standards being applied for obtaining consent among disadvantaged Aboriginal and Torres Strait Islander communities, a failure to appreciate that access to sensitive areas would be dependent upon the researcher's social status, conflict between the mores of scientific research and Aboriginal and Torres Strait Islander cultural and social values, and the increased vulnerability of Aboriginal and Torres Strait Islander groups to exploitation by researchers. The highest standards of ethical conduct in research should apply to research concerning the Aboriginal and Torres Strait Islander people, who must set their own research priorities rather than merely responding to those set by non-Indigenous people (Johnstone 1991). Indigenous people have the power to set their own ethics guidelines and insist that these be enforced because they now control access to their communities by researchers.

In some states, organisations controlled by Aboriginal and Torres Strait Islander people have established their own HRECs. In addition, some ethics committees have an Indigenous subcommittee, for example the Top End Ethics Committee in the Northern Territory. These committees and subcommittees can decide or recommend on research proposals that relate to research on Aboriginal and Torres Strait Islander people, whether internally or externally developed. It is now very difficult if not impossible to obtain access to Indigenous participants without an Indigenous co-researcher.

The NHMRC (1991) recommend that an HREC should satisfy itself that a proposal concerning research on Aboriginal and Torres Strait Islander communities should demonstrate that:

- the researcher has sought advice from Aboriginal and Torres Strait Islander health agencies and local community controlled Aboriginal and Torres Strait Islander health services and agencies
- the Aboriginal and Torres Strait Islander community, or the agency representing the community, has indicated that the research will be potentially useful to the community or the people in general
- the research will be conducted in such a way that it is sensitive to the cultural and political situation of the community

- the researcher has written consent from the community concerned or has documented the reasons why this is not possible.

In the process of obtaining informed consent from Indigenous communities, the researcher should provide information concerning collection and analysis of data, the drafting and publication of reports in a format understandable by the community, and the potential costs and benefits of the research. The researcher should have face-to-face discussions with the people concerned, where possible, or document reasons for lack of success. Sufficient time for the community to absorb and reply to the information should be allowed. There should be a demonstrated process for obtaining free consent from individuals as well as written evidence of consent from the whole community. There should be provision for informing participants of their right to withdraw consent at any time (NHMRC 1991).

Aboriginal and Torres Strait Islander communities must have involvement in research on their own people. They must be given decision-making power at every stage of the research project and receive appropriate financial recompense (NHMRC 1991). This approach will help to compensate for past injustices and enhance Indigenous control and participation in research. However, the guidelines unquestionably make it difficult to do research in Indigenous health, which may lead to less research and consequently militate against improving Indigenous health.

Human Research Ethics Committees

A Human Research Ethics Committee (HREC) is a committee that is constituted to conduct research surveillance in an institution. It is composed of persons inside and outside the institution. The HREC should be distinguished from a Clinical Ethics Committee (CEC) whose job it is to oversee ethics pertaining to client care. If you are reading overseas literature, this can be confusing, as in British terminology an HREC is called a Research Ethics Committee while in American terminology it is an Institutional Review Board and a CEC is called an Institutional Ethics Committee (Berglund 1998). To confuse the issue even more, an IEC was until recently what HRECs used to be called in Australia.

Role

The role of the HREC is to deal with ethical matters pertaining to research on human participants. All institutions in which research is carried out must have an HREC. The HREC considers the ethical implications of all proposed research projects and decides whether they are ethically sound, monitors ongoing research projects to ensure continued conformity with ethical principles, maintains records of all research proposals, and communicates with the NHMRC's Medical Research Ethics Committee (NHMRC 1992c).

A researcher who wishes to carry out a research project that involves humans or access to confidential records must obtain an ethics clearance from the

HREC. The researcher submits a research proposal that will provide information about the design of the project, the participants, and provisions for data handling. Preparation of such a proposal is discussed in Chapter 6.

The HREC will consider the proposal, giving due weight to compliance with ethical principles, institutional procedures, measures to protect the participants from harm, maintenance of cultural safety, and data storage procedures. If the HREC gives approval, the research may proceed. During the life of the project, the researcher submits a report on its status and either seeks renewal of the clearance or informs the HREC that the project has been completed. At the conclusion of the project, the HREC signs it off.

Composition

The HREC must comprise at least five men and women representing different age groups. As of the year 2000, the minimum membership as set out by the NHMRC (1999) is:

- a layman and a laywoman neither of whom is associated with the institution or closely involved in medical, legal, or scientific work
- a minister of religion or a person such as an Aboriginal elder who performs a similar role in the community
- a member with knowledge of and current experience in the professional care, treatment or counselling of people
- a lawyer
- a person with research experience in the areas of work that are usually dealt with by the NHMRC.

There is no specific requirement for a nurse. However, a nurse can be the person with the expertise in care, treatment or counselling. The list above states the minimum requirements and the HREC can co-opt others as it sees fit.

Most members of HRECs have had no training in ethics and are not likely to be as able as an ethicist to judge the ethical aspects of a research proposal. The lay and minister members are not likely to be as influential as the medical doctors.

There has, to date, been no specific position for a nurse member on the Australian Health Ethics Committee. However, in recent times an allied health professional has been designated and the first one was a nurse. At the moment, the only way to secure specific nursing representation on local HRECs is through co-option onto the committee, which does not often happen. Given that nurses are the primary carers and care co-ordinators of most potential participants and are capable of being advocates for the client, nurses have questioned this omission. This lack of nursing representation has also meant that only non-nurses were judging the ethics of nursing research.

The composition of the HREC as it is has been constituted usually means that it applies the logical-positivist model of research to all types of research, regardless of its suitability. Nursing often needs to use a qualitative research design to answer significant questions. The present application forms of many HRECs assume a scientific experimentation model. This makes it awkward for nurses to frame ethics clearance proposals in a naturalistic paradigm. Nurses need to ask who is constructing the ethical standards for nursing research, are these appropriate for nursing research, and whose interests are really being served by these standards (Johnstone 1999).

However the Report of the Review of the Role and Functioning of Institutional Ethics Committees (Review Committee 1996) recommended that the minimum membership should be increased to seven members: a chairperson; a person with knowledge of and experience in research involving humans; a person with knowledge of and experience in the professional care, counselling or treatment of humans; a minister of religion or equivalent; a layman; a laywoman; and a lawyer. The Committee also recommended that in the case of a hospital HREC a nurse should be a member.

The composition of HRECs as recommended in the Report (Review Committee 1996) does not address the imbalance of qualitative and quantitative researchers although it does remove the dominance of the medical profession. It also does not include an ethicist who is independent of the institution, perhaps because these would be in short supply outside large cities.

Functions

HRECs scrutinise and approve the applications that come before them and monitor the progress and conclusion of the projects. They are concerned to uphold ethical principles and protect the public from harm. They must ensure that proposed research conforms to the relevant guidelines (NHMRC 1992c). HRECs are concerned to protect the institution's own researchers from inadvertently committing unethical practices. HRECs are also required to conform with the NHMRC's Statement on Human Experimentation and Supplementary Notes on research in particular fields such as research on human embryos. Madjar and Higgins (1996) have suggested that ethics committees tend to err on the side of overprotecting research participants in their desire to protect themselves and their institution.

At present, the HREC must review all proposals. Although there is a mechanism for 'fast tracking' a proposal, it is time for the introduction of a set of guidelines for exemption from HREC review. Studies involving educational research, surveys, existing records, or evaluation programs could be exempt from review provided that the principles of provision of anonymity, confidentiality and privacy are maintained and there is no risk to the participants. A mechanism for expediting review by means of delegation has been recommended by the Report (Review Committee 1996).

The HREC has the responsibility of monitoring approved projects to ensure continued compliance with ethical requirements. It also monitors the researchers to ensure that they practise responsible science and thus maintain the good reputation of their institution (NHMRC 1992c). The HREC incorporates confidential mechanisms for receiving complaints on the conduct of projects from participants, research workers or others. It requires that the researchers provide a written report to the HREC about the status of the project and compliance with the conditions imposed. In addition, the principal investigators are responsible for notifying the HREC immediately of any factor that might affect the ethical status of the project.

Research ethics in the practice of nursing

With the research explosion of recent years, clinical nurses are more likely than ever to be involved in nursing or medical research in various ways. They may collect or transport specimens for research, for example foetal tissue. They may be responsible for administering experimental medications in research protocols in the course of their client care. Or they may be involved as members of a research team. If you are involved in a research project, whatever your role, you have certain rights and responsibilities.

As a participant in research, you have the rights of voluntary and informed participation, and of withdrawal without penalty. You should also be able to withdraw from a project without being put at a disadvantage.

If you participate in a research project as a part of the research team, you must assure yourself about the ethical aspects of the project. You have the responsibility for being aware of relevant research guidelines and codes of conduct and for ensuring that you are not taking part in illegal or unapproved research. You must ensure that the researchers protect the clients' rights. You need to understand the aims and design of the project, including whether it has ethics clearance. You should also assure yourself about the credentials of the investigator to conduct the research.

As a nurse-clinician with clients involved as participants in research projects, you also have certain responsibilities toward those clients. If you give clients experimental drugs the effects of which are not completely known, you should know the action, possible side effects and expected clinical outcomes of the drug and should observe the client for reactions to it. You will need to be competent in assessment of clients undergoing clinical trials so that you can recommend that the clients be removed from the trial if they are being adversely affected in any way.

You also have certain rights as a clinician requested to be a data collector for others' research projects. You have the same rights as clients to refuse to participate without fear of reprisal. One situation that may arise is a conscientious or religious objection to a particular type of research such as that on foeti. No-one should be required to participate in a project against their will or suffer reprisals because of their objection.

Scientific misconduct

Scientific misconduct is an act of deception or misrepresentation of one's own work. It can take the form of fraud such as fabrication of data to report nonexistent research, or falsification of data such as changing records. It also includes irresponsible authorship such as plagiarism, and false attribution of authorship. Furthermore, it includes publishing the same article in more than one journal and fragmenting a study unnecessarily to increase the number of publications (AVCC *Code*). Scientific fraud usually occurs when a researcher desires a short cut to rewards such as promotion, or is convinced that the desired outcome justifies altering the results to achieve the 'correct' findings.

Scientific fraud comprises both unintentional fraud in which the researcher makes an honest mistake, and intentional fraud in which there is a deliberate deception. Unintentional fraud can involve failure to recognise the important factors that affect the observed evidence or can involve misinterpretation of data. Intentional fraud, however, is a more serious matter. It usually involves the data management phase of the research process. The three most common ways of faking data are smoothing out irregularities, discarding results that don't fit the theory, and inventing the data. The publishing process is supposed to detect fraud through the process of peer review. However, peer review is inadequate as a control mechanism because reviewers generally assume that other researchers are honest and even if they do suspect fraud may be reluctant to report it because of considerable risk to their own careers.

There have as yet been no reported instances of scientific fraud in nursing but there has been anecdotal evidence that data fabrication and unjustified authorship have occurred (Chop & Silva 1991). This is not surprising given that nurses are now under the same pressures to publish as are other scientists. Adequate supervision, tenure and promotion guidelines that emphasise quality of research publications as opposed to quantity are strategies to encourage intellectual honesty. Replication studies, which may show up unsound research, are difficult to secure funding for and are not commonly published.

In Australia, there have been two documented cases of scientific fraud in the area of medical research, one on birth control pills, and one on hyoscine. Both took place in the early 1980s. The first was the case of Dr Michael Briggs, a Professor of Human Biology at Deakin University, who had faked research on the effects of contraceptive pills on blood metabolism in women using the pill for longer than 18 months and in a study on progesterone and breast tumours in beagle bitches (Kohn 1986). Briggs resigned from the university and went to Spain where he died a short time later.

The second case concerned Dr William McBride, who was lionised for discovering that the drug thalidomide could produce phocomelia, a congenital malformation or absence of limbs. McBride is alleged to have made a habit of duplicity in research, including the use of unauthorised data in his MD thesis, taking more than his share of the credit for the thalidomide discovery, stealing the neural crest theory of thalidomide action, giving false witness at a trial of a drug company in the United States, and fabricating data on a study of the effects of hyoscine on birth deformities (Nicol 1989). A medical tribunal that lasted four years found McBride guilty of 24 charges of medical research fraud and he was struck off the medical register as being not of good character in the context of fitness to practise medicine (Humphrey 1994). An appeal has since been dismissed.

A nurse may discover a case of scientific misconduct or unethical research processes and must decide whether to become a 'whistle-blower', or one who reports suspected misconduct to the authorities. Or a nurse may be the first to observe the deleterious effects of a drug in a clinical trial. Should the nurse report it, and if so to whom? On one hand, the nurse has a duty of care to the client. On the other hand, repercussions may result if the nurse reports the incident. Nevertheless, the nurse's moral duty to put the protection of the patient above other considerations is clear. However, anyone in such an invidious position would do well to read the literature on whistle-blowing and take account of protective mechanisms before 'blowing the whistle'.

How can scientific fraud be prevented? The Australian Vice-Chancellors' Committee states in their guidelines that a principle of research is the validity and accuracy in the collection and reporting of data (NHMRC/AVCC 1997). Institutions should have in place policies to deal with prevention of scientific fraud, including maintenance of records and retention of data. Nurse-researchers should be familiar with those policies. Institutions should cultivate an ethos that discourages scientific fraud. Established nurse-researchers should serve as role models and/or mentors to less experienced researchers. Finally, institutions should reward quality rather than quantity of publications, although this is not likely to happen while university funding gives precedence to quantity.

Reading a research report: ethical considerations

You will probably need to read research reports in the course of professional practice and you should be familiar with ethical aspects so that you can evaluate these reports. Nursing research papers frequently do not address ethical aspects very well but an informed reader is able to critique the implied ethical aspects. Most journals have a policy of publishing only research that conforms to ethical standards. As a reader, you will ask questions about appropriateness of topic or participants, research design, approval by an HREC, treatment of participants, and ethical procedures. The advanced reader may examine the results for evidence of propriety: results that are too good to be true may not be! Criteria for critique of ethical aspects of research reports can be found in Chapter 3.

Summary

In this chapter, I have presented the ethical issues that nurses need to know to be effective consumers of research, participants in research projects and researchers. Historical instances of unethical medical research have set the scene for understanding ethical issues and the need for codes of ethical conduct in research. The rights of participants and the responsibilities of researchers have been discussed and ways in which researchers can protect the rights of participants have been outlined. The role, composition and function of HRECs has been discussed. The issues of ethics affecting clinicians have been presented. Scientific misconduct has been outlined and the reader has been given a set of guidelines for evaluating the ethical aspects of nursing research.

Main points

- Ethics is concerned with moral questions and behaviour; it asks what ought to be done and is a guide for research procedures.
- All research should be carried out with the highest moral standards.
- There are examples of unethical research conduct in all times including the present.
- Codes of ethics and research ethics guidelines are based on the Nuremburg Code and the Helsinki Declaration as is the NHMRC Statement on Human Experimentation, which forms the ethical standard for human research in Australia.
- Ethical principles on which the codes are based comprise beneficence, non-maleficence, respect for human dignity, and justice.
- Participants have the right to informed consent, anonymity, privacy, confidentiality, not to participate or to withdraw at any time and not to suffer harm.
- Special cases such as embryos, foetal tissue, vulnerable subjects/participants and Indigenous participants have extra protection under the guidelines.
- Human Research Ethics Committees are charged with scrutinising and approving applications and monitoring progress and conclusion of projects involving research on humans.
- Scientific misconduct is an act of deception or misrepresentation of one's own work and includes fraud, fabrication or falsification of data, plagiarism, irresponsible authorship, and false attribution of authorship.
- Whether conducting or assisting with research, nurse-clinicians ought to uphold the highest ethical standards.

Review Questions

1 In relation to gaining participants' permission when undertaking qualitative research, it is
   a unnecessary for participant observation
   b necessary when people know they are involved
   c always necessary in every instance
   d unnecessary for photographs and videotaping

2 The main concern in applying ethical standards to research is:
   a ensuring the validity of the findings
   b detecting problems of scientific rigour
   c preventing harm to participants
   d applying the principle of beneficence

3 You are a researcher wishing to test out a new nursing intervention. Which design would be the most ethical?
   a new treatment group, untreated placebo group, normal treatment group
   b untreated placebo group, new treatment group
   c placebo group, old treatment group
   d normal treatment group, new treatment group

4 Not allowing anyone except the researcher access to data is an example of applying participants' right to:
   a privacy
   b confidentiality
   c anonymity
   d justice

5 Not having respondents write their names on questionnaires is an example of applying participants' right to:
   a privacy
   b confidentiality
   c anonymity
   d justice

6 If a participant chose not to disclose information, this would be an example of the application of:
   a privacy
   b confidentiality
   c anonymity
   d justice

7 Two nurses who are conducting a study in a mental institution discover that some of the nurses on Ward D are physically abusing clients. The appropriate course of action in the first instance would be to:
   a do nothing that would put the project in danger
   b report the nurses to the charge nurse and let her/him deal with it
   c report the incident to the director of nursing
   d convene a meeting of the nurses involved and express their concern

8 You are a member of a Human Research Ethics Committee. A nurse is planning to research clients' healing responses to prayer. She plans to have a group of Christians pray over half of the clients in ICU that have been randomly allocated to a prayer group, but will not be aware of the prayer. The other half will be allocated to a control group who do not receive prayer. She will then compare their rates of healing to see if the prayer makes any difference. Your main concern about the ethics of this experiment is:

   a the patients who do not receive prayer will be disadvantaged
   b the patients cannot give informed consent
   c some patients might object to being prayed over by Christians
   d other people outside the study might be praying over people in the control group

9 Intentional scientific fraud can involve:

   a smoothing out irregularities
   b discarding results that don't fit the theory
   c faking data
   d all of the above

10 If you are planning to carry out the research in the hospital, you will also have to get ethics clearance from the:

   a hospital Institutional Ethics Committee
   b director of nursing
   c hospital Human Research Ethics Committee
   d all of the above

Discussion Questions

1 With what is ethics concerned and how does this relate to nursing research?

2 Discuss the role of research standards in maintaining research ethics.

3 State the four principles of human ethics and discuss how these relate to the rights of research participants.

4 State four types of people who may require protection.

5 Describe the role of Human Research Ethics Committees.

References

Anon. 19 Sep. 1999, 'Doctors store child cardiac victims' hearts without parents' consent', *Sunday Age*, as cited in *Monash Bioethics Review*, 1999, vol. 18, no. 4, 7.

Australian Nursing Federation 1997, *Standards for Research for the Nursing Profession*, ANF, Melbourne.

Australian Vice-Chancellors' Committee undated, *Guidelines for Responsible Practice in Research and Dealing with Problems of Research Misconduct*, AVCC, Canberra.

Australian Vice-Chancellors' Committee undated, *Code of Ethics for Researchers*, AVCC, Canberra.
Berglund, C. 1998, *Ethics for Health Care*, Oxford University Press, Melbourne.
Caplan, A. 1992, 'How did medicine go so wrong?' in *When Medicine Went Mad*, ed. A. Caplan, Humana Press, Totowa, New Jersey.
Chop, R. & Silva, M. 1991, 'Scientific fraud: definitions, policies and implications for nursing research', *Journal of Professional Nursing*, vol. 7, no. 3, 166–71.
Davis, A. 1990, 'Ethical issues in nursing research', *Western Journal of Nursing Research*, vol. 12, no. 3, 413–16.
Dodds, S. 2000, 'Human research ethics in Australia: ethical regulation and public policy', *Monash Bioethics Review*, vol. 19, no. 2, Ethics Committee Supplement, 4–21.
Hicks, C. 1992, 'Of sex and status: a study of the effects of gender and occupation on nurses' evaluations of nursing research', *Journal of Advanced Nursing*, vol. 17, 1343–9.
Humphrey, G. 1994, 'Scientific fraud: the K McBride case – judgment', *Medicine, Science and the Law*, vol. 34, no. 4, 299–306.
Johnstone, M.-J. 1991, 'Improving the ethics and cultural suitability of Aboriginal health research', *Aboriginal and Islander Health Worker Journal*, vol. 15, no. 2, 10–13.
Johnstone, M.-J. 1999, *Bioethics: A Nursing Perspective*, (3rd edn), Harcourt, Sydney.
Kohn, A. 1986, *False Prophets: Fraud and Error in Science and Medicine*, Basil Blackwell Ltd, Oxford, UK.
Madjar, I. & Higgins, I. 1996, 'Of ethics committees, protocols, and behaving ethically in the field: a case study of research with elderly residents in a nursing home', *Nursing Inquiry*, vol. 3, no. 3, 130–7.
McNeill, P. 1993, *The Ethics and Politics of Human Experimentation*, Cambridge University Press, Cambridge, UK.
Milgram, S. 1963, 'Behavioral study of obedience', *Journal of Abnormal and Social Psychology*, vol. 67, no.4, 371–8.
National Commission for the Protection of Human Subjects of Biomedical and Behavioral Research 1978, *The Belmont Report: Ethical principles and guidelines for research involving human subjects*, US Government Printing Office, Washington DC.
National Health & Medical Research Council 1985, *Report on Ethics in Epidemiological Research*, Australian Government Publishing Service, Canberra.
National Health & Medical Research Council 1991, *Guidelines on Ethical Matters in Aboriginal and Torres Strait Islander Health Research*, Australian Government Publishing Service, Canberra.
National Health & Medical Research Council 1992a, 'NHMRC Statement on Human Experimentation', in *NHMRC Statement on Human Experimentation and Supplementary Notes*, ed. NHMRC, Canberra, 2–4.
National Health & Medical Research Council 1992b, Supplementary Note No. 4: 'In vitro fertilisation and embryo transfer', in *NHMRC Statement on Human Experimentation and Supplementary Notes*, ed. NHMRC, Canberra, 14–15.
National Health & Medical Research Council 1992c, Supplementary Note No. 7: 'The human fetus and the use of human fetal tissue', in *NHMRC Statement on Human Experimentation and Supplementary Notes*, ed. NHMRC, Canberra.
National Health & Medical Research Council 1995, *Ethical Aspects of Qualitative Methods in Health Research – an Information Paper for Institutional Ethics Committees*, Australian Government Publishing Service, Canberra.
National Health & Medical Research Council 1999, *National Statement on Ethical Conduct in Research Involving Humans*, NHMRC, Canberra.
National Health & Medical Research Council/Australian Vice-Chancellors' Committee 1997, *Joint Statement and Guidelines on Research Practice*, Canberra, NHMRC/AVCC.

Nicol, B. 1989, *McBride: Behind the Myth*, Australian Broadcasting Commission, Crows Nest.

Review Committee 1996, *Report of the Review of the Role and Functioning of Institutional Ethics Committees*, Australian Government Publishing Service, Canberra.

Roberts, K., Brittin, M. & deClifford, J. 1995, 'Boomerang pillows and respiratory capacity in frail elderly women', *Clinical Nursing Research*, vol. 4, no. 4, 465–71.

Robertson, J. 1992, 'Standards for nursing research: a WA initiative', *Australian Nurses Journal*, vol. 21, no.9, 14–15.

Royal College of Nursing, Australia 1992, *Nursing Research Targets into the Twenty-first Century: A National Statement*, RCNA, Melbourne.

Silva, M. & Sorrell, J. 1984, 'Factors influencing comprehension of information for informed consent: ethical implications for nursing research', *International Journal of Nursing Studies*, vol. 21, no. 4, 233–40.

Spriggs, M. 1999, 'Human subjects research: review of the NH&MRC National Statement on Ethical Conduct in Research Involving Humans', *Monash Bioethics Review*, vol. 18, no. 4, Ethics Committee Supplement, 5–13.

Thomas, S. & Quinn, S. 1991, 'The Tuskegee syphilis study, 1932 to 1972: implications for HIV education and AIDS risk education programs in the Black community', *American Journal of Public Health*, vol. 81, no. 11, 1498–505.

Vessey, J. & Gennaro, S. 1994, 'The ghost of Tuskegee', *Nursing Research*, vol. 43, no. 2, 67.

Weekend Australian, 1990, 'Guilty medic', Oct. 11, 27–8.

CHAPTER 6

Obtaining approval and support for your project

chapter objectives

The material presented in this chapter will assist you to:

- understand the reasons for preparing a research proposal
- identify the intended recipients of the research proposal
- develop a research proposal
- write a research proposal
- submit a research proposal
- evaluate a research proposal
- understand some funding mechanisms and processes
- gain entry to data collection sites
- gain access to research participants.

Introduction

In this chapter, we will discuss writing a research proposal. Some research proposals are written for the purposes of assessment of student progress in a unit on research methodology. However, others are written for the purpose of gaining support and approvals required to carry out a study. In the latter case, formal approvals, including ethics clearance, must be gained from the university. If clinical research is involved, approval must also be gained from the appropriate authorities in the clinical field. Informal support is also needed from key people in these areas. Financial support may be gained from funding bodies. The process is carried out by writing a research proposal and by approaching key people for approval and support.

The research proposal

A research proposal is a written account of the plan for the research project. It presents an argument as to why a particular problem should be investigated and what the appropriate methodology is to investigate it. It sets out what the researcher intends to do – how, why, where, when and at what cost. For quantitative research, the research proposal is like a pattern for a garment or a blueprint for a building in that it assists the researcher to follow a process that has been laid down. For qualitative research, the research proposal is much more flexible because the method tends to evolve with the research.

You may ask yourself why it is necessary to have a plan for the research as long as you know what you are doing. Just as a dressmaker would not start to cut into fabric without a pattern, or a builder to lay bricks without knowing where the walls were going, a researcher does not begin to carry out a research project without a plan. A plan helps you, the researcher, to design and organise the project. A plan allows you to see and think through the relationships between different parts of the proposal, for example the purpose, methodology and expected outcomes. It helps you to foresee potential problems, and to solve them at the planning stage rather than the implementation stage. It also allows you to consult other researchers before the study is carried out so that they can comment and make constructive suggestions for improvement – they may be able to view your proposed research more objectively than you and be more able to see the pitfalls of your project. A research plan is the best way to ensure that you avoid mistakes when carrying out the actual project.

Once you have formulated a rough plan, the next step is to write a formal research proposal. The purpose of writing a formal proposal is to communicate to a reader in a clear and concise style exactly what you propose to do in your research project. The process of writing down your ideas helps you to clarify them. It is almost always necessary to write a proposal for any intended research project because approval to carry out the research must be gained from the appropriate authorities such as a university research committee, a human research ethics committee (HREC) or a funding body. This mechanism protects the researcher because if there are any repercussions from the research, such as a lawsuit, the researcher has had the appropriate approvals. The committees giving the approvals would have to take some of the responsibility in the form of legal liability. This mechanism also protects participants, as they are assured of anonymity, confidentiality and privacy. It is therefore essential for the beginning researcher to learn how to write a satisfactory research proposal.

Preliminary steps in preparing the proposal

Before you write the proposal, you must have identified what your research problem is, regardless of what type of proposal you are doing. You will usually have read and reviewed the literature, unless you are working using a qualitative methodology such as grounded theory in which this may not be appropriate. You will have identified your research design. These processes have all been discussed in previous chapters. Unless you have identified these aspects, you will not be able to complete a satisfactory research proposal.

Another step which you must take before commencing is to identify the audience at which the proposal is aimed, usually individuals or committees that have the power to approve your proposal. It is important to direct the proposal to their concerns. Naturally, all committees will be concerned with the quality of the proposal. However, different committees have specific concerns. HRECs will be most concerned with protection of the people from whom you intend to collect data, the risk/benefit ratio, and scientific rigour. Research committees will be especially concerned with the adequacy of the research methodology and with budgetary aspects. Clinical research committees or gatekeepers will be concerned with the impact on the institution, such as how your proposed project will impact on other projects and if it will interfere with the agency's routine. Funding bodies will be concerned that the proposal is consistent with their identified objectives and priorities and whether the proposed budget is appropriate. Indeed, where there is a competitive process, for example for scholarships or funding, committees often will have developed a points system for scoring proposals. If you are submitting a proposal under those conditions, it is wise to direct the bulk of your energies to where the most points can be scored.

The formal approval mechanisms may be simple or complex, depending on your situation. Undergraduate students in a beginning research unit may have to submit a proposal only for assessment, with an indication of the approvals that they would have to acquire should the project be carried out. All projects undertaken under the auspices of the university in which data collection is involved will require the approval of university committees. In addition, all projects carried out in the clinical field must have the approval of the relevant committees in the clinical facility. Furthermore, an approval will have to be given from each clinical facility involved, unless there are joint committees operating. Table 6.1 shows the committees required for approval and under what conditions you must seek their approval. Remember that a proposal is a contract and cannot be altered substantially without agreement from the persons or agencies giving the initial approval.

Table 6.1 Necessary approvals for different types of projects

	Student in course unit: full project		Honours/postgraduate student		Clinical nurse researcher
	Laboratory	Clinical field	Laboratory	Clinical field	
Lecturer/supervisor	✓	✓	✓	✓	
University research committee			✓	✓	
University human research ethics committee	✓	✓	✓	✓	
Clinical site human research ethics committee		✓		✓	✓
Clinical field research committee		✓		✓	✓

As Table 6.1 shows, clinical field projects require the most approvals. Most funding bodies will require a letter of approval from all of the relevant committees above, plus an application for funding.

Many organisations and committees provide application forms and guidelines that you are required to use. Guidelines have been developed by an organisation to expedite the process and to help the reviewers make decisions about the proposal. The guidelines will be consistent with the aims and priorities of the organisation. They are there to help the readers make decisions about the proposal, so it is important to follow them to facilitate a positive outcome. Before you start to write your proposal, obtain a copy of their guidelines from every committee or agency that has to give approval. This is usually a matter of a telephone call or an email to the secretary of the committee. Although this can seem like a lot of forms to fill in, you will find that most forms follow the NHMRC model, so it is often a matter of a judicious cut and paste from the word processor. Some committees make their guidelines and application forms available on electronic media as a word processor file that can then be transferred straight into your word processor. Some of the application forms are quite brief, but some committees will require a full scientific protocol, or detailed research proposal, as well.

Generally, you will acquire the necessary university approvals first, so any errors are addressed 'in house' before the proposal goes out to external committees. The proposal should first be assessed and approved by your supervisor and then be sent through the appropriate university committees, followed by external committees. Figure 6.1 shows the approval process.

Allow plenty of time to prepare your proposal: it can take you up to six months to develop a proposal and get all of the necessary approvals. It is wise to find out each committee's approval process, meeting schedule and deadlines for submission

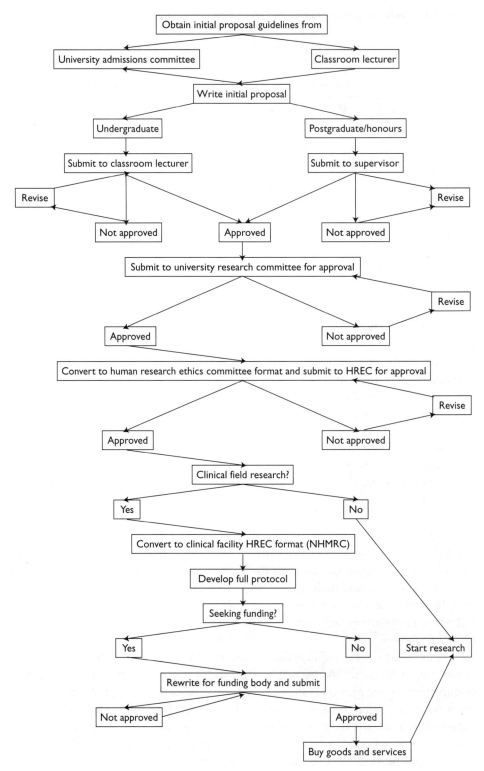

Figure 6.1 The approval process

of proposals. Meetings can be four to six weeks apart, or even longer over the summer holidays or mid-year break. Most committees require submission at least 10 days before the meeting to allow time to circulate the papers to members before the meeting. Make sure that you get your application in on time or even early – committee managers like to send the papers out all together and will not take kindly to sending your proposal out individually because it is late. If you cannot meet the deadline, it is better to wait for the next meeting than to put in incomplete papers that waste the committee's time. If you put in incomplete papers, the committee will send your application back to you for revision, so you are no farther ahead.

Content of a research proposal

The overall structure of a research proposal is fairly standard. The proposal begins with the title, then an abstract or summary, an introduction section, and a methodology section. At the end, there are references and appendices. The proposal should develop a logical flow of ideas from problem to budget and should be laid out in the correct order. This may be set by guidelines of the committee or agency reviewing the proposal. Shown below is a sample of a format for a standard research proposal.

Elements of a quantitative research proposal

In this section, we shall use as an illustration a research proposal for an experiment to compare the effectiveness of kangaroo mother care (KMC) and conventional cuddling care.

```
Preliminary pages
  • Title page
  • Abstract
Body of proposal
  • Introduction
      • Background to the study
      • Purpose statement
      • Statement of significance
  • Review of the literature
  • Methodology
      • Design
      • Setting
      • Participants
      • Instruments and materials
      • Procedures
  • Ethical implications
  • Dissemination of results
  • Work plan
  • Resources and budget
  • Details of researchers
Supporting material
  • References
  • Appendixes
```

Figure 6.2 Sample format of a research proposal

Preliminaries

The first part of the proposal is the 'preliminaries', the pages that precede the body of the proposal. The preliminaries comprise a title page and an abstract.

The title

The title of the proposal should convey the gist, or meaning of the proposal. This can be achieved by using key words. The title should be no longer than 20 words. Some agencies require both long and short titles. An example of a title for a quantitative proposal is: *A comparison of kangaroo mother care and conventional cuddling care.*

As well as the title of the proposal, the title page gives the author's name, position and qualifications. If the proposal is being submitted for ethics, funding, or other outside approvals, the author's postal and email addresses should be given, as well as telephone and fax contact numbers. The date should be placed somewhere on the page, and this can be done easily as a footer if you are using a word processor.

The abstract

The abstract is a brief summary of the proposal. It gives the reader an overview of the project, and should include the major themes or threads of the project. Primarily, it should focus on the objectives and methodology of the project. It should be concise, with a word limit of 250–300 words. Some application forms specify a limit of seven lines. An example of an abstract is as follows:

> In this study, kangaroo mother care (KMC) and conventional cuddling care (CCC) will be compared in two neonatal nurseries in Darwin, Northern Territory, Australia. Fifty mother-infant dyads will be randomly assigned to the KMC group or the CCC group. Both groups of mothers will cuddle their babies for a minimum of two hours per day, five days a week while in the study. The KMC group will have skin-to-skin contact while the CCC group will have contact only through normal clothing

You can find more information about writing abstracts in articles by Sheldon and Jackson (1998, 2000) and Kachoyeanos (1998).

Body of proposal

The introduction

The body of the proposal begins with the introduction. The purpose of the introduction is to acquaint the reader with the problem, and the background and purposes of the study. The introduction should answer the questions 'what?' and 'why?' It should explain the importance and relevance of the proposed research, that is, it should 'sell' the research project to the reader. At the end of the introduction, the reader should be convinced that the study should be carried out.

In constructing the introduction, you begin with more general 'big picture' aspects and move to the specific 'little picture' aspects. You begin with the background to the study, setting it in the context of some important previous research. You then move to the purpose of the study, and its significance.

The background to the study is a brief section that establishes the rationale for doing the study. It answers the question 'why?' This rationale should be developed logically. The rationale may be that previous research has left questions unanswered; that you may be able to devise an improved way to answer a question; that a theory suggests such line of inquiry; or that it is a new line of inquiry that may be justified by logical argument. The rationale should show why your study will provide a solution to the problem.

The background to the study begins by orienting the reader to some previous key research in the area or key theoretical issues. It should show how the problem was identified, mentioning any key theoretical issues. It should show how the proposed research builds on what has already been done in the area. An example of a background statement is:

> KMC is the positioning of a near-naked infant at or between the mother's breasts so that there is skin-to-skin contact. KMC has been reported in the literature since the mid-1980s as a method of caring for premature infants. It was initiated in South America – in Bogota, Columbia – in order to overcome the lack of staff and equipment to care for premature infants and small infants (Whitelaw & Sleath 1985; Anderson 1989; deLeeuw et al. 1991). It has further been reported in use in Scandinavia, (Anderson 1989), California (Drosten-Brooks 1993) and Mozambique (Mondlane, de Graca & Ebrahim 1989). It has even been implemented safely with intubated infants of over 700 gm that are physiologically stable (Gale, Franck & Lund 1993). The advantages of KMC for the infant are that skin temperature is maintained, there is no apnoea or bradycardia, no change in transcutaneous oxygen level (Drosten-Brooks 1993) and no increase in sepsis (Whitelaw & Sleath 1985). There are longer quiet sleep periods and the hospital stay is shorter (Drosten-Brooks 1993). Quiet sleep frequency is increased and activity level is reduced (Ludington 1990).
>
> The researchers understand that KMC is being implemented on a trial basis in Adelaide and Melbourne. The staff at the Royal Darwin Hospital Special Care Nursery have used KMC for several individual cases and have observed some of the above reported advantages. To date, no research has been reported in the Australian setting. Furthermore it is not known whether KMC will be effective in Darwin with its specialised cultural and environmental conditions.

The purposes or objectives section should give the purposes of the study, or what the study proposes to find out, in general terms. In other words, you should state the problem that you propose to investigate. This section should provide the reader with a comprehensive and coherent statement of what you hope to achieve. It should be stated concisely. Specific aims should be stated in terms of the objectives and the research question and, if it is a quantitative study, should lead to the hypotheses. An example of a purpose statement is:

> The purpose of this study is to compare the use of kangaroo mother care (KMC) with standard or conventional cuddling care (CCC) in premature and low-weight for age infants. The study will explore both maternal and infant outcomes.

The statement on significance of the study follows. It should show why this study is worth doing. It should answer the question 'so what?' A good research proposal will contain a significant research problem. It should show how the results of this study could advance knowledge or practice in nursing and/or health. If there are possible applications of the results of this study, state them. You should have reflected on these points already, when you were selecting your problem to study. An example of a statement of significance is:

> Previous research has shown that there are positive maternal and infant outcomes for KMC. However, these findings have been produced by research that was exploratory and frequently characterised by lack of a control group. As far as we have been able to determine, there has been no adequately designed and implemented experiment published that has investigated both maternal and infant outcomes. Therefore it is anticipated that this study will make a contribution to knowledge in this area.
>
> If the outcome is positive, it is intended to implement KMC in the Special Care Nursery (SCN) for all mothers who wish to carry it out. This could result in increased parental satisfaction with the care given, longer duration of breastfeeding and decreased length of stay for many infants. It is beyond doubt that breastfeeding is of great benefit to infants in terms of nutritional suitability, improved immunity from infection and fewer allergies. Therefore increased duration of breastfeeding will be beneficial to infants. The establishment of breastfeeding is especially important at Royal Darwin Hospital, which acts as a centre for childbirth for mothers from outlying communities. Indigenous mothers and others in isolated areas without proper sanitation and refrigeration facilities need to breastfeed their babies because infant formula feeding is not nearly as practicable.

In order to highlight the importance of the problem, you may incorporate relevant statistics about the incidence, distribution, relevance to health, impact on morbidity or mortality related to the problem, for example:

> In addition, there are considerable potential savings on the total cost of Special Care Nursery care where the daily rate is hundreds of dollars per infant.

The review of the literature

A good quantitative research proposal will contain an adequate review of the literature. The review of the literature section of the proposal comprises two sections: the review of the theoretical literature that constitutes the theoretical framework for the study, and the review of the empirical literature, or research findings, that are relevant to the study. The literature review demonstrates that the researcher has a command of the current empirical and theoretical knowledge concerning the proposed problem. The literature review should give the theoretical framework that is used for your study. The theory should be congruent with the question being asked. For example, if the study is about energy conservation, Levine's model would be appropriate. If it is about adaptation, Roy's model would be appropriate, and so forth. The conceptual framework should define the concepts used that arise from the theory and then lead to the variables. Relationships among the concepts should be explained. A concept map, or flow chart showing the relationships between the concepts may be helpful. An example of a brief theoretical statement is:

> The conceptual framework for this study was Levine's Conservation Principles (Levine 1991). This model states that a nursing action is to assist the client with conservation of energy, structural integrity, personal integrity and social integrity. It may be that the act of KMC will assist the infant to conserve energy because the heat transferred from the mother to the infant will conserve the infant's body heat, which in turn will free up energy for growth. In addition, the cuddling will assist with conservation of social and personal integrity through promoting mother–child bonding.

The review of the empirical literature is an outline of previous research findings that are directly relevant to the present study. It provides a background or frame of reference for the reader. The intention is to show how much is already known about the problem and how the proposed study is related to previous work on the subject and is trying to address questions not answered by previous research. The literature review should summarise the previous relevant findings and it should also critique them. The research studies chosen should relate to each hypothesis or question that you are trying to answer. An example of a brief review of empirical literature is as follows:

> Several studies have been reported in the literature, some of which dealt with maternal outcomes, and some with infant outcomes. In terms of infant outcomes, various researchers have found that KMC is equal or superior to CCC. Ludington (1990) found infants' average temperature rose significantly after KMC and that average oxygen saturation was not decreased significantly. In terms of infant activity and sleep state, Ludington (1990) found that the amount of time in quiet regular sleep increased and activity states significantly decreased after KMC. However, Whitelaw et al. (1988) found that by six months of age there was no difference between KMC and control groups in the duration of sleeping, feeding, being held, and playing but the KMC group spent significantly less time crying. Several researchers have found that KMC decreased the length of stay in the incubator and the hospital (Whitelaw et al. 1988; Ludington-Hoe et al. 1992; Wahlberg, Affonso & Persson 1992), possibly related to increased weight gain as reported by Wahlberg, Affonso & Persson (1992).
>
> KMC has also been found to have better outcomes for breast feeding. Affonso, Wahlberg & Persson (1989), Wahlberg, Affonso & Persson (1992) and Affonso (1993) found considerably higher participation rates of breastfeeding in KMC than CCC mothers, while Whitelaw et al. (1988) found that the mean duration of lactation was considerably longer in the KMC group than the normal contact group.
>
> Finally, KMC has been found to result in improved maternal confidence. Affonso, Wahlberg & Persson (1993) and Smith (1996) found that mothers who had given KMC bonded better to the infant and had increased maternal confidence. Curry

(1982), however, found that the control group and KMC did not have significant differences in attachment behaviours or self-concept scores.

In summary, previous research has demonstrated that there may be positive maternal and infant outcomes for KMC. However, these findings have been produced by research that was exploratory and sometimes characterised by lack of a control group.

The depth of the review varies according to the purpose of the proposal. For an undergraduate research proposal, half a dozen decent papers will suffice, and you may need to include only the most recent research on the topic. For a doctoral degree, the complete literature on the topic must be reviewed. For proposals for ethics committees, a few recent relevant papers will suffice.

The breadth of the review varies according to the topic itself and the amount of literature acquired. If the topic is a complex one, much literature will be needed to cover the area properly. If it is a narrow one, much less will be required. The breadth of the review also relates to the amount of literature available. If you have found a lot of literature on your topic, you will have to be selective, but not biased. Your literature review should include only research findings, and only findings that are pertinent to your topic. A common mistake that writers make is to fail to limit themselves and to present a huge mass of material in a haphazard manner (Gething 1995). Original references should be used where possible rather than citations. If there is very little or no literature on the subject, you may need to bring in literature that is related to the topic, but is more peripheral. For example, if you want to study the effects of negative ion therapy on cancer patients, but the only research has been on children with asthma, you may use this. At the end of this section you should summarise the main findings of the literature. You should show how your proposed study will extend the previous research, if any.

Writing a literature review is not easy. The review is meant to integrate the research findings on the topic and critique any weaknesses in the previous studies so that they can be taken into account in the design of your study. The process of critiquing individual studies was detailed in Chapter 3. However, developing a literature review requires more than just piecing together separate studies. A literature review is a logically constructed argument. An effective way to organise the review, particularly if you have several independent variables, is according to the independent variables, or questions being asked, and write about all of the findings on each variable, with a summary at the end. You can find an example of a review of the literature on performance indicators for discharge planning in an article by Hedges and Grimmer (1999).

At the end of the literature review, you should lead into and express your specific research question. An example of a research question is:

> Will KMC result in more weight gain, better temperature maintenance, shorter hospital stay, longer breastfeeding duration for infants and less stress and more confidence in parenting skills for mothers than CCC?

The methodology

The methodology section describes in detail the methodology for the study. This includes the design of the study, the setting, participants, instruments, and procedures proposed for the study. This section should answer the questions: 'on whom?', 'how?', 'when?' and 'where?' Each choice should be justified. A good research proposal will have a methodology that is suitable to answer the research question.

The methodology that you will choose depends entirely on the question you are trying to answer. It is impossible to overemphasise the importance of this point. If you are trying to answer a question about the lived experience of a person, a qualitative approach such as phenomenology is more suitable. If, however, you are trying to investigate the relationship between a treatment and outcomes, a quantitative methodology is more appropriate. Within each paradigm you will have to choose the appropriate methodology. For example, for studying a subculture within a community, an ethnographic approach is useful. Or, for studying the effects of a new treatment, an experimental approach is appropriate.

In writing the methodology section, you begin with the design of the study, for example, experimental, correlational, phenomenological, or grounded theory. Quantitative designs are discussed in Chapter 7, and qualitative designs are discussed in chapters 12 and 13. You should explain why you have chosen the method, that is, why it is appropriate to the research question. If it is a complex design, a diagram or flow chart may assist the reader to understand it. In deciding how much detail to give in the design of the study section, consider the level of the question. If it is a descriptive design, less detail will be required than for an experimental design. You should give enough detail to enable a reader to understand how you intend to answer the research question.

A statement of study design is as follows:

> This will be an exploratory experimental study in which at least 50 infants will be assigned randomly to two groups, the KMC group who will receive kangaroo mother care, and the control group, the CCC group, who will receive conventional cuddling care. The KMC group will be exposed to an average of a minimum of two hours per day for five days per week of skin-to-skin contact with their mothers while the CCC group will be exposed to two hours of normal contact. The subject pairs will be enrolled for four weeks or until discharge from the SCN, whichever is the lesser period. The only difference between the groups will be that the KMC group has skin-to-skin contact while the control group has contact through clothing. That is, both groups of infants will receive on average equal amounts of cuddling.

The hypothesis should be stated as a description of the anticipated outcomes. It should be well-defined, logical, clear, and necessary to answer the research question. It should show the relationships between the variables, stated in measurable terms. Examples of hypotheses statements are:

The researchers' hypotheses were that

1. KMC infants would have gained more weight on average by the date of discharge from hospital, then at six weeks and at three months compared with CCC infants
2. KMC infants would have equal or better temperature maintenance during KMC than CCC infants would have during CCC
3. KMC infants would have a shorter hospital stay than CCC infants

It was also hypothesised that KMC mothers would:

4. breastfeed for longer than CCC mothers
5. report less stress than CCC mothers
6. feel more confident of their parenting skills than CCC mothers.

The independent and dependent variables should be identified and stated in measurable terms. These are sometimes called 'operational definitions'. In the above examples, the weight gain in mean grams per day, body temperature variation in degrees Celsius, duration of breastfeeding in days, parental confidence as measured by the Parental Expectations Survey (Reece 1992) and stress as measured by the Parental Stressor Scale – NICU (Miles, Funk & Kasper 1993) in centimetres are the dependent variables, and the type of cuddling (KMC versus CCC) is the independent variable, because differences in the weight gain and so forth are dependent on the type of cuddling received.

Sometimes the variables are defined and operationalised in a list:

Definition of variables

Length of stay: birth to discharge from SCN

Weight gain: average daily weight gain during period of KMC/CCC and average daily weight gain from birth to discharge from hospital

Duration of breastfeeding: time in weeks

Stress levels: as measured by an appropriate stress questionnaire

Parenting skills: as measured by an appropriate questionnaire

Attitudes to the SCN experience: as measured by questionnaire developed by researchers

After defining the hypothesis and variables, the setting for the research should be given. For example, say whether it will take place in a laboratory or hospital or in the community. In a proposal, it is quite appropriate to give the names of agencies in which you will carry out the research. You should show that the agency is capable of supplying sufficient participants for the study by giving the numbers of potential participants that the agency has. An example of a statement concerning setting is as follows:

> The setting for the research will be the Special Care Nursery at Royal Darwin Hospital and the nursery at the Darwin Private Hospital. It will be necessary to use two different hospitals in order to achieve an adequate sample in a reasonable time.

The participants or subjects should be described next. State the characteristics of the group from which they will be selected and where they are to be found. State your rationale for selecting this particular group of participants. You should give the size of sample you wanted to end up with and say how you arrived at this figure. If it is a design that has the potential for participant mortality, you should address participant attrition and build in extra participants, usually about 10 per cent, so that you will end up with enough participants. A good research proposal will include plans to acquire sufficient participants to make the results meaningful.

It is customary to state the type of sample that you intend to use, for example a random sample, convenience sample, stratified random sample, and so on. Types of samples will be discussed in Chapter 8. If it is a convenience sample there will not be much to say except the basis of the convenience, for example they were the patients on a ward. If it is a random sample or a stratified random sample, say how the sample was drawn from the population. You should describe the criteria for participant selection and give the rationale for the criteria. You should give the details of how they were recruited, for example by letter, telephone, or personal contact. Here is an example:

> This study will be done on at least 50 premature and low-weight for age infants and their mothers. The mother must be willing to spend the required time with the infant. To be enrolled in the study, the infants must meet the criteria adapted from Ludington-Hoe et al. (1992).

30 or more weeks gestation or corrected age

Apgar at 5 minutes is 5 or more

Temperature stable for 24 hours prior to commencing study

No Phototherapy for 24 hours prior to commencing study

Nasogastric or oral feeds 1–4 hourly

Mild apnoea or bradycardia requiring mild stimulation only

No bag and mask resuscitation

May have nasal CPAP in situ, nasal cannula < 0.2L/min

Extubated > 48 hours, ceased cot or headbox oxygen > 24 hours

Nursed in an open cot or isolette

May have IV in progress

May be on course of antibiotics, theophylline, dexamethasone, or other drugs not maintaining systemic function

No maternal history of drug use

No congenital abnormalities or CNS impairment

Medically stable with clearance from unit specialist

Informed consent from participants for inclusion in study

Participants must be resident in the Darwin/Palmerston area and be prepared to spend a minimum of 2 hours/day for 5 days over maximum of 4 weeks

Participants must have a good understanding of English language

Furthermore, subjects will be prohibited from enrolment in the study if they have any of the following:

Intubation and IMV/IPPV

Hypertension

Umbilical artery/venous line in situ

Active sepsis

Bradycardia/apnoea requiring strong stimulation within 24 hours before study

Desaturation less than 88% > 3 minutes caused by anything other than artefact within 24 hours before or during KMC

The use of medications to maintain systemic functioning within 24 hours of inclusion in study

Intraventricular haemorrhage Grade III or IV confirmed by ultrasound

History of maternal substance abuse diagnosed by maternal history or neonatal examination

Once you have described your sampling procedures, you should state the number of groups, the number of participants in each group, and how they were allocated to the groups. Any special procedures such as matching participants on criteria, should be described, for example:

The subjects will be allocated randomly to two groups of approximately 25 subject pairs each, to allow for subject attrition. The groups will be stratified by gender to achieve an equal number of male and female infants in each group. One of the researchers (Roberts) will randomise the subject schedule prior to the study, and the assignments will be recorded in envelopes to be opened on enrolment of the infant in the study.

In the instruments and materials section, you will describe the instruments or materials that you will use. An instrument is any tool, including questionnaires, that you use to collect the data. The instrument should be the best possible one to assist you to answer the research question. It is not necessary to explain any standard tests, but you should explain any unconventional techniques, tests or instruments. You should state or describe any questionnaires that you propose to use, and refer the reader to an appendix, where you will include a full copy of the questionnaire. If the questionnaire is subject to copyright, you should obtain permission from the author to use it. If you propose to use a physical instrument it should be named if it is well known, for example a sphygmomanometer, or described if it is unusual or new. You should say how the instrument is scored or measured, for example on a Likert Scale or in millimetres of mercury. You can use diagrams or photographs of an instrument to avoid a long description. You should include a brief discussion of how the instrument has been used previously, according to the literature. You should justify your choice of the instrument in terms of its appropriateness to the research question or design. You should discuss the strengths and weaknesses of each instrument in terms of its reliability and validity. These concepts are discussed in Chapter 7.

It is always wise to use an instrument that has been developed already, but if you are developing your own instrument, you will need to show why no existing instrument meets your needs.

In the procedures section, you describe the procedures for the study. If it is an experiment, you describe how an experimental treatment will be applied. You state how, when and where you will collect the data. This information should be given in enough detail to allow someone to replicate your procedures. You will give your procedures for collecting the data in terms of what you intend to do to the participants. This will include procedures such as observing subjects or participants, administering a questionnaire, applying an instrument or administering an experimental treatment. Any lengthy instructions to the participants may be included in the appendix, but summarised here. Describe any calibration of the instruments or training to be given to the data collectors.

You should say when you will carry out your procedures and how long they will take so that each participant's time commitment is clear. If there is a particular time of day, week, month or year involved, this should be made clear. If the timing is complex, a diagram or flow chart may be helpful.

In this section, you should also state how you will record your data. If it is quantitative data, you can include a sample data roster as an appendix, or you can state that one is being devised. An example of a procedure section is as follows:

> The researchers working in the SCN (McEwen and Paynter) will identify prospective subjects who are physiologically stable and meet the criteria. The researchers will obtain approval from medical staff for enrolment of the subjects in the study and then approach the mothers to request their participation in the study. The researchers will explain the study and obtain informed consent. Participants will be told that they have only a 50 per cent chance of being in the KMC group. The infants will be enrolled in the study as soon as practicable after admission to the SCN.
>
> On enrolment, the mothers will be instructed by the SCN researchers on the care of the infant during the study. The KMC group will be exposed to skin-to-skin contact with their mothers who will be positioned in a suitable, comfortable chair in privacy. The infants will be dressed only in a nappy and possibly a bonnet for smaller babies, placed on the mother's skin and covered with a cloth. Appropriate variables will be measured before, during and after the research treatment. The CCC group will be swaddled in a bunny rug and fully dressed, including singlet and matinee jacket. Temperature will be taken before and after KMC or CCC cuddling. Gentle rocking may be permitted. Infants in both groups will be held for a minimum of two hours per day. Any monitors will be left in situ on the infant during the period of care. The mother may listen to music, enjoy hot or cold drinks etc. during KMC. Breastfeeding will be permitted *ad lib*. Few visitors will be permitted during the period.

Infants are normally weighed naked on the nursery scales once a day at approximately the same time. During the stay, the mothers will be given the questionnaires on stress and on attitudes to the SCN experience. Six weeks after discharge, or three months after birth, whichever is the later, the mothers will be contacted by telephone to determine whether they are still breastfeeding and given the perception of parenting skills questionnaire. Six months after birth, the mothers will be contacted to determine whether they are still breastfeeding, and if not, when they ceased.

Chart audit will be used to determine data on maternal control variables, infant weight gain and length of stay in the SCN, and breastfeeding. Data on the weight gained will be averaged across the length of stay. The length of stay will be calculated as the time between admission to and discharge from the SCN. Data will be recorded on the amount of cuddling time for the participants.

Data may be gathered from infants who do not receive cuddling from their mothers or close relatives during the study for purposes of baseline comparison of length of stay and average weight gain.

Prior to the commencement of the study, data will be collected by chart audit from 50 previously discharged SCN babies to determine more accurately a standard deviation of the weight gain and length of stay for the purposes of adjusting the sample size upwards if indicated.

Data on enrolled infants will be collected on gestational age, gender, birthweight, and apgar at 5 minutes. Data on enrolled mothers will be collected on age, parity, mode of delivery, previous neonatal death, ethnic group and duration of breastfeeding. These data will be collected by the SCN researchers by means of chart audit and the two groups will be compared to establish their initial equivalence.

Next, you should state your procedures for managing the data. These include co-ordination of data management if a multiple site is involved; data entry into the computer; and storage of original data, including how, where, and for how long it will be stored. You should also consider the ethical aspects of data management, including confidentiality of the data, previously addressed in Chapter 5. You should address the aspects of data coding: who will do it and how will it be done? Provision should be made for checking the data for errors in data entry. An example of a data management statement is as follows:

> The principal researcher will manage the data and will collect them from the midwives at both sites. The consent form will be separated from the questionnaire, thus protecting the anonymity of the subjects. Data will be entered into the computer by the researcher, using code numbers for subject identification in the computer. Data will be stored under lock and key in the researcher's office or another similar site for five years after collection.

A good research proposal will show a strong, clear, rigorous program for analysing the data. The methods of data analysis should follow from the research question, research design and hypotheses. In the proposal, you should state how you intend to analyse the data. You should say whether you intend to analyse the data by hand or computer, and if the latter, you should name the data analysis package that you intend to use.

You should justify your data analysis by showing which tests you intend to do to describe the variables and to check the validity of each hypothesis, including a restatement of the hypothesis. This allows the reader to assess the appropriateness of the data analysis in terms of the hypotheses and research questions. If the data analysis is complex, a flow chart may help. An example of a data analysis statement is:

> Data will be analysed by computer, using a suitable statistical package. One-tailed independent t-tests, analysis of variance, chi squares or other appropriate tests will be done to detect statistically significant differences in the two groups. A level of significance of 95 per cent will be set.

If you are planning to do a pilot study, which you should if at all possible, give the details here. If you have done a pilot study already, you should also give an outline of the methods and results here; it gives the reader confidence in your expertise and gives an indication of the feasibility of your study.

Ethical implications

Now that the reader knows how your study is going to be carried out, it is appropriate to discuss the ethical implications inherent in the study procedures. For a general research proposal that goes to a university research committee, this section can be brief. You will need to state your proposed procedures to obtain ethics clearance from university ethics and/or clinical ethics committees.

A proposal for an ethics committee is somewhat different. An ethics committee asks about the general design of the study not only to assess its scientific merit but also to determine the ethical implications of the study. Therefore, you should outline any ethical implications and how you propose to deal with them. These include prevention of harm to participants, and protection of the participants' rights to confidentiality, anonymity, and privacy. These were covered in Chapter 5. You should state whether a written consent is to be obtained from the participants, and justify the reasons if it is not to be obtained. For a discussion of when consent is necessary, see Chapter 5. If informed consent is being sought, you should satisfy the reader that you have made provision for the participants to be informed as to what will be required of them and the risks and benefits of participating in the study. You should include with your application a copy of your proposed plain language statement and consent form. In the consent form, make sure that you say that the participants will not be pressured into being in the study, will not be discriminated against if they do not take part in the study, and that they have the option of withdrawing from the study at any time without any penalty. An example of a statement about ethical considerations is as follows:

> While the literature has shown that KMC may be a superior method to conventional care, the conventional care provides a satisfactory standard of care so that no infant will be harmed by participating in the study. Any possible disadvantages to the conventional care group will be outweighed by the potential gains to many future infants and parents should the KMC method be shown to be superior and subsequently be adopted by the hospital as standard procedure.

Permission will be sought from the consultant paediatricians for each infant to be enrolled in the study. A mother will provide informed consent (see attached consent form) and can withdraw from the study at any time without penalty.

Since there is no invasive intervention in the study there should be no harmful effects on the infants or mothers from participation in the study. Medical practitioners will be consulted if in the opinion of the midwives there is any possibility that continuation in the study would not be in the best interests of the infant. If an infant's health deteriorates, the infant will be withdrawn from the study, either temporarily or permanently depending on the permission from the medical practitioner for the infant to re-enrol in the study.

Data will be collected in a data book that will be accessible only to the researchers. Subjects will be identified in the computer by subject number only. The master list linking the subject numbers and the hospital numbers will be kept in a filing cabinet in a locked office. Consent forms will be attached to the charts and will be filed as above on discharge. Consent will be sought at this time from mothers for further information concerning behavioural and physical milestones to be obtained from the charts at a later date for follow-up purposes.

This study does not involve any Indigenous communities directly nor does it consider Aboriginality in any way as a variable. Indigenous mothers and infants from the urban areas may well be enrolled in the study considering the population profile of the Royal Darwin Hospital. Given the design of the study, there should be an equal number of these subjects in each group. Indigenous mothers who return to their communities while the infant remains in the hospital will not be able to enrol in the study since they will not be able to adhere to the protocol.

There are some special considerations that may have to be dealt with in some studies. If you are using vulnerable participants, you must justify the choice of these, describe the procedures you intend to put in place to protect their rights, and state who will give consent on their behalf. If you are seeking to observe participants without their express individual consent, you must justify why you have selected this method and you must show that the costs in terms of potential invasion of privacy are less than the potential benefits of such a study.

At the end of the methodology section, it is customary to acknowledge any weaknesses of the theoretical or methodological approaches that you have chosen. Remember that the reader may be an experienced and distinguished scientist who will spot flaws in your design. It is better to acknowledge the flaws in your design, that is, the threats to validity, and explain how you will deal with them than to try to gloss over them and hope no-one will notice. Remember that no-one expects your study to have a perfect design and what counts is that you are aware of the limitations and can deal with them.

Dissemination of results

The proposal should include a plan for the dissemination of results and the implementation of the findings. For example, it could state that you will be giving a presentation on the results of the study and/or a written report to the institution, you will be presenting a paper at a conference or you intend to submit the results for publication in a journal. You could also state any plans for implementing your findings to change ward practice.

Work plan or time frame

A work plan may be included in a proposal for university or funding committees. This is an overall description of the sequence and duration of tasks that must be carried out. It indicates to the reader how realistic the research plan is, and how thorough the researcher has been in considering all that needs to be done to carry out the research project. The work plan incorporates the tasks, personnel requirements, estimate of time required to carry out each part of the project, and date by which each part should be done. It is often shown as a schedule or as a flow chart. For an example of a work plan, see the section in this chapter on qualitative research proposals.

Resources and budget

A good research proposal will show that the physical and human resources available are sufficient to carry out the project satisfactorily. A section on the background of the researcher, the physical resources and the budget required to run the project will be required by granting agencies and universities. In the budget section, you will give the costs for all of the materials, personnel and equipment that you will require to carry out the project to a successful completion. The major cost components are direct costs, that is, costs that are specific to the project, and indirect costs, or infrastructure costs that are incurred by the institution as a result of supporting your project.

Direct costs are usually broken down into salary costs and costs for equipment, materials and procedures. Salary costs would include salaries of secretaries, research assistants and the researcher. They should also include nursing time if nurses in the clinical area are involved as data collectors (Haller 1988). Salary costs also include a component for extra costs such as annual leave, payroll tax and the like. Your financial services personnel can advise you as to the appropriate costs to charge. There may also be costs for work carried out by non-salaried personnel such as typing, consulting, data entry, and data transcription services. Costs for equipment would include any instruments, computer software, equipment such as video cameras or tape recorders, and purchase or rental of computers. Materials would include stationery, videocassettes, audiocassettes, postage, report preparation and dissemination. Procedure costs would include printing, photocopying and laboratory analysis of data. There may also be other incidental costs such as travel and accommodation if you are collecting data out of town.

Indirect costs are usually referred to as 'infrastructure costs'. These include use of the telephone, fax, office, computing time etc. Students carrying out projects for a qualification will not usually have to include infrastructure costs in a proposal because it is taken for granted that the university supplies these as a part of the student's educational package. However, proposals for grants from outside the institution will normally be required to include an infrastructure component in the budget. Infrastructure costs are usually calculated by a formula devised by the institution and you should use this formula to calculate any such costs. For an example of a budget statement, see the qualitative proposal section of this chapter.

Details of researchers

For proposals other than classroom projects, you should include the curricula vitae (CVs) of the researchers involved in the project. The CV is included so that the person evaluating the proposal can judge whether the applicant has the necessary credentials and experience to carry out the project successfully. In organising the CV, you should emphasise your qualifications and relevant experience by putting them first. You should include a list of publications, if any, and any other research projects you have done.

Elements of a qualitative research proposal

To some extent, there are similarities in quantitative and qualitative research proposals. For example, the preliminary pages are much the same and within the body of the report the introduction has a similar structure. However, the rest of the body of the proposal may be substantially different from a quantitative proposal. Indeed, qualitative proposals may differ from one another depending on the kind of approach they intend to take.

Because qualitative proposals have to be scrutinised by academic departments, health agency organisations, funding bodies and ethics committees that are often composed of people with backgrounds in quantitative research, qualitative proposals must conform to some extent with these people's expectations of what constitutes a 'proper' research proposal. Too much creativity at this stage of the research may result in obstruction to the research at the outset. Therefore, it is important that qualitative proposals are written carefully, clearly and with a sound rationale for all of the proposed steps in the project.

To demonstrate how to prepare a qualitative proposal, we will work through an example of a proposal, pointing out how other qualitative proposals may differ. The example given is of a proposal that was submitted to a funding body (Taylor 2000c), in which there were no nurses deciding on the merits of various proposals; therefore, it was important to be clear about the focus and methodology of the project, as it would have to 'stand alone' without the benefit of 'insider knowledge' at the meeting.

The title

Be clear about what it is you want to know and why you want to know it, so that you will be able to give the research a title. The title should clarify the research approach, what the research is about and the people and setting involved. For example it might read:

> Improving the quality of hospital ward nursing care through reflective practice and action research with Registered Nurses.

Research summary

Sometimes called an abstract, the research summary provides an overall picture of what the project hopes to achieve as well as when and how. It is important to be concise. For example:

> This one-year action research project aims to facilitate reflective practice processes in experienced Registered Nurses, in order to raise critical awareness of practice problems they face every day, to work systematically through problem-solving processes to uncover constraints against effective nursing care, and to improve the quality of care given by hospital nurses in light of the identified constraints and possibilities. Convenience sampling will be used to target intentionally those research participants who are interested in reflecting on their practice in order to improve it. The nurses will meet weekly to discuss clinical problems raised by them in their journal writing and discussion, and to work through action research cycles to plan, assess, act and reflect on thematic concerns.

Research significance, aims and objectives

Aims are overall intentions and objectives are specific subsets of the intentions. At this point, a statement may be made about the significance of the project. For example:

Significance

> The significance of the project is in improving nursing care and in educating nurses in a process that they can use for any clinical problems that emerge in their practice well after the completion of this project. Nurses need to think quickly and carefully in the course of their everyday work to make accurate clinical decisions. Reflective processes will allow them to reflect effectively in and on action. Also, nurses work under complex historical, economic, cultural, social and political constraints that they need to identify and work towards changing. Working through this project will give nurses the 'tools' they require for changing anything they may face in the future. Therefore, the project will not only serve as a medium for immediate improved practice, but also as a lifelong educating process for nurses for future practice improvements.

Aims

> This project aims to facilitate reflective practice processes in experienced Registered Nurses, in order to raise critical awareness of practice problems they face every day, to work systematically through problem-solving processes to uncover constraints against effective nursing care, and to improve the quality of care given by hospital nurses in light of the identified constraints and possibilities.

Research questions

Specific questions related to the research objectives may be posed at this point. These questions will indicate the problem focus you are taking in the research. Questions of this nature may not be appropriate to all qualitative proposals, as some critical approaches may intend to use participatory processes in which the participants work collaboratively to raise questions as the research moves through cycles and group processes. However, if a proposal chooses to pose questions they may resemble the following examples:

- What practice problems do nurses face every day?
- What constraints weigh against effective nursing care?
- How can the quality of nursing care given by hospital nurses be improved, in light of the identified constraints and possibilities?

Background and literature review

Sometimes a background statement precedes the literature review, to set the context for how the ideas for the research came into being. For example:

> The idea for the research arose from a conversation with a local Director of Nursing, who indicated that nurses need the means of working through situational constraints to improve nursing practice in hospital wards. Although nurses may intend to give quality care, this is not always possible given the complex historical, cultural, social, economic, political and personal factors that may be operating in any care setting at any time. This is particularly so in hospitals where unquestioned rituals, practices and procedures may have been etched into the fabric of the bureaucracy, thereby becoming resistant to change.

The reasons for the literature review are similar to those already outlined in this chapter in 'Elements of a quantitative research proposal'. You may choose to refer to these comments to refresh your memory of them. However, there are some areas that need to be highlighted in a general approach to writing a literature review for qualitative proposals.

First, the suggestion to base the project in a nursing model is a good one, but it is not one all researchers may choose to take up. If the model fits well, use it. If not, do not. Also, it will be important to choose a model that fits with the particular methodological approach you are taking. For example, the model put forward by Parse (1987) may suit some phenomenological projects.

Secondly, there may not be much empirical literature in a highly unusual area of interest as is the case with many qualitative projects that try to push the boundaries of what can be known about phenomena. In this case, the literature may need to be linked indirectly to the main ideas in the research. Allied, nonspecific information may be shown through the proposed methods and processes to be related to and informative for the research interest.

Lastly, some approaches such as grounded theory may claim that their inductive style suggests that literature not be amassed at this stage. This is a good enough stance if it can be substantiated. However, be aware that some people reading the proposal may assume that the failure to present a literature review is a 'cop out' and that the prospective researchers may not even be aware of literature in the area.

With these disclaimers in mind, the rules of a thorough literature review still apply just as much to qualitative proposals as they do to quantitative proposals.

Continuing the proposal in this section, an example of a literature review may be:

> Nurses work in settings that have a direct bearing on the quality of the care they give. Reflective practice and action research are the methodological approaches for the proposed project. Therefore, the literature reviewed included areas relating to the nature of nursing practice in hospitals, reflective practice and action research in nursing.
>
> **The nature of nursing practice in hospitals**
>
> Nursing in hospitals involves negotiating complex interpersonal relationships, and working in a social and political context within economic constraints, while balancing a multiplicity of tasks and roles. Nurses are busy practitioners who need to have a broad range of clinical knowledge and skills, and they are accountable to many people (Benner 1984; Benner & Wrubel 1989; Taylor 1997). Authors agree on the chaotic nature of nursing practice (Holmes 1992; Pearson & Vaughan 1989) and the constraints nurses face every day in delivering quality care (Cox, Hickson & Taylor 1991; Pearson & Vaughan 1989; Street 1995; Taylor 1994, 2000a, 2000b).
>
> Nurses in hospitals work within the possibilities and constraints of bureaucratic organisational structures. This means that nurses work in political contexts where powerful people compete for scarce health care resources. Hospital doctors occupy high positions in terms of power and prestige and their roles have been described according to 'the biomedical model'. The biomedical model can be traced back to Descartes (1970 trans) who described the mind–body split and thereby reduced people to parts with machine-like functions. These reductionist criteria are bound up in the power of knowledge held by medical practitioners and their ability to dispense it, for a fee, to people who require their assistance (Friedson 1970). Pearson and Vaughan (1989) claim that, in adopting the biomedical model, nursing has resulted in routinisation with a focus on physical care and getting the work done. This is in contrast to holistic nursing models, which favour viewing patients as people in relation to their illness circumstances (Parse 1987; Watson 1988). Hospital nurses are caught up in the contradictions of how patients are viewed and managed by members of the health team. According to Street (1995) reflective process will allow them to work through these differences and to negotiate nursing care in light of them.
>
> Added to these considerations, the New South Wales College of Nursing (1992a, 1992b) asserts that there has been a tendency of health care organisations to use standardised systems to quantify health services in terms of effectiveness and efficiency. This has resulted in a tendency to value nursing in relation to its measurable outcomes (Sydney Metropolitan Teaching Hospitals Nursing Consortium 1992) resulting in a relative underestimation of the interpersonal nature of nursing and its therapeutic effects. Some commentators have assigned the need for the quantification of roles and functions, within nursing specifically, to biomedical tendencies within the health care system generally (Johnson 1980; King 1981; Beckstrand 1987). In contrast, others have argued that nursing needs to be

judged by quantitative and qualitative criteria, given that its nature and effects relate to health and healing (Kitson 1984; Kleiman 1986; McMahon & Pearson 1991; Taylor 1992; Roberts & Taylor 1998). The proposed research would satisfy the need for quantification and offer opportunities for qualification of nursing practice, given that its methods would include a combination of both approaches.

Reflective practice

In Australian universities teachers of nursing courses have adopted reflective practitioner concepts and strategies (Reid 1994). This tendency can be traced to 1988, when educationists offering postgraduate courses in education to nurses introduced some principles of critical theory and connected them to reflective practice. In essence, reflective practice is the systematic and thoughtful means by which practitioners can make sense of their practice as they go about their daily work. The need for reflection in action as it happens (reflection in action), and on action after the event (reflection on action), is built on the supposition that practitioners know more than they realise and they need ways of bringing that knowledge to their active awareness (Schon 1983).

Reflective practice was introduced to nurses and midwives in a way that encouraged them to reflect on and in their practice worlds, to develop ways of changing them (Schon 1983, 1987; Boud, Keogh & Walker 1985; Carr & Kemmis 1986; Smyth 1986). This intention carried with it a strong critical theory flavour derived from Marxist politics, which encouraged nurses and midwives to assess the status quo to find the constraining factors within it. Having done this, they were encouraged to find strategies for freeing themselves from these forces, to be liberated to more empowered and effective practice (Habermas 1973; Bernstein 1978; Giroux 1983; Schon 1983, 1987; Boud, Keogh & Walker 1985; Carr & Kemmis 1986; Smyth 1986).

Another underlying principle of reflective practice is that practitioners have a tendency to take their knowledge and skills for granted, and when talking about their mode of employment, they tend to preface their comments with: 'I'm just a nurse'. Blumberg (1990, p. 236) argues that practitioners need 'to change how they think about their work', in that they need to value themselves as practitioners and the knowledge and skills of their day-to-day practice. Research has shown that reflective practice offers nurses a stronger sense of personal and professional worth (Blumberg 1990; Boykin 1998; Johns & McCormack 1998; Lumby 1998; Taylor 1998) although caution has been emphasised about the high degree of personal investment required by nurses for successful practice outcomes (Taylor 1997).

Unfortunately, systematic and purposeful reflection is not necessarily 'second nature' to people. Schon (1987) argues that practitioners need coaching to deal with practice problems. Other writers agree that coaching is necessary and that it promotes collaborative knowing (Greenwood 1993; Conway 1994). Coaching in reflective processes also encourages co-operative communication between the instructor and participants (Belenky et al. 1986). Newell (1992) and Von Wright (1992) claim that education is needed in the art of reflection. Emphasising the need for purposeful and systematic reflection, Newell (1992) argues that mentors and support persons need time in training and support themselves, in order to be of service to others on coaching them in reflective skills. In the case of practitioners of mature age, however, it might be expected that without too much effort adults can build on their life experiences to make sense out of what happens at work (Knowles 1980). One of the aims of the proposed research is to provide expert coaching in reflective processes so nurses will be able to achieve systematic and purposeful reflection.

There are various means by which practitioners may undertake reflective practice. Methods for reflection include journal writing, metaphor analysis, storytelling and portfolio development (Caffarella 1994). Schon (1987) suggests the use of reflective diaries for personal reflections. Nurses have a rich oral tradition and they have many stories to tell, therefore personal reflections in diaries or on audiotape about interesting, and possibly disturbing, events may be a favoured means of assisting reflection. Shared in a trusting group setting, some authors claim that these stories have even more potential for raised awareness and change (Glaze 1998; Graham 1998).

Action research

Action research grew out of the effects of the Second World War and it had a social change agenda. Kurt Lewin (1946) first used the term 'action research' and in the mid-1940s he used group research processes for community projects in post-war America. Lewin's work is the basis of contemporary versions of action research including those forwarded by Australian educationists (Carr & Kemmis 1986; McTaggart 1991). Action research goes to the site of the concern or practice and works with the people there as co-researchers to generate solutions to the problems with which they are keen to deal. This type of research involves action that is directed at showing the problems in the present situation and facilitating improvements and sustaining changes to them.

The theoretical assumptions underlying action research can be traced to critical theory. McTaggart (1991, p. 25) makes the point that 'many authors in both Europe and Australia have used the theory of knowledge-constitutive interests proposed by the German critical theorist Jurgen Habermas (1973) to describe three different forms of action research: technical, practical and emancipatory'. Technical action research aims to improve techniques and procedures, by having practitioners work collaboratively to test the applicability of results generated elsewhere. Technical action research nursing projects include approaches to solve problems associated with the effective use of double staff time (Ramudu et al. 1994), problems associated with incontinence (Frey-Hoogwerf 1996) and problematic telephone orders (Retsas 1994).

Practical action research aims to improve existing practices and to develop new ones. The emphasis here is in reflecting and interpreting to take deliberate strategic action. Nursing projects using this orientation are the expanding role of the nurse consultant (O'Brien & Spry 1995), and the nature and effects of midwifery practice (Taylor, King & Stewart 1995).

Emancipatory action research involves a group of practitioners taking responsibility for freeing themselves from the constraints of their practice through understanding and transforming the political, social and economic conditions that keep them from doing their work as they would choose ideally. An important nursing project of an emancipatory nature relates predominantly to improving paediatric nursing practice (Street 1995). The research describes the collaborative processes undertaken by the nurses and researcher based on the liberating assumptions of emancipatory action research. This project will facilitate all kinds of action research, depending on whether nurses have technical, practical and/or emancipatory interests.

Although action research has been used extensively by teachers in Australian education since the early 1980s, it has only been taken up since the mid 1980s by Australian nurses studying education off campus through Deakin University, who introduced it into mainstream nursing research. Even so, there are few published reports of action research in nursing practice relative to the anecdotal evidence that many projects are being undertaken throughout Australian nursing. The proposed research fills a need for documented evidence of reflective processes used in action research while addressing directly the constraints of everyday nursing practice in hospital settings.

The references may be included immediately after the literature review, or may appear in an appendix attached to the proposal. You will find the references for this literature review at the end of this chapter.

Research plan, including methodology, methods and processes

A research plan is roughly equivalent to the methodology section of a quantitative proposal, in that it includes information about the study setting, participants and methods to be used. However, there are differences that relate mainly to the use of specific language. For example, generally speaking when qualitative researchers refer to methodology, they are referring to the theoretical assumptions underlying the choice of methods. This means that in the proposal under the word 'methodology' there will appear a short description of the theoretical tradition informing the project. For example:

Methodology

In the context of this research approach, methodology means the theoretical assumptions of how knowledge is generated and validated, which underlie the choice of methods. Given the collaborative nature of the project, a qualitative approach has been chosen, informed by reflective practitioner concepts and the technical, practical and emancipatory intentions of action research.

Methods and processes

Qualitative research often differentiates between the ways of organising the research and collecting and analysing the information (methods) and the interpersonal processes that are used in accessing, informing, maintaining and closing relationships with participants throughout the research (processes). With these differences between methods and processes in mind, it is still important to give a full account of all your intentions in doing the research. For example:

Number of participants and access arrangements

> Full ethical clearance processes will precede the commencement of the project. Ten experienced Registered Nurses working in a large local rural hospital will be invited by the researcher to participate. A spoken and written explanation of the project will be given by the researcher at a regular meeting of Clinical Nurse Specialists.

It may be necessary to provide a rationale for the number of participants, especially if the proposal is likely to be judged against empirico-analytical criteria. Committee members may not be aware of the assumptions of the nature of knowledge generated and validated through qualitative research. The extent to which you produce a strongly referenced rationale will depend on the likelihood of its being needed. It may be worthwhile checking on the composition of certain committees judging research proposals to see if they are open to and aware of the assumptions of qualitative research. For instance you might to decide that it is advisable to write a few (non-patronising, non-jargonistic) sentences about the relative and context-dependent nature of knowledge.

You may also decide that it is wise to give a sound set of reasons for what may be construed by some commentators as a 'small sample size'. You might also need to justify your 'sampling' methods, that is, how you will go about accessing the participants. Be clear about what you write. For instance, you might consider statements such as: '*This research approach is interested in accessing participants who have experience in the research interest. They have been sought intentionally for their ability to inform the research from their personal perspectives*'. In the case of the example in this section, I wrote:

> Convenience sampling will be used to target intentionally those research participants who are interested in reflecting on their practice in order to improve it. The number of participants is appropriate for this qualitative project because of the duration of this research and its potential to generate rich data sufficient to bring about changes in work practices. The number of participants is also congruent with the assumptions of qualitative research, which emphasise the context-dependent quality of process, experience and language. Therefore, this project does not seek high numbers to generalise results or use them for predictive purposes. Also, in collaborative research of this nature, the process becomes as important as the potential outcomes, because the focus is on what people learn as they experience the research itself.

You will need to decide whether it is advisable to compare and contrast quantitative and qualitative methods of accessing participants. If you choose this option be careful not to overdo the teaching angle. Intelligent people do not necessarily like to feel they are 'being hit over the head' with details that make them feel ignorant. However, they may respond to a clear and succinct synopsis that justifies qualitative research activities that differ from those to which they are most accustomed.

Data collection

Be sure to include all of the points about what data you will collect and how you will collect it. Provide examples of the questions you intend to ask. Even if they are open-ended to facilitate a spontaneous conversation, they need to be included. For a collaborative project it may not be possible to predict questions that may arise from group processes. Nevertheless, this should be explained at this point of the proposal, so that people who are uninformed about the methodology you are using will be able to understand why the questions are not given in this instance.

If the methodology you are using allows for questions to be posed, be sure that you intend to ask questions that will give you the information you need. For example:

> The nurses will meet weekly to discuss clinical problems raised by them in their journal writing and discussion. The initial meeting will be facilitated by the researcher, who will explain the project materials, including reflective practitioner guidelines and action research aims, processes and strategies. After a few weeks and at a time when the group feels confident, the researcher will hand over the chairing of the meeting to group members, who can refer to her at any time for guidance and advice.

Introduction and overview of methods and processes

The methods and processes used will be appropriate for reflective practice strategies and action research. 'Methods' refers to the kinds of activities that will be done. 'Processes' refers to how certain activities will be done. Although these methods and processes are difficult to separate, this will be attempted in this description so that the intentions can be stated as clearly as possible.

For the reflective practice component, methods will include becoming familiar with some reflective practitioner literature and with the activities outlined in the project materials (Taylor, King & Stewart 1995; Taylor 2000b). Processes to enable effective reflection will include coaching and practice in writing and speaking descriptively, in confidential and facilitative group meetings. Confidence will be bolstered in undertaking reflection in practice (during practice) and reflection on practice (after practice) through individual and collective storytelling, journalling, critical analysis and discussion.

The methods of action research involve a four-stage problem-solving approach of collectively planning, acting, observing and reflecting. This phase leads to another cycle of action, in which the plan is revised, and further acting, observing and reflecting is undertaken systematically, to work towards solutions to problems of a technical, practical or emancipatory nature (Kemmis & McTaggart 1988). The planning and acting stages may include any appropriate methods of gathering and analysing data, such as participant observation, surveys and interviews. Cycles of action research will lead to further foci and members could keep an action research approach to their work for as long as they choose, given that clinical nursing practice is fraught typically with many challenges on a daily basis.

Action research processes include attracting nurses to the project who are willing to work together over time on collective practice problems. The group would need to understand some basic principles of action research, in terms of its intention to change existing conditions to make them better. Members of the group would also need to be willing to share the workload and responsibilities of the research project and to assist one another to create effective co-researcher processes. Having established the working rules of the group, attention will be given to maintaining effective and trusting group processes, so that members continue to be facilitative and focused on the problems at hand.

The research processes will begin with nurses locating in their practice issues and constraints that they want to change. It is important that the nurses 'own' the research questions they generate and the intervention strategies, so time will be taken initially to deal with some issues in the group and in their own practice. Such issues may include power relationships and gender mix in the group if, for instance, the group includes relatively senior and/or male nurses, who may have the potential for a silencing effect on the others.

Common concerns will be identified and reconnaissance will be conducted, which means that an initial investigation of specific situations will be undertaken to get an overall idea of what is happening there. Members will then focus on a specific concern of interest to them all. They will write down their stories about the focus of concern and share these accounts in the weekly meeting of the group. The first action cycle will occur after the reconnaissance and a literature review, and it will address itself to questions about the situation. The questions will be: 'What is happening here?' 'Why is it happening?' 'What do we want to change about the situation?' Data collection strategies will include quantitative and qualitative approaches, depending on what is needed and what would best serve the purposes of the research. The findings will be pooled and discussed and the appropriate action will be taken. Observation of the effects will follow, before further reflection leads to further action. In this way, the nurses will evolve a collaborative working process for managing clinical issues of concern to them.

As explained in the previous section, the planning and acting phases may include any appropriate methods of gathering and analysing data. Data sources and instruments may include journalling, participant observation, surveys and interviews, depending on whether the methods are needed to quantify or qualify findings. Surveys may be necessary to ascertain mathematical incidences and relationships of variables in certain clinical problems. Methods such as journalling, participant observation and interviews may be required to describe the nature and effects of clinical experiences.

Nurses may maintain a journal of their experiences, the non-confidential parts of which they will be expected to share with peers in a weekly group meeting. As reflective practice may be undertaken in many ways, the kind of reflection may be determined to some extent by the kind of knowledge nurses are seeking to generate in and through their practice. If nurses intend to increase their understanding of things of interest in their practice, they might lean towards technical and practical reflective strategies. The types of questions they could pose when engaging in interpretive reflection might include: 'What is happening here?', 'What is the nature of … ?', 'What is the experience of … ?' If nurses intend to change the constraining nature and effects of political, economic, cultural, social and/or historical elements in their practice, they will require emancipatory reflective strategies. The types of questions that they could pose when engaging in critical reflection might include: 'What is happening here?', 'What factors have made it this way?', 'How might this be different?'

Participant observation will be during practice in ward areas. Notes and/or journal entries may be made during or after the nursing activities, although, given the immediacy of ward situations, note-taking/journalling is more likely to occur afterwards. Structured observation using checklists of frequently occurring behaviours may also be used if these are deemed to provide the kind of data required.

Simple surveys may be needed when nurses want to canvass a sample of people's attitudes to identified nursing and health care issues. Interviews may be needed when in-depth responses are required to describe people's experiences of nursing and health care. The choice of method will depend on what information is required, in what form, and for what purposes.

Ethical requirements

It is necessary to provide a full account of ethical considerations to be given to participants, including informed consent to ensure their privacy and anonymity, and the assurance that they can choose to withdraw from the research at any time, without penalty. Full ethical clearance will need to be sought from participating institutions. It is usual to submit a full research plan, including ethical statements, a plain language statement and a consent form for each category of participants. Ethical considerations may include these sorts of statements:

> Research participants have the right to consent freely and without coercion. They will be offered the right to refuse to participate, or to withdraw at any time, without penalty or coercion of any kind.
>
> Measures taken to ensure that research participants have the capacity to understand the research project will be to ascertain that each participant can comprehend English, and to provide the services of an interpreter should this be necessary.
>
> The forms given to participants will be relative to their comprehension. Participants will receive detailed explanations, orally and in writing, of what the research involves, the aims and the processes of the research, and participants' commitments in it. Nurses are the main participants in this research, so the plain language statement and the consent form will be written relative to their comprehension, bearing in mind that nurses are professionals conversant with

language used in higher education institutions and health care settings. Even so, any words and sentences which may cause confusion will be paraphrased into simple English so that the meaning is clear and unambiguous. The project will also be explained orally in plain language by the researcher. Participants will have opportunities to ask questions, make comments and voice any concerns that they may have concerning the project at the outset and throughout the duration of the project.

As this research encourages nurses to share their practice stories, likely risks are that the privacy and confidentiality of patients may be breached and that nurses may feel vulnerable in sharing their experiences, leading to embarrassment or possible emotional catharsis such as tearfulness or anger.

Nurses are educated in the need for patient confidentiality and they practise it daily in their work. Even so the researcher will ensure that privacy and confidentiality measures are instituted and maintained. Stories written in journals and shared in group meetings will be devoid of information that could identify patients, relatives and staff. Pseudonyms will be used and identifying material will be omitted or rewritten to protect the identities of people within the transcripts of the stories. Reflective journals will remain the personal property of participants and they will not be read or sighted by the researcher, unless it is the participants' expressed wish that this occurs. Reports and published material will describe the participants' stories and interpretations according to the issues they raised and the practice improvements they caused, rather than to identify specific people, places and situations. All data collected in the course of the research will be secured in a locked storage compartment for five years and the responsibility for the safety and security of it will reside with the researcher.

With respect to risks associated with emotional catharsis, the group will offer support to its members and the researcher is an experienced nurse with 30 years of group management and support. Should any member become emotionally upset beyond the ability of the group to offer support, he or she will be offered professional counselling. Two supporting counsellors are (name, phone number) and (name, phone number). They are aware of the project and have indicated their willingness to act as counsellors should their involvement become necessary.

The forms will indicate a clear explanation of the benefits of the project – the facilitation of reflective practice to improve nursing care.

As mentioned, the risks of the project are breaches of confidentiality and emotional catharsis, and these risks will be communicated to participants at the outset of the project and repeated as often as necessary so that participants remember the need for patient confidentiality and the availability of group and professional support. Benefits to participants include knowledge and practice of reflection and the improvement of nursing care.

Participants will be informed orally and in writing that they are at liberty to withdraw from the project at any time, without penalty or coercion of any kind.

As this project involves nurses who are healthy, consciously aware adults, they are able to consent for themselves. The issue of special cases does not apply to patients in this research, because oral consent from legally competent adults is sufficient for the simple surveys that may be used as part of the data collection phases in action research.

Analysis and interpretation

The proposal must set out clearly the methods for sorting (analysing) and making sense (interpreting) of the data. This is the main way the project will be judged as trustworthy when completed. Therefore, the proposal should be very clear about how you intend to analyse and interpret the data, so the people judging the merits of the proposal can consider whether your plans for this phase are reasonable in relation to the rest of the project.

Continuing the example in this section, the analysis and interpretation part of the proposal may include statements such as:

> The data analysis methods will depend on the types of data collection used. Analysis of journal experiences will be managed by individual and group critical reflection and problem-solving strategies. Group discussion will also be used to identify the specific nature and determinants of problems as well as the most appropriate methods to investigate problems further and the most practical and useful plan of action. Descriptions of participant observation and interview audiotapes and notes will be analysed by manual thematic analysis techniques (Roberts & Taylor 1998). Surveys will be analysed by manual or computer techniques according to their depth and scope, although it is envisaged that most quantitative measures will be relatively brief and simple, and therefore will be analysed effectively by manual estimation of the frequency and extent of identified variables. If descriptions and measurements of relationships between variables are required a computer-based program will be used, such as factor analysis and/or ANOVA.
>
> As mentioned previously, in each action research cycle the findings will be pooled and discussed and the appropriate action will be planned and taken. Successive observation of the effects will follow, before further reflection leads to further action and analysis.

Dissemination of findings

The proposal should contain a plan for the dissemination of findings. This will show that you are aware that the research will be rendered meaningless if the results are not shared with the people who may benefit from them. For example:

> The researcher will use this phase of the project to teach nurses how to plan for oral presentations to peers, and how to write for publication in refereed journals. A potential target for national presentation is the annual clinical practice conference organised by the Department of Nursing at the University of Adelaide. Local venues for speaking about the research may also include nurses' seminars at local hospitals and various nurse interest groups in the region. National refereed journals that could be targeted for publication include *Contemporary Nurse* and the *Australian Journal of Advanced Nursing Practice*. International refereed journals for which the project is suitable include the *International Journal of Nursing Practice* and *Advances in Nursing Science*. These journals will

be targeted with articles written by a combination of group members, depending on who is interested and willing to expend time and energy in getting quality articles ready for publication. In all presentations and articles each member of the group will receive acknowledgement, although they may not necessarily be listed as contributors if they have not taken a share of the workload for the oral presentation or the written article.

Of course, participants' first point of dissemination may be in thesis form to the tertiary organisation in which they are enrolled. The organisation will deposit the thesis in the library for access by borrowers. It is also a good idea for students to make plans to disseminate the research findings at professional conferences, and in journals and monographs. These avenues for dissemination will be discussed later in this book.

The project time frame

The proposal needs to show that you are organised as far as time is concerned and that you have allowed enough time to complete the project within the prescribed period. The funding body and/or your organisation will want to know what you are going to do, and when, so that they can be assured that the project will be completed on time. An example of a time frame might be:

(Year)

January–February	Finalise ethics approval
	Decide on group membership
	Begin reflective and action research methods and processes
March–September	Continue and document action cycles of planning, acting, observing and reflecting
October–November	Facilitate tuition and practice in preparing for professional presentations and publication
December	Submit the final report
	Finalise plans for the dissemination of results

Budget

If you are applying for a research grant to assist you in completing your research award, you will need to give careful consideration to the costs involved. Most grant bodies require a detailed budget, outlining costs for the research personnel (research assistants, desktop publishers, clerical assistance and so on); equipment (computer data analysis system, audiotapes and so on); travel at x cents per kilometre; and other costs, such as photocopying, mailing and so on. The grant application form will make it clear what the funding body will or will not fund, so be sure to read the information carefully.

Although the following example (Figure 6.3) was used to procure funds for a project not done as part of a research award, it may give you some idea of what is expected in an itemised budget and justification of the need for funds.

Detailed budget items	Priority	Amount requested		
		2000	2001	2002
Research assistant Paid at HEW Level 5/1, at a base rate of $22.01/hour (includes 16.5% on-costs) for 240 hours, to assist CI in arranging access, consent, and conduct and evaluation of cycles, including sequential data collection, analysis, and interpretation over a 9-month action research period	A	$5282.40		
Transcription assistant costs 40 half-hour tapes × 1.5 hrs/tape, equals 60 hrs @ $18.76/hr (includes 16.5% on-costs)	A	$1125.60		
Maintenance 40 TDK audiotapes ($32 × 4 boxes of 10)	B	$128.00		
Total	(n/a)	$6536.00		

Figure 6.3 Example of a budget

Funding bodies want to know about each item of research expenditure in your budget, to know that the money is justified and that you will use it prudently. You need to be as clear as possible in writing this section. For example:

Justification of the budget

Although I will be responsible for the conduct and evaluation of the project, I will need the help of an experienced Research Assistant (RA), who is also a Registered Nurse with an honours degree. My role as an academic has many research, teaching and community liaison facets; therefore, I need to delegate some of the practical aspects of research projects to an RA. Duties will include assistance in arranging access and consent, and helping in the conduct and evaluation of cycles. Specific duties will include the preparation and sequential data collection of surveys and interviews in the clinical area. 240 hours of work are needed to assist me in these duties over a nine-month action research period (seven hours per week for 34 weeks). The HEW Level 5/1 reflects the level of qualification and experience of an RA with established clinical competence and a high degree of confidentiality, capable of working with minimal supervision in a sensitive area of research.

The transcription assistant costs reflect the lengthy and tedious process of transcribing audiotapes. It takes three hours to transcribe a one-hour tape, and it must be done by a proficient and reliable person to maintain the integrity of the data. The number of tapes is an estimate for a nine-month data-gathering period in a wide variety of nursing settings with a range of people, including patients, relatives and health care workers.

High-quality audiotapes are required for safe recording and storing of interview data for analysis.

Summary

There are similarities in quantitative and qualitative research proposals; however, there are also differences. The similarities are in the structure of the format of a proposal. The differences relate to the use of words in the body of the report to describe the chosen research methodology, methods and processes. Qualitative researchers also need to be discerning in presenting their proposals to committees who may come from an empirico-analytical background, as criteria from that background may be used as a frame of reference for judging the merits of a qualitative proposal.

Common final elements

The final pages of any research proposal contain supporting materials – information that relates back to the material in the body of the proposal. Principally these materials are a full reference list and any appendixes containing additional material not central to the proposal but providing additional information and examples.

References

The list of references should come at the end of the proposal but before the appendixes. You should follow the referencing system recommended by your institution. Usually it is only the university that will have requirements for a particular referencing system. If you have a choice, you should use a user-friendly referencing system such as the author–date system (Harvard) unless your guidelines stipulate a different one. The Harvard system is economical in terms of time and is very flexible, as entries can be added, deleted, or changed with a minimum of disruption to the rest of the document. In addition, the reader is able to tell immediately who the author is and when the reference was published. Other systems, such as the endnote system or the footnote (Oxford) system require an adjustment of all following reference numbers whenever a reference is inserted or removed.

The Harvard system has been used in this book, so for details on how to apply it, consult the references here. References for the two proposals in this chapter can be found in the reference list on pages 170–4. For further details, consult the Australian Government Printing Service *Style Manual for Authors and Editors*, 5th edn (AGPS 1994). The Harvard system puts the author(s) and date of the work being referred to at the appropriate point in the text, rather than using a number. This is called a 'citation'. All of the works cited are then listed at the end of the paper in alphabetical order according to author. The reader can then refer from the text to the reference. It is not necessary to reference well-known facts.

Textual references should be given in a consistent manner throughout the document. Each citation in the text should refer to a reference in the reference list and each reference in the list should be cited in the text, that is, they should match. The list of references is alphabetical, by author's surname. It contains only works cited in the text; others are listed as a bibliography, if used. The reference list must contain all of the works cited in the text.

Appendixes

Appendixes are included if it is necessary to provide material that is too cumbersome for the main text, for example questionnaires and so forth. Use appendixes judiciously to avoid filling the proposal with unnecessary detail and interrupting the flow of the main text. Include only material that supports or expands on the information in the body of the text. Examples of things that are best put in an index are questionnaires, instruments, or tests, diagrams of instruments, consent forms and letters of support. Start each appendix on a new page and name them alphabetically, i.e. Appendix A, Appendix B and so on. You should be aware that it is common committee practice for the committee secretary not to copy appendixes to the committee but to have them available on the day. However, if you supply enough copies for the committee members you can ensure that they receive the appendixes.

Writing the proposal

Style

The style of a research proposal is fairly prescribed. It is not like an essay, and creativity is inappropriate in writing a research proposal (Barnard 1986). In writing the research proposal, aim for clarity, coherence, conciseness and completeness. Remember that the reviewers are busy people who want a succinct proposal because they have to read a lot of them. You should use the formal scientific style in a quantitative paper, but in a qualitative paper, the personal style is appropriate. Construct the proposal in a logical order, such as the one given above. Avoid preaching or adopting a value-laden stance since you are supposed to be an objective researcher and bias is considered to be poor science.

Aim for using good English, with short, crisp sentences. It is important to use language that can be understood by lay strangers and/or members of other disciplines. The reason for this is that some of the people on an ethics committee will fall into that category. You should avoid jargon, especially that of your nursing specialty, but where you must use specific terminology define the terms that you use clearly. Use terms consistently and do not attempt to change terms to make it read more like a novel.

It is important to avoid sexist language: never use the pronoun 'he' to refer to everyone. It is possible to avoid sexist language by using the plural rather than the singular, for example 'participants will have their blood pressure taken before and after the treatment'. However, be specific about the gender of the participants where it is relevant. For example, if your study is going to be done with females only, say so.

Using the correct tense can be difficult. Use the future tense for the parts of the proposal that state what you intend to do. Use the past tense for the literature review and the section on the pilot study if it has already been completed. Write statements of everyday knowledge in the present tense.

There are specific books on writing research proposals and reports, for example *Assignment and Thesis Writing* (Anderson & Poole 1998). Pro formas from ethics committees or funding agencies may set out sections for your guidance. If you are writing a full scientific protocol, use the format suggested above.

Use of headings

Headings assist the reader to understand the structure of the proposal and to prepare the reader for what is to come. While the use of headings is inappropriate in creative writing or an essay, it is mandatory in a research proposal. Whatever system you use, you should use headings and subheadings generously to guide the reader. However, use your common sense. If you find that every paragraph has a heading, you are probably using too many headings.

There are two major systems of headings. One uses differences in the physical appearance of the heading and the other uses a numbering system, with or without differences in physical appearance. For longer reports such as theses, the numbering system is better because it makes it easier to see the structure of the proposal. However, for shorter proposals, such as student classroom projects, the other system is quite adequate. In a thesis, a combination of the two systems can be used, but the heading system should be consistent. Modern word processors include a function that allows you to build in a heading style.

The physical appearance system

This system relies upon differences in the appearance of the letters. It uses a combination of lower-and upper-case letters in the headings, position of the headings, and underlining or boldness (heaviness) of the font. This system is suitable for only about three or four levels of headings in addition to the title. Variations can be done with italics, or different colours if you have a colour printer. A simple example of a heading format using physical appearance of lettering is seen in Figure 6.4.

> **MAIN HEADING**
> **MAJOR SIDE HEADING**
> *SECOND-ORDER SIDE HEADING*
> **Third-order side heading**
> *Fourth-order side heading*

Figure 6.4 Physical appearance system of headings

Note that the centred heading, and the major and second-order side heading are all upper-case/capital letters. The second-order side heading is italic. The third- and fourth-order side headings have only the first word capitalised and the fourth-order side heading is also italic. This system can be varied by using normal-face as well as bold-face (heavy black) and italic fonts.

The numbering system

This system relies on numbered sections. As stated earlier, it is used usually for larger proposals and in theses. Each section is given a number, and the number is used as the beginning of each heading in the section. The second-order headings begin with the number 1, and go up from there, and the third-order headings begin with 1, and so on. An example is seen in Figure 6.5.

> **SECTION 2**
> **METHODOLOGY**
> 2.1   Setting
> 2.2   Participants
> 2.3   Instruments and Procedures
>   2.3.1 Instruments
>   2.3.1.1 The questionnaire
>   2.3.1.2 The physical instrument
>   2.3.2 Procedures for data collection
> 2.4   Data Analysis

Figure 6.5 Numbering system of headings

Notice that this system may also use physical characteristics. The numbers at the same level are indented the same amount. The disadvantage of this system is that an alteration to the text may require changing subsequent numbers within the section.

The process of writing a proposal

Before starting to write your proposal, see if you can acquire both a good proposal and a weak one and compare them. This allows you to see the difference and implement the good points while avoiding the bad ones. When you are ready to begin writing, tackle what you see as the easiest part first. You do not need to write the proposal in the order in which it finally appears. The abstract is usually written last.

After you are satisfied with the structure and content of your draft, you should polish it. Check the spelling. Use the spellchecker on your word processor by all means, but don't rely on it. Check the grammar, punctuation and style using a book such as *The Elements of Style* (Strunk & White 2000) or the AGPS *Style Manual*. You can also use the grammar checker on your word processor but remember that you cannot rely exclusively on it either. You must proofread all your documents, but especially your final copy, to eliminate grammatical errors; the spellchecker is unable to pick up some errors such as 'their' when you meant 'there'.

When you are satisfied with the first draft of the proposal, leave it for a fortnight or longer. Then read it critically and analytically, and from the point of view of the lecturer, supervisor, or committee member who will be reading it. Then revise it. At this point, you should if possible get an objective colleague, friend, or relative to critique it, then revise it again. Finally, proofread it again and ask someone else to proofread it as well.

Your next task is to transfer the final draft of your proposal onto the application form, or pro forma specified by the organisation. It should be typed or word processed. This is worth an investment of your time and effort in learning to type yourself, or paying someone else to do it. You may have an electronic copy of the application form on your word processor, in which case make a duplicate and use that, retaining the blank original for future use. If you do not have an electronic copy, you may type the forms into the word processor yourself: most organisations will accept facsimiles without the fancy boxes as long you respect the page limit and keep the format and the font size the same. You may have to type the material onto a paper copy, in which case use a photocopy of the form and save one clean copy in case you have to make revisions.

The document itself should be double-spaced (unless on a pro forma with limited space) and printed in black. Use A4 bond of at least 80 gsm weight. Print the document on white paper since coloured paper doesn't provide enough contrast for photocopying. Ideally the font should be 12 point if you are typing on blank paper. However, the size on the pro forma should be matched if you are using a pro forma. Use a legible font such as Palatino, Times New Roman or Bembo (the font used in this book). Make sure that the pages are numbered. At the very end, check that the submission is complete, that is, it contains all pages including appendixes and references.

Submitting the proposal

Having completed the proposal, your next step is to submit it to the committee or agency. Make sure you provide the exact number of photocopies required – you may be required to provide one copy for each member of the committee. Or you may be able to submit the application electronically. In any event, make sure that you retain a copy of the document, in case of loss. In the case of a word-processed document, make sure that you have a backup copy. Better yet, keep two backup copies in different places in case of fire or theft.

It is possible but by no means usual that you may be asked to appear before a committee, most likely an institutional ethics committee, to explain or defend your proposal. If so, you will be notified that you are required to attend. You may bring your supervisor. In preparation for the meeting, you should rehearse a concise overview of your study because you will probably be asked to describe it. You should know the proposal thoroughly. You must be able to justify the value of your study and its impact on practice. You should also be aware of any ethical aspects that you think the committee could raise. Make sure your supervisor is well briefed. On the day, make sure you have a copy of your application with you and provide one for your supervisor too. Remember to dress appropriately and present a cool and confident manner. You can expect about 10 people to be there. During the meeting, ask for a question to be repeated if you don't understand it. You can refer to your supervisor if you get out of your depth.

You can expect that you will receive a written response from the committee, usually at least a fortnight after its meeting. Only if you are under pressure of time should you telephone the committee chair or secretary. An informal approval over the telephone would permit you to start making arrangements for carrying out your study. However, under no circumstances should you ever commence data collection without a written approval from the appropriate committees.

If your proposal is not successful, you can use any feedback provided by the assessors of your application to improve the proposal. Often the committee may require only minor modifications, or may stipulate that approval is granted subject to certain conditions. It is then your job to respond in writing to the committee stating how you will fulfil the conditions. If the response from the committee was very discouraging, you may need to rethink the entire proposal from an objective point of view. If it is appropriate, you may consult with members of the committee to clarify their points of concern.

Funding

Frequently, the cost of a project makes it imperative to acquire funding from a source other than the researcher. For student projects, you, the researcher, will have to bear the costs in excess of any funds granted by your institution. For graduate students, the university may give a stipend or you may be able to get a grant from an outside body. In addition, the university provides the infrastructure described earlier. Some graduate students may do work that is funded by their supervisor's research grant.

For clinicians, the sources of funding are from their own institution's research fund or from collaborative projects with university staff, who may be able to get a grant from the university. Alternatively, the other source of funding is from independent organisations, government or corporate bodies. The NHMRC controls government funds for clinical research, while the Australian Research Council controls funding for non-clinical nursing research such as nursing systems or nursing education. The amount given by various bodies may vary from a few hundred dollars to many thousands of dollars. Often grants are advertised in the prominent newspapers such as the *Sydney Morning Herald* and the *Australian*. If your institution has a research management unit, it will probably have the details of funding sources and may be able to advise you of them.

It is important when identifying a possible source of funds for your grant to match the aims of your research project with those of the granting body, and to make sure that the amount of funding given by the body is in line with the amount you are seeking (Hamilton 1994).

Obtaining informal approvals

The formal approval for the research project given by the ethics committee and research committees will gain you entry to the institution for the purposes of your research project. However you will also need to secure informal approvals from other parties in the clinical field in order to gain access to participants. If you plan to do a research project in a hospital, for example, you will need to see the director of nursing and the appropriate administration staff to brief them and get their approval. If you are going to use the patients of medical practitioners, it is courteous to acquire their approval. These people function as gatekeepers and it is as well to get them on side. Similarly, you will need the approval of the staff concerned, for example the nursing staff on the hospital ward. A wise researcher gets this approval and arranges to brief the staff on the project and get their co-operation. All this may seem like a lot of work, but it pays dividends in staff co-operation. Staff who feel resentful at your presence or who feel that they have not been consulted can sabotage your research project.

You can improve your access to participants by gaining credibility within the institution, and attending to the social amenities. You can enhance your credibility by promoting the benefits of the study to the staff, being visible in the clinical area during the course of the study, and by minimising the intrusions and demands that the project makes on the daily operations of the site. Social amenities include keeping key people informed of the progress of the study, acknowledging staff participation and behaving with professional courtesy at all times. If you want more detail on access, consult Foreman and Smeltzer (1991).

If the study is carried on over a period of time, it is essential to implement strategies to ensure continued access to participants. If staff turnover is a problem, you may need to do more than one briefing session. Continuing to carry out the above strategies will help to ensure continued access. In addition, at the end of the project, you should thank the nursing and other staff formally with a letter. You may also wish to thank them with a small gift, such as a box of chocolates or an afternoon tea, depending on your budget. This helps to keep the channels open for further research. Above all, don't forget to send the ward staff, as well as any other key persons, a written summary of your findings. It is also appropriate to present your findings at an inservice session as well.

If your research is being carried out at the university, you will need to brief the key people there, such as the head of the nursing department, and the academic staff. If you are using the nursing laboratory you will need to organise this with whoever handles the bookings for using the laboratory. You will also need to liaise with the laboratory technician, who may be able to help you with setting up and returning the laboratory to its previous state. The above principles with regard to social amenities and feedback apply in the university setting as well as the clinical field.

Summary

In this chapter we have discussed the mechanisms for gaining approval for your research project, including those from your supervisor, the university, and the clinical field. We have shown you the process for constructing a research proposal and the content of the proposal. In addition, securing funding for the project and gaining the necessary approvals from the clinical field have been discussed briefly.

Now that you have the necessary approval, you are at last ready to move to the next exciting part of the process: collecting your data!

Main points

- A research proposal is a written account of a plan for a project that argues why a particular problem should be investigated and what the appropriate methodology is to investigate it; and it sets out what the researcher intends to do – how, why, where, when and at what cost.
- A plan helps to design and organise a project, allows you to see and ponder relationships between different parts of the proposal, helps to foresee potential problems and solve them at planning stage, permits consultation with other researchers before the study is carried out and is the best way to prevent mistakes occurring when you are carrying out the project.
- Proposals are written to gain approval of funding bodies, university research committees, ethics committees and other bodies giving approval.
- The preliminary steps in writing a proposal are to: identify the research problem, read and review the literature, identify a research design, identify the proposal's audience, acquire protocols and guidelines from institutions and identify pathways for approvals.
- All proposals consist of preliminary pages, the body of the proposal and supporting materials.
- The body of a quantitative research proposal has a particular structure: introduction (including a literature review that elucidates the theoretical framework for the study), methodology (including participant recruitment, and data processing and analysis), ethical requirements, dissemination plan, work plan and budget.
- Qualitative research proposals have a title page and a research summary or abstract but in the body of the proposal the use of words is specific to describe the chosen research methodology, methods and processes.
- Qualitative research proposals contain clear and concise statements about: the research summary; the significance, aims and objectives of the study; the research questions; background and literature review; the research plan, including methodology, methods and processes of participant recruitment; data collection, analysis and interpretation; ethical requirements; dissemination of findings; the project time frame; and the budget.
- The writing style of the proposal should aim for clarity, coherence, conciseness and completeness with the proposal constructed in a logical order. The language should be understandable by non-nurses, avoiding jargon but defining specific terms.
- The proposal should be submitted according to the guidelines of the scrutinising body and a response can be expected to take at least a fortnight after that body's meeting.
- Seek informal approvals from gatekeepers of the institutions in which you will be collecting data and develop strategies for recruiting and retaining participants.

Review Questions

1. In a qualitative research proposal, the methodology refers to the:
   a. theoretical assumptions that underlie the choice of methods
   b. interpretive approach used in the project
   c. methods for data collection and analysis
   d. empirico-analytical criteria against which it is judged

2. Quantitative and qualitative proposals differ mainly in their:
   a. focus on the preliminaries
   b. ethical considerations
   c. use of language
   d. project time frame

3. Which of the following would be found in the introduction section of a research proposal?
   a. data analysis procedures
   b. description of an instrument
   c. a time frame
   d. statement of purpose

4. In which of the following sections of a research proposal would you be most likely to find the theoretical framework?
   a. the review of the literature
   b. the context of the study
   c. the abstract
   d. the methods

5. In comparison with a quantitative research proposal, the structure of a qualitative proposal is:
   a. much the same
   b. absolutely identical
   c. totally different
   d. completely the same

6. In qualitative research proposals the statements need to be:
   a. highly philosophical
   b. clear and concise
   c. in abstract terms
   d. unsure and approximate

7. Which of the following would *not* be in a research proposal?
   a. budget
   b. time frame
   c. methods
   d. results

8 A plan for disseminating the findings should appear in the proposal because:
   a it is important to share the results with colleagues
   b it will impress the committee
   c it is required by granting agencies
   d none of the above

9 From whom should the approval be secured first?
   a ethics committee
   b supervisor
   c clinical research committee
   d funding body

10 The reason for having a research plan is:
   a it assists with designing the project
   b it fosters congruence between parts of the project
   c it helps you to see potential problems
   d all of the above

Discussion Questions

1 List three types of agencies that require research proposals.
2 Discuss how you would prepare to write your proposal.
3 Describe the preliminaries section of a research proposal.
4 Describe the sections of the body of a quantitative or qualitative research proposal.
5 Discuss the importance of style in writing a research proposal.

References

Affonso, D. 1993, 'Reconciliation and healing for mothers through skin-to-skin contact provided in an American tertiary level intensive care nursery', *Neonatal Network*, vol. 12, no. 3, 25–32.

Affonso, D., Wahlberg, B. & Persson, B. 1989, 'Exploration of mothers' reactions to kangaroo method of prematurity care', *Neonatal Network*, vol. 7, no. 6, 43–51.

Anderson, D. & Poole, M. 1998, *Assignment and Thesis Writing*, 3rd edn, John Wiley & Sons, Brisbane.

Anderson, G. 1989, 'Skin-to-skin: kangaroo care in Western Europe', *American Journal of Nursing*, vol. 89, no. 5, 662–6.

Australian Government Publishing Service 1994, *Style Manual for Authors, Editors and Printers*, 5th edn, AGPS, Canberra.

Barnard, K. 1986, 'Writing a research proposal', *MCN: Maternal Child Nursing*, vol. 11, January–February, 76.

Beckstrand, J. 1987, 'The notion of a practice theory and the relationship of scientific and ethical knowledge to practice', *Research in Nursing and Health*, vol. 1, no. 3, 131–6.

Belenky, M., Clinchy, B., Goldberger, N. & Tarule, J. 1986, *Women's Ways of Knowing*, Basic Books, New York.

Benner, P. 1984, *From Novice to Expert: Uncovering the Knowledge Embedded in Clinical Practice*, Addison-Wesley, California.

Benner, P. & Wrubel, J. 1989, *The Primacy of Caring: Stress and Coping in Health and Illness*, Addison-Wesley Publishing Co., California.

Bernstein, R. 1978, *The Restructuring of Social and Political Theory*, University of Pennsylvania Press, Philadelphia.

Blumberg, A. 1990, 'Toward a scholarship of practice', *Journal of Curriculum and Supervision*, vol. 5, no. 3, 236–43.

Boud, D., Keogh, R. & Walker, D. 1985, *Reflection: Turning Experience into Learning*, Kagan Page, London.

Boykin, A. 1998, 'Nursing as caring through the reflective lens', in *Transforming Nursing through Reflective Practice*, eds C. Johns & D. Freshwater, Blackwell Science, Oxford.

Caffarella, R. B. B. 1994, 'Characteristics of adult learners and foundations of experiential learning', *New Directions for Adult and Continuing Education*, vol. 62, Summer.

Carr, W. & Kemmis, S. 1986, *Becoming Critical: Education, Knowledge and Action Research*, Falmer Press, Lewes.

Conway, J. 1994, 'Reflection, the art and science of nursing and the theory–practice gap', *British Journal of Nursing*, vol. 393, 114–18.

Cox, H., Hickson, P. & Taylor, B. 1991, 'Exploring reflection: knowing and constructing practice', in *Towards a Discipline of Nursing*, eds G. Gray & R. Pratt, Churchill Livingstone, Melbourne.

Curry, M. 1982, 'Maternal attachment behavior and the mother's self-concept: the effect of early skin-to-skin contact', *Nursing Research*, vol. 31, no. 2, 73–8.

deLeeuw, R., Colin, E., Dunnebier, E. & Mirmiran, M. 1991, 'Physiologic effects of kangaroo care in very small premature infants', *Biology of the Neonate*, vol. 59, 149–55.

Descartes, R. 1970, *The Philosophical Works of Descartes*, trans. E. S. Haldane & G. R. T. Ross, The Cambridge University Press, Cambridge.

Drosten-Brooks, F. 1993, 'Kangaroo Care: Skin-to-Skin Contact in the NICU', *MCN*, vol. 18, no. 5, 250–3.

Foreman, M. & Smeltzer, C. 1991, 'Gaining support for the study', in *Conducting and Using Nursing Research in the Clinical Setting*, eds M. Mateo & K. Kirchoff, Williams & Wilkins, Baltimore.

Frey-Hoogwerf, L. 1996, 'A journey towards continence through emancipatory action research', *International Journal of Nursing Practice*, vol. 2, no. 2, 77–81.

Friedson, E. 1970, *Profession of Medicine: A Study of the Sociology of Applied Knowledge*, Harper and Row, New York.

Gale, G., Franck, L. & Lund, C. 1993, 'Skin-to-skin (kangaroo) holding of the intubated premature infant', *Neonatal Network Journal of Neonatal Nursing (NEONAT-NETW)*, vol. 12, no. 6, 49–57.

Gething, L. 1995, *How to Manage Research Effectively*, The Sydney Nursing Research Centre, The Faculty of Nursing, The University of Sydney, Sydney.

Giroux, H. A. 1983, *Theory and Resistance in Education*, Heinemann Educational Books, London.

Glaze, J. 1998, 'Reflection and expert nursing knowledge', in *Transforming Nursing through Reflective Practice*, eds C. Johns & D. Freshwater, Blackwell Science, Oxford.

Graham, I. 1998, 'Understanding nursing through reflection: a case study approach', in *Transforming Nursing through Reflective Practice*, eds C. Johns & D. Freshwater, Blackwell Science, Oxford.

Greenwood, J. 1993, 'Reflective practice: a critique of the work of Argyris & Schon', *Journal of Advanced Nursing*, vol. 18, 1183–7.

Habermas, J. 1973, *Theory and Practice*, Heinemann, London.

Haller, B. 1988, 'The costs of research to nursing', *MCN: Maternal Child Nursing*, vol. 13, 460.

Hamilton, H. 1994, 'Winning finance for your project', in *Handbook of Clinical Nursing Research*, ed. J. Robertson, Churchill Livingstone, Melbourne.

Hedges, G. & Grimmer, K. 1999, 'Performance indicators for discharge planning: a focused review of the literature', *Australian Journal of Advanced Nursing*, vol. 16, no. 4, 20–8.

Holmes, C. 1992, 'The drama of nursing', *Journal of Advanced Nursing*, vol. 17, 954–60.

Johns, C. & McCormack, B. 1998, 'Unfolding the conditions where the transformative potential of guided reflection (clinical supervision) might flourish or flounder', in *Transforming Nursing through Reflective Practice*, eds C. Johns & D. Freshwater, Blackwell Science, Oxford.

Johnson, D. E. 1980, 'The behavioral system for nursing', in *Conceptual Models for Nursing Practice*, 2nd edn, eds J. P. Riehl & C. Roy, Appleton-Century-Crofts, New York.

Kachoyeanos, M. 1998, 'Keys to research. The process of writing an abstract', *MCN: American Journal of Maternal/Child Nursing*, vol. 23, no. 1, 50.

Kemmis, S. & McTaggart, R. (eds) 1988, *The Action Research Planner*, 3rd edn, Deakin University Press, Geelong, Victoria.

King, I. M. 1981, *A Theory for Nursing: Systems, Concepts, Process*. Delmar Publishers, Albany, New York.

Kitson, A. L. 1984, Steps towards the identification and development of nursing therapeutic functions in the care of hospitalised elderly, unpublished PhD thesis, University of Ulster, Coleraine.

Kleiman, S. 1986, 'Humanistic nursing: the phenomenological theory of Paterson and Zderad', in *Case Studies in Nursing Theory*, ed. P. Winstead-Fry, National League for Nursing, New York.

Knowles, M. (ed.) 1980, *The Modern Practice of Adult Education: From Pedagogy to Andragogy*, 2nd edn, Cambridge Book Co., New York.

Levine, M. 1991, 'The conservation principles: model for health', in *Levine's Conservation Model: A Framework for Nursing Practice*, eds K. Schaefer & J. Pond, F A Davis Co., Philadelphia.

Lewin, K. 1946, 'Action research and minority issues', *Journal of Social Issues*, vol. 2, 34–46.

Ludington, S. 1990, 'Energy conservation during skin-to-skin contact between premature infants and their mothers', *Heart and Lung*, vol. 19, no. 5, 445–51.

Ludington-Hoe, S., Hashemi, M., Argote, L., Medellin, G. & Rey, H. 1992, 'Selected physiologic measures and behavior during paternal skin contact with Colombian preterm infants', *Journal of Developmental Physiology*, vol. 18, 224–32.

Lumby, J. 1998, 'Transforming nursing through reflective practice', in *Transforming Nursing through Reflective Practice*, eds C. Johns & D. Freshwater, Blackwell Science, Oxford.

McMahon, R. & Pearson, A. (eds) 1991, *Nursing as Therapy*, Chapman and Hall, London.

McTaggart, R. 1991, 'Principles for participatory action research', *Adult Education Quarterly*, vol. 41, no. 3, 168–87.

Miles, M., Funk, S. & Kasper, 1993, 'Neonatal intensive care unit: sources of stress for parents', *AACN Clinical Issues*, vol. 2, no. 2, 346–54.

Mondlane, R., de Graca, A. & Ebrahim, G. 1989, 'Skin-to-skin contact as a method of body warmth for infants of low birth weight', *Journal of Tropical Pediatrics*, vol. 35, 321–6.

Newell, R. 1992, 'Anxiety, accuracy and reflection: the limits of professional development', *Journal of Advanced Nursing*, vol. 17, 1326–33.

New South Wales College of Nursing 1992a, *Casemix and DRGs: an Annotated Bibliography of Nursing Literature*, New South Wales College of Nursing, Glebe, NSW.

New South Wales College of Nursing 1992b, *DRGs and Casemix Based Hospital Management,* New South Wales College of Nursing, Glebe, NSW.

O'Brien, B. & Spry, J. 1995, 'Expanding the role of the clinical nurse consultant', *Australian Journal of Advanced Nursing*, vol. 12, no. 4, 26–32.

Parse, R. 1987, *Nursing Science: Major Paradigm Theories and Critiques*, WB Saunders, Philadelphia.

Pearson, A. & Vaughan, B. 1989, *Nursing Models for Practice*, Heinemann Nursing, London.

Ramudu, L., Bellet, B., Higgs, J., Latimer, C. & Smith, R. 1994, 'How effectively do we use double staff time?' *Australian Journal of Advanced Nursing*, vol. 11, no. 3, 5–10.

Reece, S. 1992, 'The Parent Expectations Survey', *Clinical Nursing Research*, vol. 1, no. 4, 336–46.

Reid, J. C. 1994, *Report of the National Review of Nurse Education in the Higher Education Sector – 1994 and Beyond*, Australian Government Publishing Service, Canberra.

Retsas, A. 1994, 'Problematic telephone orders: empowering nurses through action research', *Australian Journal of Advanced Nursing*, vol. 11, no. 2, 19–27.

Roberts, K. & Taylor, B. 1998, *Nursing Research Processes: an Australian Perspective*, Nelson ITP, Melbourne.

Schon, D. A. 1983, *The Reflective Practitioner: How Practitioners Think in Action*, Basic Books, New York.

Schon, D. A. 1987, *Educating the Reflective Practitioner*, Jossey-Bass, London.

Sheldon, L. & Jackson, K. 1998, 'Special feature: preparing an abstract', *Paediatric Nursing*, vol. 10, no. 5, 36–7.

Sheldon, L. & Jackson, K. 2000, 'Demystifying the academic aura: preparing an abstract', *Journal of Orthopaedic Nursing*, vol. 4, no. 1, 47.

Smith, K. 1996, 'Skin-to-skin contact for premature and sick infants and their mothers', in *Contemporary Issues in Nursing*, eds F. Biley & C. Maggs, Churchill Livingstone, Edinburgh.

Smyth, W. J. 1986, The reflective practitioner in nursing education, paper presented at the Second National Nursing Education Seminar, South Australian College of Advanced Education, Adelaide.

Street, A. 1995, *Nursing Replay: Researching Nursing Culture Together*, Churchill-Livingstone, Melbourne.

Strunk, W. & White, E. 2000, *The Elements of Style,* 4th edn, Allyn and Bacon, Boston.

Sydney Metropolitan Teaching Hospitals Nursing Consortium 1992, *Nursing Practice and Patient Outcomes Based on PAIS, Standards for September*, Sydney Metropolitan Teaching Hospitals Nursing Consortium, Sydney.

Taylor, B. 1992, 'From helper to human: a reconceptualisation of the nurse as person', *Journal of Advanced Nursing*, vol. 17, 1042–9.

Taylor, B. 1994, *Being Human: Ordinariness in Nursing*, Churchill-Livingstone, Melbourne.

Taylor, B. 1997, 'Big battles for small gains: a cautionary note for teaching reflective processes in nursing and midwifery', *Nursing Inquiry*, vol. 4, 19–26.

Taylor, B. 1998, 'Locating a phenomenological perspective of reflective nursing and midwifery practice by contrasting interpretive and critical reflection', in *Nursing through Reflective Practice*, eds C. Johns & D. Freshwater, Blackwell Science, Oxford.

Taylor, B 2000a, *Being Human: Ordinariness in Nursing*, Southern Cross University Press, Lismore, NSW.

Taylor, B. 2000b, *Reflective Practice: A Guide for Nurses and Midwives*, Allen and Unwin, Melbourne.

Taylor, B. 2000c, Improving the quality of hospital ward nursing care through reflective practice and action research with registered nurses, unpublished research report, Southern Cross University, Lismore, NSW.

Taylor, B. J., King, V. & Stewart, J. 1995, 'Reflective midwifery practice: facilitating midwives practice insights into using a distance education reflective practitioner model', *International Journal of Nursing Practice*, vol. 1, 26–31.

Von Wright, J. 1992, 'Reflections on reflection', *Learning and Instruction*, vol. 12, 59–68.

Wahlberg, V., Affonso, D. & Persson, B. 1992, 'A retrospective, comparative study using the Kangaroo method as a complement to standard incubator care', *European Journal of Public Health*, vol. 2, no. 1, 34–7.

Watson, J. 1988, *Nursing: Human Science and Human Care. A Theory of Nursing*, National League for Nursing, New York.

Whitelaw, A., Heisterkamp, G., Sleath, K., Acolet, D. & Richards, A. 1988, 'Skin-to-skin contact for very low birth weight infants and their mothers: a randomized trial of kangaroo care', *Archives of Disease in Childhood*, vol. 63, 1377–82.

Whitelaw, A. & Sleath, K. 1985, 'Myth of the marsupial mother: home care of very low birth weight babies in Bogota, Colombia', *Lancet*, vol. 1, 1206–8.

Quantitative research methodology

chapter objectives The material presented in this chapter will assist you to:

- outline the different types of research designs
- compare the strength of various types of research designs
- discuss the advantages and disadvantages of the different types of research designs
- choose an appropriate design for a research project.

Introduction

A research design details the methodology to be used in the study to answer the research question. It guides the researcher in carrying out the study, much the same way in which a recipe guides the cook in preparing a dish, or a blueprint guides the engineer in constructing a bridge. A research design tells the researcher exactly what must be done. It answers the questions 'how?', 'when?' and 'where?'

In this chapter, we will be concerned with quantitative descriptive designs, correlational designs and experimental designs. These answer questions at various levels. A descriptive design only describes a phenomenon, while a correlational design looks for relationships in the data and an experiment attempts to show whether one thing causes another. In this chapter, we will describe these designs as pure types although a study may combine some types, for example, descriptive and correlational.

There is no one answer to the question: 'What is the best research design?' The best research design is the one that is most likely to help you answer your research question. It is a matter of selecting the design with the best 'fit' to your question.

Major types of research designs

There are various types of research designs ranging from the simple descriptive design, through designs that compare groups, to experimental designs. Table 7.1 shows the major types of research designs and their features.

Descriptive designs

Descriptive designs are designs that describe phenomena in order to answer a research question. These may vary in complexity. Descriptive designs are found also in qualitative research where the purpose is to describe or draw a picture of

Table 7.1 Comparison of major research designs

	Simple descriptive	Comparative descriptive	Correlational	Pre-experimental	Quasi-experimental	Experimental
Describes participants	Yes	Yes	Yes	Yes	Yes	Yes
Compares groups	No	Yes	Yes	Yes	Yes	Yes
Investigates cause-and-effect relationships	No	No	No	No	Yes	Yes
Manipulates independent variable	No	No	No	No	Yes	Yes
Has control group	No	No	No	No	Yes	Yes
Random assignment to groups	No	No	No	No	No	Yes

a phenomenon, for example, what it is like to have a certain experience. That type of research will be described in Chapter 12. In this chapter, we will be concerned with descriptive research of a quantitative nature, that is, research that uses numbers to describe phenomena but does not investigate the relationships among the phenomena. Quantitative descriptive research may, however, compare the incidence of the phenomenon in different groups of people.

Quantitative descriptive designs are considered weak research designs in comparison to experiments, but nevertheless they have a place, particularly when little is known about the subject in question. They are a way to start building up knowledge about a topic and are used to conduct an initial exploration on a research question.

Simple descriptive designs

Simple descriptive designs measure known variables in a population. For example, suppose that you wanted to measure self-care capabilities in adults with arthritis. You could take a questionnaire that measured self-care abilities and administer it to a group of people with arthritis and come up with a measure of self-care ability for that group. Another example is the census, which is taken every five years in order to draw a statistical picture of the Australian population. Various methods can be used to collect descriptive data but the most common are surveys using questionnaires or interviews and observation by people or instruments. These methods will be discussed in Chapter 8.

In designing a descriptive study, it is first necessary to decide what you want to investigate. This involves selecting the group or population that you want to study and then identifying the aspects of the group that you want to study. These must be defined clearly and in sufficient detail that they can be measured. These characteristics may be found through theory, through the literature and through your own knowledge. When you have identified these factors, you may measure the variables in the sample or population being studied.

An example of a simple descriptive design is a study in which a survey was carried out to enumerate and describe manual handling practices and injuries among ICU nurses (Retsas & Pinikahana 1999). The researcher collected data about ICU nurses' handling of patients or objects and types and injury rates related to these practices. The report described the handling practices and injuries but did not explore whether there were differences in rates for males and females or different age groups.

The simple descriptive design is considered weak because it cannot determine degrees of difference between groups, relationships of characteristics or whether one thing causes another. It has the advantages of being quick, relatively inexpensive and useful for preliminary research that may lead to further research questions.

Comparative descriptive designs

A comparative descriptive design is one in which two or more groups are being compared on particular variables. For example, if you wanted to measure the relative self-care abilities of male and female arthritis sufferers, you would administer your self-care instrument to one group of males and one group of females and see if they got different scores on their self-care abilities. Of course, you would want to compare males and females of equal ages, stages of the disease, and any other characteristic that might affect the results.

An example of a comparative descriptive design is in a study in which the researchers compared male and female nursing students' perceptions of men entering the nursing profession (Lo & Brown 1999). They found relatively few differences between male and female perceptions, except that male students intended to work in specialty areas. Another example of this design is a study in which the researchers compared patient satisfaction on two wards in Brisbane (Wu & Courtney 2000). They found no difference in satisfaction between the ward using team nursing and the ward using patient allocation.

This design generally has the same advantages and disadvantages that simple descriptive design does but it has the added advantage of allowing comparison of groups.

Correlational designs

A correlational design examines the relationship of variables within one group without aiming to determine cause and effect. It examines the direction of the relationship and also the strength of the relationship. It does not have an independent variable that can be manipulated by the researcher, that is, there is no intervention by the researcher, just observation. The researcher identifies the variables of interest and chooses the most appropriate way to measure them, usually by means of observation, interviews or surveys. Then the researcher carries out a statistical analysis to determine whether there is a relationship between the variables; if so, how strong, and in what direction.

An example of a study with a correlational design is one that examined the relationship between personality and stress levels in nurses caring for interpersonally difficult patients (Santamaria 2000). The researchers used a personality inventory and a questionnaire about difficult patients to explore this relationship and found that there was some interaction between personality and stress when looking after difficult patients.

The advantage of correlational design is that it is a relatively easy, fast, and inexpensive way to acquire and process a lot of data that can be used to investigate relationships among variables. Correlational design has the advantage that it is useful in exploratory research to determine relationships that can later be tested out more explicitly by more exacting methodologies. In comparison to an experiment, a correlational design is more straightforward and easier to implement, and the data are collected more quickly, usually by a survey, or chart audit. A correlational study is also not as intrusive as an experiment.

Experimental designs

An experimental design is one in which subjects are exposed to some event or treatment, and their response to that treatment is measured to gauge the effect of the treatment on the subjects. Experiments can occur naturally by the intervention of nature (e.g. acts of 'God'), or artificially by the intervention of an experimenter. An experiment may be carried on in the laboratory or in the clinical setting. If a new type of drug or treatment is tested in the clinical setting, it is called a clinical trial.

Experimental designs are considered the most advanced type of quantitative research design. They are the most likely to be able to show the strength of an association between variables and can show whether changes in one variable cause effects in the other. The researcher actually sets up a situation in which one component or variable can be manipulated. This variable is called the independent variable, treatment variable or causal variable. It is expected that the manipulation of the independent variable will have an effect on another variable, called the dependent variable, outcome variable or effect variable. This variable is called the dependent variable because any changes in it are dependent on changes in the independent variable. The experimental design is characterised by the use of a control group to which an experimental group is compared. The control group does not get the treatment that the experimental group gets. A design without a control group is called a pre-experimental design. A design that has a control group but does not allocate the subjects to the control and treatment groups randomly is called a quasi-experimental design.

In nursing and health research, independent variables are usually such things as nursing interventions, nurse-prescribed drugs, or educational programs. The independent variable may be varied by giving it to one group, called the experimental group and not giving it to another group, called the control group. For example, one group may receive pre-operative teaching while another group does not. Or the researcher may give different amounts or types of the independent variable to two or more different groups. For example, suppose that you wanted to test out a new dressing technique on the rate of infection in clients. The use of the dressing technique would be the independent variable while the rate of infection would be the dependent variable because it is dependent on the dressing technique.

Although the experimental design is considered to be the classic research design, most nursing research is not experimental, for a number of reasons. First, experimental research assumes that the relevant variables have been identified so that they can be controlled but nursing is not in such an advanced state that all variables have been identified. Secondly, there are many social variables of importance to health and nursing outcomes that cannot be manipulated. Thirdly, it is difficult to carry out experimental research in the clinical setting where random assignment to groups and standardisation of research procedures may be impossible to achieve. And finally, the ethical questions concerning the best care of the patient cannot be ignored. For those reasons, most nursing research does not meet the criteria for a true experiment.

Validity in scientific research

Before we can understand why the different types of experimental research design have developed, we need to understand certain concepts related to validity. A study is said to be valid if it measures what it claims to measure. Validity in research is usually of two kinds: external validity and internal validity.

External validity

The findings of a study have external validity to the extent that they can be generalised, or applied, to the population. In order to achieve external validity, the subjects should be selected at random from the population so that they are as representative as possible. This allows the researcher to be confident that the results found from the sample would be the same as those that would be obtained if a different part of the population, or the whole population, were tested. Random sampling is often used in social science research. However, it is frequently not possible to select randomly from a whole population in health science research. If participants are not sampled randomly from the population, the results cannot be applied to the whole population, but only to that portion of the population from which the sample was taken. For example, suppose that you had done a study using 40-year-old females in a country hospital. Your findings could then only be generalised to 40-year-old females in that country hospital, and not to the entire population of 40-year old women in the state or the country.

Internal validity

An experiment is said to have internal validity if it measures what it is supposed to be measuring and the effects measured are therefore attributable to the manipulation of the independent variable. For example, if you wanted to measure the effects of a new method of mouth care on the state of the oral mucosa, you would want to be sure that it was the effects of the mouth care that you were measuring and not some other factor that came into effect during the study, for example the introduction of vitamin therapy.

Threats to validity

There are various problems that can arise to threaten the internal validity of a study. In their classic treatise on experimental design, Campbell and Stanley discussed various threats to validity, some of which are outlined here (Campbell & Stanley 1966).

Changes related to subjects
Experimental mortality

Experimental mortality does not refer to death of the subjects during the study! It refers to the loss of subjects from the study. Subjects may drop out from the experimental and control groups at different rates, leaving an imbalance in the number of subjects in the two groups. Different kinds of subjects may drop out from the groups, leaving an imbalance in the composition of the groups. If this happens, comparisons between the groups may be invalid.

History

History refers to events that happen during the course of the study, specifically between the introduction of the independent variable and the measurement of the dependent variable, that were not a part of the study design and that may affect the study results. For example, if you were studying the effects of an educational program on attitudes to use of contraceptives and during the course of the study, there was a major television campaign about contraception, that could affect the attitudes of the subjects. Therefore the results of the study could be attributed to the television campaign and not the educational campaign.

Maturation

During the course of the study the subjects change in such a way as to affect the results. This can be important in longitudinal studies because of the length of time that the study runs. It can also be important in studies in which children take part because of their physical, mental and social growth. Even in short studies, effects such as fatigue and hunger can affect certain results. However, this effect can be countered by using shorter intervals between observations.

Testing effect

Taking an initial test can affect the results of a second test. The testing effect can result from learning from a test and may be a problem when testing learning or skills. Suppose that you wished to test whether an educational program in diabetes management had any effect on control of blood sugar. You decide to measure the subjects' pre-program levels of knowledge and so you test their knowledge before you give them the education program. This then stimulates them to learn about diabetes, which interferes with your measurement of the effects of the educational program.

Selection effects

The selection effect is found after non-random selection of subjects from the comparison groups. For example, if subjects are allowed to choose the group they enter, the groups may be unequal, which may make comparison invalid. This effect can be avoided by random allocation of subjects to control and treatment groups.

Placebo effect

The placebo effect is the effect on a person's mind or body from a belief that a treatment works. If the participant believes that the treatment works, this can result in artificially high ratings of the effectiveness of the treatment. This can be a problem for a researcher testing out a treatment that has not yet been shown to work. The placebo effect can be controlled for by administering to a control group a placebo or inert substance that looks exactly like the active drug. Any change in this group will demonstrate the effect of belief and can be subtracted from the ratings of the group that receives the active treatment. The recipients must be 'blind' to whether or not they are receiving a placebo or the active treatment. The data collectors should also be 'blind' if possible.

Changes related to measurement
Changing procedures and instrumentation
If the measurement procedures change during the course of the study, then the readings will change and the comparison will be invalid. This can be controlled by ensuring that the exact procedures to be followed are written down and all data collectors are trained to follow them precisely every time measurements are taken. The major method of dealing with this problem is by running a rigorous trial on a small group, that is, a 'pilot study' to iron out the problems and develop an adequate procedure before embarking on the full experiment.

Differences in instruments
If several instruments are used, they may measure differently and this can affect the results. This can be avoided by calibrating the instruments so that they measure a standard unit in the same way, and to the same degree of accuracy. For example, if you wished to measure body temperature during a study, you should calibrate all thermometers to be used in a liquid that was a known temperature to check the accuracy and similarity of the thermometers' measurements. Any defective thermometers could then be eliminated and you could have confidence in your equipment.

Differences in measurement
If several data collectors are used, they may make measurements differently. This can be controlled by training the data collectors to take the measurements in the same way and testing them until they can achieve inter-rater reliability to a set standard. Conditions must be kept the same during the study. For example if temperature is an important condition, it must be kept controlled. Laboratory conditions may be preferable to the clinical setting because more control can be exerted over the conditions during the study.

Changes related to observation
Hawthorne effect
The Hawthorne effect (Robbins 1994) was named for a study that was done in the Hawthorne Electric plant many years ago. Researchers were attempting to measure the effects of light levels on worker productivity. They found, to their surprise, that whether they raised or lowered the light, the productivity levels increased. The workers produced more, perhaps because they were being watched, or because they perceived that the management cared about them. This suggests that people behave differently when they know they are being observed. It is difficult to control for this variable without violating ethical principles. The researcher is in a dilemma: it is unethical to watch people without their knowing it but if they know they are being watched they may behave differently, thus producing invalid data. The only way to surmount this problem, aside from deception, is to use unobtrusive observation.

Experimenter effect
The experimenter may consciously or unconsciously affect the results of the experiment. For example, a researcher who is convinced of the value of a

treatment may consciously or unconsciously 'sell' the treatment to the recipient and cause artificially high ratings of the new treatment, augmenting the placebo effect. For this reason, in placebo trials of new drugs, the person prescribing or giving out the drug should also be 'blind' to whether the client is receiving the placebo or the active treatment.

Extraneous variables

Extraneous variables are those that may affect the outcome but are not central to the question. For example, age and sex may be extraneous variables. It is important to control for extraneous variables. This can be done by making the subjects very similar on those variables, for example only studying men or people of a certain age. The problem with this approach is that the results will apply only to the sub-group selected. Another way is to build in the variable by including it in the study and measuring it to see if the sub-groups are different on the dependent variable. However, this will require more subjects. Subjects can be matched on these variables for assignment to control and treatment groups in lieu of random assignment.

Types of experimental designs

Experimental design is shown diagrammatically, using symbols. This method was developed by Campbell and Stanley (1966), who developed the typology of designs explored here.

R = random allocation to groups
O = observation or measurement
E = experimental group
C = control group
X = exposure of the group to the experimental variable

The Xs and Os in any line apply to the same specific participants
Left to right indicates time sequence
Xs and Os directly above each other indicate events taking place at the same time.

Pre-experimental designs

A pre-experimental design is one that does not use a control group. It is therefore considered weak. However, pre-experimental design can still be useful, particularly in exploratory research or where there are limitations on the numbers of subjects that preclude the use of a control group. These include one-shot case studies, pre-test post-test design and static group comparisons.

One-shot case study

In a one-shot case study design, the effect of an event or phenomenon, or the administration of a substance, or other treatment is tested on a group after it has occurred. The conclusions are based on the general expectations of what the findings would have been if the experimental event had not occurred. Usually, this design is used for events that have happened without warning, or a situation in which it is not possible to design a scientific experiment. In this design, subjects are selected because they have been exposed to some experience or substance; frequently they are self-selected. They are then measured on a selected variable to see if it is different from normal. This design is diagrammed as follows:

$$X \quad O1$$

An example of a one-shot case study is a study carried out by Armstrong, Barrack and Gordon (1995), in which a convenience sample of 30 subjects was given an educational program in taking blood pressure at home. After the educational program the subjects were tested for their ability to meet a criterion of accuracy as measured against an instructor. Subjects were recruited into the study only after the educational program was given so that a pre-test was not used, and the researchers did not use a control group from whom the educational program was withheld. The researchers claimed that patients 'can be taught to accurately and confidently measure their blood pressure'. This claim rests on the assumptions that the subjects did not know initially how to take a blood pressure and that their ability to do so after the educational program was a direct result of it.

The advantage of this design is that it does permit investigation of phenomena to explore whether or not a phenomenon may have had an effect on some characteristic of the participants. This type of design can point the way to more sophisticated designs to measure the same effects. However, it is considered a very weak design because the researcher has no control over the intervention and there is no control group

One group – pre-test post-test design

In this design, a pre-test and post-test are both done but the measurements are only made on one group. This design is used where it is not possible to use a control group, for example where there are too few subjects available. This design can be diagrammed as:

$$O1 \quad X \quad O2$$

This type of design was used in a study by Roberts, Brittin and deClifford, which measured the effects on respiratory capacity of frail elderly women lying on boomerang pillows for 10 minutes (Roberts, Brittin & deClifford 1995). This design was chosen because there was a shortage of subjects and a previous study had shown that there was no difference between respiratory capacity in well women on boomerang and ordinary pillows. The subjects were first made comfortable on ordinary pillows, and given a trial on the instrument to accustom them to it, then their pre-test breathing capacity was done. The subjects were then placed on boomerang pillows for 10 minutes and the post-test was carried out. The pre- and post-test respiratory capacities were compared and it was found that there was a decrease between the two readings.

The advantage of the pre-test post-test design over the one-shot case study design is that it allows comparison of the measurement of the dependent variable after the experimental treatment with the results before the treatment. This then allows you to draw some conclusions about the effect of the treatment.

However, there are several threats to the validity of the findings in such a design. For example, suppose you wanted to test the effect of hyperbaric pressure on the size of pressure sores. You do a pre-test measurement of the size of the sores, and then apply the hyperbaric pressure treatments, and then measure the size of the pressure sores again. If the average size of pressure sores at the end of the program was lower, you might conclude that the hyperbaric pressure treatment had reduced the rate of pressure sores. The validity of the findings of your study may be challenged on the grounds of history, for example if other events occur during the course of the study, such as increased mobility of the patients. The findings can also be challenged by the problem of maturation, or changes in the subjects that occur spontaneously during the course of the experiment, for example spontaneous remission of the pressure sores. This challenge could have been avoided easily by comparing the results to another group who had not been exposed to hyperbaric pressure but had shared all of the other experiences of the experimental group: in other words, a control group.

This type of design can be weakened by a testing effect where learning or skills are involved. It is known that people being tested for a second time tend to do better on the test. Furthermore, just taking the test may serve to stimulate the effect you are looking for. For example, suppose you want to test the effect of an anti-smoking campaign on people's rate of smoking. You decide to do a pre-test on your group of smokers selected for this campaign so you ask them to keep track of the number of cigarettes they smoke during the week before you start the intervention. You then find that after your campaign many of the smokers decide to quit and you conclude that your campaign is successful. However, it may have been that it was not your campaign that led your participants to the decision to quit smoking but the realisation of the number of cigarettes they smoked. Again, this challenge to validity could have been avoided by the use of an equal group who did measure their cigarette usage but was not exposed to your intervention.

There can also be a problem of instrument decay in which changes in the assessing instrument can affect the results. This is more of a problem where physical instruments are used over a longer period of time. This can be avoided by recalibrating the instruments against a known stable reference.

The static group comparison

The static group comparison is a design in which, in order to determine the effect of an event, a group that has experienced the event is compared with a group that has not. In the previous two examples, only one group was used. In this design, two groups are used but they are groups that occur naturally.

There is no pre-test. This design can be diagrammed as follows, with the broken line indicating that the groups are not equivalent:

$$X \quad O1$$
$$\overline{}$$
$$O1$$

The advantage of the static group comparison design is that two groups are being compared so that different practices can be compared and conclusions can be drawn. However, the problem with this design is that there is no way to establish whether the groups were initially equivalent and so you do not know whether the differences in the two groups are caused by the event, **X**. Or, put another way, you have no way of knowing if the groups would have measured the same if not for **X**. This is especially worrisome if the subjects have been allowed to select whether they are going to have **X** or not.

True experimental research designs

Because of the difficulty in drawing valid conclusions from the pre-experimental designs, research designs have tried to address these concerns by developing more sophisticated designs that address the threats to validity. A true experimental design has three major features: use of an equivalent control group to control for extraneous variables, random assignment to experimental and control groups, and the ability to control the independent variable.

Use of control group

A control group is one that is equivalent in every way to the experimental group except for the experimental variable. The group controls for extraneous variables and thus allows significant comparisons. The use of a control group allows the researcher to control for extraneous variables because anything that is going to happen to the experimental group that might affect the results will happen to both groups and this can be accounted for in the interpretation of the results. For example, the problem of history is removed since both groups have exactly the same experiences and a comparison of their results on the variable **X** will represent a true effect of **X**. In the same way, maturational differences will be accounted for because both groups will grow, or become tired at the same rate.

A placebo, or substance that has no physical effect but mimics the experimental treatment, will usually be included for trials of new drugs. This ensures that the control group receives the same psychological effects of the treatment that the experimental group receives, without actually being treated. Any differences in the post-treatment outcomes of the two groups can then be explained by the treatment alone. The reason for a placebo trial is that with new drugs it is imperative to be absolutely sure that any treatment effects are caused by the new drug and not by the placebo effect.

Subjects are 'blind' to the treatment if they do not know which drug they are receiving. If the person who prescribes and/or administers the drug also does not know which drug is being given, the design is said to be 'double blind'.

The use of an untreated control group in clinical therapeutics allows the researcher to see what would happen without the treatment. For example, if you wished to test out the effect of treatment **X** on outcome **Y**, if you only applied treatment **X** and measured the outcome **Y** before and after the treatment, you would not know at the end whether any effect was from the treatment or from other factors such as attention or spontaneous remission. If a control group is used that does not receive any treatment at all, you can eliminate spontaneous remission as a problem because it could occur in both groups but you still might be measuring the psychological effects of treatment. However, you can avoid these problems in most studies if you use an equivalent control group that receives a placebo, with both participants and those administering the treatment being 'blind' to which group gets the active treatment and which gets the placebo. If the groups are treated the same, and are measured at the same time and in the same way, any differences between the two groups could be attributed to treatment **X** and not other factors. However, in some studies it is difficult to find a placebo, for example aromatherapy studies, so another design must be used to overcome this difficulty.

The use of a control group does not preclude unforeseen events happening to one group and not the other. It is important in the design and implementation of the study to ensure that the groups have the same experiences. For this reason, it is recommended that both groups are studied at the same time.

Random assignment to groups

The subjects must be randomly assigned to the treatment and control groups, that is, they must have an equal probability of being in either group. This eliminates any systematic bias in the groups that may affect the variable being studied. It therefore allows the researcher to be confident that any other variables would be evenly distributed between the groups so that they should be alike except for the independent variable. An example of the need for random allocation to groups is as follows: suppose the researcher allowed the mothers to choose which group they went into in a comparison of the effect on duration of breastfeeding of early discharge from hospital or normal discharge. The mothers that were going to breastfeed longer might have been more confident and therefore more likely to choose the early discharge. If this group then had a longer duration of breastfeeding, it might have reflected the initial attitude of the mother rather than the time of discharge. If the subjects are not randomly assigned to groups, the design becomes quasi-experimental.

There has been more emphasis on randomisation with the recent development of evidence-based practice, which is discussed more fully in Chapter 19. Randomised controlled trials are considered by advocates of evidence-based practice to be the epitome of research evidence on which to base practice. Examples of randomised controlled trials are a study on the effect of pressure bandaging on complications and comfort in patients undergoing coronary angiography (Botti et al. 1998), a study of postural management for breech births (Smith et al. 1999), and a study of kangaroo mother care (KMC) in comparison with conventional cuddling (Roberts, McEwan & Paynter 2000).

Manipulation of the independent variable

In a true experiment, the researcher must be able to manipulate the independent variable or variables. The manipulation of the independent variable by giving the intervention to only one group ensures that, provided all other things are equal, any change in the group receiving the independent variable is then attributable to the effects of that variable.

This manipulation should ensure that the levels of the independent variable are as different as possible to pick up different findings of the groups. For example, using KMC as the independent variable, if the treatment group receives KMC for two hours on one day and the control group receives none, there would probably not be as much difference in the findings for the dependent variable as if the treatment group received KMC for two hours on 20 days.

The experimental design has the advantage that it is the only one that can truly demonstrate a causal relationship between variables because of its tight control over the experimental conditions. On the other hand, this very degree of control can create an unrealistic situation.

Types of true experimental designs
Equivalent control group pre-test post-test design

This design features random allocation of subjects to the control and experimental groups, pre-testing of both groups on the dependent variable, administration of treatment to the experimental group but not the control group, and measurement of the dependent variable on a post-test.

RE	O1	X	O2
RC	O1		O2

The results of the experiment are established by a set of comparisons. The pre-test measurements of both groups (**O1**) are compared to establish whether the groups were in fact initially equivalent. Pre-test measurements will also establish a baseline measurement. The post-test measurements for both groups (**O2**) are compared with the pre-test measurements to establish if there has been a change and if so in what direction. If the treatment has been successful, the experimental group should achieve a significantly different post-test measurement from its pre-test measurement. It should also achieve a significantly different post-test measurement from the control group not receiving the treatment. The control group may also demonstrate a slight change in the same direction because of the placebo effect.

An example of this type of design is one in which a cabbage extract ointment was tested for its effectiveness in treating breast engorgement (Roberts, Reiter & Schuster 1998). The active ointment was compared to a placebo, an inert cream that could not be distinguished from the active cream. The clients were randomly assigned to the control and treatment groups. The midwives and the clients were blind to the type of cream. The subjects were pre-tested for chest circumference, pain perceptions and hardness of breast tissue. The cream was then applied and subjects were tested after it had been on for two hours. Then the measurements were repeated. The pre-test readings of the two groups were compared to establish if they were in fact equivalent. Post-test readings were compared with the pre-test readings to see if there was any change. The post-test readings of the two groups were then compared to see if there was any difference in them. This design enabled the researchers to have confidence in the validity of the findings.

This design is considered to be the best because it controls for any changes during the course of the experiment.

Post-test only control group design

This design is often used when a pre-test is not possible or desirable. There are still two groups, a control and an experimental group. A post-test is given to both groups. A control group is used and subjects are allocated randomly to the two groups. The advantage of this design is that it eliminates any testing effect so may be used where the measurement is a test of learning or skill. This design can be diagrammed as follows:

$$RE \quad X \quad O1$$
$$RC \quad \quad O1$$

An example of this type of design is a study on the effects of Swedish massage on post-operative pain (Nixon et al. 1997). The experimental or treatment group was given the massage, while the control group was not. There was, however, a deviation from this design in assignment to groups as during the study the assignment was random at the beginning but not later. The researchers found ambiguous results. This design was appropriate for this study because the researchers could not do a pre-test since they were measuring post-operative pain. The use of a control group that did not receive the massage ensured that any effect of receiving attention was controlled.

A potential problem with this design is using it where the pre-test post-test design should be used instead. As we have seen above, sometimes it is not possible to do a pre-test. However, if you use a control group with randomisation to groups, you can reasonably assume that the groups were the same to start with and that the results were due to the treatment. If the treatment was effective, there should be a significant difference between the two groups' readings. On the other hand, if you do not do a pre-test when you should, you are not really sure whether the groups were in fact equal before the treatment so you do not know how much change might have occurred or in what direction.

Solomon four-groups design

This is a special type of experimental design that is used when the experimenter is worried that the use of a pre-test would affect the post-test readings, but is concerned to achieve equality of the groups. In this design, there are two control groups and two experimental groups. One control and experimental set is given the pre-test and the other is not. This design could be diagrammed as follows:

RE1	O1	X	O2
RC1	O1		O2
RE2		X	O2
RC2			O2

The results of an experiment with this design would be interpreted as follows. If the pre-test did not have any effect, the two experimental groups should have the same result on the post-test. If the pre-test did sensitise the subjects, the two experimental groups would have different results on the post-test. The comparison of the control with the experimental groups should be interpreted in the same way as for other experiments.

This design is a powerful design to control for testing effect and intervening variables. However, its disadvantage is that it requires many more subjects.

Factorial designs

Factorial designs involve the measuring of two or more independent variables on a dependent variable. For example, if you wanted to measure the effects of both type and timing of back care on the development of pressure sores, either you would have to do two different studies or you could develop a design that had two different independent variables, or factors. Type of back care – e.g. alcohol rub versus back cream – would be one factor, while frequency of back care – e.g. four-hourly versus two-hourly – would be the second factor. This design would have four cells, to which subjects would be assigned randomly. More complex designs with more factors and levels are possible.

	Four-hourly care	Two-hourly care
Alcohol rub	Group 1	Group 2
Back cream	Group 3	Group 4

Thus, one group would have two-hourly back care with alcohol rub, one would have two-hourly back care with back cream, and so on. This would be called a two by two factorial design because there are two factors and two levels of treatment.

Quasi-experimental designs

The word 'quasi' means 'almost' in Latin. Quasi-experimental designs are so called because they do not quite meet the requirements of classic experimental design. Quasi-experimental designs fall short of the standards set for experimental designs because there is no random allocation to control and experimental groups. Much nursing research is of this type, because random allocation in the clinical setting is often impossible. Often a control group uses a conventional treatment and the experimental group uses a new treatment. This design is susceptible to the placebo effect.

Campbell and Stanley (1966) point out that an inability to conceive and execute the perfect experimental design should not cause a sense of hopelessness in the researcher. They state that it is important to do the research but to be aware of which specific variables your design fails to control so that you interpret the findings accurately.

Non-equivalent control group designs

The most common design of the quasi-experimental type is the non-equivalent control group design. While this design does use a control group, it varies from the classic experimental design by using groups that either have been established already or are going to be established but not randomly. The subjects are self-selected into the groups or selected on some criterion. Therefore the non-equivalent control group design does not meet the criterion for random allocation to groups. The biggest problem with a non-equivalent control group design is that you cannot be absolutely sure that the groups were equal to begin with because subjects were not randomly assigned to the groups. Collection of data about possible extraneous variables such as gender, age and educational levels will help to establish whether or not the groups were equivalent on these variables. A pre-test will help to establish whether or not the groups were initially equivalent on the dependent variable.

For example, suppose that you wanted to test out the effect of a new dressing technique on wound healing compared with a traditional technique. If subjects were randomly allocated to control and experimental groups, each group must always have the same type of dressing technique. This would mean that the nurses probably would have to do dressings using the two different techniques because of changing patient allocations, which would be confusing and difficult to manage. By the same token, randomly allocating the nurses to two different techniques on one ward would not work because of shifting patient allocations – patients would most likely end up in both groups because you couldn't guarantee the continuity of nurse–client allocation. For these reasons, you would probably have to settle for using two wards, an experimental and a control ward, and introduce the new technique into the experimental ward. This then becomes a non-equivalent control group design.

Sometimes where random allocation to groups is not feasible and the groups are therefore not equivalent, subjects in the experimental group are matched with subjects in the control group on critical variables and their results are compared. This is not considered as tight a design as random allocation. An example of this type of design is a study in which pairs of clients were matched on variables identified in a pilot study, for the purposes of comparing post-operative pain in groups receiving and not receiving massage (Nixon et al. 1997).

Within the non-equivalent control group design, there are two types, the pre-test post-test type and the post-test only type. The pre-test post-test design can be diagrammed as follows:

$$
\begin{array}{cccc}
E & O1 & X & O2 \\
\hline
C & O1 & & O2
\end{array}
$$

This design has the advantage of establishing whether or not the groups were equivalent on the experimental variable before the treatment.

Another quasi-experimental design is the post-test only non-equivalent control group design. This design is similar to the pre-test post-test non-equivalent control group design except that it has only a post-test. This design can be diagrammed as follows:

    E   X   O2

    C   O2

Without the pre-test, normally you have no way of knowing whether the groups were initially equal on the experimental variable. However, as noted earlier, not all studies are suited to a pre-test.

An example of a non-equivalent groups post-test only design can be found in a study by Logan (1999), in which babies in two different regional Victorian hospitals were subjected to two different types of newborn screening test: heel prick and venepuncture in a superficial vein of the dorsal surface of the hand (VSVDH). One ward was the experimental ward, in which the VSVDH was carried out, while on the other, the control ward, the heel prick was done. This design avoids the confusion of trying to carry out two different procedures in the same ward. The post-test only design was chosen because the outcomes of crying parameters and time taken to collect the sample were not susceptible to pre-testing and one could assume that the babies started out equivalent at birth. Logan found that VSVDH was superior to the heel prick on all variables measured. Another example is a study in which the rate of Caesarean section was compared in women presenting to a birth centre and a conventional labour ward (Homer et al. 2000). The researchers found no significant difference in rate of Caesareans but that the women in the birth centre were less likely to use analgesia in labour.

Longitudinal designs

In longitudinal designs, the primary objective is to see whether a phenomenon changes over time by identifying time-dependent patterns in data. Longitudinal designs can be used with correlational experimental and quasi-experimental designs. The time period in a longitudinal design may be several years. A cohort is a group of people that enter the study at the same time.

Time series designs

A time series design is one in which the experimenter makes several measurements, both before and after the treatment. This helps to measure any variations in the data that are dependent on time. A simple pre-experimental time series design is diagrammed as follows:

    E   O1   O2   O3   X   O4   O5   O6   X   O7   O8

Time series designs can help show that any changes that occur just after the institution of the treatment are related to the treatment. Nevertheless, without the use of a control group, it is a weak design because it does not control for other events that happen during the course of the study. With the use of a non-equivalent control group, this design can become quasi-experimental, or with the use of random assignment to control and experimental groups it can become experimental.

A cross-sectional design is one in which the effects of time are established by comparing groups at different points on the phenomenon of interest. For example, the effect of time on a clinical treatment could be established by comparing groups at different points in their treatment. The advantage of this design is that it can measure the effects of time relatively quickly. The weakness of this design is that it does not establish the initial equivalence of the groups studied. An example of a cross-sectional design is a study by Tang and colleagues in which students in Year 11 and Year 12 were surveyed on their intention to study nursing (Tang et al. 1998).

Counterbalanced designs

This is a group of designs that attempt to achieve control by entering all subjects into all treatments. It is usually used where pre-tests are not advisable and control groups are not available. As noted earlier, counterbalanced designs can be used in true experiments as well. This design can be diagrammed as:

$$X1 \quad O \quad X2 \quad O$$

An example of a counterbalanced design is a study in which electrocardiographic tracings were compared on the same subjects using both tap water and electroconductive gel (Birks et al. 1993). In all subjects, the first tracing was done using water and the second using the gel. No significant difference was found.

This group of designs includes crossover designs. This can be diagrammed as:

$$\text{Group A} \quad X1 \quad O \quad X2 \quad O$$
$$\text{Group B} \quad X2 \quad O \quad X1 \quad O$$

An example of a crossover design is a study by Roberts and colleagues (1995) in which well female subjects had their respiratory volumes measured before and after spending 20 minutes on boomerang pillows and before and after spending 20 minutes on ordinary pillows. The women were randomised as to which treatment they had first to control for history in the form of fatigue. The treatment did not affect lung volumes. Another example is a study comparing povidone iodine and chlorhexidine gluconate solution and alcohol for pre-cannulation skin disinfection (Wellard & Palaster 1996). The researchers found no difference in effectiveness but the latter method was preferred by patients and was also cheaper.

Sometimes in clinical trials using placebos, there is a refinement called a 'crossover' effect built into the design. This means that at a certain point in the experiment, persons on the experimental drug are switched over to the placebo and vice versa. If the outcome data vary with the crossover, then this is additional evidence that the drug is effective. This design could be diagrammed as follows:

RE   O1 X – active   O2 \ Crossover / RC O3 X – placebo O4
RC   O1 X – placebo O2 / Crossover \ RE O3 X – active   O4

The advantage of counterbalanced designs is that in the absence of an equivalent control group of different subjects, some degree of control is achieved because the same subjects essentially serve as their own equivalent control group. This design, however, has the weakness of possible testing effects.

Summary

In this chapter, we have discussed the three major types of quantitative design: descriptive, correlational and experimental. We have examined the advantages and disadvantages of each type, with references to examples from the Australian nursing literature. You should now be able to carry out one of the most interesting parts of the research process: choosing a research design that will give you the best possible opportunity of answering the research question that you set out to ask.

Main points

- A research design guides you in carrying out your study, tells you exactly what must be done, and answers the questions 'how?' 'when?' and 'where?'
- Types of designs include descriptive designs, which only describe phenomena; correlational designs, which look for relationships in the data; and experimental designs, which attempt to show causality by testing hypotheses.
- The best research design is the one that is most likely to help you answer your research question.
- Simple descriptive designs measure known variables in a population, often by questionnaire surveys, interviews, and observation. They are inexpensive and relatively quick to administer. They are useful for preliminary research but they cannot determine the amount of difference between groups, relationships of characteristics or causality.
- Comparative descriptive designs compare two or more groups on particular variables. They have the same advantages and disadvantages as simple descriptive design but allow comparison of groups.
- Correlational designs examine the relationship of variables within one group without aiming to determine cause and effect. They can examine the direction and the strength of the relationship but they do not have an independent variable that can be manipulated.
- The researcher identifies the target variables and chooses the best way to measure them, usually by observation, interviews, or surveys. The researcher then carries out a statistical analysis to determine if there are relationships between the variables, and if so, how strong, and in what direction they are.

- A correlational design is relatively easy, fast, and inexpensive to use, and it is useful in exploratory research to determine relationships for later, more rigorous testing. However, it too does not show causality.
- In an experimental design, the subjects are exposed to the event or treatment, and the response is measured. A control group can receive a standard treatment or be untreated. An experimental design can show whether changes in one variable cause effects in the other and has the potential to show the strength of an association between variables. However, it is usually unnatural and not always suitable for answering important nursing questions.
- Broadly, experimental designs can include many types of designs, including pre-experimental and quasi-experimental designs. A true experimental design is characterised by the use of an equivalent control group, with subjects allocated to the two groups by random methods.
- Internal validity in scientific research is that the research measures what it claims to measure. External validity refers to generalisability to the population.
- Threats to validity can include changes to the participants, changing procedures and measurements, changes in observation and extraneous variables.

Review Questions

1. A design that compares two or more groups on particular variables is:
   a comparative descriptive
   b quasi-experimental
   c experimental
   d correlational

2. A design that is able to determine cause and effect is:
   a one-shot case study
   b correlational
   c experimental
   d action research

3. Which of the following refers to people changing their behaviour when they know they are being observed?
   a maturation effect
   b Hawthorne effect
   c placebo effect
   d testing effect

4 A researcher intends to investigate whether there is a relationship between passive smoking and coughing. The design to be used would probably be:
   a experimental
   b action research
   c critical ethnography
   d correlational

5 A researcher wants to examine whether the application of cold decreases tissue swelling. The best design would be:
   a experiment with equivalent control groups
   b time series
   c Solomon four-groups
   d phenomenology

6 A researcher wants to find out whether clients who have low mobility have longer healing periods for decubiti. The most appropriate type of design would be:
   a ethnographic
   b correlational
   c experimental
   d comparative descriptive

7 The advantage of a crossover design in an experiment is that it:
   a shows the effect of both treatments on both groups
   b is easy to measure
   c eliminates the need for an untreated control group
   d a and c

8 A factorial design has:
   a only one independent variable but more than one dependent variable
   b one independent and one dependent variable
   c more than one independent variable and one dependent variable
   d more than one independent variable and more than one dependent variable

9 A researcher wants to study the effects of pre-operative teaching on post-operative stress. The most appropriate design for this would be:
   a equivalent groups pre- and post-test design
   b equivalent groups post-test only design
   c correlational design
   d comparative descriptive design

10 A researcher wants to study the effects of the refugee experience on self-caring abilities in refugees from Malagonia. The most likely design to be used in the first instance would be:
   a correlational
   b comparative descriptive
   c one-shot case study
   d experiment

Discussion Questions

1 What is the purpose of a research design?
2 Distinguish between a descriptive, a correlational and an experimental design.
3 Distinguish between a pre-experimental, a quasi-experimental and an experimental design.
4 What it the reason for using a control group?
5 What is meant by random assignment to groups and why is it necessary?

References

Armstrong, R., Barrack, D. & Gordon, R. 1995, 'Patients achieve accurate home blood pressure measurement following instruction', *Australian Journal of Advanced Nursing*, vol. 12, no. 4, 15–21.

Birks, M., Santamaria, N., Thompson, S. & Amerena, J. 1993, 'A clinical trial of the effectiveness of water as a conductive medium in electrocardiography', *Australian Journal of Advanced Nursing*, vol. 10, no. 2, 10–13.

Botti, M., Williamson, B., Steen, K., McTaggart, J. & Reid, E. 1998, 'The effect of pressure bandaging on complications and comfort in patients undergoing coronary angiography: a multicenter randomized trial', *Heart & Lung: the Journal of Acute and Critical Care*, vol. 27, no. 6, 360–73.

Campbell, D. T. & Stanley, J. C. 1966, 'Experimental and quasi-experimental designs for research on teaching', in *Handbook of Research on Teaching*, ed. N. L. Gage, Rand McNally, Chicago.

Homer, C., Davis, G., Petocz, P. & Barclay, L. 2000, 'Birth centre or labour ward? A comparison of the clinical outcomes of low-risk women in a NSW hospital', *Australian Journal of Advanced Nursing*, vol. 18, no. 1, 8–12.

Lo, R. & Brown, R. 1999, 'Perceptions of nursing students on men entering nursing as a career', *Australian Journal of Advanced Nursing*, vol. 17, no. 2, 36–41.

Logan, P. 1999, 'Venepuncture versus heel prick for the collection of the newborn screening test', *Australian Journal of Advanced Nursing*, vol. 17, no. 1, 30–6.

Nixon, M., Teschendorff, J., Finney, J. & Karnilowicz, W. 1997, 'Expanding the nursing repertoires: the effect of massage on post-operative pain', *Australian Journal of Advanced Nursing*, vol. 14, no. 3, 21–6.

Retsas, A. & Pinikahana, J. 1999, 'Manual handling practices and injuries among ICU nurses', *Australian Journal of Advanced Nursing*, vol. 17, no. 1, 37–41.

Robbins, P. R. 1994, *Management*, 4th edn, Prentice-Hall International Inc., USA.

Roberts, K., Brittin, M. & deClifford, J. 1995, 'Boomerang pillows and respiratory capacity in frail elderly women', *Clinical Nursing Research*, vol. 4, no. 4, 465–71.

Roberts, K., McEwan, B. & Paynter, C. 2000, 'A comparison of kangaroo mother care and conventional cuddling', *Neonatal Network*, vol. 19, no. 4, 31–5.

Roberts, K., Reiter, M. & Schuster, D. 1998, 'Effects of cabbage leaf extract on breast engorgement', *Journal of Human Lactation*, vol. 14, no. 3, 231–6.

Santamaria, N. 2000, 'The relationship between nurses' personality and stress levels reported when caring for interpersonally difficult patients', *Australian Journal of Advanced Nursing*, vol. 18, no. 2, 20–6.

Smith, C., Crowther, C., Wilkinson, C., Pridmore, B. & Robinson, J. 1999, 'Knee–chest postural management for breach [sic] at term: a randomized controlled trial', *Birth: Issues in Perinatal Care and Education*, vol. 26, no. 2, 71–5.

Tang, K., Duffield, C., Chen, J., Choucair, S., Creegan, R., Mak, C. & Lesley, G. 1998, 'Predictors of intention to study nursing among school students speaking a language other than English at home', *Australian Journal of Advanced Nursing*, vol. 15, no. 2, 33–9.

Wellard, S. & Palaster, L. 1996, 'An evaluation of two methods of pre-cannulation skin disinfection', *Australian Journal of Advanced Nursing*, vol. 14, no. 1, 3–7.

Wu, M. & Courtney, M. 2000, 'Models of nursing care: a comparative descriptive study of patient satisfaction on two orthopaedic wards in Brisbane', *Australian Journal of Advanced Nursing*, vol. 17, no. 4, 29–34.

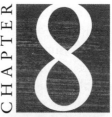

Quantitative methods

chapter objectives The material presented in this chapter will assist you to:

- identify a suitable setting in which to collect data
- choose an appropriate sampling method
- choose a data collection method that is suited to the design of the study
- outline the advantages and disadvantages of triangulation.

Introduction

In this chapter, we are going to talk about the types of methods that can be used in carrying out quantitative studies. In previous chapters, you learned how to select a problem that you want to investigate, review the literature on the problem, choose a broad methodological approach that suits the problem, and design the study. This chapter will narrow down the focus into the methods that need to be considered in order to implement the study. We will consider the appropriate setting, and types of sample. We will also explore methods of obtaining data by measurement and instrumentation, observation, and collecting information. Finally, we will examine the concept of triangulation.

Choosing a setting

The setting for the study is the place in which you, the researcher, carry it out and in which you can observe the phenomenon in which you are interested. It may be a range of places, varying from a naturalistic setting to a laboratory.

A naturalistic setting is a place in which people carry out their activities of daily life such as working, playing, or whatever phenomenon is under investigation. For example, in nursing research, a naturalistic setting might be a clinical field setting such as a hospital ward, a clinic or a nursing home. You would choose a naturalistic setting if you wanted to observe events as they occur naturally.

Data acquired from a natural setting have the advantage of increased ecological validity since the phenomenon was observed in its real situation. Other researchers will be able to compare your setting with theirs and make judgements about whether they think your findings would be valid in their setting. The disadvantage of natural settings is that they are difficult for the researcher to control. For example, there are many things in a hospital ward that you cannot control, such as routines for care, intervention of staff, presence of visitors, noise levels and so forth. Furthermore, in the natural setting it may be more difficult to make observations and to use the equipment that you need. Since the environmental factors in the clinical field cannot always be controlled it is often advisable to measure any of these factors that you think may have an effect on the study and then see if they affect the findings.

An example of a study carried out in a naturalistic setting was one in which the researchers studied the effects of timing and sites on blood volume during blood letting for blood sugar levels in diabetics in an outpatient clinic (Daniels, Poroch & DeRoach 1995). They found that neither the time elapsed between lancing and collecting the blood nor the site from which the blood was collected affected the amount of blood obtained.

A laboratory setting may be used instead of a natural setting. A laboratory is a place that is specially constructed for the purposes of practice or research. A laboratory setting is used when the researcher needs to have a great deal of control over the research situation, which often gives greater internal validity to the study. The advantage of using a laboratory is that you can control such environmental factors as temperature and procedures. You can also control who has access to the laboratory and can often prevent unforeseen events from affecting your investigation. Because experimental designs require manipulation of the independent variable they are often done under the more controlled conditions in a laboratory. Another advantage of a laboratory setting is that the equipment may be easier to use and observation methods may be easier. The disadvantage is that while the study may have greater internal validity, it may have less ecological validity because the conditions are artificial. That is, you cannot guarantee that the findings would be the same if the study were carried out in the actual clinical setting.

An example of a study carried out in a laboratory is a study in which the researchers compared the lung volumes of well women on boomerang pillows and on straight pillows, with the women serving as their own controls (Roberts et al. 1994). No significant difference in the tidal volumes of the women on the two types of pillows was found. No other example was found in the literature since 1994, indicating that laboratory research is not often done in nursing.

It is important to decide which setting to use while planning the study. You need to go back to your research question and ask yourself what setting will best help you answer the question. You should also ask yourself whether it is more important to observe the phenomenon in its natural setting or to be able to control the variables. Despite the advantages of a laboratory setting, most nursing studies are carried out in the clinical setting. This may be because it is more realistic or because it is cheaper to use readily available facilities than it is to set up a laboratory.

Defining the population

A population is a group whose members have specific common characteristics that you wish to investigate in your research study. It is important to select the population that will enable you to answer your question. A single unit of the population under study is an element. The elements do not have to be people, although often they are. The elements of the population can also be places, such as hospitals; objects, for example syringes; or events, such as immunisations. You identify your population by reviewing the literature, the conceptual framework for your study and the definition of the problem that you wish to investigate.

The population that you wish to study or to which you would like to generalise your findings is called the target population. For example, the target population in a study investigating remedies for breast engorgement would be 'all lactating women with breast engorgement'. The target population is sometimes called a 'universe'. However, one is not usually able to include the whole target population because of limited money and time. Furthermore, the members of the population may be geographically dispersed or unwilling to participate. The part of the target population that you are able to access is the accessible population. For example, the accessible population might be only those women with breast engorgement who live in a particular geographical area.

Sampling

For various reasons, one cannot usually collect data on all of the target population of a particular study. First, it is unlikely that the whole population would agree to be in the study. Secondly, there are also usually limitations of time and budget. It is better to use limited resources to acquire a smaller amount of accurate data rather than a lot of thin data. It is therefore customary to study only a part of the target population. This part of the population is called a sample. Using a sample often allows you to carry out all of the data collection yourself, thereby increasing your control and avoiding the complication of differences among data collectors. The part of the population used for sample selection is a sampling unit, for example a hospital, a person, or a patient's chart. Figure 8.1 shows the process of sampling.

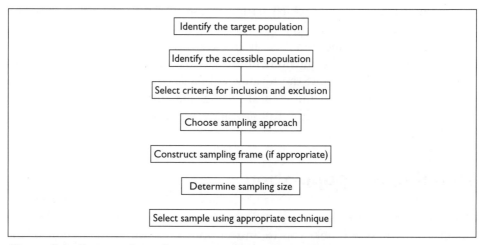

Figure 8.1 Process of sampling

Before actually drawing a sample, it is important that you make a sampling plan, which you devise in relation to the question that you want to answer and the variables of interest in your study. This allows you to be methodical about the sample and consider the various choices that you can make. By devising a plan, you will be able to see how feasible is your desired method in terms of money and resources and you will be able to get the most precise sample possible under your particular constraints. The sampling plan will help you to justify your choice of a particular sampling technique in the research proposal and in the research report. It will include the type of sample, the size of sample and the process for choosing the elements of the population that take part in the sample.

It is important to determine the characteristics of the sample before you select it. You need to ensure that the characteristics of the sample are linked to the variables that you want to measure. A simplistic example is that if you want to measure gender, it is not appropriate to confine your sample to only men or women.

It is important to determine the size of the sample before you collect your data. There are scientific and ethical considerations concerning the size of the sample. It must be sufficiently large to yield valid data or else the study will lack internal validity. However, where there is the possibility of harmful effects from participating in the study, the size of the sample should be the minimum sufficient to answer the research question. There are formulas available to assist with calculating the size of the sample to give sufficient power to the results. Applying such a formula is called a power analysis. One useful discussion of this can be found in Dawson-Saunders and Trapp (2001). The size of the population for a potential survey can be taken into consideration. For large groups, for example where there are thousands of potential respondents to a questionnaire, often a 10 per cent sample will be enough. Another consideration concerning the size of the sample is the number of variables. The more sub-groups you want to compare, the greater the size of the sample must be. For example, if you merely wanted to compare males and females, there would need to be only a minimum of data. However, if you wanted to compare males and females of three ethnic groups, this would require considerably more data to be able to draw meaningful conclusions.

The most common mistake of beginning researchers is to attempt a study that is too comprehensive and tries to answer too many questions. The process of determining the sample size is very effective in bringing home the idea that it is better to have a manageable sample size and answer one significant question than it is to assemble masses of data on a great many things and thus learn very little about anything.

Types of samples

The main types of samples and their advantages and disadvantages have been described by Henry (1990) and will be outlined briefly here. The two major types of samples are probability samples and non-probability samples. A probability sample is one that resembles the population as closely as possible and is usually selected randomly from the population. It is used to calculate the probability that the results can be generalised to the population. A non-probability sample is one that does not attempt to portray the population in miniature and the results cannot be generalised to the population. As a researcher, you will have to make a judgement about which approach will fulfil the objectives of your research.

Probability sampling

A probability sample is one that attempts to portray the target population in miniature. The distinguishing characteristics of a probability sample are, first, that each element in the population has a possibility of being chosen to take part and, secondly, the probability of its being included in the sample is known. An equal probability sample is one in which every element of the population has an equal chance of being chosen. If some elements of the population have a greater chance of being chosen than others, it is an unequal probability sample.

The probability sample is chosen by objective techniques rather than by the subjective judgement of the researcher in order to prevent sampling bias. Sampling bias occurs when the researcher, either consciously or unconsciously, selects some participants in preference to others. Only if the sample is without bias can findings be generalised to the entire population. The sample is never actually identical to the population and there is always a sampling error, which is the difference between the sample and the population. Statistical analysis can show to what extent the sample actually is representative of the population by calculating the standard error. Larger-sized samples have less sampling error.

Probability samples include the simple random sample, the systematic random sample, cluster sampling and multi-stage sampling. For a probability sample, all members of the population are physically present or listed in a sampling frame. Each element appears once and only once in the sampling frame. If all of the elements of the population are not known, the sample cannot be a probability sample. For example, you could not use the telephone book to draw a probability sample from a city population since not all people have telephones. An example of a study using a sampling frame is one in which the total population of nursing staff in the Western Sydney Health Area were in the frame and a random sample was drawn from the population (Lam, Ross & Cass 1999).

Random samples

A random sample is a sample drawn at random from the target population. Each element in the sampling frame can be selected independently of any other element. A technique for selecting elements randomly must be used in order to prevent any bias in the selection of the sample. This can be done in several ways, for example by lottery, by random number table or by a computer program. In the lottery method, names or numbers can be drawn out of a container after thorough mixing. If the numbers are not well mixed at the end, the last ones in have a greater probability of being drawn. A random number table can also be used. Random numbers can be generated by a computer spreadsheet program. In this method, each element in the population is assigned a number. The researcher, with eyes closed, then points to any number in the random number table and moves in any systematic fashion selecting every nth number until the correct number of potential participants has been reached. The third method is to use a computer program that will generate a random list of units from the list of elements.

The simple random sample is, as its name suggests, the least complicated type of sample. For a simple random sample, you choose elements at random according to the selected method until you attain the previously determined number of elements. Once selected, an element is not replaced in the sample. The best-known example of selection of a simple random sample is a lottery. Throughout Australia we have lotteries where the draw is conducted on television. The 50 numbers are placed in a bowl and a given number of balls, usually six, are selected at random. Each number has an equal chance of being selected. A computer-generated random sample was used by Grindlay, Santamaria and Kitt (2000) in their study of nurse safety in the 'hospital in the home' program.

The systematic sample is a variation on the simple random sample. You take the population list and randomly select the starting point. Then you select every nth element. For example, if you wanted a 10 per cent sample, you would select every 10th element. This is called a sampling interval. To find the sampling interval, you divide the population by the number in the sample. For example, if you want a sample of 75 in a population of 3000, you would divide 3000 by 75 and take every 40th person. This method is easier to apply than a simple random sample but the start must be random in order for every element to have a chance of selection. In addition, it is important to avoid any situation that could interfere with the randomness of the selection process.

Stratified samples

Stratified sampling is the selection of elements from a target population that has previously been divided into groups called strata. For example, a group of university students could be divided into undergraduate and postgraduate strata. Each element is placed into one stratum only. Then you select elements randomly from each stratum in the same way as for a simple or systematic random sample. If you take the same proportion from each stratum, the sample will have elements of each stratum in the same proportion as in the population. If you want to increase the numbers of a particular group in the sample, you can select proportionally more of them. This is then called a disproportionate stratified sample. The analysis of data from a disproportionate sample requires the weighting of elements to compensate for the disproportion of the sample.

Cluster sample

In cluster sampling, groups of elements in a cluster are sampled rather than individual elements. The population is divided prior to sampling into unique, non-overlapping groups, or clusters. These can be naturally occurring groups of elements such as schools, hospitals or health areas. Then the clusters are chosen randomly and each member of the cluster is studied. For example, if you wished to study the attitudes of nurses working in hospitals in a particular state but were not able to take a random sample of all of these nurses, you could divide the population into hospitals, which would be your clusters. Then you could randomly select a percentage of the hospitals. You would then survey every nurse working in the selected hospitals. The cluster is the unit of sampling. Cluster sampling is useful where you cannot get lists of the whole population. It can reduce transportation and training costs.

Multi-stage sample

Multi-stage sampling is an extension of cluster sampling. In multi-stage sampling, you first select clusters randomly according to the above method. Then you randomly select units to sample within those clusters. Sometimes there are two stages of cluster sampling before the random sampling. For example, suppose in the above example of wanting to study the attitudes of all nurses in the state hospital system, it was a very large state with hundreds of hospitals. You might, as a first stage, take the health service areas and randomly select a percentage of those. Then you might take the clusters of hospitals within the selected health service areas and randomly select a percentage of those hospitals. Then you could randomly select a proportion of the nurses on the payroll of those selected hospitals. That would be a three-stage sampling process. In addition, it is possible to add stratification to the process to make sure that you include representatives of different-sized hospitals, or nurses working different shifts, or other variables of interest.

Non-probability sampling

Non-probability sampling is sampling in which subjective judgements contribute to the selection of the sample. It is carried out where it is not possible or advisable to use probability sampling. You may have limited resources, you may be unable to identify the members of the population, or you may just need to do exploratory research that will establish whether or not the problem exists. In all of these cases, non-probability sampling is acceptable. However, the disadvantage of non-probability sampling is that, because the sample is not known to be typical of the population, you cannot generalise the results or make conclusions concerning the population from your findings about the sample.

The types of non-probability sampling are convenience sample, typical case sample, critical case sample, snowball sample and quota sample.

Convenience sample

A convenience sample is one that uses any available elements of the population that meet the criteria to enter the study. Convenience samples are very common in clinical nursing research where there may not be enough people to form a probability sample. An example of the use of a convenience sample is a study by Gerdtz and Bucknall (2000) of Australian triage nurses' decision-making and scope of practice. There is also a growing trend to acquire convenience samples from the Internet, using access to discussion lists. Client support groups can be accessed in this manner (Wilmoth 1995).

Case-based samples

Some samples are case-based. Typical case and critical case samples contain elements that are chosen specifically by the researcher. That is, the researcher selects cases that are thought to best represent the phenomenon under study in the population. These are also called purposive samples. A typical case sample is one in which the researchers choose a few cases that they judge to be normal or typical. The validity of this type of sample rests on the ability of the researcher to select typical cases. A critical case sample is one that has previously been found to be, or can be argued to be likely to be, generalisable to the population. For example, certain electorates in an election are thought to be indicative of the overall election result. This type of selection is also seen in the Delphi technique.

Snowball sample

A snowball sample is one in which the initial members of the group identify other possible members, and those members in turn identify other members. Thus the sample grows like a snowball. This type of sampling is used when the researcher is unable to identify the elements of the population in advance, for example with homeless people or illegal aliens. A snowball technique was used by Pelletier and colleagues (2000) in a study of cardiac educators and clinicians. The cardiac educator panel was determined first, and then each educator was asked to identify two suitable clinicians. Other examples of the use of snowball samples in Australian nursing research are in studies on the work of nurse-practitioners (Offredy 2000) and a study on the perceptions of Thai women of prenatal testing (Rice & Naksook 1999).

Quota sample

A quota sample is one in which elements that meet the criteria are chosen until the subsections of the sample are full. Quota sampling is used in research in which it is desirable to access different sub-groups of the population. For example, you might decide that it was necessary to interview a certain percentage of people from different ethnic groups. The interviewer would keep selecting people who fit the criteria until the quota was filled. The problem with quota sampling is that the researcher selects the participant and may unconsciously select certain types of people. Thus quota samples are considered to be biased. However, this is not of concern in qualitative research. A study that used a quota sampling technique to investigate teaching metaphors of student nurses in a phenomenological study was carried out by McAllister and McLaughlin (1996).

Quantitative methods of obtaining data

Data are obtained in quantitative research by a variety of methods that fit in with the variety of research designs. In this chapter, I have grouped them into three major groups: instrumentation, observation, and information. In addition, triangulation involves the combination of methods. There is some overlap with qualitative research methods, particularly in the areas of observation and information. However, before we discuss these methods, we are going to talk about measurement because it is a concept that can apply to all three areas.

Measurement

Measurement is the determination of the size or range of an object, characteristic or phenomenon. Measurements are carried out using instruments. Nurses are very familiar with instruments and measurements as they use them in their daily practice, but they tend to think of them as equipment and procedures. For example, as a nurse you would know how to measure body temperature using a thermometer, blood pressure using a sphygmomanometer, and blood glucose using a glucometer. When these procedures and pieces of equipment are used in research they are called measurement and instruments.

Measurement is important in quantitative research. By measuring the phenomenon of interest, we can produce data that describe phenomena and show the relationship of variables to each other. We can evaluate nursing actions to see how they affect client outcomes. We can obtain data that are reliable and valid. By having common procedures of measurement and common units of measurement, we can compare our findings with those of other researchers. For example, a thermometer is an instrument that always measures in degrees, which are standard units. Thus, the meaning of a degree in one study is the same as that in another study. Even if different temperature scales, such as Celsius and Fahrenheit are used, data can be converted to the other scale for purposes of comparison of findings. Measurement also allows us to get an accurate determination of an effect. As a nurse, you will be familiar with the concept of accuracy in measurement. For example, when giving medications it is important to measure the dose accurately, and when taking a urinalysis, blood pressure or blood glucose it is important to carry out the procedure properly to get an accurate reading. In both clinical practice and research, the conclusions reached are only as good as the accuracy of the data on which they are based.

Before deciding on a method of measurement, it is essential to identify what is to be measured. What is the characteristic or measurement in which you are interested? This is determined by the research question, the hypothesis that has been drawn and the variables that have been identified and operationally defined. You may need to measure the independent variable and/or the dependent variable. Measurements may be used in various designs such as experimental, quasi-experimental, correlational or comparative descriptive designs.

Measurement is usually carried out by instruments. The word 'instrument' is used in research terminology to describe any tool that measures, whether a sophisticated piece of machinery, a questionnaire or a simple checklist on a piece of paper. Even the researcher can be considered an instrument, for example where observation is the method of choice. The advantage of using instruments is that they can increase the accuracy of the measurement and can allow measurement in more detail. In addition, they facilitate recording of data and analysing it by numerical methods such as statistical analysis on computers. The disadvantages are that they may be expensive, mechanical, and prescriptive. Furthermore, the person using the instrument may require special skills to operate it and/or the researcher may require special skills to interpret the data that come out of it.

Direct and indirect measurements

A direct measurement measures an actual characteristic directly, without having to make an inference. The measurement of height by a ruler, temperature of the mouth by a thermometer, weight by a scale, and tidal volume of the lung by a spirometer are all examples of direct measurement using instrumentation. An example of a direct measurement in a research study is the measurement of intracranial pressure using a Siemens monitor in a study on the effects of patient repositioning on intracranial pressure (Jones 1995). Other aspects of the client such as gender, race, religion and marital status can also be measured directly without using instrumentation.

Where direct measurements are not possible, an indirect measurement of one characteristic or phenomenon is taken and the value of another is inferred. These may be done where it is not possible or feasible to take direct measurements. Pain is a phenomenon that cannot be measured directly. It is therefore necessary to use indirect measurements such as a visual analogue scale in which the research participants indicate the level on the scale that corresponds to the amount of pain that they are suffering. Indirect measurements may also be done where the concept is abstract rather than concrete. For example, cardiac status is an abstract concept that has to be inferred from other measurements such as an electrocardiogram.

An example of an indirect measurement from a clinical trial comparing the effectiveness of water and conductive gel in electrocardiograms was the inference of the effectiveness of the conductive medium from the height of the R-wave on the ECG (Birks et al. 1993). The researchers found no difference in the height of the R waves in the two media and concluded that there was no difference in the effectiveness of the two media. If you are using indirect measurements it is important to have an operational definition of what is being measured. There is considerable scope for error in indirect measurement. For example, only part of the characteristic may be measured, or irrelevant measurements may be made unintentionally.

Some phenomena or characteristics may be measured either directly or indirectly. For example, suppose you wanted to measure blood pressure. You could measure it either indirectly by a sphygmomanometer, or directly by an arterial line.

In vitro *and* in vivo *measurements*

Biophysiological measurements may also be classified as *in vitro* or *in vivo*. In Latin, *vitro* means glass (i.e. a test tube), while *vivo* means living person. Thus, *in vitro* means a measurement that is done on a sample taken from the participant, but analysed after it has been removed from the participant. *In vitro* tests usually measure chemical components carried out as hormone assays or blood components such as cholesterol; microbiological components such as infection carried out in microbiological cultures; and tissue or cell components carried out in pathology or cytology tests. *In vitro* tests may be done at the patient's bedside, for example a glucometer reading. However, many *in vitro* tests are sent to the laboratory for analysis. If you are involved in collecting *in vitro* specimens involving body fluids you should be aware of the dangers of infection. As a researcher handling *in vitro* specimens, you should ensure that appropriate procedures are carried out for labelling specimens, sending them to the laboratory and storing them.

An example of an *in vitro* measurement is the measurement of blood volume in a study done to test for the effect of sites and timing on blood volume in samples taken for analysis from diabetics in a clinic (Daniels, Poroch & DeRoach 1995). The blood samples were taken to the laboratory for analysis, so were *in vitro* measurements. The researchers found no effects of timing or sites on blood volume.

In vivo measurements are those taken directly on the participant and the value is obtained at the time of measurements. *In vivo* measurements are usually physiological characteristics of participants. Examples of *in vivo* measurements are blood pressure recordings, and temperature, pulse and respiration recordings. An example of an *in vivo* measurement from a research study is the use of the Siemens monitor to measure intracranial pressure in the study described above (Jones 1995).

Measurement-related error

Whenever measurements are carried out, there is the potential for error. As a researcher, you will need to be aware of possible errors in order to prevent, control or take account of them in the design and conduct of the research. This will diminish the threat to the validity of your findings. We have considered already error in the design of a study. Errors can also result from the measurement phase of the study.

One of the major errors in the measurement phase can result from mistakes made by the researcher in carrying out the measurements. The researcher may make mistakes in administering the instrument in such a way as to cause a false reading.

Errors can also result from variations in the participants, the environment and the procedures. The participants may be tired, hungry or emotionally affected, which could affect their response to an instrument. The environment may vary, for example, noise, temperature or electric current could cause an error in measurement. The procedures may vary from one participant to another. There could be mistakes in processing specimens – for example, laboratory specimens can be improperly collected or labelled. In the laboratory, some measurements can be made inaccurately.

Error in measurement terms means 'how accurate is a particular measurement?' It has to do with the resolution and repeatability of the measurement and this concerns both the instrument and the object being measured. Errors can be classified as random or systematic.

A group of researchers could use a micrometer to measure the thickness of a piece of steel and everyone would probably get the same answer within ± 0.01 mm. But if the same researchers tried to measure the thickness of a piece of skin with the same micrometer the tolerance might well be ± 0.1 mm. Such errors are random and can be readily determined as the standard deviation of the observations.

There may also be systematic error in an experiment. Systematic error refers to errors within the system that generate bias. Systematic error is an error that occurs whenever a procedure is carried out or at regular intervals. Systematic error may result from faulty equipment, for example a thermometer that always reads one-half of a degree too high. Pulling too hard on a tape measure around someone's chest results systematically in a measurement that is too low. Systematic error can also result from the use of multiple instruments that have not been calibrated and are thus not measuring the same. Finally, there may be a regular effect of a stimulus that changes the reading of the instrument, for example an electric current that interferes with an electronic reading. Systematic error can be avoided by taking multiple measurements and comparing the results.

Instrumentation
Selecting an appropriate instrument

In choosing an instrument, whether biophysiological or not, it is necessary to consider several factors. You should consider primarily whether the proposed instrument is the most appropriate one to help you answer the research question. The primary consideration is the validity of the instrument, or the extent to which it measures the characteristic that you are trying to measure. If the instrument is not the right one, other considerations are not important. This is easy with known factors; for example everyone knows that the correct instrument for measuring temperature is a thermometer. However, it is less easy with instruments such as questionnaires that measure more abstract concepts. When you are choosing an instrument, it is useful to consult previous studies to see how they have evaluated the validity of an instrument.

You should also consider the sensitivity of the instrument or how precisely it measures. It must be sensitive enough to pick up the amount of change that you want to measure. For example, if you wanted to measure temperature change in tenths of a degree, a thermometer that measured only fifths of a degree would not be sensitive enough. For a known instrument, you can check the manufacturer's specifications to see how sensitive it is.

You should also consider how accurate you need the measurement to be. Invasive instruments may be more accurate but they have a greater potential for injury. The accuracy of an instrument may be affected by the quality control in the manufacturing process, by wear and tear and by environmental factors such as the temperature or humidity of the environment. Before they are used many instruments will need to be calibrated against a known measurement so that their accuracy is established. The manufacturer's specifications will usually give the accuracy, or tolerance of the instrument.

You need to consider also the reliability of the instrument. It should measure consistently over time, that is, measurements should not vary very much with subsequent recordings or an error may creep in and the data will not be very accurate. Reliability can be checked by calibrating the instrument periodically.

You need to consider the cost of the instrument and the extent to which specialised training will be required. Although research budgets are limited, the validity and accuracy of the instrument should be a primary consideration. It is worth approaching the manufacturer of the instrument; sometimes a manufacturer will be willing to donate an instrument for research purposes.

Availability and suitability for the participants may be considerations too. You will need to check that the instrument is available when you want it. You should also ascertain that the instrument will be suitable for your proposed participants.

If a suitable instrument is not available, you may have to develop one, although this is not to be undertaken lightly by the beginning researcher. In developing an instrument, it is important to ensure that it is valid. This can be done by exposing it to a proven developmental process. The instrument is scrutinised by experts in the field for face validity in terms of the effectiveness of the structure, and its validity. Then it is put through a trial to see if it measures what it is supposed to be measuring. It should also be checked for reliability to see if it consistently measures the same on repeated measurements. Finally, it is revised. If there have been a lot of revisions, it would be wise to trial it a second time.

An excellent, comprehensive book on instruments for clinical health care research is by Frank-Stromborg and Olsen (1997). If you are seeking a particular type of instrument, you should look it up in such a book.

Biophysiological instrumentation

In recent times, there has been an increase in clinical nursing studies which tend to use biophysiological instrumentation to measure biophysiological variables such as body temperature, blood pressure, biochemical values, blood gases, and types of infection. However, not all data in clinical research are obtained by biophysiological instrumentation. Observation, questionnaires, chart audits and direct questioning of the patient are also used. Biophysiological instrumentation may be combined with other measurements in the same study to validate the data. For example, in our study on cabbage leaf extract (Roberts, Reiter & Schuster 1998), direct physical measurements of chest circumference and breast tissue hardness were combined with the Bourbonnais (1981) pain scale. To measure hardness, we used the Roberts Durometer, which was developed especially for the study by Dr R. B. Roberts, then trialled and evaluated (Roberts 1999).

There are many biophysiological research instruments that have been developed and tested. In addition, there are many biophysiological instruments already used in clinical management of the patient that can also be used for research purposes, such as cardiac monitors, spirometers, pulse oximeters and so forth. Ethics approval must be gained for the use of instruments in research, even if they are already in place for treatment purposes.

Biophysiological measurements as a means of data collection have various advantages. They are objective because they are not normally sensitive to errors on the part of the person who measures: if the instrument is properly calibrated any two readers should get the same reading on it. Biophysiological instruments are usually sensitive; they can record relatively small changes. They are also accurate and they have the advantage that they give quantitative, numerical data that are comparatively easy to analyse.

Biophysiological instruments also have disadvantages. They are usually expensive to purchase, and the data collector has to have the appropriate training in the use of the instrument. Biophysiological instruments may be adversely affected by changes in the environment such as the temperature. They may also be affected by the Hawthorne effect since the participant usually knows that a test is being made. In addition, biophysiological instruments may be invasive so there is a potential for harm to the participant in the study.

Observation

Observation by the human eye is a way of obtaining data about people's behaviour when and where it actually happens. We can observe how often behaviours occur, how long they last or how long it takes to carry out an action or achieve an objective. Observation can be used in both qualitative and quantitative research. It can be used as a method of obtaining data in various research designs. It is carried out by observers who are objective, reliable and trained in the skills and techniques of observation. Observation is not useful if the intention is to study people's thoughts, values, attitudes, beliefs or feelings.

Observation may be objective or subjective. In quantitative research, the observer is aiming for objectivity. However, total objectivity is unattainable; for example, observers tend to rate behaviour more positively if the person observed is someone who is attractive or whom they like. However, you aim to be as impartial as possible by putting aside your own values, attitudes and emotions. Objectivity can be enhanced by being a total observer rather than a participant observer.

Observation may be covert or overt, depending on whether the participants are aware that they are taking part in a study. Overt observation entails the observed being aware of the observation while covert observation conceals the act of observation from the observed. A discussion of the ethics of covert observation can be found in Chapter 5.

Observation may be obtrusive or unobtrusive depending on whether the observer is visible to the observed. Obtrusive observation is observation in which the participant cannot help but be aware of the observer. Unobtrusive observation is observation in which the observer is either not visible or keeps a low profile. It is less likely to result in the effect of the participants changing their behaviour because they know they are being observed. Obviously covert observation must be unobtrusive in order to remain covert. However, overt observation may be either obtrusive or unobtrusive. If you are trying to be unobtrusive, it is helpful to observe in a busy area in which you will be less noticeable. It can also be helpful to keep out of the line of sight of the observed.

There are various dimensions of observation depending on the amount of involvement of the researcher, the degree of structure, the extent to which the observation is known to the observed and the extent to which the observer is visible to the observed.

There may be varying degrees of involvement of the researcher in what is being observed. The researcher may be a complete non-participant, engaged only in observing the scene, and not involved in it at all. An example of a study using non-participant observation was one in which Borbasi (1999) observed a group of nurses in a large New South Wales teaching hospital as they went about their daily work to determine advanced practice and expertness. Another is the use of observation in the development of competency standards for specialist critical care nurses in which more than 800 hours of specialist critical care nursing practice were observed and classified into domains of practice (Dunn et al. 2000). At the other extreme, the researcher may be a participant in the situation and therefore a participant-observer. An example of a study using participant observation is by Rice (1999), who studied the cultural construction of miscarriage among the Hmong women in Australia. Proctor (2000) also used participant observation to study the impact of the Balkan conflict on the culture and emotional health of a community of Serbian Australians.

Observation may range from the unstructured, in which the observer is attempting to observe the scene without imposing any structure on the observations, to the highly structured, in which the observer categorises observations using a tool such as a checklist with pre-determined categories. In quantitative research, the observation will be highly structured because the observations are used to generate measurement rather than to describe situations or generate meaning as in qualitative research. However, structured observation has the disadvantage of not accommodating unexpected behaviours.

Observation as a research tool has several advantages. It allows us to see what people actually do in a situation. Observation allows us to see the finer nuances of behaviour, for example body language. It can be used with participants who cannot give verbal data, such as unconscious patients and infants. For the purpose of studying behaviour, observation is considered better than relying on participants' verbal accounts of their behaviour, which they may edit or distort, consciously or subconsciously, to give a positive picture.

Observation also has disadvantages. If it occurs in a laboratory setting, it may be somewhat artificial. However, if you want to observe naturalistic behaviour it is necessary to go to the natural setting and wait for the behaviour to happen, which may involve extra time and expense. Access may be a problem if the activity under observation is not something that people want to be observed doing, for example sexual behaviour. Furthermore, it is not possible for the observer to see everything in a situation or to record everything that is seen. The data are therefore limited by the amount that can be seen and recorded. Nor is it possible for the observer to be completely objective since the observer's frame of reference is superimposed on what is seen. Two observers may see the same thing differently. The data are therefore limited by the accuracy or framework of the observer.

Structured observation

Structured observation is the predominant observational method in quantitative research. It is characterised by systematic planning, and recording the data according to a framework. Imposing such a structure is intended to improve the accuracy of the observations. This framework is pre-determined by the researcher and will reflect the research question, the conceptual framework, the hypotheses and the operational definitions of the variables. The researcher needs to know what will be observed and how it should be recorded. To design this framework, the researcher needs to know what behaviours to expect. This can be determined from the literature on the subject, and/or a preliminary pilot observational study in the setting to observe and categorise the behaviour.

Structured observation normally involves an instrument. One type of instrument used in structured observation is a 'paper and pencil' instrument. A simple example is a checklist in which the observer simply indicates whether or not an explicit behaviour, for example crying, happens. Another such instrument is a set of mutually exclusive categories in which to sort the observations. Such an instrument was used in observing and categorising pedestrian behaviours of children en route to primary school, for example running, walking, skipping and so forth (Batterham 1996). Another type of paper instrument is a rating scale in which an observer rates a type of behaviour on a continuum, for example rating aggression on a scale of one to ten.

Automated methods may be used in place of or in addition to paper and pencil instruments. These include such instruments as stopwatches, audiorecordings and videorecordings. Stopwatches can be used to determine how long a behaviour lasts. Audiorecordings are not, strictly speaking, observation, but they can be used to analyse verbal behaviour or augment visual observation. Videorecordings are becoming popular because they offer a visual record of behaviour.

Automated methods such as audio- and videorecordings are used when the action is too rapid or too complex to analyse *in situ*. They are also convenient because they allow researchers to capture the data at the time of the behaviour but analyse it at their convenience. They also improve accuracy of data analysis as they allow the data to be played over and over until a decision is reached. However, these methods also have some drawbacks. Good-quality equipment and consumables are expensive. Editing videotapes is time-consuming. Furthermore, the videorecording process requires special skills of filming and editing, which may not be in the researcher's repertoire.

The process of observation

Before undertaking observation, it is necessary to decide exactly what is going to be observed and when. Do you want to observe according to time, for example a set amount of time per hour? Do you want to observe a whole event, for example the changing of a dressing? You will also need to consider questions of whether the observation is structured or unstructured, covert or overt, obtrusive or unobtrusive, and the degree of involvement that you will have in the activity being observed.

You will also need to decide how many observers are needed to collect the data. If you do it all yourself, you will not have the problem of differing observations of different data collectors. However, the use of more than one observer may improve the validity of the data if they both agree on the observations. If more than one data collector is being used, their measurements can be compared. Multiple data collectors must practise until they achieve the same or similar measurements, thus ensuring inter-rater reliability.

Before observing, you will also have to train yourself and/or other data collectors in order to ensure accurate observations. This can be done by familiarisation of the observer with the instrument and practice to ensure skilled handling of the equipment or recording of the observations.

You should carry out a pilot study in the real research situation so that you or your data collectors will be able to practise the procedure using the equipment to ensure that they develop the skills. A full pilot study can also serve as a rehearsal for the main study, thus increasing the confidence of the observers. If the same participants are being used it can also help them become accustomed to being observed.

Information

When using information as data you, as the researcher, can use either data that have been collected by someone else or data that you collect yourself in the form of information from media, or information given by the participants.

Using existing information

Existing data are data that have been collected by you or another researcher but have not yet been analysed for your present purpose. Such data may include any data that have been collected either for research or clinical purposes by another researcher or an organisation. Other researchers may have data that they will make available. Organisations such as the Australian Bureau of Statistics, state and territory health services or individual hospitals often have data that they will make available for research purposes, possibly at a cost. Previously collected data might be raw data or data already entered into a database. You might use these data for exploring new hypotheses and relationships, analysing a sub-group of the data to draw inferences about that group or using a new unit of analysis or a different method of analysis. An example of use of existing information is a study of clients' bowel care management (Keatinge et al. 1999) in which a chart audit method was used to collect data for the study. The authors found various issues related to chart documentation.

The major advantage of working with previously accumulated data is that it saves you considerable time in collecting and entering data because this has already been done. It also allows the examination of data for longitudinal trends without waiting years for data to be generated. Another major advantage is that it is less expensive than collecting and entering it yourself, even if you have to pay a fee. Previously accumulated data may also provide a greater amount and range of data than you could otherwise hope to acquire on a limited budget.

However, working with someone else's data has several disadvantages. Since the data have not been collected for the purpose of your present study there are very likely to be areas in which the fit with your purposes is less than ideal. For example, hospital medical records will be unlikely to be complete.

Methodological problems may arise such as a deficiency in the sample used, or poor matching of your definition of the variable with the definition in the existing database. The tool that you might consider superior might not be the one that the original investigator used. The data themselves may not be of adequate quality; you are dependent upon the accuracy and completeness of the original data collection and entry process. Data may not be consistent over time; for example a classification system such as nursing diagnosis may have changed in the middle of the period that you want to examine.

It is important to weigh up the costs and benefits before making a decision on whether or not to use available data. If the discrepancies between the structure and methodology of the original data and your ideal data are too great, you may decide that it is preferable to collect your own data.

Content analysis

Content analysis in quantitative research means a numerical description of the appearance of specific ideas or expressions in a body of communications that use language. Content analysis was first developed during the Second World War to analyse the content of propaganda. It can be applied to oral/aural media, such as radio and television broadcasts, and written media, such as newspapers, books, articles and letters. Since content analysis is not a common technique, it will not be explored in depth here. However, the method depends on formulating rules and categories for the analysis. The unit of analysis may be a word, phrase or theme. Content analysis has been used to analyse Australian nursing journal articles to determine the proportion of different types of scholarship (Roberts 1995; Jackson, Raftos & Mannix 1996). It has also been used to analyse Australian popular press and magazines for meanings of breastfeeding representations (Henderson 1999) and menstruation (Raftos, Jackson & Mannix 1998).

Meta-analysis

Meta-analysis is the analysis of multiple research reports to integrate and synthesise the findings on a particular topic. This is an ever-increasing necessity in these days of expanding volumes of research. Meta-analysis has potential to integrate findings on a clinical research topic and to be useful in evidence-based nursing, particularly the development of clinical guidelines, which will be explored in more detail in Chapter 19. Special statistical approaches, which convert statistical findings to a comparable measurement called an effect size, are used to determine which findings are most powerful. Since meta-analysis relies on published findings it may have a bias in its results. However, it is considered superior to a conventional literature review. You can read more about meta-analysis and its application to clinical practice in an article by Beck (1995).

Self-report

Self-report is a method of obtaining data directly from the participants in the study, using them as informants. Basically, self-report consists of answers that the participant gives to specific questions asked by the researcher in order to answer the research question. This is particularly effective where you are not investigating something that can be measured by instruments, or observed. It is ideal for things such as values, attitudes, feelings or problems. Self-report methods may be written, for example questionnaires and scales, or oral, for example structured interviews. Interviews and questionnaires may be used in conjunction with other types of approaches either to generate questions or to augment them. Interview and questionnaire questions can be the same, but the methods of delivery and response are different. The instrument chosen should reflect the purpose of the study, the research question and the variables being measured.

Questionnaires

A questionnaire is the most commonly used instrument for obtaining information by self-report. It is a document containing questions to which the person responds. Questionnaires can be used to obtain a variety of information. Through a questionnaire, you, the researcher, can seek such demographic details as age, gender, income or postcode. In addition, you can ask a series of questions related to a concept, for the purpose of investigating people's attitudes, values, beliefs and stated behaviours. The answers on a questionnaire may also be used to explore relationships between variables, for example between sex and attitudes. Questionnaires are used frequently in correlational designs.

Questionnaires have several advantages over other types of instruments. They are quick to administer and receive. Although they may incur postal costs, they are inexpensive compared to more labour-intensive data collection methods such as interviewing and observation. In addition, they have the advantage of enabling you to acquire large amounts of information from the target sample. Because questionnaires can be mailed and distributed electronically, you can distribute them over a wide geographic area, much wider than you could access easily if you had to travel to do interviews. Furthermore, since most questionnaires ask for anonymous replies, the respondents are more likely to answer candidly than they are in interviews where they may give you the answers they think you expect or that they perceive as socially acceptable. Finally, the development of statistical tests have made questionnaire data relatively easy to test for reliability and validity.

On the other hand, questionnaires have several disadvantages. They are suitable for use only with people who can understand them. You cannot use them with people whose judgement may not be valid, for example the very young, the confused elderly, the illiterate or the developmentally challenged. Even with those capable of filling in a questionnaire there may be misunderstandings and misinterpretations that cannot be clarified, resulting in incomplete or invalid data. The cost of distribution, although relatively inexpensive, may still be high. For 150 three-page questionnaires with covering letters, you would need to pay for two reams of paper, 300 envelopes, photocopying or printing, and 300 stamps. Each round of questionnaires could therefore cost between $200 and $250.

The structure that is frequently needed on questionnaires imposes constraints over the content of the questionnaire. The need to confine the length of a questionnaire so that the respondent does not get tired or bored also means that it may be necessary to leave out information that could be relevant. Finally, one of the major problems with questionnaires is that they tend to have a low return rate unless they deal with a burning issue or have been distributed by personal contact. A low return rate raises questions about how well the sample represents the population. This can be overcome partially by including demographic data, which allows you to compare some characteristics of the sample with known values in the population. If the sample is demographically like the population, responses to other questions are more likely to be typical of the population than if it is unlike the population.

Selecting an appropriate questionnaire

Selection of a questionnaire gives rise to the question of whether it is better to use a questionnaire that someone else has prepared or to develop one yourself. Using an existing questionnaire has many advantages, for example you can compare your results with those of the previous studies that used it. On the other hand, using your own questionnaire allows you to tailor it to your own requirements. We shall discuss the advantages and disadvantages of each approach as well as other aspects.

You will find it much easier to use an existing questionnaire than to develop your own. In using a questionnaire developed by someone else, you will be saving time and energy by capitalising on someone else's work. The researcher(s) who developed the questionnaire will have done all of the hard thinking work in developing the questions. They will also have piloted their questionnaire and established its reliability and validity.

It is not difficult to find existing questionnaires. There are resource books with schedules of instruments in just about every discipline that uses questionnaires. You can also locate questionnaires by doing a literature search that focuses on instruments in the area in which you are interested. Other researchers in your area of interest or nurse-researchers on the Internet will probably know of relevant questionnaires, perhaps even ones that have been developed and validated but not yet published. If you are using a questionnaire that someone else has developed, you need to check that its reliability and validity have been established. If there is an existing questionnaire that is close to what you require, it may be possible to modify it to meet your needs. However, if you do, you need to re-check its reliability and validity and trial it in your situation before using it in your main study.

In using an existing questionnaire, you should ask yourself if it is suitable for the situation in which you intend to use it. A questionnaire that has been developed for university students may not be suitable for poorly educated people, for example. You need to look at the suitability of the questionnaire in terms of the instructions, language, method of scoring and so forth. Looking at the characteristics of other groups on which it has been used should give you an idea of its suitability for your proposed group. As a matter of etiquette, you should seek permission from the author to use or adapt a questionnaire.

Developing your own questionnaire
You may decide to develop your own questionnaire. There are really only two valid reasons for doing so. The first is that no existing one will serve your purpose, even with adaptation. The second one is that you want or need to learn how to do it to develop your skills as a researcher. Developing a questionnaire is regarded as a very difficult task even for seasoned researchers (Street 1995). Street (1995, p 105) entitled the section of her book that deals with questionnaire development 'How to develop a headache without really trying'. She quoted one of her participants as saying 'If anyone ever thinks, "Aha, we will do a questionnaire", forget it.' (Street, 1995, p 105). Reasons given were difficulties constructing questions and limiting the number of questions, and group decision-making problems.

A lengthy discourse on the process of developing a questionnaire is beyond the scope of a book for beginning researchers; however, some guidance and instruction will be given. If you do decide to develop your own questionnaire, you are advised to consult a book that deals specifically with questionnaire development. A useful account of development of a questionnaire and a discussion of the methodological issues involved can be found in Dunning and Martin (1996).

Your questionnaire can be as short as one page or as long as you wish. However, be warned that the length of a questionnaire affects the return rate. Indeed, the length and the response rate tend to be inversely proportional! Few people are prepared to spend hours doing your questionnaire. The length of the questionnaire should be consistent with the attention span of the respondents. A reasonable length is one that takes less than half an hour to complete.

The response rate can also be affected by the content of the questionnaire. If the respondents judge it to be unbearably intrusive (for example asking questions about their income) or too sensitive (for example asking questions about their sex life), they may choose to discard it. Fear that they can be identified, especially on intrusive or sensitive content, can lead respondents to discard the questionnaire.

The process of questionnaire development entails many steps. These are outlined as follows:

- Decide on your primary research questions. These may be at various levels, as outlined in Chapter 2. All of the content items should be congruent with and designed to answer these questions.
- Identify your hypotheses and variables. Again, all of the content of your questionnaire should be designed to test the hypotheses and explore the interactions of the variables.
- Identify relevant concepts. These can come from your own knowledge and ideas on the topic or from your reading of the literature on the topic, including previous research which may have been qualitative research that has identified themes that you now wish to explore in a questionnaire survey. The concepts will normally be abstract, and thus not directly measurable, for instance pain.

- Concepts must then be translated into items on the questionnaire. You will probably find that there are several sub-concepts that might require separate items. For example, if you are measuring stress, it might be broken down into types of stress such as physical, emotional, social and financial stress. You may wish to focus on only one of these or on all of them. You could ask a person how much stress they perceive they are under, or ask them if they suffer from some of the indicators of stress, such as headache, skin rashes and so forth.
- Ensure that each item is necessary to your study. Every item should relate to a concept, hypothesis or variable. Questionnaires often include unnecessary items such as demographic variables. If age is not one of your variables, do not include it in the questionnaire just because it might be interesting. Eliminating unnecessary items helps to keep the length of the questionnaire under control.
- Ensure that the items are neither biased nor contain an assumption. For example, 'How often do you cheat on your income taxes?' assumes that you do. It should be rephrased to 'Do you cheat on your income taxes?', which could be answered by a range of responses from 'never' to 'always'. Similarly, 'Do you think that nurses should be paid more?' invites the answer 'yes'. It should be rephrased to include options for the pay staying the same or even decreasing. Items should be framed in as neutral a way as possible if you want unbiased answers.
- Ensure that there is only one question per item. Items that contain two actual questions cannot allow for the possibility that the respondent would like to answer the two questions differently.
- Ensure that all items are worded clearly and correctly and are easy to understand in order to eliminate incomplete item response. This is likely to occur if the respondent perceives the item to be unclear or the choice of responses to be irrelevant, unsuitable or lacking. The respondent may leave that item blank and go on to the next one.
- Choose the demographic items, if any, that you need to include and what categories you will break them down into: for example, do you want age in years or to the nearest decade? Some questionnaires ask the demographic information at the beginning to get the person answering easy questions, while others leave it till later so the person will do it, having come that far.
- Pitch the language at the correct level for the respondents. The questionnaire should not contain any jargon or ambiguous language that they may not understand because this will decrease the validity of the responses.
- Cluster related items so that the respondents do not have to jump around in their thoughts. You may wish to put headings at the tops of the sections and use a relevant numbering system.
- Put the most important items at the beginning of the questionnaire so the answers will not be subject to respondent fatigue.
- Ensure correct spelling and grammar.
- Consider the data analysis. Questions that are 'closed', i.e. tick-a-box type, permit only those responses supplied by the researcher. The responses are usually numerical or capable of being transformed into numbers.

The advantage of these is that their specificity makes analysis easier – the respondent has in effect classified your data for you. However, answers to closed questions are narrow and shallow. Open questions just give the question and allow the respondent to compose the response. Open questions are more qualitative and require a lot more work in data analysis – they need to be classified and coded, and may need to be transcribed into the computer. However the data are richer and deeper.

Developing questionnaire scales

A scale is a method that asks a respondent to rate an item on a basis that is either a number or can be converted into numbers. There are various different types of scales that can be used, but the idea is to locate the respondent on a continuum with a mathematical basis. This makes for ease of analysis of data. Some common types of scales are:

The Likert Scale: On the Likert Scale, the respondents rank their attitudes or opinions on a continuum of response from 'strongly agree' to 'strongly disagree' (see Figure 8.2). There is usually an odd number of possible responses, normally five or seven. The continuum is usually phrased as 'strongly agree', 'agree', 'mildly agree', 'neutral', 'mildly disagree', 'disagree', and 'strongly disagree'. These responses are given a numerical score from 1 to 7 (or sometimes 1 to 5). This allows you to calculate a numerical value for the purposes of descriptive and inferential statistical analysis.

| Nurses should be paid more |

SA	A	N	D	SD

Figure 8.2 A five-point Likert Scale

The semantic differential scale: The semantic differential scale is a scale that asks the respondents to rate their response to an item using a pair of adjectives at opposite ends of a continuum. For example one might be asked where one would rate euthanasia on the beautiful/ugly axis (see Figure 8.3).

beautiful ——————————————————————————————— ugly
 1   2   3   4   5   6   7   8   9   10

Figure 8.3 An example of a semantic differential scale

Rating scales: On rating scales, respondents are asked to rate how often they carry out a behaviour. Responses range from 'never' to 'always', with intermediate steps such as 'sometimes', and 'often' (see Figure 8.4).

| How often do you do daily exercise? | Always | Often | Sometimes | Seldom | Never |

Figure 8.4 An example of a rating scale

Visual analogue scales: On a visual analogue scale (VAS), respondents are asked to indicate the quality of an experience on a representation of the phenomenon (see Figure 8.5). One type of VAS is a linear, ruler-like scale that appears somewhat like a thermometer. The scale has numbers, with extreme ranks at the ends. Visual analogue scales are useful for measuring stimuli such as pain. An example is the Bourbonnais pain ruler, which ranks pain on a scale from 0 to 10, with 0 representing no pain and 10 representing excruciating pain (Bourbonnais, 1981).

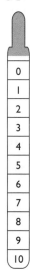

Figure 8.5 An example of a visual analogue scale

Pictorial representations of the phenomenon under investigation can be used for participants who cannot use a numerical scale, for example faces that express varying degrees of pain (see Figure 8.6).

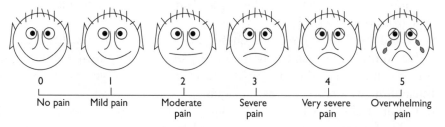

Figure 8.6 An example of a faces scale

Formatting the questionnaire

Composing the questionnaire items is the first stage. The questionnaire as a whole must be formatted and attention should be paid to its presentation. In general, you should make sure that the questionnaire looks professional and appealing so that the recipient will have confidence in your research ability. The following points can assist you in formatting and presenting the questionnaire.

- Put a title at the top of the questionnaire that reflects the overall topic. You do not need to include the word 'questionnaire' as that is self-evident.
- Make sure the pages are numbered.

- Put instructions for completing the questionnaire at the beginning. If they are brief enough, put them at the top of every page.
- Do not overcrowd the page – dense print is even less appealing than more pages and it does not conceal excessive length of a questionnaire.
- Use a readable font (12 point is best).
- Consider whether to use one side of the page or both. One side is more expensive but looks more elegant and is easier to use during data entry.
- Make sure every question is numbered to facilitate data entry.
- Put the answers near the questions but close to the edge of the page on one margin or the other to facilitate data entry.
- Make sure the pages are stapled together securely.

The draft questionnaire

When you are satisfied that the draft is as good as you can make it, the next step is to refine it and then pilot it. The next step in refining is to have the items reviewed by several experts for content validity, structure and bias. Send your draft out for comment to at least three experts in the content area of the questionnaire and take account of their suggestions for revising it. You should also ask your supervisor to vet it. Ask any colleague who has developed a questionnaire for their feedback. You will be surprised at the obvious flaws that have escaped your notice.

Once you have refined the questionnaire according to the feedback from the experts on content and structure, you are ready to trial the questionnaire with a pilot sample. The following points can help you:

- The pilot sample should be large enough to give you a realistic trial without compromising your main sample.
- Develop a covering letter (including a plain language statement) asking for participation in the study.
- You should trial all phases of the questionnaire, *including data analysis*. This will enable you to assess realistically the quality of the questionnaire and data, the time it will take and the appropriateness of the methods you have chosen for distribution, data entry and data analysis.
- You should do a statistical procedure on the questionnaire to establish reliability, for example the Kuder-Richardson test.
- Revise your questionnaire again in light of the findings of the pilot study. If there are major revisions, you will need to pilot it again.

The covering letter

Your questionnaire will need a covering letter, which can incorporate the plain language statement, as described in Chapter 6. You will not need a consent form as return of the questionnaire is implied consent. The letter should inform your potential respondents about the study. You should tell the recipients how you got their names and how they were selected, for example by random computer allocation. You should tell them what the study is about, why it is being done and who, in general, is participating. State how you plan to use the data and how your procedures will ensure confidentiality of the data. You should give them instructions for maintaining their anonymity and for returning the questionnaire. Finally, you should give a contact number for more information and thank them for considering participating in your survey.

The covering letter should be composed so that it motivates your potential respondents to return the questionnaire. You can appeal to their altruism. If possible, stress the rewards that the respondent will get for helping you. If you personalise the letters by addressing them to 'Dear Ms/Mr (Name)' instead of the impersonal 'Dear Colleague' you will improve your return rate. However, that is a lot of work, particularly if you have a large number of questionnaires to distribute. If you have secretarial resources and a word processor with a mail merge facility, it is achievable. The letter should carry your personal signature or a facsimile, which can be done by signing the original letter before photocopying. If you are using institutional stationery, you can print a letter on plain stationery, sign it, then photocopy it onto the letterhead stationery.

Building in incentives to respond

Low questionnaire return rates are one of the problems facing researchers. Not only is it disheartening after all of the work you put in; it also reduces the external validity of your findings.

In order to encourage people to return the questionnaires, you should enclose a stamped envelope with your return address on it. You might think that a stamp and an envelope are but a small cost to each participant or institution and if you could defray these costs your expenses would be significantly reduced; however, it is not the cost of the stamp and the envelope but the convenience. Even if someone fills in the questionnaire, it may take several days before they get around to buying envelopes and/or stamps or they might decide it is just too much trouble and end up not posting the letter at all. Furthermore, it is not ethical to expect institutions to unknowingly bear the cost of the postage for your research project. One way of reducing costs of postage is to arrange for a 'reply paid' billing at your end rather than putting a stamp on each envelope. This means that the envelope indicates to the participant that postage will be paid by you. Under this system you pay the post office only for the questionnaires that are returned. However, you need to make it clear in your letter that the reply paid envelope precludes the need for a postage stamp. You can consult the appropriate people to see if your institution will provide this service as part of your student stipend, if you have one.

Giving an incentive such as a small monetary reward, e.g. a lottery ticket, might seem like a good inducement. However, this can be expensive and it is difficult to administer unless you can arrange to give it out when the questionnaires are returned. In the case of postal questionnaires, postage for just this purpose is also expensive and unworkable unless the respondents can identify themselves, in which case their anonymity is not safeguarded. I recently heard of one researcher who included a tea bag in the questionnaire packet and suggested that the respondent sit down and have a cup of tea while doing the questionnaire.

Perhaps you can think of something equally creative, but beware of giving out a reward unless the questionnaire is returned.

Follow-up rounds

Unless you get your target return rate (which should be at least 66 per cent) on the first round, you will need to plan for a follow-up round of questionnaires. Basically, there are three methods you can use to determine who will receive your follow-up questionnaires and they all have advantages and disadvantages in terms of anonymity. Before choosing one of these methods, you need to ask yourself if you really need to know the identities of the respondents for any reason other than following up the non-responders.

One follow-up method is to send a new questionnaire to everyone on your original list with instructions to discard it if they have already replied. This has the disadvantage of potential double returns if some respondents forget they have already done it and do it again. You will not be able to tell if a person has sent it in twice unless the person is identified by a code number. The time involved may also be a consideration. However, the major disadvantage of sending a full second round of questionnaires is the expense of stationery, printing and postage. You will need to pay for a full set of postage to send out this round but return postage costs can be minimised by using the reply paid method.

The second follow-up method is to sacrifice anonymity and give every potential respondent a code number that you put on both your primary list of names and the questionnaire or envelope. This allows you to identify respondents and eliminate them from the follow-up round. This is much cheaper than the first method but it will almost certainly reduce the return rate, perhaps even to catastrophic levels of less than 20 per cent. This occurs because people are suspicious of strangers and will probably be afraid that you will identify their data, despite your assurances that the numbers will be used only for the stated purpose. This suspicious attitude is even more likely to be prevalent if the content of the questionnaire is sensitive or intrusive.

Sometimes the design of a study requires linking two or more sets of data from each individual, for example pre- and post-tests. You therefore need to put a linking system in place. A code number can do this. However, data-linking can be achieved more readily by asking respondents to generate their own unique code and put it on all responses. The recipient can choose the numbers, for example their mother's day, month and year of birth. The advantage of this method is that you do not know who the respondent is so the response is anonymous, but if they use a unique number that can be reliably generated each time, the data can be linked. People are used to generating pin numbers so will be familiar with this concept and likely to comply provided you give them in the letter a clear explanation for the procedure and the reasons for it.

The third method, and in the author's opinion the best one unless you need to link sets of data as above, is the use of a system that allows you to determine who responded without putting any code number or identifying mark on the questionnaire or envelope. When you are having the questionnaires and reply paid envelopes printed, have postcards printed that have your address on one side and on the other a message that Ms/Mr X has sent back the questionnaire by separate post. If you use this method, make sure that you include the person's name on the card when you send it so that you are not dependent on the respondent putting it on, which they will not always realise they are meant to do. You can do this easily by generating a second set of sticky labels with the respondents' names and addresses on them and sticking them on the postcards. However, be careful to have 'To' and 'From' printed clearly in the appropriate place to avoid confusion in the post office. When you receive the postcard you can cross off the respondent's name from your list and you are left with the non-responders, to whom you send the follow-up round minus the postcard. This is clearly cheaper than the first method but more expensive than the second as you pay for printing the postcards and for their return postage. However the increased return rate compensates for the extra cost involved. An illustration of the postcard is shown in Figure 8.7.

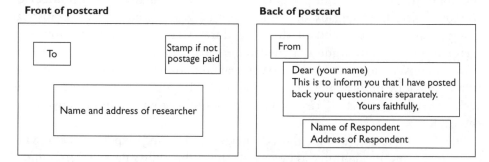

Figure 8.7 An example of a postcard used to increase questionnaire returns

Whatever method you use to follow up non-respondents, you will need to distinguish between the first- and second-round respondents so that you can compare them and see if they are any different. You can do this by making some distinction between the two questionnaires such as a slight change in format, e.g. underlining the title of one or the other, or a slight difference in colour of paper that will be obvious to you but not to the respondents.

Distribution of questionnaires
Before you can distribute the questionnaires you must determine the sample that you will use through the sampling procedures discussed earlier in this chapter. Unless you are using a convenience sample, in which you distribute questionnaires until you reach your quota of responses, you will need to identify the potential recipients of the questionnaire.

The actual process of distributing questionnaires will be discussed in Chapter 9, on data collection.

From the preceding, you can see that the art and science of questionnaires is a very comprehensive topic and requires a lot of attention to detail to be used successfully. If you wish to explore questionnaire development in more depth, read Chapter 16 in Minichiello et al. (1999) or an article devoted to questionnaire development, for example Dunning and Martin (1996), or a book on questionnaire design such as Frazer (2000).

The Delphi survey technique

The Delphi technique is a special survey method of obtaining and analysing a range of expert opinions on a topic or issue without having a face-to-face meeting of the group. It is named after the famous Greek oracle at Delphi who was thought to transmit answers from the gods. A panel of experts is repeatedly surveyed by mail or electronic means, with feedback of each round of results, until a consensus is obtained. The principle is that with each round, the experts will move closer to the prevailing view on the issue. The Delphi technique is used where the objective might be to get a consensus on policy issues, priority of goals, or forecast trends.

A classic Delphi study should meet four criteria: anonymity of panel members, iteration through presentation of a questionnaire over a number of rounds, controlled feedback of information to group members and statistical group response at the end of the procedure (Crisp et al. 1999). However, Crisp and colleagues argue that researchers have modified the classic Delphi technique over the years to the extent that sometimes little of the technique is recognisable in the method of the study. If you are interested in this technique, the article by Crisp and colleagues will provide a full discussion of the topic.

The Delphi technique has the advantage of reaching experts over a wide geographic area. In a country as large as Australia this allows people from remote areas to participate. It saves the participants the time and expense of a formal meeting. It also allows a panel of experts to achieve consensus without face-to-face interaction, which can influence the results (Pelletier et al. 2000). The anonymity of the responses allows more candid responses. However, the Delphi technique relies upon a fast turnaround time and it can be time-consuming and expensive for the researcher. The anonymity can reduce the accountability of the respondents for their responses, and responder attrition can be a problem. However, used in the appropriate situation, the advantages can outweigh the disadvantages of the Delphi technique.

An example of a Delphi survey is one of cardiac clinicians and educators in which two panels, one of educators and one of nurse-clinicians, took part in two rounds each (Pelletier et al. 2000). The Delphi technique has also been used to determine the role of the breast care nurse (White & Wilkes 1999) and research priorities for oncology nurses (Chang & Daly 1996), rural nurses (Bell, Daly & Chang 1997) and renal nurses (Daly & Chang 1996). Daly and Chang found that the research priorities of renal specialist nurses fell into four categories: that of highest value to patients, that of highest value to clinical nurse specialists and clinical nurse consultants, that which would improve community care, and that which would fulfil specialists' professional needs. The Delphi technique has also been used in nursing education to develop the Basic Intensive Care Knowledge Test (Boyle, Kenney & Butcher 1995).

In constructing a Delphi survey, one first identifies an appropriate panel of experts in the area under discussion. They should represent a range of opinion as well as be representative in other parameters such as geography and gender, otherwise the exercise will not work. After obtaining agreement from the experts for their participation in the survey, you administer the first round of questionnaires, instructing the experts not to communicate with each other about the topic. You then receive the anonymous questionnaires, analyse the data and revise the questionnaire as necessary. The tabulated results and the revised questionnaire are fed back to the experts who are asked to re-analyse the questionnaire in light of the group results. This process is repeated, usually about three times, until the desired amount of consensus is obtained. When the final results are obtained, they become the results of the study.

Q-methodology (Q-sort)

Q-methodology uses a procedure called Q-sort in which the researcher gives a participant a deck of 60–100 cards containing individual items that are developed from the literature of a particular field or discipline (Tetting 1988). The researcher asks the participant to sort the cards according to pre-determined criteria such as importance or amount of time spent on an activity. It is useful to describe and compare participants' opinions about such things as the importance of various types of nursing care or nursing behaviours, or self-perceptions, for example of personality and personal characteristics. Q-sort can also be used to sort items for inclusion in a questionnaire scale. The cards contain words, phrases, definitions or other statements about the topic being researched. Pictures could be used for special groups where language is a problem. The researcher specifies how many cards are to go in each pile, to avoid all of the cards being put into the middle or at the ends. Usually the distribution of the cards mimics a normal curve. Each statement is judged in relation to the other statements, which preserves the relationship of the statements, unlike a questionnaire where the statements are independent of each other. The participant sorts the cards into a set number of piles, usually about nine, according to some dimension such as desirable/undesirable, agreement/disagreement, and like me/unlike me. This technique is reliable although time-consuming to administer, particularly if there are numerous participants.

At the time of this edition, there was only one example in the published literature of the use of Q-sort methodology in Australian nursing research. This was a study that used the technique to compare the perceptions of patients and nurses about important nursing behaviour (Gardner et al. 2001). The researchers used the 'Care Q' instrument that measures the concept of caring, using 50 cards containing statements of nursing behaviours ranked from most to least important. They found that patients ranked technological competence first while nurses ranked listening to the patient and patient participation in care first. Several studies have also emerged from Britain, using this methodology: Caress, Luker and Ackrill (1988); Lamond and Farnell (1998); Ashworth et al. (1999) and McKeown, Stowell-Smith and Foley (1999).

Interviews

A research interview is a method in which the researcher asks the participant purposeful questions with the intention of investigating a research problem. Interviews differ from questionnaires in that the main response medium is speech rather than writing. The questions may be written down for the guidance of the researcher. There are several types of interviews, on a continuum of structure ranging from the highly structured interview, which uses an undeviating format to an unstructured interview in which only a few introductory questions may be pre-determined. In between is the semi-structured interview, which uses written questions as a guide, in order to achieve some consistency of data, but allows unscheduled exploration of topics that arise in the course of the interview. Unstructured and semi-structured interviews are used in qualitative research where the lack of structure is important in grounded theory methodology. However, in quantitative methodology the structured interview is more usual and it will be explored in more depth here.

The structured interview is appropriate when you want factual information and consistency of data across respondents. The aim of structured interviews is to get information objectively, without the interviewer influencing the process. In a sense, the interviewer tries to become as objective as a questionnaire. The structured interview is the form of interviewing that gives maximum control to the interviewer. Structured interviews allow more quantification of responses than semi-structured or unstructured interviews. The disadvantage of the structured interview is that the structure can constrain the data and you can miss things that you might pick up in a less structured format.

If you are developing a set of questions for a structured interview, it is important to undertake the same processes as when developing a questionnaire. You can refer to the section on questionnaire development earlier in this chapter for more detail, or you can consult other sources such as Minichiello et al. (1999, Chapter 16).

To implement the structured interview process, you, the researcher, develop a set script to give the initial information and instructions to the interviewee, and set questions to elicit the information. You train the interviewer to follow the set structure, asking the same questions, in the same order, and with the same tone of voice in order to promote consistency of data across participants. If there is more than one interviewer, it is essential to train them to perform the interview exactly alike, to ensure consistency across interviewers. It is important for the interviewer(s) to practise interviewing under full research conditions in order to develop their skills of interviewing and to check for consistency. Some researchers even videotape the practice interviews for critiquing.

The considerations for the actual interview process of structured interviews are similar to that of unstructured and semi-structured interviews, which will be discussed in Chapter 14.

Interviews can be carried out in different ways. The traditional way is the face-to-face interview. The most satisfactory method of conducting an interview is in person, in privacy. However, this can involve travel and accommodation expenses and can be very expensive if major distances are involved.

Interviews can also be carried out by telephone. The telephone interview is cheaper if great distances are involved but has the disadvantage of lacking visual contact between the interviewer and interviewee. This is not as important in highly structured interviews. Telephone interviews can be captured on audiotape if you arrange it with the telephone company.

In today's world of technology, the videoconference is also a possibility for a face-to-face interview. It is still relatively expensive, but could be cheaper than travel. It is relatively difficult to arrange since both parties must go to a videoconferencing centre, which may require considerable travel. Videoconferencing has the advantage of visual contact although it is not as intimate as a personal meeting. An added advantage is that it can capture the interview on videotape for future analysis of visual cues, thereby freeing part of the interviewer's attention for other matters. Researchers are also conducting 'interviews' via email on the Internet and via real-time dialogue in chat rooms. At the present time Internet technology restricts the interview to written responses, but it has the element of informality and immediate response that is associated with speech, particularly if it is done in 'real' time through a chat room. In a few years' time computers will come equipped with a camera on top that could capture interviewees' responses in both video and audio.

Interviews can be carried out with participants either individually or in groups. A method of group interview is a focus group, in which the group meets face to face and is facilitated by an interviewer. This has the advantage of several people discussing an issue, thus allowing for group consensus. However, it is possible that the participants may be less candid in a group than in a one-to-one situation. An example of a focus group is a study in which orthopaedic patients were grouped to discuss their perceptions of the acceptability of their own outcomes (Middleton & Lumby 1999). These outcomes were then compared with nurses' assessments of the outcomes.

Whatever method of interviewing you use, you will need to decide how to capture the interview data. If the interview is conducted in person, audiotape is the usual method. Some researchers feel that this interferes with the process, but today's sensitive microphones allow an unobtrusive recording process. If this is a concern, written notes can be made, although these interrupt the flow of the dialogue. Videotaping is also a possibility, but involves the presence of another person, which reduces the privacy of the process. Telephone companies offer a recording service with a teleconference call. Obviously if the Internet is used, a written record of the responses is available.

Choosing between questionnaire and interview

Sometimes, as a researcher, you will have to choose between the methods of questionnaire and interview. The advantage of interviews over questionnaires is that the data will be richer and deeper. You can access participants to whom you cannot send questionnaires, such as the homeless, or those who do not have the ability or strength to fill questionnaires in, such as the illiterate or the very ill. You will also get a better response rate since people find it harder to say 'no' in person to an interview than to throw a questionnaire in the waste bin. A questionnaire relies on the correct interpretation by the respondent, but in an interview the interviewer is present and can clarify instructions where needed and observe the interviewee's response to the questions.

The disadvantage of interviews as compared with questionnaires is that they are more expensive in terms of training, administration and travel to access the participants. You may have to pay the interviewees a small fee to compensate them for travel, child care and so on. Interviews can be difficult to arrange and are subject to cancellation if your interviewee has more pressing matters to attend to at the time. They also require more time and expense to collect and analyse the data than questionnaires do. Since it is never possible for people to be completely objective, the interviewer can inject bias into the process by tone of voice or body language, which a questionnaire cannot – unless the items are biased. Interviews require a lot of skill to carry out because you have both to conduct the interview and monitor the process at the same time. Interviewees may find it difficult to answer your questions, particularly if they have never reflected on the matter before or if the questions are on a sensitive topic. Interviewees may also give socially acceptable answers in person whereas they may give more candid responses to an anonymous questionnaire.

Triangulation

Triangulation is the use of more than one method in studying the same phenomenon, in order to validate the phenomenon. The concept of triangulation comes originally from the field of surveying where surveyors fixed one data point by taking measurements from different angles. There can be various types of triangulation, from mixing quantitative and qualitative approaches in one study design to using more than one investigator examining the same phenomenon and using several different measurement devices to measure the same variable (Sohier 1988). The goals of triangulation are to confirm data and ensure their completeness (Begley 1996). The principle is that if you collect data based on more than one observation or measurement, the data are more likely to be valid because there will be less investigator bias. There are various different typologies for classifying triangulation. One of the most well known is the one developed by Denzin, who identified data triangulation, investigator triangulation, theoretical triangulation and methodological triangulation (Denzin 1989). Data triangulation refers to the use of multiple data sources. These can be collected at different times (time triangulation), from different places (space triangulation) or from people at different levels (person triangulation). In person triangulation, the method entails collecting data from any pair of the three levels of individuals, groups and collectives (Begley, 1996). Investigator triangulation refers to triangulation occurring when two or more skilled researchers with different expertise examine the data. Theoretical triangulation refers to the use of different theories in the conceptual framework for a study. Methodological triangulation is the use of more than one research method in the one study (Begley 1996). Within methodological triangulation, between-method triangulation entails combining methods from two or more research traditions, for example, quantitative and qualitative, in one study. Within-method triangulation involves combining two or more similar data collection methods within one study to measure the same variable (Begley 1996). According to Begley (1996), Kimichi, Polivka and Stevenson (1991) have added 'unit of analysis' triangulation, in which two or more approaches to analysing the same set of data are used. Methodological triangulation of the between-method type was used by McCann (1997) in a study of nurses' and doctors' attitudes towards mainstreaming of hospital inpatient services for clients with HIV/AIDS in hospital wards. McCann used both a survey questionnaire and semi-structured interviews. Other examples of between-methods triangulation can be found in studies by Burr (1998) and Maltby (1999). Creedy and Hand (1994) used within-method triangulation, collecting journals, interviews and classroom observation data to study the conceptual changes associated with nurse-academics' adopting problem-based learning as part of their alternative teaching strategies.

Redfern and Norman (1994, pp. 51–2, cited by Begley 1996) have discussed the advantages and disadvantages of triangulation. The advantages are that triangulation:

- overcomes the bias of 'single-method, single-observer, single-theory studies'
- increases confidence in the results
- allows development and validation of instruments and methods (confirmation)
- provides an understanding of the domain (completeness)
- is ideal for complex issues
- overcomes the elite bias of naturalistic research
- overcomes the holistic fallacy of naturalistic research
- allows divergent results to enrich explanation.

Redfern and Norman (1994, cited by Begley 1996) cite the disadvantages of triangulation as:

- no guarantee of internal and external validity
- may compound the sources of error
- methods selected may not be the right ones
- unit of analysis might not apply to all methods
- cannot compensate for researcher bias
- expensive
- no use with the 'wrong' question
- replication is difficult.

As Begley points out, some of these disadvantages are applicable to any method and are not a feature of triangulation as such.

The whole concept of triangulation is based on a positivist view of the world, that it is somehow necessary to augment qualitative findings and that combining various methods will lead to finding the truth (Begley 1996). While triangulation can be useful, it is important to avoid the assumption that qualitative findings are useful only if they are supported by quantitative findings. Further debate on these issues can be found in Shih (1998).

Summary

In this chapter we have discussed the methods you can use in carrying out quantitative studies. We looked at different types of settings and sampling methods. We considered ways of collecting data by measurement and instrumentation, different types of observation, and information-collecting strategies. Finally, we examined the ways in which multiple methods, or triangulation, can be used. After choosing the appropriate methods to match your aims, question, broad methodological approach and study design, you are now ready to move on to the next exciting part of the research process, applying for the necessary approvals for your project. This was discussed in Chapter 6.

Main points

- A setting is the place in which the study is carried out, where the phenomenon of interest can be observed. It can be a naturalistic setting, or a laboratory setting.
- The population is a group whose members have specific common characteristics that you wish to investigate in your research study. The 'population' can be people, places, objects, or events.
- An element is a single unit of the population studied.
- The sample is the part of the population that you study. The sample can be selected by a variety of methods, but the two major groups are probability and non-probability samples. In non-probability sampling, subjective judgements contribute to the selection of sample and findings will lack external validity. In probability sampling, each element has the possibility of being chosen to take part and the probability of each element being included in the sample is known. This precludes the likelihood of bias.
- A random sample can be selected by a lottery, random number table or computer program.
- Measurement is the determination of the size or range of an object, characteristic or phenomenon. Carried out using instruments, measurement gives the advantages of standardisation of data, accuracy, and the ability to compare findings with those of other researchers.
- Measurement can be direct or indirect and *in vivo* or *in vitro*.
- An instrument is any tool that measures. An instrument has the advantages of increasing accuracy, allowing measurement in more detail, and facilitating recording and analysing data but the disadvantages of being mechanical,

- prescriptive and relatively expensive and possibly requiring special skills to operate.
- Considerations for choice of instrument include: validity, sensitivity, accuracy, reliability, cost and requirements for specialised training.
- Error in measurement can be random or one-off errors or systemic errors that occur whenever the procedure is carried out or at regular intervals.
- Observation is done by the human eye and comprises obtaining data about people's behaviour when and where it actually happens. It can be used in lieu of interview, can see what people actually do as opposed to what they say, allows us to see the finer nuances of behaviour (such as body language) and prevents distortion of data by the person being observed. However, observation can be artificial if done in a laboratory, must await the behaviour, and entails problems of access. Observations can be inaccurate and biased.
- Observation can be unstructured or structured, as participant or observer, covert or overt, and obtrusive or unobtrusive.
- Information can be gained from existing data, content analysis, meta-analysis, or self-report (by questionnaires or interviews).
- A questionnaire is a document containing questions to which a person responds. Questionnaires are relatively quick to administer and receive, are cheaper than interviewing or observation, can yield large amounts of information, can be distributed over a wide area and can yield candid responses if anonymous. The data are relatively easy to analyse.
- Questionnaire data can be limited by the respondents' lack of literacy, language, or misunderstandings and misinterpretations. Questionnaires can be expensive and tend to have a low return rate.
- Questionnaire design is complex and requires attention to content and format, with trials and procedures to ensure content validity and reliability.
- A scale is a tool that asks the respondents to rate their responses on a numerical basis. Common types are Likert Scale, semantic differential scale, rating scales, and visual analogue scales.
- In an interview, the researcher asks the participant purposeful questions with the intention of investigating a research problem. Interviews can be conducted by a variety of face-to-face or technological methods. Interview data are richer and deeper, the interviewer can access difficult participants, the response rate is usually good and the interviewer can clarify instructions and observe the interviewee's response to the questions.
- Interviews involve training, administration, travel, and possibly a fee to the interviewees, can be difficult to arrange and are subject to cancellation. Data collection and analysis are time-consuming. Interviews can be difficult to carry out: the interviewer can inject bias by tone of voice or body language, interviewees may find it difficult to answer questions and they can give socially acceptable rather than candid answers.

Review Questions

1. The advantage of a naturalistic setting is that it:
   a cannot be compared with other settings
   b has increased ecological validity
   c is easier to make observations
   d is easily controlled by the researcher

2. A place that is especially constructed for purposes of research is a:
   a clinical area
   b naturalistic setting
   c field setting
   d laboratory

3. A population is:
   a a group whose members have specific common characteristics under investigation
   b a group in a specific geographical area
   c a group with a particular condition that you wish to study
   d a single unit of the group under study conditions

4. A sample in which each element has an equal likelihood of taking part is a:
   a biased sample
   b snowball sample
   c probability sample
   d quota sample

5. Measurement is:
   a important in qualitative research
   b determining size or range of something
   c finding a determination by inference
   d not prone to error

6. Which of the following could be measured directly?
   a pain
   b hope
   c health
   d weight

7. The most important consideration in selecting an instrument is its:
   a validity
   b reliability
   c availability
   d cost

8   As a researcher who wishes to study nurses' dressing techniques you would select as the most appropriate method:
    a questionnaire
    b participant observation
    c pure observation
    d content analysis

9   An advantage of questionnaires is that they:
    a accurately reflect the thoughts of the respondents
    b are relatively inexpensive to administer
    c have a high return rate
    d are suitable for use with all types of respondents

10 A method in which several rounds of questions are given to a panel of experts is called:
    a Q-methodology
    b meta-analysis
    c Delphi survey
    d content analysis

Discussion Questions

1 Discuss the advantages and disadvantages of laboratory and clinical settings.
2 Compare and contrast probability and non-probability sampling.
3 Describe the different types of observation.
4 Describe the process of questionnaire development.
5 Compare structured and unstructured interviews.
6 Describe triangulation and state its advantages.

References

Ashworth, P., Gerrish, K., Hargreaves, J. & McManus, M. 1999, '"Levels" of attainment in nursing practice: reality or illusion?', *Journal of Advanced Nursing*, vol. 30, no. 1, 159–68.

Batterham, C. 1996, *The Behaviour of Child Pedestrians at Darwin Primary Schools*, Federal Office of Road Safety, Canberra.

Beck, C. 1995, 'Meta-analysis: overview and application to clinical nursing practice', *JOGNN: Journal of Obstetric, Gynecologic and Neonatal Nursing*, vol. 24, no. 2, 131–5.

Begley, C. 1996, 'Using triangulation in nursing research', *Journal of Advanced Nursing*, vol. 24, no. 1, 122–8.

Bell, P., Daly, J. & Chang, E. 1997, 'A study of the educational and research priorities of registered nurses in rural Australia', *Journal of Advanced Nursing*, vol. 25, no. 4, 794–800.

Birks, M., Santamaria, N., Thompson, S. & Amerena, J. 1993, 'A clinical trial of the effectiveness of water as a conductive medium in electrocardiography', *Australian Journal of Advanced Nursing*, vol. 10, no. 2, 10–13.

Borbasi, S. 1999, 'Advanced practice/expert nurses: hospitals can't live without them', *Australian Journal of Advanced Nursing*, vol. 16, no. 3, 21–9.

Bourbonnais, F. 1981, 'Pain assessment: development of a tool for the nurse and the patient', *Journal of Advanced Nursing*, vol. 6, 277–82.

Boyle, M., Kenney, C. & Butcher, R. 1995, 'The development of the Australian Basic Intensive Care Knowledge Test', *Australian Critical Care*, vol. 8, no. 3, 10–16.

Burr, G. 1998, 'Contextualising critical care family needs through triangulation: an Australian study', *Intensive and Critical Care Nursing*, vol. 14, no. 4, 161–9.

Caress, A., Luker, K. & Ackrill, P. 1998, 'Patient-sensitive treatment decision-making? Preferences and perceptions in a sample of renal patients … including commentary by Meyer J.', *NT Research*, vol. 3, no. 5, 364–73.

Chang, E. & Daly, J. 1996, 'Clinical research priorities in oncology nursing: an Australian perspective', *International Journal of Nursing Practice*, vol. 2, no. 1, 21–8.

Creedy, D. & Hand, B. 1994, 'The implementation of problem-based learning: changing pedagogy in nurse education', *Journal of Advanced Nursing*, vol. 20, no. 4, 696–702.

Crisp, J., Pelletier, D., Duffield, C., Nagy, S. & Adams, A. 1999, 'It's all in a name: when is a delphi study not a delphi study?' *Australian Journal of Advanced Nursing*, vol. 16, no. 3, 32–7.

Daly, J. & Chang, E. 1996, 'A study of clinical nursing research priorities of renal specialist nurses caring for critically ill people', *Intensive and Critical Care Nursing*, vol. 12, no. 1, 45–9.

Daniels, G., Poroch, D. & DeRoach, J. 1995, 'Blood letting for BSL: the effects of timing and sites on blood volume', *Australian Journal of Advanced Nursing*, vol. 12, no. 3, 11–14.

Dawson-Saunders, B. & Trapp, R. 2001, *Basic and Clinical Biostatistics*, 3rd edn, Lange Medical Books-McGraw-Hill, New York.

Denzin, R. 1989, *The Research Act: A Theoretical Introduction to Sociological Methods*, 3rd edn, McGraw-Hill, New York.

Dunn, S., Lawson, D., Robertson, S., Underwood, M., Clark, R., Valentine, T., Walker, N., Wilson-Row, C., Crowder, K. & Herewane, D. 2000, 'The development of competency standards for specialist critical care nurses', *Journal of Advanced Nursing*, vol. 31, no. 2, 339–46.

Dunning, T. & Martin, M. 1996, 'Developing a questionnaire: some methodological issues', *Australian Journal of Advanced Nursing*, vol. 14, no. 2, 31–8.

Frank-Stromborg, M. & Olsen, S. 1997, *Instruments for Clinical Health-care Research*, 2nd edn (revised), Jones and Bartlett, Boston.

Frazer, L. 2000, *Questionnaire Design and Administration: A Practical Approach*, John Wiley and Sons, Brisbane.

Gardner, A., Goodsell, J., Duggan, T., Murtha, B., Peck, C. & Williams, J. 2001, 'Don't call me Sweetie', *Collegian*, vol. 8, no. 3, 32–8.

Gerdtz, K. & Bucknall, T. 2000, 'Australian triage nurses' decision-making and scope of practice', *Australian Journal of Advanced Nursing*, vol. 18, no. 1, 24–33.

Grindlay, A., Santamaria, N. & Kitt, S. 2000, 'Hospital in the home: nurse safety – exposure to risk and evaluation of organisational policy', *Australian Journal of Advanced Nursing*, vol. 17, no. 3, 6–12.

Henderson, A. 1999, 'Mixed messages about the meanings of breast-feeding representations in the Australian press and popular magazines', *Midwifery*, vol. 15, no. 1, 24–31.

Henry, G. 1990, *Practical Sampling*, Sage Publications, Newbury Park, California.

Jackson, D., Raftos, M. & Mannix, J. 1996, 'Through the looking glass: reflections on the authorship and content of current Australian nursing journals', *Nursing Inquiry*, vol. 3, no. 2, 112–17.

Jones, B. 1995, 'The effects of patient repositioning on intracranial pressure', *Australian Journal of Advanced Nursing*, vol. 12, no. 2, 32–9.

Keatinge, D., Cadd, A., Henssen, M., O'Brien, L. & Parker, D. 1999, 'Nurses' use of patients' notes to chart bowel care management for the palliative care patient', *Australian Journal of Advanced Nursing*, vol. 16, no. 4, 36–47.

Kimichi, J., Polivka, B. & Stevenson, J. 1991, 'Triangulation: operational definitions', *Nursing Research*, vol. 40, no. 6, 364–6.

Lam, L., Ross, F. & Cass, D. 1999, 'The impact of work-related trauma on the psychological health of nursing staff: a cross-sectional study', *Australian Journal of Advanced Nursing*, vol. 16, no. 3, 14–17.

Lamond, D. & Farnell, S. 1998, 'The treatment of pressure sores: a comparison of novice and expert nurses' knowledge, information use and decision accuracy, *Journal of Advanced Nursing*, vol. 27, no. 2, 280–6.

Maltby, H. 1999, 'The common thread: health care activities of Vietnamese and Anglo-Australian women', *Health Care for Women International*, vol. 20, no. 3, 291–302.

McAllister, M. & McLaughlin, D. 1996, 'Teaching metaphors of student nurses', *Journal of Advanced Nursing*, vol. 232, no.6, 1110–20.

McCann, T. 1997, 'Willingness to provide care and treatment for patients with HIV/AIDS', *Journal of Advanced Nursing*, vol. 25, no. 5, 1033–9.

McKeown, M., Stowell-Smith, M. & Foley, B. 1999, 'Passivity vs. militancy: a Q-methodological study of nurses' industrial relations on Merseyside (England)', *Journal of Advanced Nursing*, vol. 30, no. 1, 140–9.

Middleton, S. & Lumby, J. 1999, 'Comparing professional and patient outcomes for the same episode of care', *Australian Journal of Advanced Nursing*, vol. 17, no. 1, 22–7.

Minichiello, V., Sullivan, G., Greenwood, K. & Axford, R. 1999, *Handbook for Research Methods in Health Sciences*, Addison Wesley Longman Australia, Sydney.

Offredy, N. 2000, 'Advanced nursing practice: the case of nurse-practitioners in three Australian states', *Journal of Advanced Nursing*, vol. 31, no. 2, 274–81.

Pelletier, D., Duffield, C., Adams, A., Mitten-Lewis, S., Crisp, J. & Nagy, S. 2000, 'Australian clinicians and educators identify gaps in specialist cardiac nursing practice', *Australian Journal of Advanced Nursing*, vol. 17, no. 3, 24–30.

Proctor, N. 2000, 'Cultural affirmation and the protection of emotional well-being', *Holistic Nursing Practice*, vol. 15, no. 1, 5–11.

Raftos, M., Jackson, D. & Mannix, J. 1998, 'Idealised versus tainted femininity: discourses of the menstrual experience in Australian magazines that target young women', *Nursing Inquiry*, vol. 5, no. 3, 174–86.

Redfern, S. J. & Norman, I. J. 1994, 'Validity through triangulation', *Nurse Researcher*, vol. 2, no. 2, 41–56.

Rice, P. 1999, 'When the baby falls!: the cultural construction of miscarriage among Hmong women in Australia', *Women & Health*, vol. 30, no. 1, 85–103.

Rice, P. & Naksook, C. 1999, 'Pregnancy and technology: Thai women's perceptions and experience of prenatal testing', *Health Care for Women International*, vol. 20, no. 3, 259–78.

Roberts, K. 1995, 'Early Australian nursing scholarship: the first decade of the AJAN: Part 2: Scholarship', *Australian Electronic Journal of Nursing Education*, vol. 1, no. 1.

Roberts, K. 1999, 'Reliability and validity of an instrument to measure tissue hardness in breasts', *Australian Journal of Advanced Nursing*, vol. 16, no. 2, 19–23.

Roberts, K., Brittin, M., Cook, M. & deClifford, J. 1994, 'Boomerang pillows and respiratory capacity', *Clinical Nursing Research*, vol. 3, no. 2, 157–65.

Roberts, K., Reiter, M. & Schuster, D. 1998, 'Effects of cabbage leaf extract on breast engorgement', *Journal of Human Lactation*, vol. 14, no. 3, 231–6.

Shih, F. 1998, 'Triangulation in nursing research: issues of conceptual clarity and purpose', *Journal of Advanced Nursing*, vol. 28, no. 3, 631–41.

Sohier, R. 1988, 'Multiple triangulation and contemporary nursing research', *Western Journal of Nursing Research*, vol. 6, no. 6, 732–42.
Street, A. 1995, *Nursing Replay: Researching Nursing Culture Together*, Churchill Livingstone, Melbourne.
Tetting, D. 1988, 'Q-sort update', *Western Journal of Nursing Research*, vol. 10, no. 6, 757–65.
White, K. & Wilkes, L. 1999, 'The specialist breast care nurse: an evolving role', *Collegian*, vol. 6, no. 4, 8–13.
Wilmoth, M. 1995, 'Computer networks as a source of research subjects', *Western Journal of Nursing Research*, vol. 17, no. 3, 335–8.

Quantitative data collection and management

CHAPTER 9

chapter objectives
The material presented in this chapter will assist you to:

- prepare for data collection
- collect data
- process data for analysis
- manage the data and products of analysis
- carry out a pilot study.

Introduction

For most researchers, data collection is the time when they feel as though they have finally got down to the nitty gritty of the research process. It seems as though you have spent an inordinate amount of time planning the process, but at last you are going out to collect your data! Even if all of your planning has promoted a smooth data collection process, there are pitfalls in this phase of the process and things can still go wrong. You can help to prevent problems from arising, and minimise any damage, by anticipating potential traps and managing the data collection phase effectively.

It is not easy to generalise about the data collection phase of the process because so much of the approach to it depends on the methodology – the design and methods chosen for your study. What might be appropriate for one method could be inappropriate for another. In this chapter, therefore, we will try to confine our discussion to broad principles that you can apply to most quantitative data collection and management.

Preparing for data collection and management

Preparing for the data collection phase in your research project is analogous in some degree to preparing to carry out a nursing procedure. You need to select and obtain the equipment and materials, prepare the client, set up the area where the procedure will take place and prepare yourself.

In preparing to collect data, it is a good idea to construct a data collection plan using a flow chart or some other method of laying it out and tracking the process. You can do this on anything from butchers' paper to a sophisticated computer program. You then have a 'roadmap' of the project against which you can check your progress.

Acquisition and preparation of equipment and materials

Your first task is to select and acquire any necessary equipment such as biophysical instruments, computers, modems, recording equipment, statistical packages and so forth. This may involve buying, renting or borrowing pieces of equipment. You have more security if you hire or buy equipment because you are not subject to the lender's needs. If you are borrowing equipment, you need to make sure that it will be available when you need it and for as long as you need it.

It is essential to order any equipment and materials well before you expect to need them. The reason for this is that this process inevitably takes longer than you think it will, particularly if you have to order things from overseas. If you are ordering through a university or hospital bureaucracy, you may have to wait for the purchase order to be approved, which can entail waiting for the institution's preferred suppliers to supply goods, or for expensive items of equipment to go out to tender. Furthermore, you do not want to find out at the last moment that the equipment you ordered is no longer being made, is out of stock or is sitting on a wharf due to industrial action. Nor do you want to find out at the last minute that the printery that promised to do your questionnaires by a certain date is unable to meet your deadline. Photocopiers have a way of breaking down at inopportune times. It is also a good idea to get the promised dates of delivery in writing so that there can be no misunderstandings later. For equipment or material that is not too expensive, order a few extra copies or a few spare consumables as insurance against loss or breakage.

If you are buying a statistical package, buy it in advance and learn how to use it so that you can be sure that the data you are proposing to collect will be compatible with the package and with your skills. Ask experienced researchers what package they use and why they find it useful. You can also consult a database such as CINAHL or a journal such as *Computers in Nursing* for reviews of software. The Statistical Package for the Social Sciences (SPSS 1999) is a package commonly used by nurse-researchers. It is relatively expensive to buy for a personal computer, but most universities have it available on the network. You would probably need to buy the manual. If you are buying a data analysis package for your own personal computer, StatView is a reasonably priced, user-friendly data analysis package. It is available in both PC and Macintosh form and will meet the needs of most beginning researchers. So will the data analysis functions of Excel or Lotus. Whatever you buy, it is wise to consult the manual to learn how to operate the program. Some universities may have classes in running particular statistical packages.

You will need to order, in plenty of time, any necessary consumables such as consent forms, receipts, information sheets, sticky labels, logbooks and so on. You will need to prepare your informed consent document and your plain language statement. You will need to prepare any protocols for the ward staff: that is, instructions for taking part in data collection for your study.

It is important to check your equipment after you acquire it to make sure it is complete and in running order. Do this in plenty of time to get it repaired if necessary. If you are using any equipment that has been around for some time, you would be well advised to get it serviced before you are going to use it, for example to make sure that the rubber belts that drive the spindles of the tape recorder have not perished. Do a final check of your equipment immediately before you take it to the site. Check materials such as batteries, audiotapes and videotapes to make sure that they are not defective. This is especially important if you have bought materials of lower quality. Check materials when they arrive to ensure that there are sufficient copies and that all of the pages in such items as questionnaires are there.

Finally, ensure that you have a secure place to store your equipment and materials so that no-one else can borrow them, leaving your stock empty just when you need it.

Preparing questionnaire materials

You will need to get your questionnaires printed. You can use different coloured paper to identify different sites, or to differentiate the original from follow-up questionnaires, but coloured paper is more expensive than white paper. Be sure that you have proofread the questionnaire carefully before it goes to the printery.

If you are doing a questionnaire survey you will need the names of the population so that you can access them. In some circumstances, you may need to construct your own mailing list, although this is time-consuming. Sometimes you can acquire a mailing list that has been developed already. Some organisations keep mailing lists of their memberships and may be willing to give you access to that membership for research purposes. If you need to request a mailing list do so in plenty of time to make other arrangements if your request is not granted. Many organisations will not give you a list of their members' names and addresses because they need to protect the privacy of their members, and prevent them from receiving too many mail requests. However, some of these will distribute your questionnaire packet to their members at your expense. There are also agencies that have mailing lists for sale.

If you are selecting a random sample from your population you will need to do so according to the principles outlined in Chapter 8. It is possible to arrange for a computer to select names randomly from the database, or to follow a set of instructions to select a stratified random sample. If you need to do this, you should make the appropriate arrangements with the institution involved. Be warned that there may be a charge for computer programming time for specialised requests. However, using a computer to randomise the sample has the advantages of being fast, eliminating investigator bias, and being able to generate multiple random samples from the same list without using the same name twice (Cox, Harsanyi & Dean 1987).

The best way to address your questionnaire materials is by using sticky mailing labels generated by computer, especially if you need more than one set. There are computer programs that will create a file that can be printed out on sticky mailing labels. These are worth the money if you have some computer expertise and if you have to do your own mailing list. If you are doing a set of labels, remember to do as many sets as you will need for the round. For example, you may need one set for envelopes and one set for postcards if you are using that system. If you are doing a follow-up round you will need another set of labels.

You will also need self-addressed envelopes for respondents to return the questionnaires. You can either get them printed at a printery or use sticky labels, depending on the number. The most cost-effective way is to use reply paid post because you pay only for the actual returns.

Access to the site and participants

In most sites, it is mandatory to secure permission to collect data. The exception is a public place such as a street, where it is not strictly necessary to get permission. However, it is a good idea to let the police know what you are doing. This can save you trouble if some citizen reports you as a person behaving strangely (Batterham 1996). Also, it is a good idea to let the police know if your study involves any approach to members of the public or impedance in the flow of pedestrians (Benton & Cormack 1996).

If you are doing research in a semi-public area, such as a shopping centre, a health clinic lobby, or a hospital waiting room, you must secure permission.

If you are doing research that involves access to a library beyond that to which you may be entitled, you will need to seek permission. Also remember that even in a library in which you are entitled to use the open collections there may be restrictions on access to rare books, theses and other valuable collections. Access to these may require advance negotiation. Special conditions may apply to data collection in these areas; for example some rare book rooms allow only pencils to be used for note-taking and the books must not be removed from the room.

You will need to write all necessary letters (or emails) concerning access to the site well before you are ready to carry out data collection. You will need the letters of permission before the time of data collection.

It is wise to make sure beforehand that the site is still there, still available and in a fit state to be used for your research. It would be disastrous for the data collectors to arrive on the appointed day only to find that the venue has vanished or been totally reorganised. If you are using a laboratory, you will need to book it well in advance and confirm the booking a week or two before your projected use.

Before you go to the site, and as part of preparation for your study, make sure that there are sufficient participants available for your project, including extras to provide for participant mortality. If you are in doubt, you may need to acquire access to a second setting that is similar to the first one.

Ensure that the clinicians in charge of your potential participants are going to allow you access. Before the time of data collection, you can write letters requesting access or go and see the clinicians if it is convenient. Involving clinicians in the study will improve access, particularly if they are influential. Often they will be happy to assist you, particularly if you reward them in some way, for example a box of chocolates, morning tea, or an inservice. However, sometimes clinical staff such as medical practitioners, nursing unit managers and clinicians caring for the client may deny you access to their clients. They do so because they do not understand your project, they do not approve of it personally, or they are trying to protect 'their' clients from taking part in a research project.

Just before you are due to go into the site, check and make sure that the gatekeepers are still on side. You can follow up your initial letter with another letter, email or fax asking them to acknowledge that they know you are coming, or you can make a telephone call reminding the relevant people that you will be coming and when. A personal visit near to the time is ideal if you are near the site. You should also confirm that the person that arranged for your access is still in that position and is expecting you to come. If it is another person, you will have to brief them, send them copies of the earlier approvals, and hope that they will be co-operative. It is very important to do this in order to avoid the situation in which you arrive for your data collection, only to find, say, that the very helpful nursing unit manager has been replaced by an unco-operative one who thinks research is a waste of time.

Immediate preparation of the site

You will need to get into the laboratory or clinical field well in advance to check that your equipment can be placed where you want it. Set up your equipment and check that it actually works on site. You will also need to make sure that any special conditions that you require will be fulfilled, such as a specific temperature of the room.

If you are doing interviews, you will need to set up some mechanism to ensure privacy during the interviews. Strategies could include arranging to use a vacant office, making a sign for your office door, and arranging for someone else to answer the telephone if possible. You can also warn anyone who is likely to interrupt that you will not tolerate interruptions during this period. Check again that the tape recorder is working and that you have all the needed equipment such as extension cords, batteries, audiotapes and so forth.

Preparation of people

When preparing for data collection, it is also necessary to prepare the people involved including the gatekeepers, the staff in the clinical area or laboratory, the participants, and yourself, the researcher.

Staff

If you are using ward staff, remember to brief them in person if possible – you could do one or more inservice sessions to explain your study and how it will affect the staff. In order to promote co-operation it is useful to prepare a resource folder about the study to leave in each participating clinical area. This folder could contain any procedures, protocols, patient materials (such as informed consent document and plain language statement), and any relevant previous literature. Ensuring the co-operation of the clinical staff is crucial to the success of a study. The same principles apply to any location in which you are going to collect data.

Recruitment and preparation of participants

When you get to the site, in either a clinical or non-clinical situation, it is necessary to recruit participants to take part in the study. Depending on the design of your study, you may recruit clients, members of the public or colleagues. Each of these groups has inbuilt problems. Members of the public are often suspicious of strangers. Colleagues require special consideration if they are in a junior position to you to ensure that they do not feel compelled to take part in the study. Special care is needed with participants from another culture, and participants who do not understand English. Care is also needed with vulnerable people such as the elderly, and any special types of participants that cannot give informed consent on their own behalf. Procedures with these participants were discussed more fully in Chapter 5.

You may need to recruit all the participants at the beginning of the study or as you go along, depending on the design of the study. Recruitment is done either by you, the researcher, or by your colleagues on site. Recruitment is best done by someone involved in the study personally so that you can be sure that all possible potential participants are approached.

Personal contact, either by you or by colleagues assisting you with the research, is the best method of recruitment, especially when it is done one-on-one, because people find it harder to say no to you in person than they do to less personal methods. If personal contact is not possible because of distance, you can use a telephone call, fax, letter or email. It helps to use a personal touch if possible. When approaching clients, introduce yourself and give your credentials so that they understand with whom they are dealing. Remember that the system of identification of staff that is so clear to you as a nurse may be incomprehensible to the participants.

Remember that it always takes longer than you expect to get the required sample size. If recruitment is a problem, for example where you do not have a captive pool of possible participants, you can advertise in suitable sites, for example the newspaper or, in the clinical setting, fliers. Another strategy is to offer some small reward for participation in the study; remember, this should be sufficient to recompense them for their time.

You may be unable to recruit enough participants. This can occur when your criteria are too restrictive – if so, you may need to re-examine them. Another problem of recruitment is occurring increasingly with general trends like shorter hospital stays for surgical operations and childbirth. This can both limit access to participants and decrease the number of potential data collection days for each participant. These influences have also resulted in fewer nursing staff, which means not enough time for them to assist with data collection.

One recruitment problem that can occur is that potential participants decline to participate in your study. Participants may refuse because of fear of invasive procedures required, disillusionment with research, or poor health status. Some may have been discouraged by staff who have criticised the project.

As a part of the recruitment process, you need to have procedures in place to ensure that you avoid generating a biased sample. It is necessary to approach all of the selected potential participants at a suitable time, for example when they are not heavily medicated. Explain the study in plain, simple language, avoiding the use of jargon. Most ethics committees require that you give the potential participant a statement to read that has already been approved. It is a good idea to give the potential participant time to consider participating in the study by leaving the information and coming back later for an answer. After the potential participant has consented to participate, you will need to get the consent form signed.

In making arrangements to collect your data in the clinical area it is wise to consider nursing care and other routines. With regard to individual clients you will need to consider their specific scheduled care and their conscious state. Be flexible in arranging times and rescheduling times for data collection if necessary.

Prior to collecting the data, it may be necessary to allocate participants randomly to treatment and control groups. For two groups, this can be done by a coin toss. Because you almost never end up with equal numbers of heads and tails, you will need to toss the coin about 20 per cent more times than the number of names you need to allocate. List the results of each throw. If you throw more heads than tails, say, you need to keep tossing and listing till you get enough tails. Between the first and last tail that you need, you may find too many heads, so you have to keep tossing and listing till you have equal numbers of heads and tails. You keep the part of the list that has the equal numbers and disregard the rest. You then match your list of heads and tails to your list of names to assign the participants to the two groups.

To cope with two or more groups you can put all the names, or numbers representing participants, in a hat. The first name or number drawn out goes in the first group, the second into the second group and so forth. Another method is to write each name on a card, then shuffle the cards well and 'deal' them into as many groups as you need.

If you are using a list of random numbers or heads and tails, you allocate the participants according to your list. You can do this effectively by numbering envelopes and putting a slip in each envelope that tells participants which group they were assigned to. Each new recruit is given the next envelope in the sequence.

Researcher and data collectors

It is necessary also to prepare yourself and your data collectors for the data collection. You should ensure that anyone collecting data is sufficiently practised with the equipment and materials to ensure a smooth running process during the actual data collection. You can practise trial interviews or application of instruments on friends or colleagues. Multiple data collectors must practise until they achieve inter-rater reliability. Brief data collectors about procedures, but to prevent biased data do not tell them about an expected outcome.

In preparing yourself for data collection you should remind yourself to be co-operative at all times with the clinical area. Remember that you will be there as a guest and that you are a representative of your institution. Recognise that the client care takes priority over your research needs.

It is a good idea if you are a student or if you are acting as a clinical staff member to ensure that the research activity is covered by the professional indemnity insurance of your employer or university. This is particularly important if you are using any invasive equipment or if there is any potential for harm to the participants.

Make sure that any travel and accommodation arrangements are made well in advance.

Preparation for data management

You will probably have to do some preparation for the management of your data once you get it; for example learn how to operate any data analysis software, draw up coding sheets if you are using them, set up computer files for your data and allocate participant numbers to the data. Preparing for data entry also involves testing all of your procedures on the computer prior to entering real data.

The process of data collection

Data collection can take place using a variety of methods which have been discussed in Chapter 8 and earlier in this chapter. Obviously, how you collect data will depend on which method you are using since different methods will require different techniques. You can safely anticipate that the data collection phase of the study will take longer than you expected and be more difficult than you anticipated, and will require adjustments during the process.

We will talk about some of the general principles of data collection and problems that may occur. We will then proceed to discuss some of the specific techniques of the more common quantitative methods, such as questionnaires, content analysis, structured observation, and using existing data sources. General observation and interviewing techniques will be discussed in Chapter 15 on qualitative data collection.

Managing equipment and materials

Various types of equipment can be used to collect quantitative data, depending on the design of the study, for instance biophysical instruments, audiotape recorders, videotape recorders and computers. Treatment and use of the equipment will vary, depending on what it is. Of course, all equipment should be treated with respect. Whatever hardware you are using, you must make sure that it is kept in top condition during the course of the data collection. It should be given whatever regular maintenance is suggested by the manufacturer. For example, recording heads on audio- or videotape recorders should be cleaned regularly.

If you are using a computer in data collection, it is likely to be either a laptop into which you can type your data directly, or a computer that is an integral part of another instrument. A computer may also be interfaced with a bioinstrument so that the instrument inputs data directly into the computer. Such a process was described for a study to examine the effects of early parent touch on premature infants (Harrison 1989). In that study a portable computer was interfaced with the infants' cardiac monitor and pulse oximeter and data were automatically input into the computer every six seconds. The parent–infant interactions were recorded on a videocamera that was also interfaced with the computer so that the data on the infants' physiological parameters were recorded on the videotape. This allowed the researchers to analyse the infants' physiological responses to the parents' actions. According to the researcher (Harrison 1989), the advantages of computerised data collection are: increased reliability and accuracy, ability to collect larger and more frequent amounts of data, savings of time in recording and coding, and economy over the long term. The disadvantages are the need for increased space, a lengthy set-up time, focus on the machine rather than on the client and possible measurement error related to the computer.

If you are using computers during the actual process of data collection, you should ensure that the data are put in correctly and completely. You should also ensure that you have procedures in place to protect against loss at any time during the process. The computer must be protected against power surges if it is plugged into the mains; if necessary use a surge protector in the line. If you are using batteries, make sure that the batteries give sufficient power for the period of data collection. Save the file at least every 10 minutes using an automatic save function if you have one. Make frequent backup copies of your files using whatever system you normally use, store them in safe places, and update them regularly.

Distribution of questionnaires

You can distribute questionnaires by several methods – the more personal the contact with the respondents, the higher rate of response you are likely to get, all else being equal.

You can deliver them personally to a nearby site. Then you can distribute them yourself to clients or nurses, or to a contact person to distribute for you. If you are using a self-selected convenience sample you can leave the questionnaires in a box with a flier asking people to take them. Personal delivery to the individual or the site may entail some travel costs to get to the group but this is balanced by a saving in postage.

If you are sending the questionnaires all over Australia or even overseas, postal delivery or email will be necessary. You can identify a contact person at the site to distribute them then send them to that person by post or email. Or you can send them individually by post or by email. You can even administer them by telephone or fax, which saves on the cost of postage but incurs the cost of a telephone call.

Whatever method you choose, you will need to be consistent in the distribution in order to even out external influences. That is, you should distribute them all using the same method and close together in time. You should send them all to the recipients' homes or all to their work, but not mix them.

If you are distributing your questionnaire by email to a list you will have no postage costs for either distribution or return but you may have sending and downloading costs if you are paying a commercial provider. You need to weigh the reduced cost against the quality of the sample. That is, the people on a list may not be representative of the characteristics of the population that you wish to sample. Instructions to people on email lists should include an instruction to return the reply to the individual researcher, not to the whole list. Your instructions should include in a prominent place the method of changing the address to the researcher rather than just hitting the reply button, which will send the reply back to the whole list. If the whole list can read the response, the confidentiality of the respondents is destroyed. If you send it out over the

Listserver, everyone, including yourself, will get a copy but no-one will be aware of anyone but themselves receiving the information. Getting your own copy by email from a Listserver is a good way of checking that the message actually went out to the list.

If you are compiling your own list of email addresses to which you wish to send your questionnaire, it is a good idea to select the 'Blind CC' in the header of the email. This conceals the identity of other recipients of the questionnaire. In this case, of course, replies will come directly back to you as you have not sent them out over a Listserver.

Managing the site

If you are collecting data in the field, it is important to try to keep the site as conducive as possible to smooth data collection. Make sure there are no interruptions. Just before you commence an interview take your telephone off the hook, turn off your mobile telephone and disconnect any beepers. Also ask your interviewee to turn off any mobile phone or beeper.

Collecting data on site can give rise to problems. The worst possible problem is a catastrophic change in the site during the time of data collection, for example a flood, fire, cyclone or earthquake destroying the site. Almost as bad are unforeseen institutional factors such as changes of policy that affect your study, industrial action, unplanned closure or reorganisation of a clinical area, transfer of co-operative staff out of the unit and transfer of unco-operative staff into the unit. If you are using available data, there may be a loss of charts that you were going to audit or the charts may be incomplete. In this day and age of 'downsizing', changes in institutional structures are not unusual. However, if you are lucky, they will be planned long enough in advance for you to adapt to them. If a disaster happens, you will have to decide whether you have enough data to make a worthwhile study. Alternatively, if you have partial data, you could cut your losses and use the collected data as a pilot study, finding another site for the main study.

Managing the participants

The way to manage the participants during the data collection phase is to keep them onside. Treat participants well – you are dependent on them for your data. Remember, they are not compelled to participate and they can withdraw at any time. It is important to put participants at ease as much as possible during the data collection by introducing yourself, reminding the participant of the purposes and procedures of the research, and chatting briefly about other things just to break the ice.

There may be problems with the sample that has been recruited – it may be subject to participant mortality or loss of participants from the study. Some people agree to participate and then fail to show up for the interview or do not do the questionnaire. Try phoning the day before to remind them of the interview. Sometimes clients in the clinical field are transferred to another ward or facility or discharged before your study is complete. It is a good idea to maintain regular contact with clients and keep note of their home address so that if this happens you can arrange perhaps to collect the data later.

Even if participants complete the study, some produce unusable data, such as obviously flippant or insincere responses to interview questions, leaving lots of blanks on questionnaires or failing to co-operate with clinical procedures integral to your study. Any of these can render those parts of the data useless.

If these things happen and your sample gets smaller, you can spend longer to achieve an adequate sample, you can live with the smaller sample or you can re-evaluate your criteria. If you need to live with a smaller sample you must take the sample size into consideration when analysing the results.

Managing colleagues

The people on the data collection site must be managed as well. It is important to treat them well, because you are also dependent on their co-operation. Several ways of facilitating the study by interacting with the staff have been mentioned already. It is important to continue these overtures and keep the staff onside. Perhaps make a contribution to morning tea or make other small gestures that show your appreciation for the opportunity to collect data.

Despite your best efforts, however, sometimes the staff will make it difficult for you to collect data. They can unwittingly do things that interfere with your data collection. Even worse, they can sabotage your project. They can unintentionally or intentionally 'forget' to notify you of suitable prospective participants, they can schedule other activities that interfere with data collection or they can fail to carry out properly the procedures that are crucial to your research.

Sometimes staff factors outside their control interfere, such as horrendously busy spells, roster changes and so forth. If an increased workload occurs, naturally the staff will give a higher priority to the nursing care than to your research. Keep an eye out for these kinds of problems and deal with them by strategies such as educating the staff, inducting new people into the project, securing the support of the nursing unit manager, taking over more of the data collection activity or modifying your protocols. It is important to give regular feedback to the staff concerning your project but do not give so much feedback that it influences your data in some way.

Managing the process

It is important to manage the process so that you get accurate, complete data. The importance of accuracy applies both to the measurement and to the recording of data. You or your colleagues as data collectors must be very well versed in the procedures to achieve this goal. Even then, unplanned errors can occur. You might forget to turn on the microphone of the tape recorder or you might overwrite an interview tape, thinking it is blank. Have procedures in place to prevent this sort of thing, such as routine checking and labelling of tapes before using them. In some methods, such as questionnaires, the accuracy will depend on the participant carrying out the procedure correctly, or giving the correct answers.

Sometimes researchers come up against a conflict of interest or ethical problem during the course of data collection. You might be trying to collect data as a participant observer and find that you have to choose between two functions that are both equally important. It has also been known for a researcher to discover an abuse of clients during the course of data collection. This poses a dilemma, because if the researcher blows the whistle, the institution and/or staff will probably cease to co-operate with the study and the data collection at that facility will be ruined. On the other hand, not to report the abuse would be unethical because it would harm the clients. Client safety must take precedence over research outcomes, but if it is possible to negotiate with the staff that the behaviour stops, the research project may be saved.

Keep track of events that may affect your data. We mentioned earlier the threat to validity of historical factors. Sometimes unforeseen events could affect the staff on whom you are collecting data, for example the death of a colleague or a favourite client. If this happens, you may need to suspend data collection until things have settled down. Unforeseen events can also interfere with your processes, for example industrial action or natural disasters interfering with travel arrangements or, even worse, destroying the site in the middle of the data collection period.

Monitoring the process

In every project, no matter how small, it is important to keep track of the process: that is, to keep records of what steps you have taken. It is important to keep a written record, a logbook, so that you are not dependent on your memory. Memory can be unreliable, especially over the longer periods of time involved in a large project such as a thesis. Record-keeping can be done in a simple fashion for a small project by writing in an exercise book, ideally one with divided sections to keep track of the different parts of your project. For larger projects, it may be worth keeping records on a spreadsheet, or even a computer program designed for project management. You should record a 'diary' of your visits – dates, length, impressions and problems that you encountered. Record what data you collected on each occasion. Record your expenses for future reference, and keep receipts. These records will assist you when it is time to write up the procedures for the study.

Check the entries in the logbook regularly to make sure that things are going to plan. It is crucial to ensure that the appropriate steps of the data collection process, such as collecting protocols and making telephone calls, are carried out. It is also important to document the arrival of data. It may be necessary to monitor nursing interventions during a clinical project (Gilliss & Kulkin 1991). It is also important to identify any intervening variables that have not been accounted for, and monitor their effect or revise your data collection plan.

Aftercare
Your data collection process is not complete until you have taken care of the cleaning up process. It is necessary to clean and repair any equipment and return it to its owner if it is borrowed. Leave the laboratory or clinical site at least as good as you found it if not better. Thank the staff of a clinical site in some creative way, and offer to send a summary report of your findings and any publications that ensue.

One of the most important things to do is to prevent loss of data from natural disasters, such as flood or fire, or human intervention, such as theft. The usual way is to make a set of backups and store them away from the place where your data are held.

Management of data and products of analysis
Logging the data
It is extremely important to keep good records of your data. Each piece of data should be clearly labelled and recorded. Each piece of data, whether a questionnaire, audiotape, videotape or rhythm strip, should be assigned some sort of code number or name to be used in all data pertaining to that item. A separate list of the code numbers and participant names, if any, should be kept in the logbook.

It is also important to monitor the quality and completeness of the data. Each piece of data should be checked for accuracy and completeness so that you can collect more data at the time if necessary.

Consider making a copy of all data, regardless of their format, and storing them in another secure place at a distance from the primary copy. This is important, at least until you have completed the objectives of the study, for example getting your degree. Making copies may be expensive, but it is less costly than collecting all of the data again if the originals are lost or destroyed.

A code book should be kept, either in an exercise book or on a computer program. The code book should show a map of the variables, including in which column they are in the database, the name used for each variable and element and, in the case of a program such as SPSS, how many columns each variable occupies. For more detail on the construction of code books, see Lobo (1993).

Your original data must be stored in a secure place in the institution for a set period of time. This requirement of the NHMRC is implemented by the institutional ethics committee of the university, hospital, or other institution under whose auspices you are doing the project. You should be aware of the regulations of your institution. (These restrictions would not apply to storage of data for short undergraduate research courses whose purpose is to teach about research rather than to conduct actual studies. They would apply, however, to data for honours and postgraduate theses.) The main purpose of storing the data is to allow for investigation of fraud, should it be necessary. In any case, it is worthwhile to store data to enable further analysis. The period of time for which the data must be stored may vary from institution to institution but is usually five years after publication. Consult your supervisor about data storage.

Processing data for analysis

Some data do not require any processing because they can be analysed directly from their original form. Some data require a small amount of processing, for example writing code numbers on questionnaires. Some data require a large amount of processing, for example converting text units to numbers. Most methods of data collection require the researcher to transform the raw data in some way so that they can be transferred easily from the data source into a computer data analysis program. The principle is to process the data sufficiently to facilitate data analysis. The method of analysis will determine the preparation that will need to be done.

Some data that have already been put into a computer may not require any further preparation. For example, if you are using a database that has been input into a computer already you will only have to transfer the data into your own program for analysis. Similarly, some researchers can enter their data straight into a portable computer in the field or laboratory either directly from an instrument that is hooked up to the computer, or by means of the data collector typing the data into the computer keyboard. Questionnaires that have been prepared and responded to in such a way that they can be directly scanned into a computer can be entered into the computer easily. For more detail on how to do this, see Dennis (1994).

If the data are on audiotape, most researchers prefer to have the audiotapes transcribed into word processor text before analysing the data, particularly if they are analysing the meaning of the text. Transcription of audiotapes can be done by the researcher, a research assistant or a typist who has the requisite skills. If you are planning to do much of it yourself, it is well worth acquiring a dictaphone-type audiocassette player with foot controls and automatic rewind. These features allow you to keep your hands on the keyboard and retain your place in the tape when you pause.

If you are using videotapes, they will need to be edited and the shots you are using will need to be identified using a coding system.

Most questionnaires will require some coding. Coding is the process that usually renders the data into numbers that can be entered into your database in a form in which they can be analysed easily. Data can be from open-ended questionnaires that require a lot of researcher coding, to pre-coded questionnaires that require minimal coding. For example, on a pre-coded questionnaire, the respondent must tick one of four boxes, numbered 1–4, to answer a question. The researcher enters the number into that person's data entry for that question. To illustrate, the answer 'never married' could be given a code of '1', married '2', de facto '3', and divorced '4'. Actual numbers, for example the person's age in years, temperature or oxygen saturation, do not need to be coded. Sometimes data will be from open-ended questions on questionnaires or from text that is for content analysis. If you wish to quantify these data, you will have to develop a coding schema to handle it.

The process of coding can be done in two ways. The first method is to code directly from the data source. With questionnaires, some people like to write the code on each questionnaire and some prefer to code straight into the computer.

The amount of transformation of data required depends on how the questionnaire has been constructed in the first place. If it is pre-coded by putting the numbers on the questionnaire, then there is little coding to do at this stage. The second method is to code the data onto a coding sheet and then enter it into the database from the coding sheet. Both of these methods have advantages and disadvantages. Coding directly from the data source is faster and avoids transcription errors that arise from the double-handling of the data, but is more prone to errors of data entry. The coding sheet method speeds up the data entry process and increases its accuracy but is more prone to errors of transcription during the coding process.

Direct data entry

If you are coding straight into the computer file, you must set it up first so that it will accept the data. A database file is usually a matrix of rows and columns, which intersect to form cells. Each row of the matrix is one person's data, while each column is one variable or answer to one question of the questionnaire. Thus, reading across a row will give you a participant's data, while reading down a column will give you every person's data on that one variable. You should head each of the columns with the variable name or its abbreviation to make it easier for you to recognise the variable. In addition, always put at the beginning of the row a participant number that is also on the raw data. Do not use the database row numbers instead of participant numbers. If you sort the data, the database numbers will not change with the data.

All programs will need to be instructed what your variable names are and what the values of the elements that comprise the variables are: for example, '1' equals 'never married' and so forth. Some data analysis programs let you type in the actual element name or part of it, such as 'n' for 'never married', 'm' for 'married', 'di' for divorced, 'de' for de facto and so forth. However, even though you type them in as names and they appear as names on the monitor, the computer stores them as numbers. It is useful to have a logical structure for the element labels of the variables, for example yes = '1', no = '0'. This will help later in interpreting your data correctly. It is particularly important where the variable has an underlying numerical structure, for example the Likert Scale. It is vital to keep to the same code as a pre-coded questionnaire when you are entering data in order to avoid errors in data entry. If necessary, you can re-code the data later. An example of a print-out from a database is shown in Figure 9.1.

When you have set up your data file in the computer, you are ready to enter the data into the computer. This is part of the drudgery of research, but a necessary part. You will have to decide whether to go for speed or accuracy.

Using coding sheets

If you are using a separate coding sheet, it is very important to make it the same structure as the computer file into which the data will be put, for ease of transfer. A blank coding sheet would look much like the print-out shown in Figure 9.1, only without data.

Participant	Gender	Age	Marital status	Religion	Education
1	M	30	Married	Prot	Yr 10
2	F	25	Nevmar	RC	Yr 12
3	F	45	Div	Prot	Yr 12
4	F	64	Nevmar	Buddhist	Uni deg
5	M	36	De facto	Prot	TAFE cert/dip
6	M	29	Div	Nil	Yr 10
7	F	21	Nevmar	Muslim	Yr 12
8	M	19	Married	Nil	Uni deg
9	M	53	De facto	RC	Yr 12

Figure 9.1 Print-out of data in database

It is crucial to check the finished coding sheet against the raw data. If there is only a small amount, you should check it all. If there is a large amount, you can check 10 per cent at random. If it is error-free, you could assume that the rest will probably be too, and decide to live with any errors.

During the actual processes of data coding and data entry, it is very important to ensure that they are done consistently. Changes can occur in the data because the data coder changed the code part way through coding or direct data entry. This should be resisted, but if it happens, the previous coding will have to be rectified so that it is consistent with the new code. Another source of disparity is the use of two or more different data coders. If this is the case, they should all be asked to code one section and the consistency of the coding should be checked. The accuracy rate should be one that you can live with, but it must be at least 90 per cent.

It is also extremely important to ensure accuracy during the process of data coding and data entry. If, for example, you have complicated procedures that require special care during coding and entry, you must check even more carefully. One example is that in a long questionnaire, the order of items may be reversed in half of the copies to control for respondent fatigue. Extreme caution must be exercised to make sure that all of the answers to each item are in the correct column.

Missing values are a problem that every researcher will have to deal with at some time. These occur where for some reason the data are missing: for example, a respondent has not given an answer for a question. If a whole section of data is consistently missing, you cannot enter any of it. For example, if you are collecting data on each of three days after childbirth, and most of the mothers have gone home on the second day, you can delete all data for the third day.

Some data analysis programs have a mechanism for handling missing values, giving them a code or not using that case in the data analysis. If your variable is numerical, it is important not to put zero for a missing value as this will lower the value of the mean. You can either leave it missing or put in the median value.

After the data have been entered into the computer, it is vital to proofread them. Your final results are only as good as your data. You can check them against the original source, or against the coding sheet if it has been proofread. There are various ways of doing this. One is to do it yourself; however, this does not eliminate potential for error. A better way is for two people to do it, one reading from the coding sheet and one reading from the computer print-out or monitor. Finally, some computer programs have a facility for double entry of data and checking both entries against each other and giving you a list of the mismatches. It is important to check the data for errors such as missing data, missing lines, or values that are higher or lower than those stipulated in the code.

Manipulating data

During the process of data analysis, it is almost always the case that you will want to change your data in some way. This can involve such operations as combining variables, re-coding variables to change the values, applying a weighting to a variable and/or applying mathematical formulas. It is crucial to double check that the conversion has been done correctly by checking the input with the output. If you have carried out these operations incorrectly, your data will be meaningless. Whenever you change your data, it is mandatory to note this in your logbook or record it in some way. Do not rely on your memory. When you have finished any changes and are satisfied with the result, it is imperative to make a fresh backup copy, renaming the file. Older versions of your data should be kept in an archive, either on a floppy disk or as hard copy. You should always keep backup copies of the original computer data as well as your working copy of the transformed data.

Managing the products of data analysis

When you begin to generate your data analysis, you will need to organise it in some way. A data analysis program will generate the analysis. Most programs generate output files that can be saved on your computer, or you can create a word processor file and copy the data analysis into it. These methods allow you to organise the data analysis and save it. You normally print the data analysis that you want to keep, either from an output or word processor file. The word processor file can also serve as a backup copy of the hard copy so that if you lose the hard copy you will not have to redo the analysis.

If you want to store hard copy of the data analysis, you will need to organise some sort of system. Normally, hard copy will be generated on ordinary A4 paper that can be put into an ordinary ring binder, possibly with plastic document protectors and section dividers if it becomes large enough to warrant separation into sections.

Pilot study

A pilot study 'is a miniature replica of the planned research strategy and is designed to test every aspect of it' (Hockey 1992). It is a small-scale version of the study that goes in advance, incorporating all aspects of the procedures of the main study and providing guidance for the larger study. Thus, it is like a pilot ship, a small ship that navigates a difficult, dangerous or unknown route ahead of an ocean liner in order to lead the ship safely along its course. The pilot study can also be thought of as similar to the test piloting of a new aeroplane before production models are put into service. You can read more about pilot studies in Prescott and Soeken (1989) and Hinds and Gattuso (1991). An example of a pilot study is one by Grindlay, Santamaria and Kitt (2000) in which nurse safety in the 'hospital in the home' care program was evaluated.

There is a difference in purpose, however, between a pilot study and a main study. The purpose of a pilot study is to identify strengths and weaknesses in the research plan in order to improve the main study, whereas the purpose of a main study is to develop knowledge. There is also a difference in the scale of the pilot and main studies. The pilot study is carried out on a much smaller scale than the main study.

A pilot study should be carried out in such a way as to be as close as possible to the real thing. It should, if possible, be carried out in the actual setting in which the main study will be conducted. It should use the actual procedures proposed for the main study, including such things as obtaining informed consent. It should use the same type of participants.

As a researcher, you will need to consider whether or not a pilot study is necessary in your circumstances. Experienced researchers who are very familiar with techniques and have done previous similar research may be able to forego a pilot study. Most readers of this book, however, are unlikely to be in that category. The other exception is if you are a student doing a small undergraduate student project. The reasons for this are that the major purpose of such an exercise is to learn about research rather than to produce new knowledge, and that the time frame for this type of study is usually very short. However, in the real world of research, researchers do not do pilot studies frequently enough. This may be attributed to a small amount of perceived benefit for the amount of effort. As a researcher, you should incorporate at least one pilot study in the research plan of any substantial study. It may seem like a lot of fuss and bother to do a pilot study when one has designed the perfect research study with which nothing can possibly go wrong, but most researchers can tell you stories of studies – either where they did not do a pilot study and wished they had, or where they were glad that they did. It is a wise expenditure of time and money because it can save time and money later and prevent potentially devastating mistakes.

One major purpose of a pilot study is to assess the feasibility of the main study so that you can correct any problems before carrying out the main study. A pilot study will allow you to assess whether your study design is adequate. You can see whether the methodology is going to work. You can evaluate such things as the recruitment of participants, the sampling technique, the appropriateness and effectiveness of the procedures, the time frame and the costs. You can also see whether the instruments are going to work, and if not, choose an alternative. You can see whether you need any extra equipment that you might not have anticipated. Testing the proposed study will help to identify any unanticipated variables and allow you to consider their impact on the study and ways of dealing with them. If the study design is not adequate you can repair it before you carry out the main study. It is not ethical to conduct studies that are badly flawed or to collect data that have no chance of being valid (Western Australian Research Network 1994).

Another major purpose of a pilot study is to allow the researcher or data collectors to practise with the equipment, techniques and procedures with actual participants, in the real setting. This will give confidence to the personnel conducting the research, allowing the main study to progress smoothly. It will also inspire confidence in the participants and allow multiple data collectors to achieve inter-rater reliability.

You can also assess the reaction of the people involved in the research project. You can see if your participants have understood the instructions and observe their reaction to the instruments. You can assess the efficacy of your recruitment procedures and you should find out how many participants you can expect to drop out. If it is a clinical project, you can also monitor the reaction of the staff in the setting and address any problems that arise, for example the impact of the project on any routines of nursing care. Finally, you can check the reaction of the researchers and data collectors to the project, addressing any problems that arise and incorporating any suggestions for improvement.

A pilot study will allow you to assess the adequacy of your data and adjust any instrumentation appropriately. You should enter your pilot data into your proposed data analysis program and assess the data entry procedures. You should analyse the pilot data, using the techniques that you propose to use in the main study, so that you can determine if you have collected the most appropriate form or level of data. You can save time and money if you revise or eliminate questionnaires that do not work.

After you have carried out the pilot study to the point of data analysis, you should evaluate your methodology. If you make major changes, you should do a second pilot study. Finally, you should write up the pilot study. The process of analysis involved will force you to evaluate the pilot study thoroughly.

The results of a pilot study are not normally included in the main results. The reason for this is that historical events and changes made between the pilot and the main study may render the pilot data different from those of the main study and therefore unable to be incorporated into it. If there have been no changes and if you are short of participants, you may include the pilot data in your results.

It is also not customary to publish results of a pilot study; however, there have been some exceptions such as Daly, Chang and Bell (1996), King and Wilson (1998) and Grindlay, Santamaria and Kitt (2000).

When you have carried out your pilot study and revised your research plan accordingly, you are ready to commence data collection for your main study.

Summary

In this chapter, we have covered the main points in the process of data collection and management. We have focused on strategies for managing equipment and materials, participants, staff and colleagues. We have looked at processing data, coding data, setting up computer files, data entry and managing the products of data analysis. We have explained the importance of running a pilot study as a 'dress rehearsal' for your main study. Having collected and processed your data, you can now take the next exciting step of analysis.

Main points

- Data are what the researcher collects in order to answer the research question. The data will be congruent with methodology and there may be more than one form of data.
- In quantitative methodologies, data are almost always numbers or something that is converted to numbers.
- In preparing for data collection and management, the researcher sets up a data collection plan; selects and obtains the equipment and materials; prepares the participants, setting and self; and ensures arrangements for insurance, travel and accommodation are made.
- The researcher gains access to the site and the participants by securing written permission from gatekeepers where necessary.
- Immediately before collecting data, the researcher checks the equipment on site, and the site conditions. The gatekeepers and staff are also briefed.
- Data collectors are given the necessary training.
- Participants are recruited from relevant groups such as clients, the public and colleagues, with special care to cultural safety and language considerations. Plain language statements are given out and consent forms are signed before data are collected.
- In planning times of data collection, consider nursing care and other routines in the clinical area, be flexible in arranging times and reschedule if necessary.
- In preparation for data management, learn how to operate any data analysis software, draw up any coding sheets and set up computer files.
- Treat your equipment (including computers) with respect, consider safety aspects and ensure regular maintenance.
- Questionnaires can be distributed by various methods, with personal contact preferred.
- When on site collecting data, ensure there are no interruptions; try to anticipate problems and forestall them.
- When dealing with participants, be polite, brief them, ensure good lines of communication and keep to your commitment of time.
- When dealing with your colleagues, be considerate, keep them informed and remember that client care takes precedence over research.
- Keep a logbook of visits and data collection procedures.
- After data collection, clean and repair any equipment, leave things as you found them and thank those who helped you.
- Implement sound procedures for handling, entering and analysing data and dealing with the products of data analysis. Ensure that you have backups.

- A pilot study 'is a miniature replica of planned research strategy and is designed to test every aspect of it' (Hockey 1992). It is a small-scale, dress rehearsal for the main study, incorporating all aspects of the main study's procedures.
- A pilot study is done to find strengths and weaknesses of methods, to assess feasibility, to practise with equipment and procedures, to assess the reaction of researchers and data collectors, to assess the adequacy of data and then to adjust the methods appropriately.
- A pilot study should be done in an environment as close as possible to the real thing, in the actual setting for the main study, using the actual proposed procedures and the same type of participants.

Review Questions

1 One important thing to remember about equipment is:
   a it can be counted upon to work
   b it should be ordered in plenty of time
   c it does not include software
   d all of the above

2 You do not need to acquire official permission to collect data in:
   a semi-public places
   b public places
   c institutions
   d shopping centres

3 Data collection can be commenced as soon as you have:
   a acquired permission from the gatekeepers
   b given out the plain language statement to the participants
   c acquired formal informed consent
   d a and c

4 The best method of recruiting participants is by:
   a personal contact
   b personalised letter of request
   c email
   d poster in an appropriate place

5 A process that renders data into numbers that can be entered into a database is:
   a matrixing
   b coding
   c transcribing
   d editing

6 A written record of the process of data collection is called a:
   a spreadsheet
   b database
   c logbook
   d code book

7 Advantages of computerised data collection are:
   a need for less space
   b savings of time in recording and coding
   c less setup time
   d less measurement error

8 After data have been entered into the computer, it is important to:
   a manipulate the data
   b keep a backup copy
   c print it out and file a hard copy
   d all of the above

9 A pilot study:
   a is a replica of the main study
   b is a dress rehearsal
   c aims to identify faults in procedures
   d all of the above

10 In a pilot study you would:
    a assume the equipment works
    b not be concerned about costs
    c assess the adequacy of the data
    d try unplanned methods

Discussion Questions

1 Describe how you would obtain access to a data collection site.
2 Outline three methods of allocating participants to groups randomly.
3 Discuss different ways of distributing questionnaires.
4 What information should be entered into a logbook?
5 What are the advantages of a pilot study?

References

Batterham, C. 1996, *The Behaviour of Child Pedestrians at Darwin Primary Schools*, Federal Office of Road Safety, Canberra.

Benton, D. & Cormack, D. 1996, 'Gaining access to the research site', in *The Research Process in Nursing*, 3rd edn, ed. D. Cormack, Blackwell Science, Oxford.

Cox, H., Harsanyi, B. & Dean, L. 1987, *Computers and Nursing: Application to Practice, Education and Research*, Appleton & Lange, Norwalk, Connecticut.

Daly, J., Chang, E. & Bell, P. 1996, 'Clinical nursing research priorities in Australian critical care: a pilot study', *Journal of Advanced Nursing*, vol. 23, no.1, 145–51.

Dennis, K. 1994, 'Managing questionnaire data through optical scanning technology', *Nursing Research*, vol. 43, no. 6, 376–8.

Gilliss, C. & Kulkin, I. 1991, 'Monitoring nursing interventions and data collection in a randomised clinical trial', *Western Journal of Nursing Research*, vol. 13, no. 3, 416–22.

Grindlay, A., Santamaria, N. & Kitt, S. 2000, 'Hospital in the home: nurse safety – exposure to risk and evaluation of organisational policy', *Australian Journal of Advanced Nursing*, vol. 17, no. 3, 6–12.

Harrison, L. 1989, 'Interfacing bioinstruments with computers for data collection in nursing research', *Research in Nursing and Health*, vol. 12, 129–83.

Hinds, P. & Gattuso, J. 1991, 'From pilot work to a major study in cancer nursing research', *Cancer Nursing*, vol. 14, no. 3, 132–5.

Hockey, L. 1992, *Surviving the Research Process*, Deakin University, Melbourne.

King, M. & Wilson, K. 1998, 'Diabetes health care of Aboriginal people at Nunkuwarrin Yunti', *Australian Journal of Advanced Nursing*, vol. 15, no. 2, 26–32.

Lobo, M. 1993, 'Code books – a critical link in the research process', *Western Journal of Nursing Research*, vol. 15, no. 3, 377–85.

Prescott, P. & Soeken, K. 1989, 'The potential uses of pilot work', *Nursing Research*, vol. 38, 60–2.

SPSS 1999, *SPSS 10.0 Syntax Reference Guide*, SPSS Inc., Chicago.

Western Australian Research Network 1994, 'Planning and conducting research' in *Handbook of Clinical Nursing Research*, ed. J. Robertson, Churchill Livingstone, Melbourne.

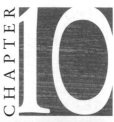

Quantitative data analysis

chapter objectives The material presented in this chapter will assist you to:

- understand the difference between descriptive and inferential statistics
- describe the various types of scales
- interpret the meaning of common statistical tests
- choose an appropriate statistical test for an hypothesis
- describe patterns in your data.

Introduction

There are two major types of data: quantitative, which requires numerical analysis, and qualitative, which seeks meaning in the content of word-based data in order to answer a research question. The majority of data in nursing research is quantitative.

The purpose of this chapter is to introduce some beginning concepts of analysing quantitative data. Whether you actually carry out quantitative research or just read about it, you will need to know something about quantitative data analysis and how it is done. You will also need to understand something about statistics because researchers use them routinely to present information about quantitative data. Many beginning researchers are frightened by statistics. Indeed, one popular book on statistics (Kranzler & Moursund, 1999) is entitled *Statistics for the Terrified*! Fear is a normal reaction when one sees what appear to be some strange numbers and symbols. However, it is possible to learn statistics at a beginning level by learning a few concepts and symbols. You will realise quickly that the symbols are just convenient representations of familiar concepts. Later, you can build on this knowledge when you need to.

Statistics have several uses in the research process. They allow us to see the patterns in the data, thus making some sense out of an otherwise shapeless mass of data. Statistics also allow us to see relationships between variables and to test hypotheses. Furthermore, it is important to be able to interpret statistical results if you are going to be able to understand what other researchers have written in their reports. It is also important to be able to decide what statistical analysis to do if you are undertaking a research project.

Most researchers now employ data analysis software to carry out statistical operations on the computer. These programs have enabled researchers to analyse data and generate statistics without the drudgery of knowing statistical formulae and how they work. But you must understand the language of statistics in order to be able to carry out the data analysis.

If you are developing a research project as a university student, it is wise to consult your lecturer or supervisor concerning statistical aspects of your project. You may also be fortunate enough to go to a university or work for an institution that provides a statistical advice service that you may use. It is worth availing yourself of these services after you have done some preliminary reading on the subject.

In this chapter, we will discuss quantitative data analysis using various statistical operations.

Quantitative data analysis

In quantitative data analysis, numbers are everything. Using numbers, you can describe amounts, proportions and patterns in the data. You can also test hypotheses by investigating the type and strength of relationships between variables. Quantitative data analysis can produce anything from simple sums to complex three-dimensional patterns.

Scales
Types of scales
A scale is a way of classifying variables (Powers & Knapp 1995). Quantitative data are measured by different types of scales, ranging from the simple to the complex. The simplest type is a nominal scale, comprising named categories. The least complicated is one with only two categories, for example 'male' or 'female'. The respondent is allowed to choose only one category; that is, the categories are mutually exclusive. Note that the categories in this scale do not have a numerical relationship and there is no allocation of a value to the categories; that is, 'female' is not considered a higher value than 'male'. A hypothetical example of using a nominal scale in nursing research is the classification of babies into breastfed and bottlefed. A more complex category scale might have several categories, for example marital status might have the categories 'never married', 'married', 'de facto' and 'divorced'.

The next type of scale is an ordinal scale in which the elements are ranked numerically or on some criterion. A ranking implies that there is an order to the categories. However, the distance between categories cannot be measured although a numerical value for it is sometimes assumed. An ordinal scale that is frequently used in research is the Likert Scale, in which people are asked to rate a concept using categories ranging from 'strongly agree' to 'strongly disagree'. Other examples of ordinal scales with which you may be familiar are the Glasgow Coma Scale and the Apgar rating for newborns.

The next type of scale is an interval scale, in which the elements are constructed in equal intervals. The amount that the interval measures is a known and defined quantity, for example a degree on a thermometer. Each degree is exactly the same as every other degree, regardless of the temperature.

A ratio scale is an interval scale in which there is a true zero that is an absence of the element. For example, height and weight are ratio scales since zero on those scales represents an absence of height or weight. In a ratio scale, the ratio of one reading to another is known. For example, a height of 40 cm is twice that of 20 cm.

Choosing a scale
When you are planning the data collection phase of your research project and choosing an instrument, you will need to consider what type of scale to use. Each type gives you a different kind and amount of information. You should consider the options carefully so that you end up with the correct data. Sometimes the choice is clear; for example gender is obviously only nominal. If, however, you are collecting data concerning your respondents' age, you could use either a set of nominal categories such as decades or you could ask them their age in years, in which case you would have interval-level data. You can see from the above that the type of scale you choose depends on the question you are asking and the hypothesis that you have.

The type of scale used for each variable will also influence your choice of statistical test. Some statistical tests can be used only on nominal data, some can be used on only interval or ratio data, and some can be used where one variable is nominal and one is interval. You must choose the appropriate test to match the type of scale on which you record the data.

In terms of advantages and disadvantages of the different types of scales, the nominal scale is the simplest and the easiest to process because the result is a set of ticked boxes. However, it gives you the least detailed amount of information about your data. It is important to realise that you can re-code interval and ratio data to nominal data but not the reverse. For example, if you have collected your data on age in decades, you do not know the exact age of the person. If, however, you have people's ages in years, you can either use the numerical age or re-scale the data into sets of decades.

Descriptive statistics

In writing up the results of a research project, you will probably want to describe the characteristics of the group or the sub-groups that comprise the group. For example, you may wish to give the total number in the group or the average score on a test. Descriptive statistics enable us to do that. We will now look at some statistics that describe and summarise data.

Sum

Frequently you want to know the total of something, for example how many patients are in a hospital or come to a clinic. You do this by counting all of the elements to get their sum.

Suppose that you wanted to test an hypothesis that patients in the respiratory clinic where you work were more likely to be heavy smokers than light smokers or non-smokers. You could, through a chart audit, come up with the following list for one day's patients (Figure 10.1).

By counting, you establish that there were 50 patients seen. This statistic is often given by the computer program in the course of other statistical analysis.

Heavy	Light	Non	Heavy	Heavy
Non	Non	Light	Heavy	Non
Light	Heavy	Heavy	Light	Light
Heavy	Non	Heavy	Light	Heavy
Heavy	Light	Heavy	Heavy	Light
Light	Heavy	Non	Light	Heavy
Heavy	Heavy	Light	Non	Light
Heavy	Light	Heavy	Light	Heavy
Light	Heavy	Non	Light	Non
Heavy	Non	Light	Light	Non

Figure 10.1 Table showing clients who were heavy, light and non-smokers

You may also wish to find out about the numbers in the different categories of smoking. To get this information, you must count the numbers of patients in the different categories to calculate the sum or total of heavy smokers to be 21, light smokers 18 and non-smokers 11. This tells you that on the day on which you collected your data more heavy smokers than light smokers or non-smokers were seen.

Percentage

A percentage is the proportion out of 100 that a group comprises. You obtain a percentage by taking the number, dividing it by the number of elements in the group and multiplying by 100. The beauty of a percentage is that it allows comparisons of groups. You cannot meaningfully compare a raw number of one group with a raw number in another group if the totals of the groups are different.

If you now want to establish what proportion of clients are in the three categories of smokers you would work out the percentage of the total clients in each category. By dividing each total by 50 and multiplying by 100, you find out that the proportion of heavy smokers is 44 per cent, the proportion of light smokers is 34 per cent and the proportion of non-smokers is 22 per cent. In the same way, you can also calculate that the proportion of smokers is 78 per cent. Again, a computer will give you this information.

Frequency distributions

If you have your data entered into a statistical computer program, you can get it to generate the number and percentage of each sub-group by generating a statistic called a frequency distribution table. This is a description of the components in a group. It tells you the number and percentage of elements in each sub-group of the main group. A frequency distribution statistic can also be used to generate both histograms and pie graphs by computer. The frequency distribution table for the client data will look something like Figure 10.2.

This table tells you that there are 11 non-smokers comprising 22 per cent of the group, 18 light smokers comprising 36 per cent of the group and 21 heavy smokers comprising 42 per cent of the group.

Using graphics to show sums and percentages

In a research report, you can show categorical information more dramatically by means of a graphic illustration or figure called a histogram or bar graph. There is a trend towards using graphics to illustrate points in reporting information about

Bar	Element	Count	Percentage
1	Non	11	22%
2	Light	18	36%
3	Heavy	21	42%

Figure 10.2 Frequency table of categories of smokers and non-smokers

data because graphics are easier to interpret than tables, thus illustrating the old saying that 'a picture is worth a thousand words'. Putting graphics into reports used to be constrained by the difficulty in generating them and the cost of printing them. However, with modern technology, computer programs can generate graphics easily and the cost of reproducing them is decreasing because of modern printing processes.

Histogram and bar graphs

Histograms and bar graphs are figures that show the numbers in groups as vertical columns or horizontal rows, which allows for easy comparison of groups. The largest group will have the longest column or bar and the smallest group will have the shortest one. A bar graph shows discrete categories, such as types of injuries, while a histogram shows numbers in different categories of a range, such as income groups. In a bar graph there will be space between the bars, while in a histogram there is no space (Hicks 1990). Figure 10.3 shows a bar graph of our group of clients broken down into its sub-groups of heavy, light and non-smokers.

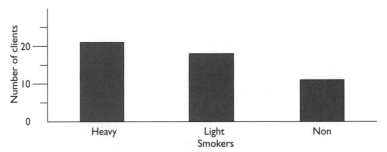

Figure 10.3 Bar graph of number of clients who are heavy, light and non-smokers

Pie chart

A pie chart is another kind of figure that shows the proportions of sub-groups in a group. It divides the total 'pie' into its components, again allowing for ease of comparison. Figure 10.4 shows a pie chart of the client data.

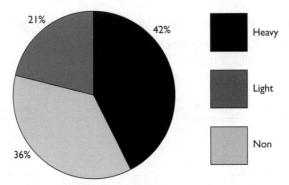

Figure 10.4 Pie chart showing types of smokers and non-smokers as percentages of the group

Table

Tables are one of the most common tools that a researcher uses when analysing data. A table is a meaningful presentation of numbers in rows and columns. Columns are the vertical arrangement of like numbers, and rows are the horizontal arrangement of like numbers. The intersection of a column and a row is called a cell. Each number will appear in both a column and a row, or a cell.

By analysing the clients in the clinic at the present time, you have taken a 'snapshot' of the data to see whether your hypothesis has any potential for a conclusion. However, you would not want to base your conclusion on data taken on only one day in case that day were atypical. You therefore decide to obtain data for a more extended period. You decide to take a random sample of one day per month and examine all of the clients on those specific days. Once again, you need to organise your data into some form that makes sense of it and allows you to see the patterns. You therefore decide to organise your data into a table showing the numbers of each group of smokers and non-smokers for each of the days that you have examined. You construct a table as follows, using the numbers that you have obtained (Figure 10.5).

Taking a look at your raw data, you see that there were 400 clients seen on the 12 selected days. Of these, 175 or 44 per cent were heavy smokers, 119, or 30 per cent were light smokers, and 106 or 26 per cent were non-smokers. This is the same pattern that you saw for the one day in January, so you can safely conclude that your January day was fairly typical. To see whether each day was typical, you would have to calculate the percentage for each group for each of the 12 days. You do this and construct the table overleaf (Figure 10.6). This allows you to compare the percentages of types of smokers and non-smokers for each month.

Month	Heavy	Light	Non	Total
January	21	18	11	50
February	18	9	8	35
March	14	10	6	30
April	19	14	10	43
May	20	9	15	44
June	7	6	3	16
July	9	6	7	22
August	10	6	9	25
September	11	9	9	29
October	15	9	6	30
November	16	16	12	44
December	15	7	10	32
Total	175	119	106	400
Total as %	44%	30%	26%	100%

Figure 10.5 Table showing number of clients, by month, who were heavy, light and non-smokers

Month	Heavy	Light	Non
January	42	36	22
February	50	27	23
March	48	33	19
April	42	30	24
May	45	20	35
June	48	30	22
July	41	29	30
August	38	25	37
September	40	30	30
October	50	30	20
November	36	36	28
December	48	22	30

Figure 10.6 Table of percentages, by month, of smokers and non-smokers

Notice we didn't work out the percentages first and then calculate the 'average' from them. Try it: you will get 48 per cent for heavy smokers, for example, instead of the 44 per cent calculated from the totals. The reason for this apparent discrepancy is that averaging the percentages gives each month's result the same 'weight' or importance. In our example, the results for January are four times as important as those for June because we had four times as many observations. It is absolutely crucial to look at the raw data before transposing them to percentages. Otherwise you run the risk of drawing conclusions that misrepresent what happened. The information in the table of percentages can also be shown in graphic form (Figure 10.7).

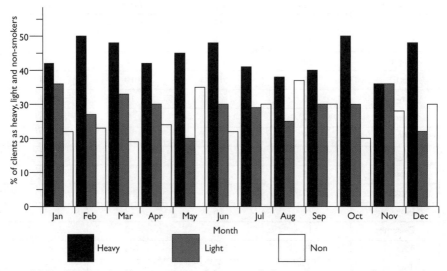

Figure 10.7 Bar graph showing the percentage of clients, by month, who were heavy, light and non-smokers

272 *Nursing research processes: an Australian perspective*

The graph above shows that on every day examined, the percentage of clients who were heavy smokers was equal to or greater than each of the other groups. However, there is some fluctuation when different months are considered. The first day you measured in January may have had a fairly high proportion of heavy smokers compared to the other days. In order to find out how typical it was, you need to look at what the general picture is. This is explored in the next section.

Measures of central tendency

Measures of central tendency are the mean, median and mode. These are statistics that let us see what the most common scores in a group are, and how the group did as a whole.

The mean

The mean score of a group is the average, a concept with which you will be familiar. The mean is obtained by taking the sum total of the elements and dividing it by the number of elements in the group. To continue our example, it would be helpful to compare the findings for January with the findings for the whole year. This would tell us whether January was a typical month for the percentages of sub-groups of clients. To do that, you calculate the average, or mean, percentage for the year for each sub-group. So, in this example, you divide the total number of clients seen by the number of days, or 400/12 = 33. The heavy smokers comprised (175/12 = 15)/33 = 44 per cent, light smokers comprised (118/12)/33 = 30 per cent, and non-smokers comprised (106/12)/33 = 27 per cent. You can now compare each month's percentage with the mean or average percentage and see how typical it was. January's figures were: heavy smokers 42 per cent, light smokers, 36 per cent and non-smokers 22 per cent. Thus, you can conclude that January's figures were a bit over-average for heavy smokers, but under-average for light smokers and non-smokers.

The median

Another useful measure of central tendency is the median. This is the score in the middle. For an odd number of scores, the middle one is the median. For an even number of scores, the median is the average of the two middle ones. In the case of heavy smokers, if the data were rearranged from smallest to largest score, they would look like this:

$$36, 38, 40, 41, 42, 44, 45, 48, 48, 48, 50, 50.$$

Since this set of figures comprises an even number (there are 12 months in the year), the median would be the average of 44 and 45, the two middle scores, or 44.5. In this case, the mean and the median are very close.

You can calculate the median of the light smokers and non-smokers in a similar fashion.

The mode

The mode is the most frequently occurring score. In the case of heavy smokers, it can be seen easily that the mode is 48 since that score occurs three times in the data set. The mode is higher than the mean or the median for heavy smokers. You can calculate the mode for light smokers and non-smokers in the same way.

Measures of variability

Sometimes you want to see how the figures are distributed in a group of scores. Measures of variability help you to do this.

The range

The range is a number that reflects the spread of the scores. It is obtained by subtracting the lowest score from the highest score. To follow our example above, the highest number of heavy smokers is 50 and the lowest number is 36, so the range is 50 − 36 = 14.

The normal curve

The normal curve is a way of showing the distribution of scores in a group of participants. If you take any group of people and look at the distribution of the scores on any characteristic, you would expect them to vary. You would expect some to be on the high end, some to be in the middle and some to be on the low end. You would also expect there to be very few extremely low scores and very few extremely high scores. Let us take an example of temperature readings in a group of people. The lowest temperature that you would expect to find would be 35° Celsius and the highest would be 39°. The temperatures are recorded to the nearest 0·5 of a degree. The data shown in their unsorted form are, as usual, difficult to interpret. If we sort them into their frequencies, we can see a pattern emerge. You can show this by doing a frequency count by simply placing a stroke next to each temperature for every person that recorded that temperature (Figure 10.8). These data can also be shown as a bar graph (Figure 10.9).

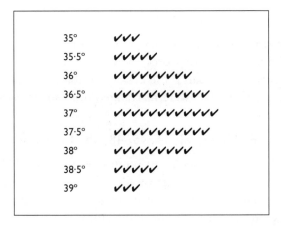

Figure 10.8 A frequency count

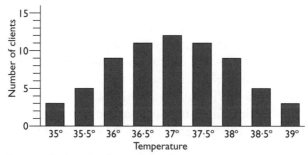

Figure 10.9 Bar graph showing frequency of temperatures

Note that if we plotted out the frequencies as points and connected the points, we would have a peaked shape. This is called a frequency polygon (many-sided figure) (Figure 10.10).

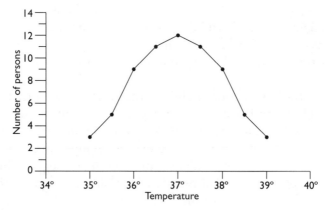

Figure 10.10 Graph of frequency polygon of temperature data

This type of curve is called a normal curve. A normal curve is bilaterally symmetric – the curve is approximately the same shape on both sides.

However, the distribution is not always bilaterally symmetric. Suppose that the observations were taken from a series of patients with a fever, so that there were disproportionately more high temperatures in the group. The data might then look like this (Figure 10.11):

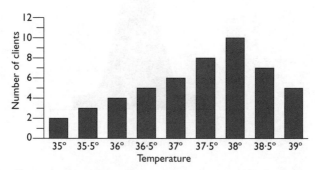

Figure 10.11 Skewed temperature data

Chapter 10 Quantitative data analysis 275

This lopsidedness of the data is called a 'skew'. And, of course, under different circumstances, it could well skew the other way.

The shape of the data is important when deciding what type of statistical analysis to use, since some statistical operations assume that the data are normally distributed. Statistics that have an assumption that the data are normally distributed are called parametric statistics. Statistics that do not require a normal distribution of the data are called non-parametric statistics. We will talk about these different types of statistics in the section on comparing groups.

Standard deviation

The standard deviation is a number that is calculated from the data to show the amount of dispersion of the data. The standard deviation is the number that incorporates approximately one-third of the scores (34 per cent) above or below the mean. In the temperature data set, the mean is 37° and the standard deviation is 1. This means that one-third of the temperatures lie between 36° and 37°, and another third lie between 37° and 38°, or two-thirds are between 36° and 38°. If the data are normally distributed, then another 14 per cent are between two standard deviations above and below the mean, so that 96 per cent are between 35° and 39°.

If the temperatures were more tightly clustered about the mean, the standard deviation would be low. For example, in Figure 10.12 you can see that there are a lot of people with a temperature on or around the mean temperature of 37° whereas there are very few people at the extreme temperatures.

The standard deviation of these temperatures is 0·6 of a degree. This means that one-third of the observations fall between 36·4° and 37° and another third fall between 37° and 37·6° and so forth.

On the other hand, if the temperatures were more spread out, the area graph would look like Figure 10.13.

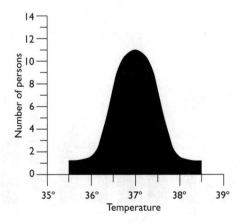

Figure 10.12 Graph showing temperature, low standard deviation

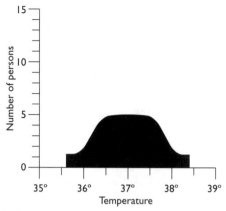

Figure 10.13 Graph showing temperature, high standard deviation

You can see that there are fewer people with temperatures on or around the mean, and more at the extreme temperatures. The standard deviation for this set of data would be higher than the previous example because the temperatures are more dispersed.

Introduction to probability and inferential statistics

Probability

Probability is a concept that you will need to understand at a basic level in order to make sense out of most research reports and to decide whether or not the findings are valid. Findings could occur by chance or be totally random. Given that there can be an error, we would not want to recommend a change of nursing procedures based on research findings in which we do not have true confidence. To take the previous example of smoking, it might be pure coincidence that there were more heavy smokers than light smokers or non-smokers in January. That is why we looked at 12 days because if we got the same pattern each time, it would be less likely to be by chance than would a pattern on one day only.

Researchers speak of the probability that a finding is statistically significant; that is, it is not very likely to happen by chance alone. Fortunately, a statistical computer program will compute the probability. Its scientific notation is 'p'. You will often see this in reports, e.g. '$p = 0.01$', or '$p < 0.05$'. The p value ranges from '0.0001' to '1' and it means the probability that the result could have happened by chance. At $p = 0.0001$, there is virtually no probability that the finding could have occurred by chance. At $p = 1$, the probability that the finding could have occurred by chance is at its highest. To give you something to aim at and to think about, what is the significance of a result if the probability that it occurred by chance is no better than flipping a coin?

Nursing research, in common with behavioural science, has accepted a probability of 0.05, which means that there is less than a 5 per cent probability that the results would have happened by chance alone. In other words, if you repeated the experiment 100 times, you would probably get those findings by chance alone on only five occasions. You can turn this around and say that you are 95 per cent sure that you will not get those findings by chance alone. This is sometimes expressed as a 95 per cent level of confidence, for example, 'the level of confidence was set at 95 per cent'. The level of confidence should be set before the data are collected, not after.

In the results section of a research report, a statement about the statistical significance will be given, for example 'Comparison between the two groups [venepuncture versus heel prick] (table 2) revealed a significant reduction in the time required to collect the NST [newborn screening test] when VSVDH [venepuncture] was performed (... $p < 0.01$)' (Logan 1999). This meant that the researchers were confident that their results were statistically significant and that their findings could have occurred by chance less than 1 per cent of the time.

Testing for statistical significance

In order to test for statistical significance, it is first necessary to define the relationship that you are testing. This is usually done by means of an hypothesis, or statement of the expected difference between scores on a variable, whether between groups or within groups. The research hypothesis may be directional; that is, the expected difference will be in one direction or another, and the direction is known or predicted from theory or previous research. One usually states the hypothesis as a null hypothesis or a statement that there will be no significant difference between the groups. Then as a finding of the research, the null hypothesis is rejected if there is a statistically significant difference ($p < 0.05$), or not rejected if there is not a statistically significant difference, that is, $p > 0.05$. At a level of probability of 0.05, it is possible that you could get the finding by chance alone five times in a hundred. This is a low level of risk that the researcher is willing to accept. This element of chance is the reason that a researcher rejects a null hypothesis but does not accept a research hypothesis.

In deciding whether the results of a study are statistically significant, it is possible to commit two types of errors, labelled 'type I error' and 'type II error'. A type I error is caused by rejecting the null hypothesis when it is true; that is, concluding that there are significant differences between the groups. This leads the researcher to conclude that a result is significant when it is not. An analogy that may be useful here is to liken the type I error to a false positive test. In a false positive test, a disease is indicated when it is not present (Dawson-Saunders & Trapp 2001).

A type II error is the opposite of a type I error. The researcher fails to reject the null hypothesis when it is false; that is, the researcher concludes that there is no difference between groups when there actually is. This leads the researcher to conclude that findings are not significant when they actually are. A type II error is analogous to a false negative in which a disease is incorrectly shown as not present when it is (Dawson-Saunders & Trapp 2001).

Relationships in one group
Correlation

Some research designs require the researcher to examine relationships between the characteristics of people in a group. For example, you might want to see if post-operative pain levels were higher for clients who had high levels of pre-operative anxiety than for those who had low levels. To do this, you would collect data on each person's anxiety and pain. If you had a numerical pain scale and an anxiety scale, you could investigate whether the amount of anxiety was related to, or correlated with, the amount of post-operative anxiety. You would expect perhaps that clients who scored high on the anxiety scale would also score high on the pain scale. However, it is possible that clients who scored low on the anxiety scale could score high on the pain scale. Finally, it is possible that there is no relationship between the two factors.

In order to test out your hypothesis, you would need to look at the numerical relationship between the clients' scores on the two scales. To do this you would do a plot of each client's anxiety level along one axis of a graph (the **X** axis) and the pain score along the other axis (the **Y** axis) (see Figure 10.14). This concept can be shown pictorially by means of a scattergram, or a graph that shows each person's data as a point on the graph. Note that both variables must be numerical in order to use this test. Each client's datum for where the pain score intersects with the anxiety score will appear as one point on the graph. (You can find what each person's score was on both scales. Find a dot and draw a horizontal line from it to the **Y** or vertical axis and a vertical line to the **X** or horizontal axis.) The idea now is to 'fit' a straight line that best represents the data. You can do this 'by eye' or ask the computer program for the 'regression line', which is the fancy name for the best-fit straight line.

The graph in Figure 10.14 shows a positive relationship between anxiety and pain. Clients who had high anxiety levels also had high pain levels and clients who had low anxiety levels also had low pain levels. This means that anxiety is positively correlated with pain for this group of clients.

The graph in Figure 10.14 also shows the regression line that has been fitted to the data by the computer program.

The extent to which the variables are related to each other is expressed as a correlation coefficient, the symbolic notation for which is an 'r' in italics. The 'r' value corresponds to the slope of the line. The most common correlation coefficient used in modern computer analysis is the Pearson Correlation Coefficient. The Pearson Correlation Coefficient has a range of scores from -1.0 to $+1.0$. The more strongly the two variables are correlated with each other, the farther the score will be from zero. A score of 0 in the middle represents no correlation at all.

–1 –0.9 –0.8 –0.7 –0.6 –0.5 –0.4 –0.3 –0.2 –0.1 0 0.1 0.2 0.3 0.4 0.5 0.6 0.7 0.8 0.9 +1

A helpful way to think of this is as similar to a pH scale. A pH reading at one end (14) is very basic, a reading at the other is very acidic (1) and in the middle it is neutral (7).

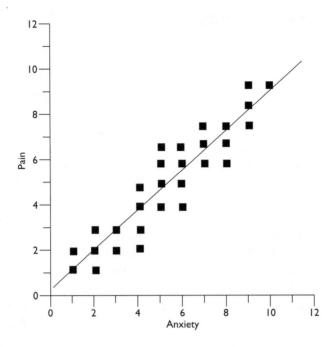

Figure 10.14 Scattergram showing positive correlation of pain and anxiety

The Pearson Correlation Coefficient has the assumption that the data are normally distributed. If they are not, you would use a non-parametric test such as the Spearman Rank Order Correlation.

Figure 10.14 shows a strong positive relationship of pain and anxiety, with the participants' scores on one scale similar to their scores on the other scale. This result would give you a Pearson Correlation Coefficient of 0·92, which is a strong positive correlation.

If, on the other hand, you had a set of data in which the anxiety scores go up while the pain scores go down, you would see a different result, as the following graph (Figure 10.15) shows.

You can see in Figure 10.15 that the data points and the regression line run in the opposite direction to those in the previous graph. The high scores on the anxiety scale are matched to the low scores on the pain scale. Participants who were very anxious had a low level of pain after the operation. Conversely, participants who had high anxiety levels before the operation had low levels of post-operative pain. The Pearson Correlation Coefficient for these data is −0·9.

The third possibility is that there is no relationship between pain and anxiety. Figure 10.16 shows the lack of a relationship when anxiety is regressed upon pain.

Note that the scatter on this graph is random: there seems to be no relationship between anxiety and pain. The Pearson Correlation Coefficient on these data was near zero at 0·01.

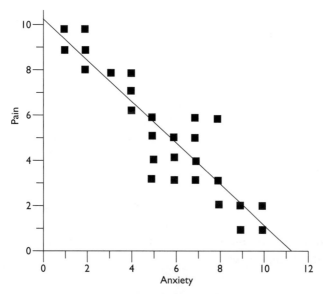

Figure 10.15 Scattergram showing negative correlation of pain and anxiety

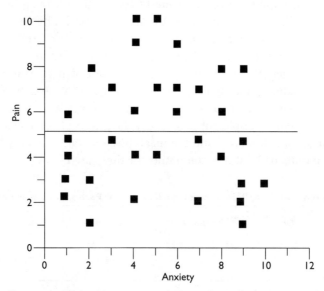

Figure 10.16 Scattergram showing no correlation of pain and anxiety

Correlation and significance

At this point in discussing the statistical nitty gritty, things get a little sticky. In the first example we saw a strong positive correlation spread over the whole range of possible responses. What if we had had only a few data and they were all grouped at one end, but showing the same 'best-fit line'? The 'r' value is the same (same slope) but our feeling about the reliability of the data is way down.

Chapter 10 Quantitative data analysis 281

Or what if the scatter is much wider? Again the slope of the best-fit line could be the same but we are not so sure of it.

At this point the statisticians give us an almost universally confusing table which relates the number of subjects in the study (the number of data points in this instance) to the value of 'r' that must be exceeded for it to pass a certain level of significance. The left-most column is usually headed 'degrees of freedom (df)' and for reasons we need not go into, is 2 less than the number of data points (so for our example 'F' or 'f' or 'df' is close enough to our number of data points, say 30. This determines which row of the table we use. It does not make sense to be too fussy here, provided you have more than a dozen points. We now compare our 'r' value (in this case 0·92) with the values in the 'F' or 'f' or 'df' = 30 row. If our value for 'r' is bigger (neglecting whether it is positive or negative) than the value in the column for our required level of significance, we have a winner! Fortunately, the computer program will work out the p value for us, taking the pain out of the process.

Paired t-test

Another test that can be done to find relationships in one group is the paired or one-group t-test. This test is done when you wish to compare two readings for each participant on the same variable. The paired t-test needs at least an ordinal level scale for this test; that is, it is done on data that are numerical. This test is useful where you have a pre-test/post-test design, or more than one post-test measurement. For example, suppose that you want to see whether pre-operative teaching results in less post-operative anxiety. You do a pre-operative pre-test of anxiety, an intervention of pre-operative teaching, and a post-operative post-test of anxiety. You then do a paired t-test to see if the post-operative anxiety scores are lower than the pre-operative scores. For example, suppose that your group of participants had a mean pre-operative anxiety level of 7 and the mean post-operative anxiety level was 4, i.e. a drop of 3. Figure 10.17 shows the results for the paired t-test.

Paired *t*-test	X: Pre-operation anxiety	Y: Post-operation anxiety	
DF	Mean x–y	Paired *t*-value	Prob. (2 tail)
20	3	14	0·0001

Figure 10.17 Table showing results of paired *t*-test

The p value shows that these results were highly significant and that your hypothesis that the post-operative anxiety would be less after the intervention of pre-operative teaching is probably correct.

Chi square test and contingency tables

The chi-square test is a test for determining within-group relationships on nominal variables, that is, variables that are measured by categories rather than numbers. In a chi-square test, there are two variables, each of which is broken down into two levels.

Let us take a simple example. Suppose that you wish to look at the relationship between bedrest and constipation in long-stay clients. You hypothesise that those who are on bedrest are more likely to be constipated than those who are not. You collect data on 40 clients, classifying each one as either on bedrest or not, and constipated or not. Each person must be classified in both categories. Note that there are now four possible categories into which you can classify your clients. They can be constipated and on bedrest, constipated and not on bedrest, not constipated and on bedrest and not constipated and not on bedrest. You then do a chi-square test. If there were no relationship between bedrest and constipation, you might expect to have equal numbers of clients in each category, and your results might look something like this (Figure 10.18):

	Bedrest	Mobile	Totals
Constipated	10	10	20
Normal	10	10	20
Totals	20	20	40

Figure 10.18 Table showing chi-square: expected values

However, if your hypothesis is correct and there is a relationship between mobility and bowel activity, your results might look like this (Figure 10.19):

	Bedrest	Mobile	Totals
Constipated	14	6	20
Normal	5	15	20
Totals	19	21	40

Figure 10.19 Table showing chi-square: relationship between mobility and bowel activity

Just looking at Figure 10.19, you can see that the clients who are on bedrest are constipated, and those who are mobile are not constipated.

The chi-square test will also give you information about percentages of clients in each category. By reading down the columns of the table in Figure 10.20, you can see that three-quarters of the clients who are on bedrest are constipated and 71 per cent of those who are mobile are not constipated.

	Bedrest	Mobile	Totals
Constipated	74%	29%	50%
Normal	26%	71%	50%
Totals	100%	100%	100%

Figure 10.20 Table showing chi-square column totals

Another type of table looks at the percentages from the point of view of the other variable (see Figure 10.21).

	Bedrest	Mobile	Totals
Constipated	70%	30%	100%
Normal	25%	75%	100%
Totals	48%	52%	100%

Figure 10.21 Table showing chi-square row totals

Figure 10.21 tells you that 70 per cent of clients who are constipated are on bedrest and three-quarters of non-constipated clients are mobile.

A computer chi-square test will also give you a p value: in this case $p = 0.01$. This means that this result probably would have happened by chance alone only 1 per cent of the time and so the findings meet a 99 per cent level of confidence.

A contingency table is an expanded chi-square used where either variable has more than two categories. In the example above, you might want to break down the variables into finer categories. For example, mobility could be broken down to 'completely mobile', 'partially mobile' and 'bedrest', while bowel activity could be broken down to 'badly constipated', 'mildly constipated' and 'normal'. In this case you would have nine categories, with a 3 × 3 contingency table instead of the 2 × 2 table shown in Figure 10.21. However, you would need many more participants to give enough data in each cell.

Testing for differences in means of two groups
Independent groups t-test

Some research designs and hypotheses call for testing to see if there is a significant difference in two different groups' means on the same variable. For example, suppose that you were not satisfied to classify your mobile and immobile clients in a long-term care facility simply as constipated or not constipated. You want to compare the actual difference in numbers of bowel motions per week for the two groups. Again, you would collect your data on whether each client was mobile or immobile and also on the number of bowel motions for one week. You could then do an independent groups, or unpaired, t-test to see whether the mean number of bowel actions per week for the immobile clients was greater than that for the mobile clients. Your results might look like Figure 10.22.

Figure 10.22 tells you that you had 25 mobile patients, with 15 bedfast ones. The mean number of bowel actions per week for your mobile patients was 6·8 while for the bedfast ones it was 3·9. The results of the t-test tell you that this finding was statistically significant ($p = 0.0001$). This means that there was a probability of less than one in ten thousand that this result could have happened by chance alone.

The independent t-test rests on the assumption that your data for bowel motions are normally distributed; that is, they approximate the normal curve

Unpaired t-test: X: mobility and Y: bowel actions

Unpaired t-value	Probability
6·8	0·0001

Group	Count	Mean	Std Dev.
Mobile	25	6·8	1·1
Bedrest	15	3·9	1·6

Figure 10.22 Table showing unpaired t-test

outlined earlier. If, however, your data were skewed, you would need to use a non-parametric test such as the Mann-Whitney U-test because it does not require a normal distribution. But how do you tell? The best way is to do a histogram to show the distribution of the data. If the data look skewed, it would be better to do the non-parametric test.

Testing for differences in means of more than two groups

Many research designs call for determining whether there is a difference in the mean score for more than two distinct groups. Suppose that you wanted to expand the earlier design, this time to look at the effect of three levels of mobility: bedfast, partly mobile and fully mobile upon the number of bowel actions. An analysis of variance (ANOVA) would allow you to determine whether the mean number of bowel motions per week was significantly different in the three groups. This test examines the mean scores and will detect whether there is a significant difference in them. The test actually detects whether there is more difference within each group than between the groups. Note that the independent variable, mobility, is nominal while the dependent variable, number of bowel actions, is numerical.

To do this test, you would need more participants since you are looking at three levels of mobility. Suppose you re-did the study with more clients, classifying them as bedfast, partially mobile and fully mobile, again collecting data on the number of bowel motions for the week. Your results, using an analysis of variance, would look something like Figure 10.23 overleaf.

Figure 10.23 tells you that you had 15 bedfast patients, 22 partially mobile patients and 23 fully mobile patients. It also tells you that there was a statistically significant difference in the mean number of bowel motions per week for the two groups. The bedfast patients had a mean of approximately three bowel motions per week, the partially mobile had a mean of five and the fully mobile had a mean of eight. This finding is statistically significant ($p = 0.0001$) with only

One factor ANOVA: X: mobility and Y: bowel actions ($p = 0.0001$)

Group	Count	Mean	Std Dev.
Bedfast	15	2.9	1.2
Partially mobile	22	5.3	0.8
Fully mobile	23	7.8	1.0

Figure 10.23 Table showing analysis of variance

one chance in ten thousand that this finding would have occurred by chance. From these results, you would conclude that, all other things being equal, mobility makes a difference to the bowel activity of patients.

Again, if your data were skewed, you should use a non-parametric test. You could use the Kruskal-Wallis test for three groups. However, these data have a reasonably normal distribution, so a parametric test is indicated.

Methods involving more than one dependent or independent variable

It is not the intention of this chapter to teach you about complex statistical analysis. However, we want to introduce you to some advanced quantitative techniques so that you will recognise the words if you see them in research reports. You can learn more about these techniques when the need arises by looking them up in books about statistics.

The advent of computers and statistical analysis programs has meant that ever-increasingly sophisticated techniques of data analysis have been demanded by researchers and devised by statisticians. The current complex techniques that we are about to introduce could not have been done by pen on paper or even by using hand calculators. This increased availability of sophisticated techniques has created a demand for research consumers to know something about them.

Condensing data into scales: factor analysis

Some research projects use questionnaires that have a considerable number of items. Using the methods so far outlined, you would only be able to test your independent variables on each item individually. This would leave you with a large mass of data out of which it would be hard to make sense. One way of handling the data is to group the items into scales. In the context of a questionnaire, a scale is a group of items that are conceptually related. There are various ways of developing scales; one common way is factor analysis. All of the items can be entered into a factor analysis program. This program tests each item to determine with which group of items it belongs conceptually and clusters the related items into 'factors', or groups of items with a similar focus. The researcher can then treat each factor as one dependent variable.

Tests in which there is more than one independent variable

If a researcher wants to test the effects of two or more independent variables upon the dependent variable, more complex tests must be done. The researcher can test each independent variable individually using the techniques outlined earlier in this chapter; indeed this is one way to eliminate from the analysis variables that have little or no effect. However, individual analysis will not tell the researcher how the variables interact with one another and which has the most powerful effect. To do this, the researcher must use a test that will allow the entry of a group of independent variables into the analysis. Some of these statistical tests are described briefly below.

Multiple regression

If the independent variables are numerical and the dependent variable is also numerical, a more complex regression called a multiple regression can be used. For example, a researcher might want to analyse the relative effects of intelligence and socioeconomic status upon the ability of clients to learn information about diabetes mellitus. The researcher could administer an intelligence test (IQ) and a test of diabetes knowledge to the participants in the study and also determine their score on an index of socioeconomic status (SES). The researcher could then use a multiple regression with the test of knowledge score as the outcome variable and the SES and IQ scores as the research variables. This would tell the researcher what effect SES and IQ have and whether they are linked.

Two-way and three-way ANOVAs

If there is more than one nominal-level independent variable and one interval-level dependent variable, the researcher would need to use a more sophisticated analysis of variance (ANOVA). A two-way ANOVA will handle two independent variables, a three-way ANOVA will handle three and so forth. Continuing our earlier example, suppose that a researcher wanted to examine the effects of both mobility and gender on mean number of bowel motions per week in nursing home clients. The researcher would use a two-way ANOVA, with three levels of mobility and two levels of gender. If the researcher wanted to examine the effect of type of diet along with mobility and gender, a three-way ANOVA would be indicated.

Logistic regression

Log-linear analysis is a type of regression analysis in which all of the variables are measured on a nominal scale (Dawson-Saunders & Trapp 2001). Logistic regression examines the relative effect of more than one nominal-level independent variable upon a nominal-dependent variable. It is a kind of expanded chi-square. For example, a researcher might want to examine the effect of both gender and mobility upon whether clients are selected for placement in a particular nursing home or not. An example of this type of statistical analysis can be found in a study by Tang and colleagues that examined predictors of high school students' intention to study nursing. The researchers found that a higher annual parental income, shorter period of settlement in Australia and less prestigious occupation of the father were predictive of intention to study nursing (Tang et al. 1998).

Discriminant analysis
Discriminant analysis is a technique that allows the researcher to use numerical independent variables to predict whether participants will belong to different groups. The independent variables must be interval level and the dependent variable is nominal level. For example, if a researcher wanted to see whether SES and IQ would predict whether a person was a smoker or a non-smoker, a discriminant analysis could do so.

Tests involving more than one dependent variable
Some research designs have more than one dependent variable. If the dependent variables are unrelated, they can be examined using separate ANOVAs. You will remember that an ANOVA allows only one dependent variable to be analysed at one time. If, however, the dependent variables are related in some way, they can be examined together, using more advanced statistical techniques. One of these is the MANOVA, or multivariate analysis of variance.

Want to learn more about statistics?
For further knowledge you can do some reading in basic books on statistics that have been written for nurses. An example is *Data Analysis & Statistics for Nursing Research* (Polit 1996). If you need further information, there are other books for health professionals such as *Primer on Simplified Statistics – for the Health Care Professional* (Swain, Burgess & Barley 1998), *Basic Statistics for the Health Sciences* (Bohneneblust 2000), *Basic and Clinical Biostatistics* (Dawson-Saunders & Trapp 2001). You could also take a course in statistics.

Summary
In this chapter, we have looked at the use of computers and various methods of analysing data using statistical analysis. We have looked at different ways of describing our data and of testing hypotheses, leading to conclusions about the validity of our findings. We have introduced the concepts of probability and type I and II errors. Finally, we have briefly introduced more complex statistical tests.

Main points
- Quantitative data analysis usually involves the use of statistics to describe the data, allow inferences about the relationships expressed in hypotheses and show the results of hypothesis testing.
- The main descriptive statistics are the sum, percentage and frequency count.
- Illustrations such as tables, bar graphs, histograms and pie graphs can be used to illustrate the composition of the data.

- Inferential statistics are used to show whether differences between groups are statistically significant and therefore whether a hypothesis is supported or not.
- The statistics chosen will be appropriate to show the trend in the data and to test the hypothesis and will reflect whether the data are parametric or non-parametric, and the number and nature of the dependent and independent variables.

Review Questions

1. Descriptive statistics are useful in quantitative research because they:
   a. always prove the hypothesis
   b. show patterns in the data
   c. allow inferences about the validity of hypotheses
   d. all of the above

2. Which of the following would be an example of a nominal scale?
   a. age in years
   b. Apgar rating
   c. faces visual analogue pain scale
   d. gender

3. Which of the following types of scales has an absolute zero point?
   a. nominal
   b. ordinal
   c. ratio
   d. interval

4. Which of the following contains a cell?
   a. table
   b. pie graph
   c. bar chart
   d. frequency distribution

5. The most frequently occurring score in a set is the:
   a. median
   b. percentage
   c. mode
   d. mean

6. Which of the following would test for a relationship between two interval-level variables?
   a. chi-square
   b. *t*-test
   c. ANOVA
   d. Pearson Correlation

7   Which of the following would test for a relationship between two nominal-level variables?

   a   chi-square
   b   t-test
   c   ANOVA
   d   Pearson Correlation

8   Which of the following would test for a relationship between a nominal independent variable comprising two groups and an interval-level dependent variable?

   a   chi-square
   b   t-test
   c   ANOVA
   d   Pearson Correlation

9   Which of the following tests requires more than one dependent variable?

   a   chi-square
   b   ANOVA
   c   contingency table
   d   MANOVA

10 Which of the following is an example of a non-parametric test?

   a   t-test
   b   ANOVA
   c   Mann-Whitney U-test
   d   Pearson Correlation

Discussion Questions

1   Describe the four types of scales and state when you would use each one.
2   What is a measure of central tendency?
3   Distinguish between descriptive and inferential statistics.
4   Discuss probability.
5   Distinguish between a Type I and a Type II error.

References

Bohneneblust, S. 2000, *Basic Statistics for the Health Sciences*, Mayfield Publishing Co., Mountain View, California.

Dawson-Saunders, B. & Trapp, R. 2001, *Basic and Clinical Biostatistics*, 3rd edn, Lange Medical Books-McGraw-Hill, New York.

Hicks, C. 1990, *Research and Statistics: A Practical Introduction for Nurses*, Prentice-Hall International (UK) Ltd, Hemel Hempstead, Hertfordshire.

Kranzler, G. & Moursund, J. 1999, *Statistics for the Terrified*, 2nd edn, Prentice-Hall, Upper Saddle River, New Jersey.

Logan, P. 1999, 'Venepuncture versus heel prick for the collection of the newborn screening test', *Australian Journal of Advanced Nursing*, vol. 17, no. 1, 30–6.

Polit, D. 1996, *Data Analysis & Statistics for Nursing Research*, Appleton & Lange, Stamford, Connecticut.

Powers, B. & Knapp, T. 1995, *A Dictionary of Nursing Theory and Research*, 2nd edn, Sage Publications, Thousand Oaks, California.

Swain, P., Burgess, E. & Barley, L. 1998, *Primer on Simplified Statistics – for the Health Care Professional*, Swain & Associates, St Petersburg.

Tang, K., Duffield, C., Chen, J., Choucair, S., Creegan, R., Mak, C. & Lesley, G. 1998, 'Predictors of intention to study nursing among school students speaking a language other than English at home', *Australian Journal of Advanced Nursing*, vol. 15, no. 2, 33–9.

CHAPTER 11

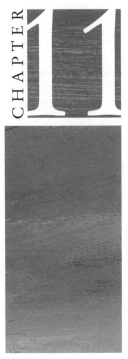

Interpreting quantitative findings

chapter objectives The material presented in this chapter will assist you to:

- keep track of your interpretations
- interpret relationship findings
- distinguish between causal and non-causal relationships
- distinguish between statistically significant and non-significant findings
- distinguish between statistically and clinically significant findings
- search for the meaning in your findings
- relate the results of your study to theory, research and practice.

Introduction

You have collected and analysed your data. Now you are about to enter another exciting phase of the research process: interpreting the results to make a coherent, meaningful interpretation of the findings. As a researcher, you are responsible for interpreting your findings. You will describe the findings, search for their meaning, draw conclusions from them, determine implications for practice and make recommendations for implementing any significant findings.

At some level, you may have started this process already if you have been doing some interpretation while you did the data analysis. Indeed, the processes of data analysis and interpretation are somewhat iterative. Some findings need immediate interpretation and some interpretations take you back to do more data analysis to answer questions that emerge from the data analysis.

Preparation

You are sitting at your desk with what will probably seem like an impossible amount of computer printout to analyse. Where do you start? First of all, make sure that you are confident about the accuracy of the data analysis. In Chapters 9 and 10, we covered techniques to ensure accuracy. If you have followed my earlier suggestions, you will probably have accurate results. I re-emphasise this point because the value of your findings and the interpretation of the findings rests on the accuracy of your data analysis, which in turn rests upon the accuracy of the data and their input into the computer.

If you have not done so already, organise your material into logical groupings so that you can tackle one section at a time. Each project will suggest its own groupings to you. It is best to start with the purely descriptive data analysis output and then work up to the more complex analyses grouped according to your conceptual framework, hypotheses or questions. You may care to refer to Chapter 9 for suggestions on methods of organising your data analysis.

Some people like to keep track of their findings on a spreadsheet so that they can see the overall picture easily. Many people also find it useful to transform their findings into graphs to make it easier to interpret them. You can do this easily with a statistical analysis program.

As you interpret your data analysis and produce findings, it is best to start writing out your account of these, which will also serve as a preliminary draft of your research report. You can do this in a logbook, or type straight into the word processor.

Interpreting descriptive findings

In interpreting your data, it is also easier to start with the purely descriptive data analysis. In looking at the descriptive statistics, you should look first at the statistics for all of the sample before progressing to any sub-groups.

You can examine the results for your general descriptive variables such as age, sex and so forth. This will give you a profile of your sample. Then you can compare your sample with the known characteristics of the population to see how typical it was. This will reinforce the earlier point that it is important to plan your data analysis so that when you come to compare it with the population you actually have the correct data for the comparison. If your sample matches the population reasonably well on the major variables of interest in the study, you are probably fairly safe in generalising about the external validity of your results. For example, in a previous study, I sent out questionnaires to the whole population of nurse-academics in Australia (Roberts 1997). The two-thirds who responded were a fairly close match for the known characteristics of the whole population, such as gender and state of employment, so I was reasonably confident that the results had external validity. However, you can never be absolutely sure whether your sample is the same for the whole population on the variables that you measured in the sample, but not in the population. Unfortunately, it is these variables that normally comprise your main findings.

If your sample is not similar to the population, or if it does not match on any one major variable of interest, you should not claim that your findings are valid for any group other than your sample. For example, if you collected data only on participants from urban areas, it would not be legitimate to claim that your results were typical of all clients in the country, or indeed the state. It is always better to err on the side of caution in generalising your findings.

Once you have looked at your descriptive data about the characteristics of the sample, you should also look at the descriptive data analysis about the variables you are investigating. For example, if you are relating the variable 'amount of tobacco smoking' to demographic data, you should also first look at the descriptive information about the smoking. This will give you a picture of the sample in relation to the major variables. Again, you can compare this picture with that of the population to look for its representativeness.

If you have created a questionnaire in which you have identified your first-round responders from your follow-ups it is useful to compare them on the various variables to see whether they are the same. If so, you can treat them as one group for the rest of the interpretation. If they are different, you will need to account for that in your interpretation of the findings.

If you are doing a clinical study or one that requires more than one data collection point, it is also useful to compare your drop-outs with your persisters on the demographic variables. This will tell you if your study has been affected by participant mortality.

Relationship findings

Hypotheses have expressed relationships between variables. Some of these may require testing for differences of variables between groups, for example males and females, control and experimental groups. You may or may not find differences in the dependent variable for the different groups. Sometimes you will want to compare the pre-test values for a control and experimental group to see if they were the same before the experiment. If not, the results of the experiment could be in doubt. Again, you need to look at the *p* value to decide whether to reject the null hypothesis or not.

You also need to check that the results are not the result of some intervening variable. For example, suppose that you found that there was a higher rate of domestic violence in one racial group than another. The violence might not be related to the race as such, but an increased alcohol intake in that group.

A correlational relationship looks at the relationship of variables within one group. It can be positive; that is, when you have a high level of one variable, you have a high level of the other. Or it can be negative, in which a high level of one variable is accompanied by a low level of the other. Of course, you may find that there is no relationship. In Chapter 10, we looked at an example of these relationships, so you may wish to refresh your memory by revisiting that section. To determine whether or not a relationship is statistically significant, it is necessary to determine whether the probability level is above or below the level of confidence that you set. Usually if the *p* value is below 0·05, we can say that the result is statistically significant at any rate.

In interpreting findings it is very important not to go beyond what the findings actually tell you. If you find a relationship between two variables, it means only that where you find one you find the other. It is very important not to assume that because one thing is related to another it is caused by the other. Both of the variables may be related to a third variable, for example, which may or may not cause the effect. For example, you may have found that there is an increase in body malfunction in people who live in a district that has a high-power transformer. It would be premature to conclude that high-power lines cause the malfunction. Perhaps the area that has a high-power transformer is a low socioeconomic area in which there is poor nutrition. It might therefore be the nutritional status of the people that underlies the malfunction, not the emissions of the transformer. Relationships such as those require further investigation before causality can be concluded.

Also, just because one thing is statistically related to another, there is not necessarily any meaningful relationship between the factors. For example, if you looked at the census data, you might find all sorts of correlations that were present but were not meaningful.

Causal relationships

You should be speaking about causal relationships only if you are sure that the one variable causes the other. In order for one thing to cause another, the causative factor must precede the effect. For example, a lightning flash always precedes electrocution from lightning. The two variables must also be specifically and strongly related to each other, for example a micro-organism and a disease. When you have a patient with syphilis, you will always find the organism *Treponema pallidum* in the body. Finally, the relationship should be reasonable. For example, if you found that two things were related but it did not seem logical that one caused the other, you would probably conclude that the relationship was correlational rather than causal.

Causal relationships can be demonstrated usually only by an experiment in which a change in the independent variable can be shown to result in a corresponding change in the dependent variable. Even then, the experiment should be so highly controlled that the independent variable is the only factor that could have caused the result. A causal relationship will almost always require the examination of differences between a pre-test and a post-test on the same group to see if the manipulation of the independent variable resulted in a change in the dependent variable.

It is normally through experimentation (see Chapter 7) that scientists have built up knowledge about causes of diseases. However, sometimes if a statistical relationship is very strong and the other criteria are satisfied we can assume causality if it is not possible to experiment. Sometimes a disease in humans, for example AIDS, is always linked to a specific micro-organism (HIV virus) that has been demonstrated to cause the disease in other primates. It would therefore be reasonable to assume that the micro-organism causes the disease despite the fact that you cannot do an experiment on people for ethical reasons. Tobacco smoking as a cause of cancer of the lung is another example of assumed causality from a naturalistic 'experiment' rather than from a controlled experiment. However, smoking tobacco always precedes the lung cancer, correlates strongly with the amount of tobacco smoked and the length of smoking, and produces cancer in animals. Furthermore, it is logical that inhaling an irritant into the lungs could disrupt cellular functioning. The case meets the criteria for causality so strongly that it is reasonable to assume that smoking causes lung cancer.

If your results suggest a causal relationship, you need to be suspicious of a placebo effect and be very cautious in your interpretation of them. For example, two groups reported equal amounts of relief of breast engorgement discomfort from cabbage extract cream and a placebo (Roberts, Reiter & Schuster, 1998). It would therefore be a false conclusion to suggest that the cabbage extract had relieved the discomfort. Similarly, many people place a great deal of belief in the power of therapeutic touch, but there has never been any evidence that it is anything more than a placebo effect.

Significance of findings
Non-significant findings
You need to examine the findings to see whether they are significant. If they do not meet the criterion set previously for significance (usually $p < 0.05$) then the findings are not significant ($p \geq 0.05$) and the null hypothesis is not rejected. You are then faced with the task of explaining why they are not significant. Before reporting non-significant findings you should look for an alternative explanation for them. Perhaps they can be explained by an inadequate or biased sample, incorrect methodology, a design flaw, errors in measurement, data collection or analysis, or even some unforeseen event that affected participants. However, results that are statistically non-significant may still be important if they add to our knowledge because the lack of difference is important.

Significant findings

If your findings are statistically significant, you get a rush of satisfaction. But wait! There are questions to be answered before you go and tell the world.

Are the findings pointing in the direction that you predicted? It is possible to have findings that are significant but that are the opposite of what you expected. Now you are left with the difficult task of explaining why, and you will have to critique your whole study to see if you can come up with an explanation. Before you do so, however, it is wise to check your data entry and analysis to see whether you carried it out correctly. For example, an incorrect step in re-coding or omitting to re-code a variable in the opposite direction could explain your results. If so, you are in the happy position of at least being able to fix your mistake and re-interpret the corrected data analysis. If not, you still have to explain why you got these results. If you are sure that your study was well designed and your methods were appropriate and carried out correctly, you might conclude that the theory is wrong.

Even if findings are statistically significant they may not be valid. It is therefore necessary to be cautious in the interpretation of statistically significant findings. You need to be sure that there is a continuity between your problem, theoretical framework, methodology, methods and findings. Remember that you have to be certain also that your findings have not been affected by any of the threats to validity that we discussed in Chapter 7. You must consider whether they could be accounted for by another explanation such as a very large sample resulting in very small differences being statistically significant. Be careful not to mistake statistical significance for meaningful differences.

Indeed, you need virtually to do a critique of your own study, using the criteria in Chapter 3, so that you can evaluate the validity of your findings and be ready to defend your findings against criticism from colleagues. Of course, if your study problem, conceptual framework, design, data collection methods and data analysis were adequate, then your findings are likely to have internal validity. However, it is easier to see the flaws in the study in hindsight and some events cannot be predicted so it is necessary to review the adequacy of every part of the study.

Difference between statistical and clinical significance

In interpreting research results, it is important to distinguish between statistical significance and clinical significance. Statistical significance is a difference in groups that is related to testing an hypothesis. It says only that the results probably could not have happened by chance alone. A small difference may turn out to be statistically significant, particularly if there are many participants. Clinical significance, on the other hand, is the substantive difference above and beyond the statistical significance (Abdellah & Levine 1994). It is a difference that is sufficiently large to recommend a change in practice. In interpreting results, it is useful to consider whether the difference justifies attaching much importance to it. Many researchers fall into the trap of mistaking statistical significance for clinical significance. In interpreting the importance of the findings it is better to be conservative, especially in clinical studies where you may be recommending a change in practice.

It is also a good idea to run another power analysis to make sure that your sample was large enough to produce a real difference. The original power analysis (See Chapter 8) will have taken into consideration the standard deviation of previous findings. If your standard deviation in your present data is larger than the previous findings, you may have needed a larger sample to achieve a true significance.

Finally, remember that with research you never actually prove anything. The best you can do is say that something is very probable.

Mixed findings

Mixed findings occur when you have rejected some null hypotheses and not others, or some findings are in the direction of the hypotheses and some are not. It is important to consider each finding carefully in the light of the methodology and the theoretical framework. It may be that the different findings reflect different methods of measurement, or different data collectors, or a faulty theory.

Serendipitous findings

Serendipitous findings are findings that are unexpected. On most projects, most researchers cannot resist doing extra analyses if they have the data, just to find out what might be there. Sometimes this will result in a finding that you were not expecting. Some of these findings may be useful and some may not. Serendipitous findings may go either in the direction of or against the hypotheses. Or they might be totally unrelated to the study but noticed by chance. A classic example is the story of the discovery of penicillin that resulted from Fleming's noticing that a culture plate contaminated with *Penicillium notatum* mould showed no growth around the bacteria. He concluded that the mould contained a bacteriostatic agent, and penicillin was born.

You need to consider very carefully how an unexpected finding could have happened – whether it is a spurious finding that occurred because of an error or whether it is genuine. If you think it is genuine, you need to arrive at an explanation for this finding. You should also consider the finding in the light of the theoretical framework. Serendipitous findings will usually need to be investigated further to determine whether or not they are valid, as another method may be more appropriate for a research project arising out of a serendipitous finding.

Searching for meaning within

In searching for meaning within the study findings, it is important to look at the patterns and connections in the total picture as well as the individual parts of the findings. For example, in the study on cabbage leaf cream we found a pattern that supported the hypothesis that cabbage extract acted as a placebo.

Although the mothers perceived relief from discomfort after the application of the cream, the physical indicator of hardness of tissue was actually showing an increase in hardness (Roberts, Reiter & Schuster 1998). The pattern of the findings, along with a lack of difference in the placebo and active treatment groups, was indicative of a placebo effect.

In interpreting patterns in your findings, particularly if you have a complex set of findings, it can be useful to use a whiteboard or butchers' paper. By grouping the findings on the paper or board and looking at them and drawing links between them you can find the patterns in the findings. It is this conceptual mapping and synthesis that is the highest point of the interpretation of the results.

In searching for meaning, you need to go beyond a description of your findings and ask 'why did this occur?' or 'why did it not occur?' Any competent researcher can look at and describe findings. However, to make a meaningful commentary, you need to go beyond documentation or narration of the results and ask 'so what?' This involves interpreting for the research consumer the real difference that these findings make. This is a difficult step because it requires much thought and reasoning, and sometimes even intuitive leaps.

You need to relate your findings to the purpose of the study and the problem that you were investigating. Did they answer the study question? If so, how? If not, why not? If they answered some other question, then you have a serious threat to the validity of your findings.

It is important when interpreting findings to relate your findings to the conceptual framework that you used to guide the study. This may be at the descriptive, correlational, explanatory or predictive level. Were your findings consistent with the theory? If not, why not?

You should also relate your findings to the results of previous research cited in your literature review. This is one of the areas that students find very difficult, because it requires a comparative evaluation and a synthesis. You need to have at least a simple concept map of previous research findings in order to see the relationships. What you need to ask yourself is how your results add to the total known picture about the findings on this topic. You need to decide whether they support previous findings or not. Again, it is also useful to group the previous findings according to an individual question or topic rather than on a study-by-study basis.

Searching for meaning beyond: implications, conclusions and recommendations

It is important to evaluate your study in terms of its implications for further theoretical development. Your findings may confirm the theory or part of it, may reject the theory or may make no difference one way or the other if they are not significant. Similarly, they may help to develop the theory further or they may help to critique the theory.

It is also important to evaluate your findings in terms of the implications for future research. It is rare for a study not to give rise to other questions that would need further research to answer them. For example our first two studies on cabbage leaves were done using a crossover design to test the difference between chilled gelpaks and cabbage leaves, and chilled and room temperature cabbage leaves (Roberts 1995; Roberts, Reiter & Schuster, 1995). A comparison of pre- and post-treatment subjective indicators showed similar levels of relief from all of these treatments. However, we were still left with the question of whether these were real or placebo effects. The only way to find out was to do a double blind placebo trial of cabbage extract cream. Similarly, the study comparing lung function in normal females on straight and boomerang pillows (Roberts et al. 1994) led to the question of whether the pillows would affect the lung function of frail elderly women (Roberts, Brittin & deClifford 1995).

It is also important to evaluate your findings for the implications for practice, assuming they are clinically significant. If they are clinically significant, how can clinicians improve practice on the basis of your findings? What would be the outcomes for clients or their families if the practice were changed? What would be the cost in poorer client outcomes if the change were not made? An example of a clinical implication is the finding that the minute volume in the lung capacity of frail elderly women was reduced after 10 minutes on boomerang pillows (Roberts, Brittin & deClifford 1995). We recommended that unless further research indicated that these pillows were safe, clinicians should use them with caution on frail elderly women.

When you have addressed the implications, ask yourself what conclusions you can draw from your findings. Conclusions may be tentative or firm, depending on the certainty you have about the external and internal validity of your findings.

You should also consider what recommendations you would make, based on the findings, implications and conclusions from any significant and meaningful results. They can be recommendations for research, practice, theoretical development or testing, and education. These recommendations will follow naturally from the implications; indeed, they are an extension of the recommendations. Recommendations are very important because they are one of the major products of your research.

Summary

In this chapter, we have discussed how to go about discovering the meaning of your findings. This is the time when you examine your findings for validity and meaning both in terms of the question that you were trying to answer and the study's place in the bigger picture. Having done so, you are ready to move on to writing up the research report and disseminating it to the professional community.

Main points
- Researchers are responsible for interpreting their data accurately and objectively to convey to the audience a coherent, meaningful interpretation of the findings.

- Descriptive data are interpreted to give a picture of your sample and findings.
- Relationship findings and hypothesis testing are interpreted using p values.
- Causal relationships should only be inferred from an experiment.
- It is important to distinguish between findings that are statistically significant and those that are also clinically significant and can be used to influence practice.
- It is important to search for the meaning behind the findings and the relationships between the findings.
- Findings should be related to the theoretical framework and previous findings set out in the literature review.
- Findings should be considered for implications for further research, theory development and practice.
- Conclusions and recommendations should be formulated, based on the findings.

Review Questions

1. In interpreting the data, it is easiest to start with the:
    a hypothesis testing
    b correlational relationships
    c descriptive data
    d conclusions

2. External validity depends on:
    a similarity of the sample to the population
    b accuracy of the findings
    c follow-up data being the same as initial-round data
    d eliminating participant mortality

3. In order to conclude that a group had changed due to the intervention, you should find that:
    a the control and experimental groups were initially different
    b the pre-test results for the control group were different from the post-test results
    c the pre-test results for the experimental group were different from the post-test results
    d the control and experimental groups were equivalent on the post-test

4. Which of the following will suggest that your results have external validity?
    a The sample is equivalent to the population on the demographic variables.
    b The sample is a non-probability sample.
    c The return rate is high.
    d a and c

5 In the social sciences, a statistically significant result is usually indicated by a *p* value of:
   a <0.9
   b <0.5
   c <0.1
   d <0.05

6 Which of the following could cause false conclusions?
   a inaccurate data
   b intervening variables
   c assumption of causality
   d all of the above

7 In order to state that a finding has clinical significance:
   a the finding should have a *p* value of >.05
   b the null hypothesis should not be rejected
   c the effect should be large enough to recommend a change in practice
   d all of the above

8 Serendipitous findings are:
   a correlational
   b mixed
   c unexpected
   d always meaningful

9 Findings should be interpreted in relation to the:
   a conceptual framework
   b previous research on the topic
   c implications for practice
   d a and b

10 Conclusions should:
   a be tentative in the absence of external validity
   b be drawn from the findings
   c lead to recommendations
   d all of the above

Discussion Questions

1. Discuss the description of the sample.
2. In what circumstances can you infer causality?
3. What are some of the reasons for a non-significant finding?
4. Differentiate between statistical and clinical significance.
5. How would you evaluate your findings for implications for practice?

References

Abdellah, F. & Levine, E. 1994, *Preparing Nursing Research for the 21st Century*, Springer, New York.

Roberts, K. 1995, 'A comparison of chilled cabbage leaves and chilled gelpaks in treating breast engorgement', *Journal of Human Lactation*, vol. 11, no. 1, 17–20.

Roberts, K. 1997, 'Nurse-academics' scholarly productivity: framed by the system, facilitated by mentoring', *Australian Journal of Advanced Nursing*, vol. 14, no. 3, 5–14.

Roberts, K., Brittin, M., Cook, M. & deClifford, J. 1994, 'Boomerang pillows and respiratory capacity', *Clinical Nursing Research*, vol. 3, no. 2, 157–65.

Roberts, K., Brittin, M. & deClifford, J. 1995, 'Boomerang pillows and respiratory capacity in frail elderly women', *Clinical Nursing Research*, vol. 4, no. 4, 465–71.

Roberts, K., Reiter, M. & Schuster, D. 1995, 'A comparison of chilled and room temperature cabbage leaves in treating breast engorgement', *Journal of Human Lactation*, vol. 11, no. 3, 191–4.

Roberts, K., Reiter, M. & Schuster, D. 1998, 'Effects of cabbage leaf extract on breast engorgement', *Journal of Human Lactation*, vol. 14, no. 3, 231–6.

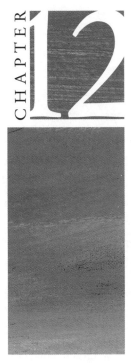

Qualitative interpretive methodologies

chapter objectives The material presented in this chapter will assist you to:

- describe research as a means of generating knowledge
- define epistemology and ontology
- clarify some common qualitative theoretical assumptions
- differentiate between quantitative and qualitative research
- describe postmodern influences on contemporary epistemology and ontology
- differentiate between interpretive and critical forms of qualitative methodologies
- describe postmodern alternatives for qualitative methodologies
- describe four qualitative interpretive methodologies in terms of their respective methodologies and methods
- recognise nursing research examples of four qualitative interpretive methodologies
- generate potential nursing research questions using these approaches.

Introduction

One of the most important points to remember in the study of research approaches is why they exist at all. This might seem a strange way to begin this chapter, but it seems timely to reiterate a simple message – research is about looking for answers to puzzles. The questions that have perplexed humans since the first conceptual conjectures are: 'What is true knowledge?' and 'What is the meaning of life?' In some respects, little has changed in that these questions are still being asked today and they still form the core of modern-day research into a wide variety of topics, albeit with infinitely finer degrees of focus and sophistication.

The history of the search for ideas through research approaches has been long and intensive. That is why it is important to 'begin at the beginning' when describing qualitative research methodologies, otherwise you may become lost along the way. Therefore, this chapter will begin by discussing research as a means of generating knowledge, then move to defining some essential terms, clarifying some common qualitative theoretical assumptions, differentiating broadly between quantitative and qualitative research, describing postmodern influences, and showing you how qualitative research methodologies can be categorised into interpretive and critical forms.

Having clarified these foundational ideas, the chapter will then exemplify a selection of four qualitative interpretive methodologies – grounded theory, phenomenology, ethnography and historical research – by describing them in terms of the key ideas contained within their respective methodologies and methods. Nursing research examples and potential nursing research questions will be presented, so that you can consider the possibilities of using some of these approaches in research areas you might like to explore.

Research as a means of generating knowledge

The basic reason for doing research is to find knowledge. This seems like a tautology in a book of this kind, but it is a point worth reiterating. The history of research is, basically, the history of ideas, or philosophy. It is not appropriate to go into a lengthy discussion here of the twists and turns in historical philosophical debate about finding knowledge. Suffice it to say that humans have adjusted their views over time to what constitutes research, and that it is, at this time, a relative matter, with no absolute answers.

From the time of Plato and Socrates and their contemporaries, through a time of dismal uninterest in the Dark Ages, to the rebirth of knowledge in the Renaissance, humans have progressed through phases of observation and conjecture about people, the planet, and the universe. Since the seventeenth century and Descartes, the scientific model has been the established approach, and there has been a reaction to that as the benchmark of all research in the last century or so, with the generation of multiple qualitative and postmodern research approaches. If you are interested in following these changes in depth, you would be advised to read an easily digestible form of philosophy in a book, such as Palmer (1988), before moving on to some of the heavier texts, such as Descartes (1970 trans.), Hume (1966; 1969, first published in 1739) and Barnes (1987). If these books excite you, you definitely need to consider studying philosophy!

The reason for raising these ideas about research as a means of generating knowledge is to have you consider from the start the possibility that there may be many approaches to finding knowledge through research that have merit, and that one kind should not be seen necessarily as being superior to another. Nurse-scholars such as Carper (1992) and Chinn and Kramer (1995) have expressed this idea succinctly in discussing the interrelatedness of four kinds of knowledge in contributing overall to nursing research.

Carper (1992) described empirical, personal, aesthetic and ethical ways of knowing. Respectively, they have basically to do with science, personal insights, a sense of the beautiful, and moral judgements. Carper also made the point that these ways of knowing need to be integrated. This argument was taken up more strongly by Chinn and Kramer (1995) who contended that knowledge should not only be integrated, but that it should also be balanced, because too much of one way of thinking and knowing about things can cause distortions; for example, too much empirical knowledge may result in control and manipulation, too much personal knowledge may result in isolation and self-distortion, too much aesthetics may result in prejudice and bigotry, and too much ethical knowledge may result in rigid doctrine and insensitivity to others. Using this reasoning, it seems fairly sensible to try to balance the kinds of knowledge generated and verified in research, to try to ensure that ideas, descriptions and explanations have the best chance of being well-rounded and comprehensive.

Defining epistemology and ontology

Two words are inescapable in understanding how knowledge is generated: **epistemology** and **ontology**. Epistemology is the study of knowledge and how it is judged to be 'true'. Inverted commas have been used intentionally around the word 'true', to show that truth is, and has always been, an uncertain concept in philosophy. The search for what counts as truth has accounted for the various interpretations of new knowledge over time. It has always been important to argue the veracity of ideas before claiming their validity in counting towards the development of new knowledge.

Ontology is the study of existence itself. Various authors have given their versions of 'the meaning of life' and their views have been debated thoroughly. For example, one philosopher named Martin Heidegger (1962) considered that ontology and epistemology were one and the same thing. In other words, he argued that by understanding the nature of the existence of anything of interest, answers were supplied automatically to the very nature of knowledge itself. Whereas a diversion into ontological thought is not warranted now, you should be aware that it is a central focus of human thought and that it has relevance for nursing research.

Questions of human knowing and existing have been posed for ages through philosophical thought. Nurses are thinking workers who need to ask questions about knowing and existing in nursing because the answers to such questions form the substance of their discipline. Whenever nurses raise questions about what they know and how they know it is trustworthy knowledge, they are asking epistemological questions. Whenever nurses are asking about the nature of the existence of something or someone in nursing, they are asking ontological questions. Therefore, these words are relevant and integral to nurses and to nursing research.

Some common qualitative theoretical assumptions

In this chapter, the word 'methodology' will be used to mean the theoretical assumptions underlying the choice of methods in generating a particular form of knowledge. Many philosophical traditions have contributed to research in that they have supplied theoretical assumptions about certain kinds of knowledge. For example, one of the bases of empirical/quantitative knowledge is that any knowledge that counts as truth should be free from the subjectivity of the researcher. In this section, we will examine some key theoretical assumptions that are common to various qualitative research approaches and that constitute some fundamental ideas about the nature of people as inquirers and research as a means of knowledge generation.

Qualitative research attempts to explore the changing (relative) nature of knowledge, which is seen to be special and centred in the people, place, time and conditions in which it finds itself (unique and context-dependent). Qualitative research uses thinking that starts from a specific instance and moves to the general pattern of combined instances (inductive), so that it grows from 'the ground up' to make larger statements about the nature of the thing being investigated.

The measures for ensuring validity in qualitative research involve asking the participants to confirm that the interpretations are correct, that they represent, faithfully and clearly, what the experience was/is like for the people acting as sources of information in the research. Reliability is often not an issue in qualitative research, as it is based on the idea that knowledge is relative and dependent on all of the features of the people, place, time and other circumstances (context) of the setting.

People are acknowledged as sources of information. Their expressions of their personal awareness (subjectivity) are valued as being integral to the meaning that comes out of the research. Qualitative research acknowledges that people and things may change according to their circumstances, so it is inappropriate to generalise research findings to the wider group of people or things being studied.

Differences between quantitative and qualitative research

It is a major oversimplification to say that, at the present time, the search for explaining human knowledge and existence has gone into two main streams, specifically, quantitative and qualitative inquiry. However, this will be asserted here, for the sake of ease, and to prevent the need for following each and every detail and detour in past and present philosophical debate. The following table might be useful for you to consider some differences in quantitative and qualitative research.

Table 12.1 Differences in quantitative and qualitative research (Taylor 1995)

Quantitative	Qualitative
Knowledge is	
absolute	relative
about finding cause-and-effect links	unique and context-dependent
deductive	inductive
Research questions are	
hypothesised	left open as tentative ideas
tested empirico-analytically	explored by a variety of means
analysed using numbers	analysed using language
interpreted as mathematical relations	interpreted as themes
Research conditions require	
validity through control of variables	participants' validation
reliability through test and retest	attention to context
objectivity without human distortion	valuing subjectivity
Problem areas for research	
are reduced to smallest parts	are part of the whole context
Findings	
are quantified in numbers	are qualified in words
need to be significant statistically	do not make absolute claims
can be predictive	provide insights to possibilities
claim to be generalisable	are specific to local phenomena
Outcomes include	
description, prediction and change	description, meaning and change

The reason for caution in thinking of quantitative and qualitative research as being categorically different is that there may be some remnants of one in the other. For example, both approaches can use deductive and inductive thinking, and both require 'scientific' designs, in the sense that they must both show that they are systematic and rigorous. Caution is necessary also in trying to set both approaches up as irreconcilable alternatives, because some researchers (Bull & Hart 1995) would argue that it is not the case, and that it is possible to combine them both and come up with richer research data and outcomes.

In summary, the features of empirico-analytical/quantitative research, also known as 'the scientific method', are to attain rigour in the reliability and validity of projects by using observational and analytic means to control and manipulate variables, and to produce objective data that can be quantified to demonstrate the degree of statistical significance in cause-and-effect relationships. This sounds like a good idea, and it is, for research in which the rules of the scientific method can be applied uniformly. Problems become apparent when researchers decide that they want to ask questions about human knowledge and existence that are outside the 'observe and analyse' domain, and when they want to value people's intentions, ideas and emotions as part of the research process.

Postmodern influences on contemporary epistemology and ontology

Nursing research has had to take into account a radical critique of modernist (positivistic and post-positivistic) notions of epistemology and ontology. In other words, nursing has been alerted to postmodern ways of thinking about what knowledge and existence might mean in an era that questions taken-for-granted quantitative and qualitative assumptions about 'truth' and 'being'. Although postmodern literature is vast, a handy guide to setting a foundation has been written by Rosenau (1992), who differentiates between a range of overlapping extreme to moderate forms of skeptical and affirmative postmodernism. Even though the book is dated, it remains the best explanation I have located of the various writings on postmodernism, up until the time of its publication. I use Rosenau's work throughout this book because of its importance as an explanatory text for those of us who are not scholars in postmodernism and need a guide to making sense of it all.

Rosenau (1992, p. 15) explains that the skeptical postmodernists offer 'a pessimistic, negative, gloomy assessment (and) argue that the post-modern age is one of fragmentation, disintegration, malaise, meaninglessness, a vagueness or even absence of moral parameters and societal chaos'. Contrastingly, affirmative postmodernists, while agreeing with the critique of modernity, nevertheless have a 'more hopeful, optimistic view of the post-modern age' (p. 15).

Extreme forms of skeptical postmodernism lambaste modernity to the extent that they leave no reasons for, or ways of, doing research, because they claim authors use their authority as writers to control and censure readers, thus the 'death of the author' halts academic inquiry. The human as subject is rejected because s/he is a humanist product of modernity representing a subject–object dichotomy, and s/he is criticised 'for seizing power, for attributing meaning, for dominating and oppressing' (p. 42). Effectively, these criticisms remove humans from the objects of their attention, such as asking or pursuing research questions. History is viewed as 'logocentric, a source of myth, ideology, and prejudice, a method assuming closure' (p. 63). This means that nothing that has gone before can be taken as fact or truth because of its association with human interpretation, rendering research methods and processes impotent as records of events over time. Time itself is rejected as chronological and linear, the modernity understanding of which is 'oppressive, measuring and controlling one's activities' (p. 63).

Truth 'claims are a form of terrorism', that threaten and provoke, silencing those who disagree (p. 78), thereby making research tantamount to a terrorist activity. Words, images, meanings and symbols constitute a 'fixed system of meaning', and, as representations, they are rejected by skeptical postmodernists because they do not allow for diversity (p. 96). The inability to place (even tentatively) some faith in language renders researchers incapable of transmitting ideas gleaned by any research means. In summary, skeptical postmodernism leaves no reasons for, or ways of, doing research, making research endeavours unnecessary and impossible.

'All is not lost', however, as affirmative postmodernists allow room for different, less pessimistic interpretations, while still holding onto some central ideas. Affirmative postmodernists do not abandon the author completely, but they reduce the author's authority, so that s/he 'makes no universal truth claims, has no prescriptions to offer' (Rosenau 1992, p. 31), and offers only options for public debate. This position allows researchers, as the authors of projects, to offer tentative insights for readers' interpretations and discussion. The human as subject returns 'not as the same subject banished' by skeptical postmodernists, but as a 'post-modern subject with a new non-identity', who 'will reject total explanations and the logocentric view that implies a unified frame of reference' (p. 57). This allows researchers to focus on humans as subjects, but in ways that do not make bold, broad theory claims. History is a source of criticism, but it is revised radically 'to focus on the daily life experience of ordinary people', akin to storytelling of small events on the margins of human existence, left open to constant questioning as possibilities rather than statements of fact and truth. Time is not linear or bounded, and truth is rejected as universal in favour of 'specific, local, personal and community forms of truth' (p. 80). This allows researchers to work with people's narratives to emphasise the relative nature of their self-understandings. Representation is permissible, but in improved political forms that assist oppressed minorities and women to find voice, leaving room for participatory and emancipatory research that focuses on the specific circumstances of participants and finds multiple and contradictory personal and local solutions. In summary, affirmative postmodernism does not sever ties with organised research; rather it can influence projects by the application of redefined ideas about people and the sense they make out of their knowledge and existence.

Differences between interpretive and critical qualitative methodologies

There are many ways of categorising qualitative research; however, a useful and reasonable way is to think of them as essentially interpretive or critical. Essentially, interpretive research is about making meaning and critical research is about causing change. Some examples of qualitative methodologies (used here as meaning 'the theoretical assumptions underlying the choice of methods') are presented in Table 12.2.

Table 12.2 Differences in interpretive and critical qualitative methodologies (Taylor 1995)

Qualitative interpretive examples	Critical qualitative examples
Grounded theory	Action research
Phenomenology	Feminist research
Historical research	Interpretive interactionism
Ethnography	Critical ethnography

The major difference between interpretive and critical qualitative research is the main intention of what they hope to achieve through the research process. Interpretive research aims mainly to generate meaning; in other words, it tries to explain and describe, in order to make sense out of things of interest. Critical research aims to bring about change in the status quo, by working systematically through research problems to find answers and to cause change activity in light of those answers. In doing what they intend to do as their first priority, interpretive and critical research also manage to do other things; for example they both generate meaning and they can bring about change, but they differ in the intensity of their intentions.

Postmodern alternatives for qualitative methodologies

Although postmodernism does not fit into the categories of interpretive or critical qualitative research approaches, and by its own admission repudiates grand narratives and would not be seen as one itself, it needs attention because it is related to interpretive or critical qualitative research by extending their ideas into greater realms of relativism, contradiction and deconstruction. Leaving aside skeptical postmodernism (which rejects the intentions, methods and processes of research), alternatives for qualitative methodologies exist, if one takes qualitative methodologies in this case to mean post-positivist (after quantitative) theoretical assumptions underlying the choice of research methods.

Grand theories (narratives) are rejected by postmodernists as statements that claim universal truth, and that can be applied in all like cases. As grand theories are indefensible, so also are the research methods by which these theories can be developed and validated. The words 'strategies' or 'struggles' may be used in preference to the word 'method', which has typically taken on the meaning of the rules and procedures of modern science (the scientific method). By association, the whole idea of grand theories is suspect when the rules of rigour or trustworthiness are used to test the legitimacy or 'truthfulness' of knowledge. This thinking can lead to a methodological void if it is not tempered with some affirmative postmodern redefinition.

The turn against absolute truth claims is pulled back from the brink of extreme relativism by affirmative postmodernists who argue that some realities are brutal and some causes matter. Rape, poverty, violence, starvation and diseases are real, and the plights of women and other minorities matter. If it were otherwise, society would disappear into a moral morass and the vulnerable would be left to the wiles of more powerful groups, who would be left to their own political devices.

Extreme contradiction and deconstruction of texts negates and questions the thinking of all authors and leaves the way open for 'anything goes' to the point of creating multiple paradoxes, never-ending questions and a multiplicity of answers. The problem in this is best described by Rosenau (1992, p. 137) who suggests that postmodern social science (by which nursing is influenced in its delivery of care):

> ... rejects the Kuhnian model of science as a series of progressive paradigms and announces the end of all paradigms. Only an absence of knowledge claims, an affirmation of multiple realities, an acceptance of divergent interpretations remain. We can convince those who agree with us, but we have no basis for convincing those who dissent and no criteria to employ in arguing for the superiority of any particular view. Those who disagree with us can always argue that different interpretations must be accepted and that in a post-modern world one interpretation is as good as another. Post-modernists have little interest in convincing others that their view is best – the most just, appropriate or true. In the end the problem with post-modern science is that you can say anything you want, but so can everyone else. Some of what will be said will be interesting and fascinating, but some will also be ridiculous and absurd. Post-modernism provides no means to distinguish between the two.

What does this all mean for nursing research? Just as postmodernists reject paradigms as being legitimate solely on the basis of the claim that they are progressive in thought, researchers can choose to be influenced by postmodern ideas, but not constrained or directed by them. This leaves open the possibilities of multiple choices for nurse-researchers, who can choose to be influenced by postmodern variations of thought about human knowledge (epistemology) and existence (ontology) and adjust their projects to take account of the diversity, difference and contradiction of life on the margins as everyday ordinary history told in people's narratives and interpreted by them as their self-understandings. Researchers who do not choose postmodern influences can be guided by methodologies that claim tentatively the legitimacy of relative degrees of local theories that are trustworthy by virtue of their context-dependence and the ways in which they resonate with their readers. A detailed account of trustworthiness in qualitative research is in Chapter 14.

The methodologies of grounded theory, phenomenology, ethnography and historical research will now be discussed as examples of qualitative interpretive research approaches. Each approach will be discussed in terms of methodology, methods, nursing research examples and potential questions that you might ask, should you be considering such approaches for your nursing research interests.

Grounded theory

Grounded theory gets its name from being a research approach which starts from the ground and works up in an inductive fashion to make sense of what people say about their experiences and to convert these statements into theoretical propositions. Because it is close to, yet different from, quantitative research, grounded theory retains some of the terms that are characteristic of quantitative research, such as hypotheses and variables. This is important to remember, because it is the only qualitative approach which does this, and it might be tempting to think that the use of these words makes it more rigorous somehow, and that would be an erroneous assumption, based on general principles of qualitative research. Just remember that grounded theory 'lies on the cusp' between quantitative and qualitative research when you are wondering why some of the terms sound so much like quantitative research.

The methodology

Grounded theory, a qualitative interpretive approach, grew out of the symbolic interactionist tradition (Robrecht 1995), which is a form of social psychology. Polit and Hungler (1995, p. 643) define grounded theory as

> an approach to collecting and analysing qualitative data with the aim of developing theories and theoretical propositions 'grounded' in real-world observations.
>
> Grounded theory also bears the remnants of empirical-analytical influences, in that the language that is used by grounded theorists is reminiscent of that used by researchers who use forms of 'the scientific method.' The point of departure, however, lies in the assumptions of grounded theory, that participants' subjective and objective perspectives emerge from analysis of the data and that these perceptions are worthwhile information for describing research interests.

Grounded theory is useful when little is known or experienced about the problem under scrutiny (Stern 1985; Hutchinson 1986). The approach identifies and relates factors that might be used to define and explain relatively unknown situations; thus the methodology is based on the assumptions that problem identification and solution generation are within the realms of interpretive research. This means that practical solutions can be found to problems generated by nurses.

Grounded theory is generated solely from the data and thus the participants' perspectives are reflected in the findings (Glaser & Strauss 1967). Existing theory is not imposed on the data, but it is utilised to support the emergent theory, creating possibilities for multiple theoretical frameworks to be applied to the research interest (Stern 1985; Hutchinson 1986).

The method

Glaser and Strauss (1967) used the term 'grounded theory' to refer to the generation of constructs (or theory) from the data, so that theory remains connected to or grounded in the data. As a research method, grounded theory involves searching out and relating factors to the research problem being studied.

The grounded theorist is involved in looking for processes, rather than being concerned with static conditions. Observational, interview and document-analysis methods generate data through a system of constant comparison until hypotheses are generated. During the research process, existing theories are consulted as hypotheses are generated to find relationships between existing ideas and those that are emerging. However, a theory is not imposed on the research, because grounded theory comes from the data. Hypotheses are linked together so that the integrated theory has the potential to explain the problem being researched. The theory is developed when the related variables are ready to be tested. This is dissimilar to theory-driven research, such as quantitative research, which normally begins with statements about relationships between variables and then sets out to disprove or prove them.

The means of checking the validity of the findings in grounded theory is through the participants, whose positive responses testify to their own truth contained within the research document. Qualitative researchers rely on participants' validating processes as the most effective way of ensuring the validity of qualitative studies, because they claim that '... truth is subject-oriented rather than researcher-defined' (Sandelowski 1986, p. 30)

Grounded research requires 'bracketing' to eradicate or minimise researcher preconceptions and the bias in effects they can have on the data (Sandelowski 1986). Researcher presuppositions about the area of interest are acknowledged at the outset and set aside to allow the data to speak for themselves. The word 'bracketing' comes from its use in mathematics, in which numbers are put to one side in brackets to be attended to separately. In research bracketing occurs when the researcher's presuppositions about the area of interest are acknowledged at the outset and set aside to allow the data to speak for itself. For example, registered nurses would need to acknowledge their previous knowledge and experience of any area of nursing they might choose to research.

After ethical clearance for the research is obtained, theoretical sampling is used to select participants who are considered to know a great deal about an area of interest. Various modes of data collection may be used, for example unstructured interviews, media items, personal observations and informal conversations. Of these methods, Swanson (1986) and Stern (1985) explain that an unstructured interview is considered the most fitting means to elicit the personal viewpoint of the participants, to preserve the flexibility required to follow themes and clear up inconsistencies arising from the data.

The interviews are transcribed by the researcher as soon as possible after the interview and data analysis commences within the first interview to facilitate the simultaneous collection, coding and analysis of the data, and to provide a focus for subsequent data collection (Glaser & Strauss 1967; Stern 1985; Swanson 1986).

The identification of a central theme or social process is the focus of analysis. Coding of the data occurs on three levels:

1 Substantive codes are derived from the language of the participants and describe actions such as relating, thinking or feeling.
2 Categories are a condensation of level 1 codes. In developing categories the researcher hypothesises as to which coded data may be subsumed by an emergent category. Comparison of emerging categories allows the development of higher order categories which are mutually exclusive and which explain several other categories. The literature is reviewed to identify information which substantiates the emergent fit of categories and leads to the development of a conceptual framework (Stern 1985).
3 Theoretical constructs conceptualise the relationships between the three levels of coding. They relate to academic and clinical knowledge, but are grounded in substantive or category codes and not abstract theorising (Hutchinson 1986).

Following this, a constant comparative analysis is employed, which involves beginning data analysis as soon as the information is at hand, and comparing it constantly to all new data that emerge. The reason for this is to identify similarities in codings and categories, and to facilitate conceptualisation of higher order categories by comparison of codings, categories and their properties. Interpretations and codings arising from the data analysis are clarified during the interview, or at a later time, and are substantiated during subsequent interviews. Indicators including causes, contexts, contingencies, consequences, co-variance and conditions, are utilised to clarify the nature and validity of emergent categories and theoretical constructs (Stern 1985; Corbin 1986).

Category saturation is reached when there are no new codes or categories identified during analysis of subsequent data. That is, no new ideas are raised in the data. As the research progresses, written memos produced by the researcher may document hunches and ideas related to patterns, themes and relationships identified in the data. The memos may provide an additional focus for further sorting of codes and categories and to identify interrelationships between the potential social processes, and may provide a basis and reference for the emergent theory.

If you are considering a grounded theory approach to your research, you would be well advised to return to some of the original writing to help you with the steps in the method (Glaser & Strauss 1967), and to some well-known writing by Spradley (1979) to give you hints on how to do a successful ethnographic interview.

According to Skodol Wilson (1993, p. 235) a good grounded theory is one that

- results from formulating and discarding hypotheses if they are not supported by the data
- has included a look for contradictory occurrences
- is based on a variety of slices of data, direct observations, interviews and document analysis
- can transcend the substantive area and have broader reference
- specifies the conditions under which it was developed and to which it can be generalised

- fits the data
- works to explain the variations in behaviour in a given area and to predict what can occur when conditions change
- is relevant and comprehensible to people in the study setting
- is modifiable, dense, and integrated into a tight analytic framework.

Nursing research examples

An example of grounded theory research is that of an Australian nurse Dr Winsome St John, who explored the role of community health nurses in relation to Situated Health Competence, defined as requiring 'families, groups and communities to address their own illnesses, health problems, health issues and health behaviours; and seek out and access appropriate health resources on an ongoing basis' (St John 1999, p. 30). She collected data from 17 'excellent' community health nurses in various health care settings in three Australian states, including transcripts of in-depth interviews, questionnaires, group discussions, job descriptions, agency and professional organisation documents and focus group discussions.

Data were analysed using a constant comparative technique (Glaser & Strauss 1967) and theoretical concepts were developed (Corbin 1986), assisted by constant memoing and the qualitative computer analysis program NUD★IST (Qualitative Solutions and Research 1995). In her research article St John gives a clear explanation of how she managed the data by open coding and axial coding to identify major themes, and then undertaking selective coding to 'identify central concepts within the data, particularly in relation to the purpose of the community health nurse' (St John 1999, p. 31). Central themes pointed 'to the issues of client self care, client self-responsibility and assisting the client to manage their own health problems, situated in their own context, within a wellness perspective' (p. 31). Seven properties related to the ways nurses aimed to promote Situated Health Competence – contextuality, scope, meaning, allocation of responsibility, client focus, responsiveness and a recognition of a continuum in possible patient achievement.

Contextuality refers to the ways in which community nurses considered the various and unique features of place, time, culture, social setting, power and responsibility in providing nursing care. Nurses worked within clients' everyday realities, and identified their roles as dealing with well, not ill, people, who assigned their health a priority in line with their everyday lives.

Scope refers to a primary health care model that focuses on

> ... individual, family, group or community clients' ability to: cope with and manage their own illness on a longer term basis; have the knowledge and ability to manage not only their diseases, illnesses and rehabilitation, but also incorporate preventative or health enhancing behaviours into their daily lives; question and make decisions about their health; appropriately seek out and use health and community resources; and to do this while going on about their daily lives' (St John 1999, p. 32)

Client focus considered clients' needs to be broader than the individual – they expanded to the clients' families, groups and communities.

Health competence was understood in responsive, flexible ways, linked to clients' perspectives and contexts, being 'sensitive to clients' views, resources and specific social, cultural and physical environments, drawing on their special knowledge' (p. 33).

Responsibility shifts from the nurse to the client in Situated Health Competence, allowing the individual, family, group or community to make decisions and deal with health issues according to their own 'at home' situation.

Responsiveness to clients' most recent social, cultural and political changes allows nurses to facilitate Situated Health Competence, responding with appropriate action according to clients' unique needs.

Nurses addressed clients' needs across a continuum of identifying, intervening and enabling activities, in facilitating possible patient achievement. 'At every stage of Identifying, Intervening and Enabling, the aim is to move clients towards greater health competence' (p. 35).

St John concluded that the study made 'the intangible motivations of the community health nurse more explicit' and that the 'aim of facilitating Situated Health Competence results in an expanded view of nursing practice' (p. 35). She reiterated the nature of the community nurse's situated role with a health focus, based on negotiated understandings and 'a shift in responsibility and control from the nurse to the client' (p. 35)

Other recent examples of nurses who have undertaken grounded theory research projects include Watt (1997), Brennan and Stevens (1998), Hawley and Irurita (1998) and Irurita (1999a, 1999b).

Irurita (1999a, 1999b) used grounded theory methodology to explore the adult patient's perspective of quality nursing care in acute-care hospital settings in Western Australia, by seeking the factors patients perceived to influence high-quality nursing care. Patients identified broad environmental factors, such as ageism and staffing levels, which further influenced factors at organisational and personal levels, that in turn facilitated the process of preserving patients' sense of integrity, thereby influencing their perceptions of quality care. Irurita concluded that factors 'enhancing the quality of nursing care were incorporated in, and facilitated by soft-hand care' in addition to technical competence and an effective nurse–patient relationship. (Irurita 1999a, p. 93). The core problem shared by clients was vulnerability, relating to 'an inability to retain control of their life situation and/or protect themselves against threats to their integrity (physical and emotional wholeness, intactness)' (Irurita 1999b, p. 10).

Brennan and Stevens (1998) used grounded theory to explore with cancer sufferers and their partners the use and perceived effects of meditation. A number of theories were generated from the analysis of semi-structured interviews, regarding the use of meditation in the oncology domain. The theories fell into two main categories: theories about the cancer experience; and theories about meditation in the treatment of cancer. Theoretical statements about the cancer experience highlighted the value of storytelling and the participants' inability to remember aspects of their chemotherapy, and motivation to change behaviour was strongest when the client was actually feeling the effects of the disease. Theories regarding meditation in cancer therapy made statements about: clients using meditation in taking control of their pain, reducing the severity of side effects, and slowing the disease process; the absence in clients' accounts of nursing staff; and not informing oncologists about using meditation, making incomplete the measures for judging treatment success.

Hawley and Irurita (1998, p. 9) used grounded theory to 'discover the experience and meaning of prayer in hospital when undergoing coronary artery bypass graft surgery'. During interviews 13 participants expressed how they sought comfort through prayer. Constant comparative analysis of the transcripts showed three stages in seeking comfort: re-establishing or maintaining their relationship with God; making peace with God; and asking God to be with them during their hospitalisation. Levels of prayer when asking God to be with them were: acquiescence (not being able to pray and needing to rely on others for prayer); instinctive prayer (making innate pleas to God in a few words); surviving (one sentence or so about wanting to survive the experience); confiding (conversing with God through long prayers); and honouring (deep prayers reflecting the unconditional acceptance of God's will).

The purpose of Elizabeth Watt's (1997, p. 119) study 'was to provide a beginning exploration of the way in which registered nurses perceived the concept of patient advocacy'. Using the techniques of grounded theory she interviewed, in a semi-structured format, eight registered nurses working in an acute care setting in a major Melbourne hospital, and explored with them their personal definitions of advocacy, the advocate role and the reasons why nurses act as patient advocates. Data analysis started after two interviews and emerging themes were coded, that gave direction for further interviewing. As analysis continued themes were grouped into clusters and categories. Conditions that were perceived by participants to be the basis of patient advocacy were basic beliefs about the person and the quality of the nurse–patient relationship. Three processes involved in advocacy were informing, supporting, and representing.

Other Australian studies using grounded theory research include Irurita (1992), Armitage and Kavanagh (1995), McCabe (1995), Muir-Cochrane (1995) and Barclay, Donovan and Genovese (1996).

Potential nursing research questions

In deciding on the kinds of questions you might like to pose, which may be answered well by a grounded theory approach, you need to think of any nursing situations involving people, in which very little is known. The question(s) may be about anything at all, the knowledge of which can be communicated to you best by talking with people who know it well. To assist you in choosing some areas of possible exploration through grounded theory, begin with specific areas of nursing practice, and people/conditions/circumstances/events you would like to know about related to each of them.

For example, clinical settings may include an Accident and Emergency Department, a Medical Ward, a Surgical Ward, a Paediatric Ward, a Community Health Clinic and so on. People of interest within these clinical areas may include patients, nurses, and/or allied health staff. Conditions, circumstances and events may include a wide range of possibilities, such as specific interpersonal relationships and interactions, routines, procedures, rituals and policies. Any area of patient concern may be explored, such as reactions to illness and hospitalisation, the need for education, and so on. As you can see, the possibilities are many for interesting and practical research using a grounded theory approach.

Phenomenology

A phenomenon is a thing, or entity. Defined simply, 'phenomen - ology' is the study of a thing. In the human sciences, phenomenology concerns itself with the study of things within human existence, because it acknowledges and values the meanings people ascribe to their own existence. Its prime intent is to discover, explore and describe 'uncensored phenomena' (Spiegelberg 1970, p. 21) of the things themselves, as they are immediately given. There are many kinds of phenomenology although they all propose to explore the nature of a thing directly, by going to its source (Spiegelberg 1976). Therefore, phenomenology will allow nurses to explore the lived experience of any person involved in nursing practice of any kind.

The methodology

Much has been written about the theoretical assumptions of phenomenology (Husserl 1960 trans; Heidegger 1962; Husserl 1964 trans., 1965 trans., 1970, 1980 trans.; Kockelmans 1967; Gadamer 1975 trans., 1976 trans.; Krell 1977; Hekman 1986; Dreyfus 1991). You would be well advised to leave these references until you are ready to embark on an in-depth study of phenomenology. However, if you are keen to get started, Spiegelberg (1976) is worth reading, because he will give you a good introduction to the many kinds of phenomenology and point out some important differences between them.

Because there are so many approaches to phenomenology, it is difficult to know where to focus when considering theoretical perspectives. Probably, the most useful approach might be to look at a few ideas of two well-known philosophers, Husserl and Heidegger, before reverting to some of the ideas of Max van Manen, who is a contemporary phenomenologist cited often in nursing circles.

Husserl (1970 trans.) suggested that it is necessary to suspend one's ideas about what you know, when you try to see it as it really is. This phenomenological reduction, or 'bracketing', is supposed to be helpful in narrowing one's attention in such a way as to be able to discover rational principles underlying the phenomenon of concern. In contrast to this idea, Heidegger (1962) was concerned with Being-in-the-World. Therefore, instead of trying to lay presuppositions to one side, Heidegger explored them as legitimate parts of finding out about the nature of a thing of interest. In other words, Heidegger suggested that humans live in a body and that the experiences of living in the world could give them clues to the nature of human existence.

Max van Manen (1990) applies a mixture of phenomenological concepts, such as bracketing and the value of understanding lived experience. Derived from Husserl's work, bracketing means suspending one's own knowledge about a certain phenomenon. Lived experience refers to the knowledge people have of things of interest, because they have experienced them through the daily activities of living their lives. Bracketing and lived experience are two of many key concepts that may underlie a phenomenological approach to research.

The theoretical assumptions presented in this section are simplistic explanations of relatively complex concepts, so it should be remembered that if you want to undertake research informed by phenomenological thought, you will need to grapple at some time with these and other philosophical ideas.

The methods

Phenomenological methods differ according to the kinds of theoretical assumptions on which they are based. Some people advocate that there should be no structured steps in a method (Psathas 1973; Morris 1977; Schwartz & Jacobs 1979), while others, such as Patton (1980), feel that the inquiry must proceed as the experience unfolds, the only methodological consideration being that inquirers use some form of bracketing to minimise presuppositions.

Some authors claim that researchers need some framework to assist their inquiries and thus some adaptations of 'the phenomenological method' for analysing particular phenomena by intuiting, analysing and describing (Spiegelberg 1976) have been suggested. Some of these include the Van Kaam method (1959), the Giorgi method (1975) and the Colaizzi method (1978) and a method of transformation of interpretations (Langveld 1978). The methods range in specificity for guiding the researcher in a method, which will uncover, supposedly, the nature of the phenomenon of interest.

Max van Manen (1990) has been accredited with a method that may be useful to you in understanding how to go about phenomenological research. It involves:

1 turning to the nature of the lived experience
2 investigating experience as we live it, rather than as we conceptualise it
3 reflecting on the essential themes which characterise the phenomenon
4 describing the phenomenon through the art of writing and rewriting
5 maintaining a strong and oriented relation to the phenomenon
6 balancing the research context by considering the parts and the whole.

If you still think that this section on phenomenological methods has not been so helpful, you would not be alone in thinking this way. Many of the so-called phenomenological methods leave prospective researchers wondering just what to do. This was the dilemma I faced in my PhD research (Taylor 1994; 2001); therefore I devised my own phenomenological method based on selected theoretical assumptions. In the section that follows, this research will be described as an example of phenomenological research.

Nursing research examples

In my research: 'The Phenomenon of Ordinariness in Nursing', I was a participant observer of six registered nurses in a Professorial Nursing Unit (PNU) in Australia. I was present at 24 nurse–patient interactions, as each nurse interacted with four patients. Following each interaction, I wrote my impressions in a personal-professional journal and audiotaped conversations with the respective patients and nurses to gain their impressions. I then analysed and interpreted the recorded impressions.

Many qualities and activities emerged within each interaction and they have been described in detail in the thesis. They included such things as: appreciating skilful nursing care; appreciating help; facilitating independence; facilitating learning; and facilitating coping. The categories of the qualities and activities were grouped into eight main parts. I gave the term 'aspects' to these groupings, to denote their identities as parts of the phenomenon itself.

In the second phase of the analysis and interpretation eight 'actualities' of the nature of the phenomenon emerged, such as: 'allowingness,' 'straightforwardness,' 'self-likeness,' 'homeliness,' 'favourableness,' 'intuneness,' 'lightheartedness' and 'connectedness.' Interested readers are referred to the book (Taylor 1994, 2000) for a fuller description of the research, but a synopsis of it is that nurses and patients revealed themselves to one another through the embodiment of their ordinary human qualities, or being human. The shared sense of ordinariness between nurses and patients made them as one in their humanness and created a special place, in which the relative strangeness of the experience of being in a health care setting could be made familiar and manageable.

Catherine Jones and Ysanne Chapman (2000) used methods consistent with hermeneutic phenomenology to explore seven people's lived experience of being treated with autologous bone marrow/peripheral blood stem cell transplant. Based on the assumption that 'lived experience is central to the phenomenological view of the person', Jones and Chapman (2000, p. 154) identified seven people from one metropolitan teaching hospital's databank to interview 12 months or more after their experience of receiving the transplant.

Using van Manen's method (van Manen 1990), the researchers analysed the interview transcripts and by 'hermeneutically engaging with the text, interpretation of commonalities as well as differences were articulated in and through themes' (Jones & Chapman 2000, p. 155). The main themes that illuminated the participants' experiences of bone marrow transplant were changing concepts of self, the significance of relationships, being different from the past and temporality.

Changing concepts of self included the sub-themes of being in a different world, changing appearance, and changing emotion – thoughts of surrender. Being in a different world of the treating hospital caused trauma because of its unfamiliarity, having to negotiate trust with strangers. Changes in physical appearance were frightening for participants and confirmed for them daily how dreadful they felt. Changing emotions coincided with extreme physical weakness and caused recognition that death may have been imminent.

The theme of significance of relationships highlighted how participants maintained close relationships with friends and family. 'As the participants were able to go home, many relied heavily on their relationships with others to negotiate the transition between the world of suffering and their previous familiar world' (Jones & Chapman 2000, p. 157).

The theme of being different from the past reflected how the physical and emotional changes participants had undergone meant that it was difficult to go back to their 'normal' lifestyles. Some people described having to learn to use a wheelchair and to walk again, and of fitting into previous roles, in the face of incredible weakness and emotional changes. The theme of being different had within it the sub-theme of an altered outlook on life, to express feelings such as of the treatment being a form of punishment, or the sense of valuing life more and purposely altering their outlooks believing stress was an important factor in developing the cancer.

The theme of temporality alluded to the ways in which people lived time. For these people time suggested that thoughts of imminent death were part of everyday existence. As the researchers mention at the end of the section on themes the 'people who participated in the study had survived post-transplant for up to 12 months. In contrast, others who died during or shortly after the treatment may have told different stories' (Jones & Chapman 2000, p. 158). This statement shows the relative nature of knowledge gained from qualitative research, in this case, projects influenced by phenomenological thought.

Other recent examples of nursing research using phenomenology include Borbasi (1996), Kellet (1998), Hemsley and Glass (1999) and Zeitz (1999). Sananda Hemsley and Nel Glass (1999) used a hermeneutic phenomenological approach to explore the lived experience of five nurse healers. In the analysis of the transcribed interviews it was revealed that participants described 'super presencing', responding, evolving and weaving. 'Super presencing' refers to experiences beyond the ordinary. Responding refers to the strong negative and positive ways in which others perceived the nurse healers. Evolving connotes the personal healing journey the nurse healers were on, and weaving refers to the seamlessness between healing work and nursing work.

Kathryn Zeitz (1999) used a hermeneutic-phenomenological approach to facilitate an enhanced understanding of the experience of four registered nurses who had had uncomplicated surgery at least six months prior to the unstructured interview. Nurses told their stories of receiving nursing care and the transcripts were analysed using a composite method influenced by Colaizzi (1994), Munhall (1994) and Streubert and Carpenter (1995). Ten themes 'uncovered the voice of the nurse in being in the experience of being a patient' and 'provided insight into the value of the relationship between the nurse and the patient and insight into the significance of the nature of care delivery' (Zeitz 1999, p. 64).

Ursula Kellett (1998) took an ontological hermeneutic approach to highlight the importance of family caring within a nursing home context. In-depth audiotaped conversational interviews and observation with 14 family carers who continued to care within a nursing home, revealed a sense of family life past, a sense of break, a sense of change in engaged involvement, a sense of worth, a sense of concern, and a sense of continuity. A sense of family life past 'was described in terms of valuing commitment to kin, experiencing a sense of family closeness and belonging, and recognising the importance of sharing and facing life situations together' (p. 115). A sense of break refers to facing the adaptations in experiencing the relative's transition from home to hospital. A sense of change in engaged involvement refers to ways in which carers searched 'for new possibilities in everyday caring' (p. 116). A sense of worth 'was experienced in terms of possessing special knowledge about the older relative which qualified family caregivers as experts in the care of their relative' (p. 116). A sense of concern expressed 'being out of control and not being heard' (p. 116) and a sense of continuity 'was characterised by a fear of change, a loss of continuity, and a fear of being forgotten' (p. 117), leading to the desire to pursue active involvement in the relative's care.

Sally Borbasi (1996) used van Manen's (1990) method to analyse the text of interviews with 26 patients who were asked to comment on the nurses they perceived as being more expert than others, what this nurse did that was special for them, what they looked for in advanced nurses, what expert nursing meant to them, what nurse 'busyness' meant to them, and to give one account of an instance in which a nurse did something special for them. 'There was a perception by patients of differing types of nurses, that is, of "experienced", "better", and/or "special" nurses as opposed to "lesser" ones, and a high value was placed on the advanced practice nurse' (Borbasi 1996, p. 222).

Other examples of nursing research using phenomenological approaches include Wilkes and Wallis (1993), Kermode (1995), Owen (1995), Smyth (1995), Walters (1995, 1996) and Gorman (1996).

Potential nursing research questions

Any questions which ask: 'What is the nature of ...?' and 'What is it like to experience ...?' can be considered to be research interests that may be illuminated by a phenomenological approach. This means that nurses can raise questions about the nature of nursing, in whatever practice and theory areas they choose. Nurses might also want to know about what it is like for certain people to experience various phenomena, such as patients' experiences of particular illnesses, nurses' experiences of specific clinical practices, and/or relatives' perceptions of all sorts of things related to being a loved one of someone who is ill or hospitalised. Therefore, the possibilities are many and varied for using phenomenological research in nursing.

Ethnography

Ethnographic research is derived from anthropology, and as the word 'ethnography' suggests, it seeks to provide a 'portrait of people'. The intention is to 'describe a culture through describing various cultural characteristics' (Burns & Grove 1993, p. 71). This means that an ethnographic researcher needs to spend time in the place the people of interest inhabit, so that 'on the spot' observations can be made about the ways in which they interact with one another and create their own rituals and practices in their own setting and circumstances.

The most prolific writer of all nurses publishing in the area of ethnography is Madeleine Leininger, a noted American nurse anthropologist. She defines ethnography as 'the systematic and process of observing, detailing, describing, documenting, and analysing the lifeways or particular patterns of a culture (or subculture) in order to grasp the lifeways or patterns of the people in their familiar environment' (Leininger 1985, p. 35). Ethnographic research has become so prevalent in American nursing, that it has been coined by Leininger (1985, p. 238) as ethnonursing, which 'focuses mainly on observing and documenting interactions with people of how these daily life conditions and patterns are influencing human care, health, and nursing care practices'.

The methodology

According to Leininger (1970, pp. 48–9), culture is:

> a way of life belonging to a designated group of people, a blueprint for living, which guides a particular group's thoughts, actions and sentiments, all of the accumulated ways a group of people solve problems, which are reflected in the people's language, dress, food and a number of accumulated traditions and customs.

Research into transcultural nursing can be managed well by an ethnographic approach. The Australian counterpart of Madeleine Leininger is Olga Kanitsaki, who has published widely in transcultural nursing perspectives (Kanitsaki 1988, 1989, 1992, 1993). Awarded the Order of Australia in the Australia Day Honours List in 1995 for outstanding professional leadership in the field of nursing, especially in the area of multicultural care services, Olga provides a fresh and clear view of issues and challenges faced by nurses who seek to consider transcultural aspects of their work.

Although the kind of knowledge generated from an ethnographic research approach may have particular reference to a specific group of people, it may also be informative for others. For example, in her research Kanitsaki (1989, p. 102) described the importance of family to Greek people in Australia and how 'the rituals of eating, play, work, conversation, birth, baptism, marriage, health crisis, illness, death, and so on, are family rather than individual events'. These are important insights for nurses when Greek people are admitted to their nursing care, and on a wider perspective, research findings such as this are important to alert nurses generally to the need for culturally sensitive care of all people.

The method

Ethnography has adopted two basic research approaches from anthropology, emic and etic. Behaviours are studied from within the culture in an emic approach, and behaviours are studied from outside the culture and across cultures in a wider etic approach (Burns & Grove 1993, p. 72). For example, nurse-researchers interested in describing the culture of the people interacting in a particular clinical setting would take an emic approach, whereas a comparison of American and Australian nurse education institutions would take an etic approach.

Ethnographies can vary according to the scope and nature of the research. Leininger (1985) uses the practical distinction of 'maxi' and 'mini' ethnographies, so that large, comprehensive studies, and smaller scale studies, with a narrowed focus of inquiry, can be done.

According to Burns and Grove (1993, p. 72), the steps of ethnographic research involve:

1 identifying the culture to be studied
2 identifying the significant variables within the culture
3 reviewing literature
4 gaining entrance
5 cultural immersion
6 acquiring informants
7 gathering data
8 analysing data
9 describing the culture
10 theory development.

The result of attention to these steps is a thick description of the culture of the group of people being studied, so that a deep understanding is gained of the activities and ideas that comprise the culture of that group.

Each of the steps in the method outlined above has further subsets to ensure that the process is thorough and results in the best possible accounts of culture of the group of interest. If you are interested in pursuing this kind of research, you will need to spend some time reading extra sources of information that will help you undertake ethnographic research. Some 'older yet evergreen' references to get you started include: Germain (1979), Leininger (1978; 1981; 1984; 1985) and Spradley (1980). After these, it might help to read some accounts of ethnography in more recent journal articles such as Rosenbaum (1989) and Allen (1990), and research texts such as DePoy and Gitlin (1994), LoBiondo-Wood and Haber (1994) and Streubert and Carpenter (1995). As always, it is a good idea if you are undertaking honours or postgraduate research to acquire copies of theses using the particular approach you want to use. Copies of theses may be obtained through the various universities to which they were submitted for the award.

Nursing research examples

Some nursing research projects that are ethnographic in design (Fiveash 1998) or influence (Rossiter & Yam 1998; Josipovic 2000) will now be described. Barbara Fiveash (1998) used an ethnographic approach guided by the work of Spradley (1980) to explore with eight key informants their experiences of nursing home life. Her study aimed to 'describe, interpret, understand and question the experiences of nursing home residents and ... to offer the nursing home resident an opportunity to reflect on their experiences and voice their opinions of the situation' (Fiveash 1998, p. 167).

Data were collected from two New South Wales 80-bed nursing homes that were similar in size and mix of residents. Barbara used participant observation for two hours once a week for six months, and in-depth, semi-structured, open-ended interviews with articulate residents. The selection criteria were 'their broad knowledge of the cultural experience; their ability to critically examine, express and communicate their thoughts and feelings about the experience; the rapport between the researcher and the informants; and their willingness to participate in the study' (p. 167). Key 'informants decided what was legitimate and relevant within the cultural scene' and data 'were collected and analysed simultaneously, until the context had been described and no new data informed the focus of the study' (p. 167).

According to Fiveash (p. 168) four 'themes emerged from the data: (i) against my will, (ii) living in a public domain (iii) cultural implications of living with others, and (iv) the impact of nursing home residency'. The theme of 'against my will' reflected some residents' experiences of not being involved in the decision by family members to relocate them to a nursing home, so that they felt their admissions were against their wills. 'Living in a public domain' suggested the restrictiveness of the public nature of living in a nursing home, where time is ordered and other people make decisions for you. Cultural implications of living with other sick and disabled elderly people reminded participants of 'their own inevitable decline' (p. 169). The impact of nursing home residency involved living with patients, staff and the organisational features of the home, which may be affected by cost cutting or nurses who expected residents to be subservient and compliant.

In discussing the findings of the study Fiveash (p. 171) noted that 'despite government regulation some residents still experience some of the harmful effects of institutionalisation'. She cited literature from other studies with similar findings, that elderly people experienced boredom (Gibb & O'Brien 1990); loss of contact with the outside world; enforced idleness; loneliness; staff bossiness; loss of personal friends and family possessions, independence and privileges; and physical and psychological abuse. She also referred to work by Sarantakos (1989), and to Nay's (1995) research themes of: there was no choice; everything went; devalued self; and the end of the line. The concluding words of the article (Fiveash 1998, p. 174) are:

> The findings of this study indicate that, whilst for some residents the nursing home experience is acceptable, for others the experience is both constraining and

dehumanising. The issue of lack of choice for access and lifestyle in aged care accommodation will not resolve itself spontaneously, and the voices of the articulate residents who participated in this study may well be the tip of the iceberg of consumer opinion.

Two other projects show an ethnographic influence inasmuch as they are about cultural interests, but they do not use participant observation as one of the methods (Rossiter & Yam 1998; Josipovic 2000). Although definitions of methodologies are broad in this postmodern research age, the derivation of ethnography from anthropology suggests a need to include some type of observation in data gathering.

Patricia Josipovic (2000, p. 146) based her project on a descriptive ethnographic approach to explore 'how nursing curricula can be modified to adequately incorporate transcultural nursing practices, so that nurses can meet the challenges of caring for Australia's multicultural population'. From 150 questionnaires to five educational institutions, 16 overseas-qualified registered nurses from non-English-speaking backgrounds agreed to be interviewed, all of whom participated in migrant nurses' pre-registration programs in Melbourne from 1991 to 1993, and were thus culturally and linguistically diverse (CLD). 'The findings from the questionnaire and interviews were analysed for emerging themes that linked the questionnaire and interview data with the major categories identified from the literature review' (p. 147). The thematic analysis revealed themes of the need to recognise and facilitate the importance of: language issues; cultural understanding; prior learning; communication skills; cultural adjustment; overseas nursing practice; nursing ethics and law; the status of nursing; innovations in nurse education; and government/employing institution initiatives. The researcher concluded that CLD nurses 'are a very useful resource that has been largely untapped to meet the cultural needs of multicultural patients' (p. 152).

Joh Chin Rossiter and Bernard Yam (Rossiter & Yam 1998, p. 213) used an ethnographic approach to explore 'the perceptions of nursing among the non-English-speaking background high school students in Sydney' and described 'how the nursing profession could be promoted to them'. A convenience sample of 31 students was recruited, consisting of four groups of male and female students (Years 10, 11 and 12) with parents from Lebanon, Vietnam, Korea and China. The findings from the transcribed interviews 'indicated that there is a recruitment problem in recruiting NESB (non-English speaking background) high school students into nursing', and that students with high TER scores were not contemplating studying nursing (p. 217). As Rossiter and Yam (1998, p. 217) explained, although 'some students are aware of the knowledge and skills that nurses use in clinical areas, many of them still regard nursing as a low status occupation, an adjunct to medicine, with minimal economic power and autonomy to manage nursing service'.

For further examples, you can read an abundant and easily accessible source of ethnographic research by locating the *Journal of Transcultural Nursing* in a library near you that is well stocked with American nursing journals.

Potential nursing research questions

You could use an ethnographic approach in nursing research for any instance in which you want to get to know what the culture is like within a particular group. This could be from a broad, comprehensive 'maxi' approach if you have time and resources to undertake such an initiative, or a smaller focus, to fit in with constraints of time, funding, length of research degree and so on. Broader questions for a 'maxi' ethnography may be posed about comparisons between nursing practices in different countries or clinical settings, or nursing care of specific cultural groups. 'Mini' ethnographies might frame questions about the people and practices in the culture of a ward or unit, and how they relate to nursing and health.

Remember, you do not have to undertake a project with an ethnic flavour to undertake ethnographic research. You could use this approach to study the culture of any group of people in any place, so in nursing this might be aged people in a nursing home, children in a ward, or nurses in a specialist unit. The choice is entirely up to you, if ethnography serves your research purposes, and you need close and systematic observation and description of people and their customs, symbols, rituals and habits of daily life.

Historical research

History documents the events and trends of human activity as they have taken place over time. History is a form of research, because its methods seek to discover new knowledge about what has happened in times past in relation to specific portions of time and foci of interest. Allemang (1987, p.2) contends that history is 'all that has been thought and said and come to be since human beings inhabited the planet'. This being so, there is wide and deep potential for the generation of historical knowledge.

Yuginovich (2000, p. 70) suggests that history 'is probably a stronger force than language in the moulding of social consciousness' and that it is inextricably connected with power and political systems. Interestingly, this would not be denied by skeptical postmodernists, who would argue that the immersion of history in power is one of the reasons it should be discounted as representing bias, domination and oppression (Rosenau 1992).

The methodology

Certain theoretical assumptions are forwarded as to the value of historical knowledge, including the need for the representation of historical accounts through interpretation. The retrospective nature of the documentation of history has been open to the interpretations of the historian, because 'facts, events, ideas, institutions and societal trends do not speak for themselves, but must be interpreted by a human mind hard at work trying to analyse the continuity, diversity and change involved in the complex interrelationships that characterise human history'(Ashley 1976, p. 30).

The issue of how to represent the past objectively has been a perplexing question for some historians, given that only remnants of the past exist (Iggers 1971; Dray 1978, 1980). Such clues to the past are through documents, art works and artefacts, memorabilia and the oral tradition.

Historical research and historiography are terms which are used interchangeably in nursing literature (Sorensen 1988; Sarnecky 1990; Daisy 1991). Sarnecky (1990, p. 2) claimed that 'most nurse historians define historical research from the standpoint of process', which are the ways in which the researcher 'subjectively synthesises and weaves together a diversity of facts'.

The compilation of a valid history relies on the legitimacy of its sources. The two kinds of historical sources are primary and secondary (Schafer 1980). Primary sources are provided by the original sources of the information, such as participants and observers. Secondary sources are all other accounts, once removed from participation.

According to Yuginovich (2000, p. 70) history is of political significance, as she claims that

> Against a background of an expanding and increasingly literate electorate, history has come to be seen as a unifying element in any country's political culture. To know about the past is to know that things have not always been as they are now and by implication that they need not always be as they are now. History has a social role in a society that requires an understandable past in order to learn and progress or to become whatever it is that is aimed for both on an individual as well as a national level ... does history have value as a body of independent knowledge?

In answering generally in the affirmative, she describes the form of historical research she uses as historical comparative research, 'that reconstructs what occurred from available evidence but cannot have absolute confidence in the reconstruction because it depends on the survival of accurate data from the past and must take into account the bias or contextual meaning of the original recorder of the original data' (Yuginovich 2000, p. 72).

The methods

A systematic set of steps is advocated in doing traditional historical research, fashioned on the rules and procedures of empirical science (Schafer 1980) including: defining a topic by using an hypothesis or a set of questions; locating texts and compiling a bibliography; researching other sources; analysing and compiling information; and writing a research report. The researcher decides on the appropriate means of presenting the data. The completed historical research document may appear deceptively simple to the reader, who is unaware of the painstaking work needed to create the final product of historical research. The intention is to reconstruct from primary and secondary sources, with due attention to a rigorous research process, a faithful historical account of the area of interest that can be judged to be an accurate and 'truthful' record of events over time.

Historical comparative research is a form of historical research that compares social arrangements and policies in various societies, and explores the differences (Goldstone 1998). As such, the method is useful in studying commonalities, uniqueness and long-term changes in entire social systems. Researchers using this method employ an inductive process similar to grounded theory and akin to fieldwork in that they begin with the data and analyse information to build up to theories about relationships and silences (Neuman 1994). Silences are the significant historical events that have not occurred through a repression of possibilities and people's ability to speak out about injustices (Skopcol 1995). Historical comparative research method is guided by a set of specific characteristics (Goldstone 1998) and needs to be recorded with careful attention to sequence, comparison, contingency, origins and sequences, sensitivity to incompatible meanings, limited generalisation, association, part and whole, analogy, and synthesis (Neuman 1994).

Another form of historical research is oral history, which provides 'a picture of the past in people's own words' (Robertson 1990, p. 2). Oral evidence is gathered from a primary source whose accounts act as raw historical data, that can stand alone as their own account, or be synthesised with other sources for further analysis and interpretation. The benefits of oral history include the validity of the primary oral source as the person who has lived the experiences, and the potential for the historian to cross-check interpretations with the person providing the oral history. Plummer (1983), however, notes that oral history has been viewed by some historians as marginal, suspect and trivial, because it deals with accessible people in recent times, it relies on people's accounts of the past that may be coloured by the present, and huge amounts of data may be gathered for no useful purpose.

Reflective topical autobiography is an autobiographical method that can be used by nurses to retrace the events of their lives and the sense they have made of them through reflection. Johnstone (1999, p. 24) suggests that this form of historical research 'is an important research method in its own right, and one which promises to make a substantive contribution to the overall project of advancing nursing inquiry and knowledge'. She explains that ' "re-visioning" of an original topical self-life story demonstrates the enormous creativity of the reflective topical autobiographical method' and 'leaves open to the self-researcher the opportunity to return at will to his or her life story again to re-read, re-vision and re-tell the story in the light of the new insights, understandings and interpretations of meaning acquired through ongoing lived experience' (p. 25). Such a suggestion situates reflective topical autobiography in the interpretive paradigm in a place that integrates storytelling with history. Johnstone (p. 25) cautions that when 'utilised as a research method, the aim is not to render a "true" account of the self (as some researchers subscribing to the tenets of positivistic research expect ...) but to render an account of the lived experience of self that advances shareable understanding of common human experiences'. In this aim, reflective topical autobiography contributes postmodern influences to the traditional practice of historical research (see the discussion of postmodern influences on contemporary research in this chapter).

Nursing research examples

An example of historical research (Pearson, Taylor & Coleburn 1997) is *The Nature of Nursing Work in Victoria, 1840–1870*. The researchers were interested in documenting how the nursing role evolved and was socially constructed in early Australia. The history addressed the absence of accounts of nurses between 1840 and 1870, and a lack of comparative analysis of male and female roles in nursing care in this period. In so doing, it explored some of the social, political and economic influences on the delineation of nursing work and the relevance of these factors to the relationships between hospital staff.

An example of oral history is *50 Years of Influence: An Oral History of Marjory Taylor* (Taylor 1996), which traces the life of Marjory Alice Hamlet Taylor in her own words. Born in 1920, in Corowa, New South Wales, Marjory Taylor and her family moved to Geelong, Victoria in 1925, where she was to grow up to become one of the most influential members of that community. She is known best for her role as the matron of the Geelong Hospital from 1956 to 1981. Marjory's lifetime has been devoted to humanitarian service, and the oral history of her life relates her stories of growing up in Geelong, her nurse training days, her work with the RAAF nursing service in Sydney, her work with the Red Cross as an organiser of nursing services in refugee camps in Germany from 1947 to 1950, the health and nursing care advances of the 1950s to the 1980s and her present-day social and political community activities.

Other examples of literature and historical approaches to nursing research are Russell (1990), Silins (1993) and Cushing (1995). Lynette Russell's book *From Nightingale to Now: Nurse Education in Australia* might be particularly interesting for you to read. The publishers provide a synopsis of the book by writing:

> This unique historical overview of the education of the general nurse in New South Wales and Australia is a valuable text for nursing students, other health professionals and all those with an interest in nursing history. Beginning with the introduction of the Nightingale model of nurse training in the second half of the nineteenth century, it examines the development of the hospital-based apprenticeship system of training and traces in detail the factors and events that led to the eventual transfer of nurse education into the tertiary sector' *(back cover)*

Potential nursing research questions

Any questions relating to exploring the facts, events, ideas and people's lives in history can be answered by an historical approach. In nursing, this means that the entire history of nursing is accessible though this approach. This creates incredible potential for nursing research projects, which may choose to focus on certain times in history to document the events and trends in nursing, or on specific people who have been of particular influence.

Summary

This chapter has described some qualitative interpretive research methodologies and some postmodern influences on them. It began by reminding you that research is a means of searching again for knowledge, as a basic premise on which all research is based. Generating knowledge is about using certain approaches to find information of a certain kind, which extends what is known, or says something new and different about what has been known previously. Some essential terms were defined such as epistemology and ontology, in order to clarify some common qualitative theoretical assumptions about what constitutes useful and valid knowledge.

A broad differentiation between quantitative and qualitative research approaches assigned certain assumptions to either 'camp' and the caution was sounded that these artificial distinctions are not as clear cut and poles apart as they might at first appear. For ease of definition, qualitative research methodologies were categorised into interpretive and critical forms, the latter being the focus of the next chapter. In a postmodern world, distinctions such as paradigms and methodologies may have questionable use, but they are presented here for you in your present role as a novice researcher, knowing that you have a vast body of research knowledge to work through that requires some categorisation into manageable parts for easier explanation and understanding.

Four qualitative interpretive methodologies were described in this chapter, specifically: grounded theory, phenomenology, ethnography and historical research. They were described in terms of the key ideas contained within their respective methodologies and methods. Nursing research examples and potential nursing research questions were presented to allow you to consider the possibilities of using some of these approaches in research areas you might like to explore. You need to remember that the choice is yours. There are many approaches that you might take and the decision on a particular approach may be influenced by the research questions you are asking, and how you intend to answer them.

Main points

- Epistemology is the study of knowledge and how it is judged to be 'true', and whenever nurses raise questions about what they know, and how they know it is trustworthy, they are asking epistemological questions.
- Ontology is the study of existence itself, and whenever nurses are asking about the nature of the existence of something or someone in nursing, they are asking ontological questions.
- Qualitative research attempts to explore the relative nature of knowledge, often by inductive processes, and by valuing the subjectivity of people's experiences, as being unique and context dependent.
- Postmodern ways of thinking question what knowledge (epistemology) and existence (ontology) might mean by critiquing taken-for-granted quantitative and qualitative assumptions about 'truth' and 'being'.

- Interpretive research aims mainly to generate meaning by explaining and describing, thereby gaining insights into areas of interest.
- Critical research aims to bring about change in the status quo, by working systematically through locally generated research problems to find answers and create change in light of identified constraints.
- Postmodernism does not fit into the categories of interpretive or critical qualitative research approaches, because it repudiates grand narratives and would not be seen as one itself; however, it is important for nurse-researchers as it encourages deconstruction that emphasises relativism, diversity, difference, contradiction and everyday ordinary history told in people's narratives and interpreted by them as their self-understandings.
- Grounded theory starts from the 'ground' of an area of human interest and works up in an inductive fashion to make sense of what people say about their experiences, and to convert these statements into theoretical propositions.
- Phenomenology ('phenomen - ology') is the 'study of things' within human existence, by discovering, exploring and describing the essence of phenomena through attending towards them directly.
- Ethnography provides a 'portrait of people' by describing and raising awareness of a group of people's cultural characteristics, such as their shared symbols, beliefs, values, rituals and patterns of behaviour.
- Historical research reconstructs from primary and secondary sources (with due attention to a rigorous research process) an accurate and 'truthful' record of events over time, thereby amending previous knowledge and discovering new knowledge in relation to specific portions of time and foci of interest.

Review Questions

1. The study of knowledge and how it is judged to be 'true' is:
   a. ontology
   b. epistemology
   c. philosophy
   d. scientology

2. Qualitative research questions are:
   a. tested empirico-analytically
   b. analysed using numbers
   c. left open as tentative ideas
   d. interpreted as mathematical relations

3. Qualitative research findings:
   a. provide insights to possibilities
   b. need to be significant statistically
   c. claim to be generalisable
   d. can be predictive

4   Qualitative interpretive methodologies aim mainly to:
    a   enable emancipation
    b   generate meaning
    c   predict outcomes
    d   permit generalisation

5   An example of a qualitative interpretive methodology is:
    a   critical ethnography
    b   grounded theory
    c   action research
    d   feminist research

6   Grounded theory gets its name because it:
    a   starts from the ground ideas and works up inductively
    b   is grounded in the scientific method and is deductive
    c   starts from the ground ideas and works up deductively
    d   is grounded in the critical paradigm and emancipation

7   The researchers who coined the term 'grounded theory' are:
    a   Polit and Hungler
    b   Glaser and Strauss
    c   Roberts and Taylor
    d   LoBiondo-Wood and Haber

8   In phenomenology, the knowledge people have of things of interest, because they have experienced them through daily activities, is:
    a   bracketing
    b   Being-in-the-world
    c   understanding
    d   lived experience

9   Ethnography means a:
    a   portrait of people
    b   critique of ethnicity
    c   study of ethics
    d   survey of minorities

10 Data collection for historical research includes:
    a   surveys and questionnaires
    b   double blind trials
    c   structured interviews
    d   primary sources

Discussion Questions

1. Discuss the relationship between epistemology, ontology and research.
2. What are the main theoretical assumptions about knowledge generation and validation in qualitative research approaches?
3. Describe postmodern influences on contemporary epistemology and ontology.
4. Differentiate between interpretive and critical forms of qualitative methodologies.
5. Name four qualitative interpretive methodologies and describe for each one example of a nursing research project.

References

Allemang, M. M. 1987, 'Oral historiography', *Recent Advances in Nursing*, vol. 17, 2–11.

Allen, J. D. 1990, 'Focussing on living not dying: a naturalistic study of self-care among seropositive gay men', *Holistic Nursing Practice*, vol. 4, no. 2, 56–63.

Armitage, S. K. & Kavanagh, K. M. 1995, 'Continuity of care: discharge planning and community nurses', *Contemporary Nurse*, vol. 4, no. 4, 148–55.

Ashley, J. 1976, *Hospital Paternalism and the Role of the Nurse*, Teachers College Press, New York.

Barclay, L., Donovan, J. & Genovese, A. 1996, 'Men's experiences during their partner's first pregnancy: a grounded theory analysis', *Australian Journal of Advanced Nursing*, vol. 13, no. 3, 12–24.

Barnes, J. 1987, *Early Greek Philosophers*, Penguin Books, London.

Borbasi, S. 1996, 'Living the experience of being nursed', *International Journal of Nursing Practice*, vol. 2, 222–8.

Brennan, C. & Stevens, J. 1998, 'A grounded theory approach towards understanding the self perceived effects of meditation on people being treated for cancer', *Australian Journal of Holistic Nursing*, vol. 5, no. 2, 20–6.

Bull, R. & Hart, G. 1995, 'Clinical nurse specialist: walking the wire', *Contemporary Nurse*, vol. 4, no. 1, 25–32.

Burns, S. & Grove, N. 1993, *The Practice of Nursing Research: Conduct, Critique and Utilisation*, W. B. Saunders Company, Philadelphia.

Carper, B. 1992, 'Fundamental patterns of knowing in nursing', in *Perspectives on Nursing Theory*, 2nd edn, vol. 1, ed. L. Nicholl, J. B. Lippincott Co., Philadelphia.

Chinn, P. & Kramer, M. 1995, *Theory and Nursing: A Systematic Approach*, 4th edn, Mosby Year Book, St Louis.

Colaizzi, P. 1978, 'Psychological research as the phenomenologist views it', in *Existential Phenomenological Alternatives for Psychology*, eds R. S. Valle & M. King, Oxford University Press, New York.

Colaizzi, P. 1994, 'Psychological research as the phenomenologist views it', in *Existential Phenomenological Alternatives for Psychology*, eds R. S. Valle & M. King, Oxford University Press, New York.

Corbin, J. 1986, 'Qualitative data analysis for grounded theory', in *From Practice to Grounded Theory*, eds W. C. Chenitz & J. M. Swanson, Addison Wesley, Menlo Park, California.

Cushing, A. 1995, 'An historical note on the relationship between nursing and nursing history', *International Journal of Nursing History*, vol. 1, no. 1, 57–60.
Daisy, C. 1991, 'Searching for Annie Goodrich', *Western Journal of Nursing Research*, vol. 13, no. 3, 408–13.
DePoy, E. & Gitlin, L. 1994, *Introduction to Research: Multiple Strategies for Health and Human Services*, Mosby, St Louis.
Descartes, R. 1970, *The Philosophical Works of Descartes*, translated and edited by E. S. Haldane & G. R. T. Ross, The Cambridge University Press, Cambridge, UK.
Dray, W. 1978, 'Point of view in history', *Clio*, vol. 7, 265–83.
Dray, W. 1980, *Perspectives on History*, Routledge & Kegan Paul, London.
Dreyfus, H. L. 1991, *Being-in-the-world: A Commentary on Heidegger's Being and Time, Division 1*, The MIT Press, Cambridge, Massachusetts.
Fiveash, B. 1998, 'The experience of nursing home life', *International Journal of Nursing Practice*, vol. 4, 166–74.
Gadamer, H.-G. 1975 trans., in *Truth and Method*, eds G. Barden & J. Cumming, Seabury, New York.
Gadamer, H.-G. 1976, 'The universality of the hermeneutical problem', in *Philosophical Hermeneutics*, translated and edited by D. E. Linge, University of California Press, Berkeley, California.
Germain, C. P. 1979, *The Cancer Unit: an Ethnography*, Nursing Resources, Wakefield.
Gibb, H. & O'Brien, B. 1990, 'Jokes and reassurance are not enough: ways in which nurses relate through conversation with elderly clients', *Journal of Advanced Nursing*, vol. 15, no. 1, 1389–401.
Giorgi, A., Fischer, C. L. & Murray, E. L. 1975, *Duquesne Studies in Phenomenological Psychology*, Duquesne University Press, Pittsburgh.
Glaser, B. & Strauss, A. 1967, *The Discovery of Grounded Theory: Strategies for Qualitative Research*, Aldine, Chicago.
Goldstone, J. 1998, *Sociology and History: Producing Comparative History*, Working Papers in Economic History No. 108, Australian National University, Canberra.
Gorman, L. 1996, 'I'm on edge all the time: residents' experiences of living in an integrated home', *Australian Journal of Advanced Nursing*, vol. 13, no. 3, 7–11.
Hawley, G. & Irurita, V. 1998, 'Seeking comfort through prayer', *International Journal of Nursing Practice*, vol. 4, 9–18.
Heidegger, M. 1962, *Being and Time*, Harper & Row, New York.
Hekman, S. J. 1986, *Hermeneutics and the Sociology of Knowledge*, Polity Press, Cambridge, Massachusetts.
Hemsley, S. & Glass, N. 1999, 'Nurse healers: exploring their lived experience as nurses', *Australian Journal of Holistic Nursing*, vol. 6, no. 2, 28–34.
Hume, D. 1966, *An Enquiry Concerning the Principles of Morals*, reprinted from the edition of 1777, Open Court Publishing Company, La Salle, Illinois.
Hume, D. 1969 (first published 1739), *A Treatise of Human Nature*, Penguin Books, London.
Husserl, E. 1960 trans., *Cartesian Meditations: An Introduction to Phenomenology*, Martinus Nijhoff, The Hague.
Husserl, E. 1964 trans., *The Idea of Phenomenology*, Martinus Nijhoff, The Hague.
Husserl, E. 1965 trans., *Phenomenology and the Crisis of Philosophy*, Harper & Row, New York.
Husserl, E. 1970, *The Crisis of the European Sciences and Transcendental Phenomenology*, Northwestern University Press, Evanston, Illinois.
Husserl, E. 1980 trans., *Phenomenology and the Foundations of the Sciences*, Martinus Nijhoff, The Hague.

Hutchinson, S. A. 1986, 'Chemically dependent nurses; the trajectory towards self annihilation', *Nursing Research*, vol. 35, no. 4, 196–201.

Iggers, F. 1971, 'The new historiography in historical perspective', *Australian Journal of Politics and History*, vol. 17, 44–55.

Irurita, V. 1992, 'Transforming mediocrity to excellence: a challenge for nurse leaders', *Australian Journal of Advanced Nursing*, vol. 9, no. 4, 15–25.

Irurita, V. 1999a, 'Factors affecting the quality of nursing care: the patient's perspective', *International Journal of Nursing Practice*, vol. 5, 86–94.

Irurita, V. 1999b, 'The problem of patient vulnerability', *Collegian*, vol. 6, no. 1, 10–15.

Johnstone, M.-J. 1999, 'Reflective topical autobiography: an underutilised interpretive research method in nursing', *Collegian*, vol. 6, no. 1, 24–9.

Jones, C. & Chapman, Y. 2000, 'The lived experience of seven people treated with autologous bone marrow/peripheral blood stem cell transplant', *International Journal of Nursing Practice*, vol. 6, 153–9.

Josipovic, P. 2000, 'Recommendations for culturally sensitive nursing care', *International Journal of Nursing Practice*, vol. 6, 146–52.

Kanitsaki, O. 1988, 'Transcultural nursing: challenge to change', *Australian Journal of Advanced Nursing*, vol. 5, no. 3, 4–11.

Kanitsaki, O. 1989, 'Cross cultural sensitivity in palliative care', in *The Creative Option of Palliative Care*, eds P. Hodder & A. Turley, Melbourne City Mission, Melbourne.

Kanitsaki, O. 1992, *Transcultural Nursing: a Teaching Package for Lecturers*, La Trobe University, School of Health Sciences, Department of Nursing, Melbourne.

Kanitsaki, O. 1993, 'Transcultural human care: its challenge to and critique of professional nursing care', in *A Global Agenda for Caring*, ed. D. A. Gaut, National League for Nursing Press, New York.

Kellett, U. 1998, 'Meaning-making for family carers in nursing homes', *International Journal of Nursing Practice*, vol. 4, 113–19.

Kermode, M. 1995, 'Patients' experiences of nursing interventions during hospitalisation with an AIDS defining illness', *Australian Journal of Advanced Nursing*, vol. 12, no. 3, 20–30.

Kockelmans, J. J. (ed.) 1967, *Phenomenology: the Philosophy of Edmund Husserl and its Interpretation*, Anchor Books, Doubleday & Co., Garden City, New York.

Krell, D. F. 1977, *Martin Heidegger: Basic Writings*, Harper & Row, New York.

Langveld, M. J. 1978, 'The stillness of the secret place', *Phenomenology and Pedagogy*, vol. 1, no. 1, 181–9.

Leininger, M. 1970, *Nursing and Anthropology: Two Worlds to Blend*, John Wiley & Sons, New York.

Leininger, M. 1978, *Transcultural Nursing: Concepts, Theories and Practices*, John Wiley & Sons, New York.

Leininger, M. 1981, *Caring: An Essential Human Need*, Charles B Slack, Thorofare, New Jersey.

Leininger, M. 1984, Reference Sources for Transcultural Health and Nursing, Charles B Slack, Thorofare, New Jersey.

Leininger, M. 1985, *Qualitative Research Methods in Nursing*, Grune and Stratton, New York.

LoBiondo-Wood, G. & Haber, J. 1994, *Nursing Research: Methods, Critical Appraisal, and Utilisation*, Mosby, St Louis.

McCabe, P. 1995, 'Exploring the phenomenon of healing: healing as a health capacity', *Australian Journal of Holistic Nursing*, vol. 2, no. 1, 13–24.

Morris, M. 1977, *An Excursion into Creative Sociology*, Columbia University Press, New York.

Muir-Cochrane, E. 1995, 'An exploration of ethical issues associated with the seclusion of psychiatric patients', *Collegian*, vol. 2, no. 3, 14–20.

Munhall, P. 1994, *Revisioning Phenomenology: Nursing and Health Science Research*, National League for Nursing Press, New York.
Nay, R. 1995, 'Nursing home residents' perception of relocation', *Journal of Clinical Nursing*, vol. 4, 319–25.
Neuman, W. 1994, *Social Research Methods: Qualitative and Quantitative Approaches*, 2nd edn, Allyn and Bacon, Boston.
Owen, M. 1995, 'Challenges to caring: nurses' interpretations of holism', *Australian Journal of Holistic Nursing*, vol. 2, no. 2, 4–14.
Palmer, D. 1988, *Looking at Philosophy: the Unbearable Heaviness of Philosophy Made Lighter*, Mayfield Publishing Co., Mountain View, California.
Patton, M. G. 1980, *Qualitative Evaluation Methods*, Sage Publications, Beverly Hills, California.
Pearson, A., Taylor, B. & Coleburn, C. 1997, *The Nature of Nursing Work in Victoria, 1840–1870*, Deakin University Press, Geelong, Victoria.
Plummer, K. 1983, *Documents of Life: An Introduction to the Problems and Literature of a Humanistic Method*, George Allen & Unwin, London.
Polit, D. & Hungler, B. 1995, *Nursing Research, Principles and Methods*, 5th edn, Lippincott, Philadelphia.
Psathas, G. 1973, *Phenomenological Sociology: Issues and Applications*, John Wiley & Sons, New York.
Qualitative Solutions and Research 1995, NUD*IST (Non-Numerical Unstructured Data: Indexing Searching & Theorising), application software package, QSR, Melbourne.
Robertson, B. M. 1990, *Guide to Oral History*, 2nd edn, Oral History Association of Australia (South Australian Branch), Adelaide.
Robrecht, L. C. 1995, 'Grounded theory: evolving methods', *Qualitative Health Research*, vol. 5, no. 2, 169–77.
Rosenau, P. 1992, *Post-Modernism and the Social Sciences: Insights, Inroads and Intrusions*, Princeton University Press, New Jersey.
Rosenbaum, J. N. 1989, 'Depression: viewed from a transcultural nursing theoretical perspective', *Journal of Advanced Nursing*, vol. 14, no. 1, 7–12.
Rossiter, J. & Yam, B. 1998, 'Promoting the nursing profession: the perceptions of non-English-speaking background high school students in Sydney, Australia', *International Journal of Nursing Practice*, vol. 4, 213–19.
Russell, R. L. 1990, *From Nightingale to Now: Nurse Education in Australia*, Harcourt Brace Jovanovich, Sydney.
Sandelowski, M. 1986, 'The problem of rigour in qualitative research', *Advances in Nursing Science*, vol. 8, no. 3, 27–37.
Sarantakos, S. 1989, *For a Caring Care*, Kean Publications, Sydney.
Sarnecky, M. T. 1990, 'Historiography: a legitimate research methodology for nursing', *Advances in Nursing Science*, vol. 12, no. 4, 1–10.
Schafer, R. J. 1980, *A Guide to Historical Method*, The Dorsey Press, Homewood, Illinois.
Schwartz, H. & Jacobs, J. 1979, *Qualitative Sociology: A Method to the Madness*, The Free Press, New York.
Silins, E. 1993, 'Looking back by listening: reflections on an oral history', *Contemporary Nurse*, vol. 2, no. 2, 79–82.
Skopcol, T. 1995, *Social Revolutions in the Modern World*, Cambridge University Press, New York.
Smyth, D. 1995, 'Healing through nursing: the lived experience of therapeutic touch, Part One', *Australian Journal of Holistic Nursing*, vol. 3, no. 1, 15–25.
Sorensen, E. S. 1988, 'Archives as sources of treasure in historical research', *Western Journal of Nursing Research*, vol. 10, no. 5, 666–70.

Spiegelberg, H. 1970, 'On some human uses of phenomenology', in *Phenomenology in Perspective*, ed. F. J. Smith, Martinus Nijhoff, The Hague.

Spiegelberg, H. 1976, *The Phenomenological Movement* (vols 1 and 2), Martinus Nijhoff, The Hague.

Spradley, J. P. 1979, *The Ethnographic Interview*, Holt, Rinehart & Winston, New York.

Spradley, J. P. 1980, *Participant Observation*, Holt, Rinehart & Winston, New York.

St John, W. 1999, 'Beyond the sick role: situating community health nursing practice', *Collegian*, vol. 6, no. 1, 30–5.

Stern, P. M. 1985, 'Using grounded theory method in nursing research', in *Qualitative Research in Nursing*, ed. M. M. Leininger, Grune & Stratton, New York.

Streubert, H. J. & Carpenter, D. R. 1995, *Qualitative Nursing Research: Advancing the Humanistic Imperative*, J B Lippincott Co., Philadelphia.

Swanson, J. M. 1986, 'The formal qualitative interview for grounded theory', in *From Practice to Grounded Theory*, eds W. C. Chenitz & J. M. Swanson, Addison Wesley, Menlo Park, California.

Taylor, B. 1994, *Being Human: Ordinariness in Nursing*, Churchill Livingstone, Melbourne.

Taylor, B. 1995, *Qualitative Research Data: What it can Offer Women's Health Centres*, Centre for Professional Development in Health Sciences, Southern Cross University, Lismore, NSW.

Taylor, B. 1996, *50 Years of Influence: an Oral History of Marjory Taylor*, Centre for Professional Development in Health Sciences, Southern Cross University, Lismore, NSW.

Taylor, B. 2000, *Being Human: Ordinariness in Nursing* (adapted), Southern Cross University Press, Lismore, NSW.

Van Kaam, A. L. 1959, 'The nurse in the patient's world', *American Journal of Nursing*, vol. 59, no. 12, 1708–10.

van Manen, M. 1990, 'Beyond assumptions: shifting the limits of action research', *Theory into Practice*, vol. 29, no. 3, 152–7.

Walters, J. 1995, 'The lifeworld of relatives of critically ill patients: a phenomenological hermeneutic study', *International Journal of Nursing Practice*, vol. 1, no. 1, 18–25.

Walters, J. 1996, 'Being a nurse consultant: a hermeneutic phenomenological reflection', *International Journal of Nursing Practice*, vol. 2, no. 1, 2–10.

Watt, E. 1997, 'An exploration of the way in which the concept of patient advocacy is perceived by registered nurses working in an acute care hospital', *International Journal of Nursing Practice*, vol. 3, 119–27.

Wilkes, L. & Wallis, M. 1993, 'The five c's of caring: the lived experiences of student nurses', *Australian Journal of Advanced Nursing*, vol. 11, no. 1, 19–25.

Wilson, H. S. 1993, *Introducing Research in Nursing*, Addison-Wesley Nursing, Menlo Park, California.

Yuginovich, T. 2000, 'More than time and place: using historical comparative research as a tool for nursing', *International Journal of Nursing Practice*, vol. 6, 70–5.

Zeitz, K. 1999, 'Nurses as patients: the voyage of discovery', *International Journal of Nursing Practice*, vol. 5, 64–71.

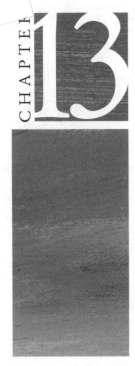

Qualitative critical methodologies

chapter objectives The material presented in this chapter will assist you to:

- clarify some common qualitative theoretical assumptions about the importance of critical research approaches
- differentiate between critical methodologies, poststructuralism and postmodernism
- define key terms associated with critical methodologies, such as empowerment, emancipation, hegemony and praxis
- describe through methodology, methods and nursing research examples, three forms of qualitative critical methodologies – action research, feminism, and critical ethnography
- generate potential nursing research questions using these approaches
- define key terms associated with postmodern thought
- describe nursing research discourse reflecting postmodern influences.

Introduction

This chapter deals with qualitative research methodologies that have social change as their 'up-front agenda' and some postmodern thought that aligns with this aim. Whereas qualitative interpretive methodologies may bring about change as a consequence of raising awareness of social and political issues, critical methodologies begin with the stated objective of questioning the status quo in order to improve things for the better. Therefore, critical research approaches have greater potential to address social and political issues in human life than interpretive approaches, which aim mainly to explore and describe.

In nursing, this means that critical approaches can address the power imbalances in nursing conditions, relationships and organisations, and turn upside down some taken-for-granted assumptions about the way things are, and the way they need to be. This is a crucial point to remember in working your way through this chapter. Many of the circumstances in which nurses now find themselves can be attributed to events and influences over time. Due to the often subtle historical changes in the events inside and outside nursing practice, nurses may develop ideas that they cannot change their work conditions and relationships, and that little can be done about the social and political injustices they face as part of their practice.

Although not intended to be a precise placement, for the sake of seeing where it fits in the scheme of methodologies, we can imagine that poststructuralism comes in between critical social science and postmodernism. Following on from the work of Habermas, other philosophers, especially Foucault (1990), reconceptualised key epistemological ideas such as power and knowledge, taking different viewpoints from critical social theorists. Some of these ideas are discussed later in this chapter and in Chapter 16.

Postmodernism reaches into all areas of life, including nursing, and nurse-researchers can benefit from being aware of some postmodern ideas, even though sorting through and making sense of the masses of literature may be difficult. Rosenau (1992) is an author who has made the reading of postmodern thought easier for newcomers to the area, by her description of skeptical and affirmative forms. Skeptical postmodernism offers 'a pessimistic, gloomy assessment' and it argues that the postmodern 'age is one of fragmentation, disintegration, malaise, meaninglessness, a vagueness or even absence of moral parameters and societal chaos' (Rosenau 1992, p. 15). Such a position leaves little room for systematic inquiry through research. In contrast, affirmative postmodernists 'have a more hopeful, optimistic view' of the postmodern age (Rosenau 1992, p. 15).

Researchers reflecting affirmative postmodern influences might agree in part with research approaches represented in this book as qualitative critical methodologies inasmuch as they repudiate social constructions of power and domination. While espousing postmodern ideas, affirmative postmodernists may nevertheless be uncomfortable with extreme objectivity or relativism that requires an uninvolved and 'anything goes' attitude to questions of human knowledge and existence. For example, feminist postmodernists agree that men have had privileged status, but they are critical of not giving special authority to women's voices (Fahy 1997; Glass & Davis 1998). Therefore, researchers reconciling their need to maintain a political consciousness for minority groups can choose a collection of methods influenced by affirmative postmodern thinking.

Common qualitative critical theoretical assumptions

In Chapter 12 you were introduced to the differences in interpretive and critical qualitative methodologies and some postmodern influences on them; the differences seem to be in knowledge-producing intentions. Whereas interpretive approaches aim mainly to generate descriptions and meaning, critical methodologies aim to address and change conscious and unconscious oppression and inequities in the status quo.

Critical methodologies are derived from some key ideas in critical social science, which emerged from the critical theory perspectives of the Frankfurt School of philosophers, who were intent on finding ways to improve social life after the defeat of left-wing working class movements during the First World War (Stevens 1989). Early critical theorists of the 1920s, such as Horkheimer, Adorno and Marcuse, were also concerned with the dominance of positivistic science and the tendency to dismiss as unnecessary the questions of reason, which had been the long epistemological tradition of philosophers. The critical theorists reacted against the taken-for-grantedness of the supremacy of the empirical-analytical paradigm and its apparent inability to quell the rising unrest in world affairs.

The concern of the critical theorists was that science was being applied to human understanding with little appeal to social conscience. Objective facts, techniques and scientific rule-following had taken over subjective knowing, critical thinking and reason. The critical theorists considered that the ideology of science was tantamount to the ideology of the aggressors who were sweeping over Europe in the name of progress. Thus, critical social science was born out of reaction to social need as well as to epistemological dilemmas.

Some of the basic ideas of that time were that people need to feel, or be assisted to feel, the effects of oppression and sincerely desire liberation. They must be able to see and understand their history and effects of their false consciousness and realise that there are alternative ways of knowing and being. There must be a social crisis, which causes dissatisfaction and threatens the social cohesion of the group. The social crisis is illuminated through an historical account of the members of the group and the structural bases of the society. The accounts will bring enlightenment and the possibility of social transformation.

The criticism levelled against critical theory has been in relation to its idealism, in that the high aspirations of critical theorists have generally not been realised in relation to securing equity for oppressed groups. The powerful still tend to flourish, even in the centre of the most stringent reasoned reflection and critique. A postmodern criticism has been that politics intended to 'free the masses' is often reduced to superficiality by candidates in public office, rendering their representation unauthentic (Baudrillard 1983). However, it has been claimed that sociopolitical and cultural critiques, when effective, can have local effects and can bring changes over time (Culbertson 1981).

Essentially, the kind of knowledge that critical methodologies generate has the potential to be emancipatory; that is, it can free people from the conditions in which they are entrenched to something that can be better for them. The need for emancipation comes from the assumption that certain people may suffer oppression and constraints of some kind at the hands of other people, and through the effects of the historical, social, political, cultural and economic circumstances in which they find themselves. Freedom from oppression comes from being aware that it is happening and in finding the motivation and means to do something about it.

Critical social science is of the view that collective social action can be successful in recognising and dealing with oppressive relationships, systems and conditions. Therefore, the critical research methodologies derived from critical social science apply to research that adopts this assumption about the nature and effects of power in human relationships. Critical research activity can be geared directly and strategically towards freeing people from forces and agents that cause human oppression and domination.

Invariably, critical methodologies involve research methods that encourage people to come together to share collaboratively, to bring forward their personal and collective concerns and to make group efforts for changes through their research efforts. The intention is to decrease possible power differences between researcher and participants so that the people in the group take on co-researcher identities, thus attempting to own more equally their research problems, processes and outcomes.

Critical methodologies compared with poststructuralism

Following on from, and in response to, the limitations of the descriptive potential of interpretive qualitative methodologies, critical methodologies have taken on a change agenda through enlightenment, emancipation and empowerment. Beyond these still, lies poststructuralism, which focuses on discourses and discursive practices constituting power relations and knowledge.

For example, critical social theorists analyse powerful cultural forces and the patterns of domination that maintain them, in order to free less powerful people from their false consciousness about the hegemonic nature of their oppression (Giroux 1983; Fay 1987). The implications in this noble intention to emancipate are that people *are* oppressed and, relatively equally, the emancipator is sufficiently informed of the levels of the false consciousness of the people to be able to free the oppressed, and that the emancipation will be to more favourable conditions devoid of other more subtle forces of domination. With these and other critiques in mind, recent critical theorists have moderated their grand claims for enlightenment, empowerment and emancipation, to 'redress injustices of race, class, ethnicity, gender, sexual preferences, age, and ability' (Best & Kellner 1991; Giroux 1992; Mohanty 1994; Jordan & Weedon 1995; in Manias & Street 2000, p. 51).

Poststructuralists reject the idea that power is possessed as a source of domination over other people; rather authors such as Foucault (1990) contend that power is exercised and it operates in all directions, not just 'from the top down'. As power is not possessed, it cannot be given to someone else in an act of empowerment and emancipation; thus empowerment needs to be 'context-specific and based on the micropractices of a particular setting' (Gore 1992, cited in Manias & Street 2000, p. 54).

Poststructuralism compared with postmodern thought

Poststructuralism and postmodernism are in some ways similar and authors have tended to use the terms synonymously, but this is not strictly correct. Rosenau (1992, p. 3) explains that

> Most of what is written ... with reference to post-modernism also applies to post-structuralism. Although the two are not identical they overlap considerably and are sometimes considered synonymous. Few efforts have been made to distinguish between the two, probably because the differences appear to be of little consequence ... As I see it the major difference is one of emphasis more than substance: Post-modernists are more oriented toward cultural critique while the post-structuralists emphasise method and epistemological matters. For example, post-structuralists concentrate on deconstruction, language, discourse, meaning, and symbols while post-modernists cast a wider net. There also seems to be an emerging difference in the status of subject and object ... The post-structuralists remain uncompromisingly anti-empirical whereas the post-modernists focus on the concrete in the form of 'le quotidien', daily life, as an alternative to theory.

Bearing in mind that postmodernism 'is stimulating and fascinating; and at the same time it is always on the brink of collapsing into confusion' (Rosenau 1992, p. 14), it is important to realise that postmodernism is derived from many '-isms' creating divergent and contradictory forms reflecting partially their theoretical roots. For example, using the qualitative methodologies in this book as a case in point, some versions of postmodernism have sprung from the work of Nietzsche and Heidegger, connected here to qualitative interpretive research, and other forms of postmodernism can be traced to the critical theorists Horkheimer and Adorno, connected here to qualitative critical research. As a consequence, postmodernism adopts the views of critical theory to suspect the validity 'of instrumental reason, modern technology, and the role of the media in a modern consumer society' (Rosenau 1992, p. 13).

Even given the historical connections to forms of knowledge named in this book as being foundational to qualitative interpretive and critical research methodologies, you need to remember that for many postmodernists, methodologies constitute in *varying degrees* grand or meta (master) narratives 'that claim to be scientific and objective, that serve to legitimate modernity and assume justice, truth, theory, hegemony' (Rosenau 1992, p. 85). The qualification of *varying degrees* lies in the opposition of qualitative interpretive research to the absolute nature of the rules of the scientific method and objectivity, and the claims critical research methodologies make in fostering processes that oppose hegemony. In so doing, however, both the qualitative interpretive research methodologies and the critical research methodologies assume some authority in addressing issues of justice, truth and theory, and thus run counter to some postmodern thinking.

What does this mean for nurses who choose to adopt postmodern thinking in their projects? Cheek (2000) argues that postmodern approaches can be used in nursing research. She suggests that, in keeping with postmodern thought, Foucault's perspectives of discourse, gaze and governmentality in relation to power (Foucault 1990) can be particularly helpful in exploring and analysing health care practices. If you are interested in what this means for your project, read more about Foucault's perspectives and how Cheek (2000) has applied these ideas in her own research. It is important to remember, however, that there are no prescriptive approaches and that research influenced by postmodern thinking should not be a 'case of attempting to replace one grand narrative with another' (Cheek 2000, p. 124).

In the absence of standard 'strategies' or 'struggles' (methods), researchers can enlist ideas derived from various sources, such as the approaches taken by Fahy (1997), Glass and Davis (1998) and Hall (1999). All of these authors combine concepts in critical theory, such as liberation and emancipation, with selected postmodern ideas. Some work of these authors is presented later in this chapter.

Defining critical terms

When you are reading literature that deals with critical methodologies you may find that certain words recur. In this section four common words will be defined so that you can recognise them readily and understand how they fit into your study of critical research approaches.

Empowerment is the process of giving and accepting power. In critical research this means that the research processes are geared towards helping people to find their own power as a means to liberate them from their oppressive circumstances and understandings of themselves in those circumstances. Empowerment for nurses may come about when they have worked through a radical critique of their personal and professional roles and conditions and they have liberated themselves to other possibilities.

Emancipation is freedom, and it implies that one is free *from* something and free *to* something. Critical research methodologies claim to be helpful in emancipating research participants from their present conditions to something better. Emancipation for nurses, therefore, can mean that they experience freedom from standardised expectations and roles, and have freedom to embrace knowledgeable, creative and intuitive practice.

Hegemony means ascendancy or domination of one power over another. In a critical social science interpretation, hegemony refers to the ways in which some social systems and the people in them give the impression that they are unassailable, and that the conditions they have produced are not only good, but also appropriate for the people over whom they have control. In nursing, this might mean that nurses come to think that the hospital bureaucracy is not only necessary, but also conducive to their welfare, and that the oppressive elements within it, such as dominating relationships and difficult work conditions, cannot and should not be changed. Thus hegemony would have nurses believe that they can do little to change their work lives.

Praxis is change through critical reflection on practice. You may find that it is easy to think of praxis as change in action, because of deliberate and systematic reflection. Praxis in nursing means change through reflection on practice, therefore praxis in critical research is collaborative processes that work with research participants to bring about change.

You may notice that the words to which you have just been introduced convey fairly familiar concepts, now you know what they mean. You may also notice that many of the ideas merge, so that they relate closely to one another and combine to bring about a common message, which is that change allowing freedom from relatively enduring oppressive forces is possible through collective social action and research activities. If you are interested in these theoretical assumptions underlying critical methodologies in nursing, you might like to read further (Dzurec 1989; Stevens 1989; Ray 1992).

Even though there has been a progression of thought in nursing research in response to philosophical debates, this does not mean that all of the methodologies that went before poststructuralism and postmodernism are eradicated, inappropriate or not useful. If that were so, there would be no use for this book, and you would be caught in a philosophical 'straitjacket' that would take away your choices. Whereas you need to remain aware of the recent epistemological critiques and trends, you can still exercise your rights as a researcher to choose any approach that may be useful for the kinds of questions you are asking and the aims and objectives you have set for your project. In other words, there is no escaping the 'fact' that if you are to do research you need to be proactive as the 'author' of the project, even in thinking up the ideas and setting the project into train, regardless of any recent philosophical thinking by which you may be influenced. With this in mind, we explore examples of qualitative critical methodologies including action research, feminisms and critical ethnography. In the section that follows, each of these approaches will be described in terms of its specific methodological assumptions and methods. Nursing research examples for each methodology will be given and you will be encouraged to generate your own potential nursing research questions using respective approaches.

Action research

As with the history of critical theory, action research grew out of the effects of a war, in this case, the Second World War (Chein, Cook & Harding 1948), and it had a social change agenda. Kurt Lewin (1946) first used the term 'action research' and in the mid 1940s he used group research process for community projects in postwar America. Lewin's work is the basis of contemporary versions of action research including those forwarded by Australian educationalists such as Carr and Kemmis (1986) and Kemmis and McTaggart (1988).

As you might expect action research goes to the site of the concern or practice, and works with the people there as co-researchers to generate solutions to the problems with which they are keen to deal. This form of research involves action which is directed to showing the problems in the present situation then facilitating improvements and sustaining changes.

The methodology

Most of the theoretical assumptions underlying action research can be traced to critical theory. McTaggart (1991, p. 25) makes the point that 'many authors in both Europe and Australia have used the theory of knowledge-constitutive interests proposed by the German critical theorist Jurgen Habermas (1972, 1973) to describe three different forms of action research: technical, practical and emancipatory'.

Technical action research aims to improve techniques and procedures by having practitioners work collaboratively to test the applicability of results generated elsewhere. In nursing, this could mean that a group of nurses might work together to research the effects of a new aseptic dressing procedure to ascertain its benefits.

Practical action research aims to improve existing practices and to develop new ones. The emphasis here is on reflecting and interpreting to take deliberate strategic action. A nursing example might be that nurses decide to work together to look at the patterns of communication and interpersonal relationships in their ward and how these patterns might be improved to facilitate more effective nursing care.

Emancipatory action research involves a group of practitioners taking responsibility for freeing themselves from the constraints of their practice through understanding and transforming the political, social and economic conditions that keep them from doing their work as they would ideally choose. In nursing, this might mean that nurses would meet to consider and work on all of the factors within their work settings that stop them from giving effective nursing care. They would then work towards changing the constraints by working within and through the influential sources in the system.

The method

Nurses conversant with the Nursing Process (Wilkinson 1992) may see some similarities in action research, in that it takes a problem-solving approach, to assess, plan and implement ideas as part of a systematic approach to reflection on research issues. The method of action research involves four stages of collectively planning, acting, observing and reflecting (Dick 1995; Stringer 1996). This phase leads to another cycle of action, in which the plan is revised, and further acting, observing and reflecting is undertaken systematically to work towards solutions to problems of a technical, practical or emancipatory nature (Kemmis & McTaggart 1988).

If you are thinking of undertaking action research, you would need to find other nurses who are willing to work together over time on collective problems. The group would need to understand some basic principles of action research in terms of its intention to change existing conditions to make them better. Members of the group would also need to be willing to share the workload and responsibilities of the research project and assist one another to create a co-researcher process.

Having established the working rules of the group, attention would need to be given to maintaining the group processes, so that they continued to be facilitative and focused on the problems at hand. Cycles of action research could lead to further foci and members could keep an action research approach to their work for as long as they chose, given that clinical nursing practice is typically fraught with many challenges on a daily basis. A helpful step-by-step account of an action research method is given by Kemmis and McTaggart (1988). Even though their main audience for the book was teachers, the method works equally well for any kind of practitioner.

Annette Street (1995) undertook action research with nurses working with the Royal Children's Hospital in Melbourne. The research began with the nurses involved, who were interested in locating issues and constraints in their practice that they wanted to change. It was important that the nurses 'owned' the research question and the intervention strategies, so time was taken at the outset for nurses to deal with some issues in their own practice. Issues about power relationships and gender mix in the group were also addressed as the group included relatively senior and/or male nurses, who may have had a silencing effect on the others.

Common concerns were identified and reconnaissance was conducted, which means that an initial investigation of the specific situation was undertaken to get an overall idea of what was happening. Members then focused on a specific concern of interest to them all. They wrote down their stories about the focus of concern and these accounts were shared in the group. The first action plan occurred after the reconnaissance and a literature review, and it addressed itself to questions about the situation, questions that began with who, what, where, when and how. The overall question arising from the first round of questions was: 'What do we want to change about the situation?' Data collection strategies included quantitative and qualitative approaches, depending on what was needed and what would best serve the purposes of the research. The findings were pooled and discussed and action was taken. Observation of the effects followed, before further reflection led to further action. In this way, the nurses evolved a collaborative working process for managing clinical issues of concern to them.

For information on getting a participatory action research group going refer to Street (1995).

Nursing research examples

Nurses have been using action research successfully in a variety of settings with differing thematic concerns (for example, Chenoweth & Kilstoff 1998; Koch, Kralik & Kelly 2000; Keatinge et al. 2000).

Keatinge and colleagues (2000) set up a participatory action research (PAR) group in a psychogeriatric unit in New South Wales, to work through a problem they had identified collectively as agitation in institutionalised residents with dementia. The nurses agreed that the care of people with dementia and agitation was a major challenge in their practice and they wanted to improve their nursing care of these people. The nurses aimed to identify manifestations, levels and patterns of agitation, the outcomes of current management practices, and nursing or contextual factors coinciding with episodes of patient agitation.

The research tools used to measure agitated behaviours were a rating scale adapted to the language commonly used by the observing nurses, and a Critical Incident Form. The rating scale was trialled for inter-rater reliability, and adjustments were made until 'within each group observers and managers rated each episode [of agitation] at the same level on all but one occasion (Keatinge et al. 2000, p. 18). The Critical Incident Form was developed to facilitate the recording of information about the situation, the manifestation of agitation, the rating, actions taken by the nurse and outcomes of the action. Nurses were requested to document details on observing the incident, and then 15 and 30 minutes later. Each nurse was allocated two residents to observe and nurses and residents were given code names for anonymity.

There were three phases over 10 months in the study, reflecting its PAR approach. Phase 1 included the initial period of observation and the use of the Critical Incident Form. Phase 2 involved the analysis and discussion of Phase 1 results and the identification and implementation of one impacting element. Phase 3 repeated Phase 1 to evaluate the impact of the change identified and implemented in Phase 2.

In recording the findings of the study the researchers concluded that the

> ... study determined that agitation in the demented elderly manifests as two distinct types of agitated behaviour, aggressive (higher rating) and non-aggressive (lower rating). It was also determined that there were peak times of agitated behaviour that coincided with those periods of increased interaction between nurses and residents, and that the majority of these interactions were associated with ADL (activities of daily living). Nursing practices used in the management of agitated behaviour were readily identifiable and varied according to the level and type of this behaviour. The change implemented as a result of Phase 1 of the study (e.g. in toileting regimes) did not impact on the frequency of episodes of agitated behaviour but may have impacted on the severity of these episodes (Keatinge et al. 2000, pp. 24–5).

Koch, Kralik and Kelly (2000) formed a participatory action research group of four men with multiple sclerosis (MS) and urinary incontinence, two continence nurse advisers and the researchers. The aims of the study were 'to redress a conspicuous absence of research literature on MS-related urinary incontinence' and to develop a 'better understanding of what it is like to live with MS and incontinence, in order to implement best practice in the management of urinary incontinence' (Koch, Kralik & Kelly 2000, p. 254). The study followed a previous pilot project with the research team and eight women with MS and incontinence, who benefited from a PAR group in gaining control over their lives in relation to the challenges of incontinence.

The men's PAR group worked with 'consensual and participatory procedures that enable the participants to set their own agendas, set issue priorities, discuss and systematically investigate problems and devise plans of action' (p. 255). The four men who volunteered to be involved met with three research members for two hours, fortnightly for five meetings. The first meeting allowed the men to talk about themselves and share their stories of when they first experienced urinary incontinence, the changes in their lives as a consequence, their strategies for urinary management and other areas they experienced that made them feel well. From these beginnings, the men set their own agendas for further discussion as the process unfolded each fortnight.

The principal researcher's handwritten notes of the meeting procedures and her reflections were typed and analysed to extract themes, which were then discussed by the research team, before being fed into the PAR process for discussion and validation. As Koch, Kralik and Kelly (2000, p. 256) explain 'there is no need to seek consensus in PAR groups; divergence of opinion is an equally useful finding' and 'it should not be assumed that people who share the objective features of a situation share a set of meanings about that experience'. The emergent themes expressed in the men's own words were 'planning your life around toilets', 'today will not be the same as tomorrow', 'managing myself', and 'motivated to make changes' (p. 259). The researchers concluded that living 'with adult incontinence can be restrictive, inconvenient' and can 'cause distress, embarrassment and humiliation' and the 'process of learning to successfully manage urinary incontinence within one's life can have a liberating effect' (p. 259).

Chenoweth and Kilstoff (1998, p. 175) undertook an action research project 'which arose out of the initiatives of people caring for clients attending a multicultural dementia day-care program'. The aims of the study were to create new ways of caring for people with dementia with a therapy program and to evaluate the process, as described by Dick (1995), that encourages participation by all group members through ongoing cycles of reflection and evaluation, leading to group decision-making and action (Chenoweth & Kilstoff 1998, p. 178). Study participants included 16 clients attending the day-care centre, their chief family carers (n = 16) and eight day-care staff, who worked together over a 12-month period, in which 12 stages evolved in the PAR process. Over this time, data were collected using focus group discussions, group memos, in-depth semi-structured interviews, client observation logbooks, the Revised Elderly Person's Disability Scale (REPDS) and field notes.

The researchers noted difficulties in the research design, the most challenging aspect of which was working with clients and family carers from multicultural backgrounds, unable to speak, read or write English. Bilingual health care workers assisted with communication in discussion groups and translation of logbooks. Other problems were associated with the dementia itself; however, those who were not too incapacitated to participate and their carers 'gained benefits through the companionship offered by others' (p. 183). The researchers noted that the flexibility of the action research process allowed them a great deal of freedom to explore issues and to deal with changes in the research plan as they arose.

The researchers concluded that the 'collaborative process helped all participants to empower themselves by designing, implementing and evaluating a new therapy program' (p. 186). Possibly the most telling statement about the success of the project in using action research was in the last sentence of their article in which Chenoweth and Kilstoff (1998, pp. 186–7) wrote that the 'successful outcomes of this study indicate that ordinary people have the capacity to determine their own health care needs and derive both empowerment and satisfaction in doing so'.

Other action research approaches in nursing have been taken to solve problems associated with the effective use of double staff time (Ramudu et al. 1994), problematic telephone orders (Retsas 1994), the expanding role of the nurse consultant (O'Brien & Spry 1995) and incontinence (Frey-Hoogwerf 1996).

Potential nursing research questions

Research questions that may use action research are those concerns and issues raised by the research participants themselves, and/or someone else's questions, possibly those of a researcher or team of researchers, that have been adopted by the research group for their collaborative research inquiry processes.

The potential is vast for raising nursing research questions using action research, because any practice issue can be managed by this approach, especially if nurses are willing to take the time and effort to work together to find strategies and solutions. Action research projects have explored the practical problems of nurses and nursing.

If you want to consider possibilities for action research, begin by spending some time thinking about your work situation and the people and situations you face there. In what ways are these people and situations problematic to you and your nursing practice? Do other nurses have similar concerns? Do you think others would be prepared to work with you to use an action research approach to working collaboratively through these problems? Ask them. You may find that you have made the first step towards setting up an action research project.

Feminisms

Feminism is a social movement concerned with women's issues and lives (Chinn & Wheeler 1985), and many kinds of feminisms reflect transitions over time in defining and addressing women's concerns, requiring multiple theories to explain the causes of women's oppression (Tong 1989). Examples of feminisms include liberal, Marxist/socialist, radical, poststructuralist, and postmodern representations. Glass (2000, p. 357) states emphatically that 'there is no one feminism; feminism is feminisms' and describes three waves of feminisms.

First-wave feminism refers to events at the beginning of the twentieth century, which identified the lack of material benefits and production for women, the viewing of women as objects, the mistaken assumptions that women should not be thinking people with voices. The first wave also ushered in women's rights to vote, and to be 'self-determining, enlightened and sexually liberated' (Glass 2000, p. 360).

The second wave includes liberal, Marxist, radical and lesbian feminists. Liberal feminism seeks equal rights within the existing social structures, through reasoning and equal educational opportunities for women. Liberal feminists seek to determine their social roles and 'compete with men on terms that ... are as equal as possible' (Jagger 1983, p. 324). Critics of this approach argue that opportunities for education that privilege men negate women's attempts for equality and their ability to reason (Cheek et al. 1996), and that women's subjectivity is not addressed in gender differences in the development of reasoning (Bunting & Campbell 1990; Doering, 1992).

Marxist/socialist feminism asserts that ownership of property and women is the basis of sexism and class division, and that women are oppressed within the family, motherhood, consumerism and class. This approach advocates the freedom to define one's own sexuality, equal sharing of child rearing and domestic roles, and the right to choose a family (Weedon 1991) thus addressing the relationships between the economy, family, class and gender (Seidman 1994). The ideas of Marxist/socialist feminism are influential with radical feminism.

Radical feminism withdraws from the dominant patriarchal system to replace it with 'woman defined systems, thought and culture' (Chinn & Wheeler 1985, p. 74). Critics who oppose radical feminism question a separatist stance, even though they may agree that women need to be free from the biological oppression of motherhood and sexual slavery, and the allocation of womanly work (Weedon 1991). Lesbian feminists 'espouse all of the values of radical feminists; however, they are concerned primarily with their sexual orientation in a feminist context' (Glass 2000, p. 362). Their issues involve 'not succumbing to male desire and rejecting heterosexuality per se' (Evans 1997, in Glass 2000, p. 362); therefore, they risk being doubly oppressed as women and lesbians.

The third wave of contemporary feminism, from the 1980s onwards, 'encompasses poststructural and postmodern feminisms' (Glass 2000, p. 363). Feminist poststructuralism responds to the idea that the division of feminisms into categories is problematic because the categories are arbitrary and socially produced (Gatens 1992; Delmar 1994) and the idea fails to address issues of power in language, subjectivity, social processes and institutions (Weedon 1991; Doering 1992). A feminist poststructuralist approach offers ways of identifying how language and discourse exercise power, showing how oppression operates by creating and affecting the possibilities for resistance (Weedon 1991), and of identifying women's participation in multiple discourses of everyday life (Davies 1994). Feminist poststructuralism allows women to recognise and change the cultural patterns of oppression inherent in dominant patriarchal society, through constantly renewed ways of seeing and repositioning themselves.

Postmodern feminists espouse 'a philosophy that supports and values the social contextual experience and difference of unique individuals and rejects the generalisation of those experiences' (Glass & Davis 1998, p. 44). For example, third-wave feminists 'have become disgruntled with the generalising theories of women's oppression' (Glass 2000, p. 363) and question whether all women are oppressed equally, resulting in the same effects.

The methodology

Pervading much of feminist literature are the key ideas of embodiment, empowerment and emancipation. Embodiment refers to living in a particular body. In relation to feminism, it means living a life through adherence to, and activation of, certain feminist principles that value the individual and collective good of women. Empowerment and emancipation have been defined previously in this chapter, but in feminist research they are of particular relevance in using participatory research processes to work towards the attainment of women's power and freedom.

Living a feminist perspective is about understanding and applying certain principles of feminism to daily life, so that it shows in the way you live. Embodying feminism means that the person is open to others, and is prepared to listen and collaborate for the collective good of women. It also means being attentive to those conditions that dominate and oppress women, through valuing women and their issues, concerns and experiences, and striving to create social change through critique and political action.

As one of the key assumptions of feminism is that women are dominated and oppressed by masculinist structures and processes, the potential for being free from these constraints features strongly in feminist literature and research. Speedy (1987, p. 23) claimed that 'the domination (or colonisation) of nursing by physicians and administrators occurred early in nursing's history, when medicine became a dominant force and hospitals proliferated'. She went on to assert that nurses did not recognise their oppression, because they became enculturated into it. In nursing, this means that women nurses need to raise their awareness to the forces that dominate and oppress them, and act to be liberated from those forces. One of the end results of empowerment in nursing can be powerful practice through a heightened sense of personal and professional worth.

As can be seen from the three waves of feminism, different theoretical emphases have evolved over time, but they have not necessarily replaced each other sequentially. For example, some feminists may align with particular views preceding the third wave and see no reason for making postmodern adjustments in their thinking. However, feminist researchers agree that 'women are the major focus of feminist research from the beginning to the end of *whole* research projects'; therefore feminist methodology 'concerns research *by* and *for* women ... putting feminist theory into practice ... by applying feminist principles directly from feminist premises' (Glass 2000, p. 368).

The methods

Feminist research uses methods that best reflect feminist principles and thereby ensure that all of the women involved are empowered by the research processes. In other words, feminist research not only emphasises *what* is done in terms of methods, but also *how* projects are done, in faithful reflection of feminist processes. Methods are not prescriptive, but they may include groupwork, storytelling, interviews, participant observation and so on, depending on the focus of the research interest. The main consideration is keeping to the important principles of feminist research, listed by Glass (2000, pp. 368–9), including the importance of a transforming and empowering focus, and research *with*, never *on* women, based on mutual respect and sharing. 'The researcher's values, beliefs and assumptions about who she is or her experiences are openly disclosed ... as a means of equalising power relations'. Interpersonal interactions are 'based on equality, reciprocity, and promote mutuality amongst all women involved'. Feminist research values women's unique experiences and stories and recognises and respects 'the inherent sensitivity in collecting data from women'. Feminist research methods and design 'benefit the women involved either whilst actively participating in the research or in the longer term'.

Nursing research examples

Nursing research examples of projects influenced by feminist thought are Glass (1994), Lumby (1997), Jackson and Raftos (1997) and Walter, Davis and Glass (1999).

The first example is of a Bachelor of Nursing (Honours) project by Ruby (Ruth) Walter, the publication of which was guided and assisted by her co-supervisors Kierrynn Davis and Nel Glass. Walter, Davis and Glass (1999, p. 12) used a feminist methodology to 'explore the role and significance that self concept plays in women nurses' experience of their beginning practice', by examining 'factors which contribute to and impact on self concept within a nursing practice environment'. The decision to situate the project in a feminist methodology was influenced by 'beliefs that women and nurses are oppressed and the desire to embed the research within a framework that recognises oppression, and offers the potential for emancipatory solutions', as well as to enable women nurses to find voice 'to speak for themselves' (p. 13).

The participants and the first-named author (researcher/participant) were all involved in a postgraduate nursing program in North Coast NSW. In Phase 1 the researcher/participant kept a journal, and in Phase 2 six participants told stories of their experiences. The research article related the findings of Phase 1, and explained how reflective journalling is 'congruent with feminist methodology as it encourages the researcher's own reflexivity through disclosure of emotion and experience, and as such works to make the research more equal and non-hierarchical' (Walter, Davis & Glass 1999, p. 14).

Thematic analysis of the transcribed journal entries identified three major themes of: exploring experiences, interconnecting personal and professional worlds, and integrating self into nursing. In exploring experiences, the researcher/participant 'was able to explore and question her own experiences related to self concept and nursing' (p. 14). The theme of interconnecting personal and professional worlds showed 'that practising nursing is inextricably linked to the lifeworld of the individual practitioner' (p. 14). Integrating self into nursing involved reflection on the idea that 'there is room in nursing for the nurse to feel able to be herself' (p. 14).

In the closing reflections, the researchers (Walter, Davis & Glass 1999, p. 15) concluded that the research

> permitted an exploration of reflective journalling as an appropriate method for the researcher/participant to situate herself within the research process, and demonstrated the effectiveness of reflective journalling as a tool in seeking to understand the interrelationship of self and nursing practice. It is the writers' belief that increasing nurses' awareness and understanding of the importance of how they feel about and experience themselves is vital to an increased recognition of the value of both the individual nurse, and the nursing profession.

In her PhD research Nel Glass (1994, p. ii) situated the project 'in the critical emancipatory paradigm using critical social science and feminist theory as the overarching methodology'. The study investigated 'hospital RNs' attitudes and reactions to nursing degrees' and aimed to 'enhance the existing theoretical base of research concerning post-registration RNs and to increase awareness of the related issues for all nurses' (Glass 1998, p. 24). Nel used a mixed method, triangulated approach, involving a survey questionnaire with 529 hospital-based (degree and non-degree) RNs, a self-reflective journal on field experiences while she was conducting the survey, and semi-structured interviews with 20 degree women nurses 'across all major classifications of RNs' (p. 25). The quantitative data were analysed by descriptive and inferential statistics using the SPSS package and the qualitative data were analysed by thematic analysis.

In presenting the results Nel makes the point that one 'of the main issues which arose in this research concerned the issue of continually working amongst tension and conflict' (p. 26) as highlighted in the open-ended question responses and in the interviews. While degree nurses felt empowered by their tertiary studies, 'they were essentially silenced by the negative environment in which they were working' (pp. 26–7).

In discussing the results, the researcher (1998, p. 30–1) concluded that:

> ... when this research was conducted, the clinical environment for both groups of nurses was hostile. Negative reactions to continual changes in university nurse education were predominating. The difficulties which both groups experienced working together were exemplified by the tension and forces that existed between and also within the groups ... Moreover, it was evident that degree nurses were aware that they were breaking a long held 'social' silence, in choosing to speak and discuss their decisions about university education. This of course was not without risk to themselves in their interactions with their peers ... It is hoped by putting the results of this research forward for public 'dissemination', that all nurses will be motivated to develop constructive strategies such as [to] (re-) examine their own attitudes to change, their associated potential fears, reactions to betrayal, and critically reflect on the issue of being 'wounded' by other nurses ...

The women nurses' empowered voices spoke of 'dialectical tensions' (Glass 1997, p. 177) within their personal and professional lives, in that they had to recognise their oppression in order to become empowered. In other words, emancipation was possible after they became empowered through their tertiary nurse education experiences to uncover and deal with the overt and subtle effects of oppression.

Judy Lumby (1997, p. 231) used critical and feminist perspectives in her postdoctoral study, of two years, which explored, with eight 'survivors', 'the paradox of facing life and death at the same time, which occurs when one has a terminal illness but is on a waiting list for a donor organ which could be life saving'. The aims of the study were: to explore and share the experiences of surviving a liver transplant, to enhance the care and quality of life of future patients, and to refine an emerging feminist method for nursing. Focus groups were used to collect stories. Within 'a focus group the synergy triggered memories for others, thus contributing to the building of the group stories' (p. 233).

The transcripts of the stories revealed the main issues of context, caring and care, control, and thanatological themes. The main determinants of a person's perceptions of care and treatment were connected to personal and professional features of the context, psychological states and the individual's well-being. 'The issue of caring and care engendered strong responses from the group both positively and negatively', but overall there was praise for the health care team. Control was expressed as a fear of loss of control while at the same time needing to relinquish control to the health care team. Thanatological issues involved facing life and death, mostly 'in terms of celebrating each day of life' (p. 236).

In reflecting on the study, the researcher (Lumby 1997, p. 237) concluded:

> The implications for further research lie in the research methods used in this study which allowed the participants to reveal their stories. Thus, while a medical team may judge an episode of illness by laboratory results and mortality rates, transplant recipients judge it in terms of personal and professional gains and losses and the quality of the experience itself.

Debra Jackson and Maree Raftos (1997, p. 35) grounded a study in feminism that 'aimed to explicate the experiences of nurses in Australia who have found themselves in the position of "whistle-blower" regarding the care and treatment of people living in residential care institutions' and to understand 'the issues that enhanced and impeded the nurses in their confrontation of institutionalised neglect and abuse'. Three experienced registered nurses with post-basic qualifications, using the pseudonyms of Gayle, Sally and Elizabeth, met with the researchers at a neutral venue over a period of weeks and shared their secrets 'to reconcile themselves with the events and their role in them in a meaningful and satisfying way' (p. 35).

Great care was taken to ensure the anonymity of the participants and their 'concern with identification has meant that certain information has been withheld from publication', however 'documents already in the public domain' corroborate participants' information (p. 35). Participants preferred not to be interviewed on audiotape, so researchers took extensive field notes that were analysed by feminist interpretive means (Reinharz 1992). Findings revealed three phases including an initial period of trepidation and optimism, confrontation of barriers and obstacles to action, and disillusionment and defeat.

Trepidation was experienced when first impressions were 'of an overwhelming despondency within the home', described as 'an inertia and a poverty of spirit affecting both staff and residents'. The physical environment was described as 'malodorous and oppressive', and there was a lack of staff and equipment (p. 36). Residents' rooms lacked privacy, were overcrowded and not suited to managing people with disabilities. Despite the initial feeling of trepidation, the participants all felt some optimism in their hope to effect change.

Barriers and obstacles faced in trying to change the conditions in the home led to intense frustration, as the women's relationships with management became strained. The women felt 'professionally disabled' as they realised 'their sense of professional autonomy was compromised by the power of management to control every aspect of care provision' (p. 36). For example, the home employed only the minimal complement of registered nurses and no enrolled nurses; thus the 'nursing care' was provided by lay people, many of whom had no prior experience or educational preparation. Registered nurses were kept busy attending to extensive documentation required by funding authorities, and in giving medications and treatments, taking phone calls and replacing staff for the next shift.

Disillusionment and defeat came when the women became increasingly demoralised, realising there was little support from management for positive change. Participants witnessed a high staff turnover, with some new staff leaving in disgust after days or even hours. 'The participants became acutely aware of the censure and reproach from others who had witnessed the poor conditions of the residents, yet had remained silent, unwilling or unable to change the status quo' (p. 37). The women were increasingly marginalised within their workplace, because attempts to effect positive change were confronting and threatening for other staff. The decision to become whistle-blowers to outside agencies came when the women realised they could not effect changes within the home. The women chose to work through government and non-government agencies rather than the media, necessitating frequent and sustained efforts; thus they became so fearful and demoralised that all of them resigned.

In concluding the research article, the researchers (Jackson & Raftos 1997, p. 38) contended that the

> nursing profession needs to examine the structures and support available to nurses who wish to challenge those organisational cultures that act to shape nursing practice in a negative and destructive way. The experiences of Gayle, Sally and Elizabeth may well be shared by others in their daily practice as nurses. As a community of health care providers, nursing must take the lead and act to defend ethical practice by providing advice and ensuring support for whistle-blowers. A specific task force could be established under the auspices of a national nursing body, which could function as referral point for nurses who find themselves in these types of situations ... The professional body, while providing practical and moral support, could take over the role of notifying appropriate authorities. Such an innovation by nurses would have an emancipatory effect, in that clinical nurses would be further empowered to act to improve practice.

Another example of a feminist nursing research project was an empirical study of first-year nursing students to examine 'their perspectives on nursing as a career, family commitments and the influence of gender equity issues on their future life goals' (Poole & Isaacs 1995, p. 100). The nursing students described 'a plurality of meanings and competing discourses' as they made sense of their experiences as students. You may enjoy locating this article and reading this interesting research.

Potential nursing research questions

If you are thinking of using a feminist approach to nursing research, you could begin by asking yourself some basic questions that relate to some underlying feminist assumptions. For example, you might ask yourself: 'What is it that I know that is of concern to women?' 'In what ways will this research attempt to value women's experiences?' 'How might this research increase the awareness of factors that oppress women?' 'How can this research assist women to create social change through critique and political action?' and 'How can postmodern thinking enhance my understanding of women's experiences and issues?' With these broad questions in mind, you need to consider specific areas of interest that may be best addressed by a feminist research perspective.

Questions for nursing and nurses may emphasise power relations between nurses and other members of the health care system. The focus might be on generating historical nursing questions about the origins of healing that readmits women to its accounts. You might like to think of ways of working with women nurses to address any issues of concern that they might have. You might prefer to start with a feminist process for research such as 'Peace and Power' described by

Wheeler and Chinn (1989) and ask yourself: 'What sort of nursing concerns could be managed best by this research process?' The questions may begin at any point and lead to multiple possibilities, but the thing to keep in mind is the extent to which they reflect some fundamental principles of feminism such as those covered in this section (Glass 2000).

Critical ethnography

The meaning of critical ethnography connotes a hybrid of ethnography and critical social science. As you might imagine, critical ethnography not only has the exploratory and descriptive mission of an ethnography, but it also has the emancipatory aims of critical research approaches. This means that it can go further than descriptive or interpretive ethnography, which seeks only to describe the cultural features of a particular group of people in order to understand their symbols, rituals and practices.

The methodology

Critical ethnography began life as ethnography and added its critical component in response to a growing critique of the perceived inability of traditional ethnography to address political questions in research. With arguments similar to those raised against other interpretive research approaches such as grounded theory and phenomenology (Fay 1975; Carr & Kemmis 1986), ethnography has been criticised for failing to recognise that all human activity is political, that shared meanings are worked out through discourse, and that researchers are not exempt from subjectivity and bias (Angus 1986; Gitlin, Siegal & Boru 1989). For an ethnography to become critical it must be 'openly ideological, socially critical, overtly political, and emancipatory in intent' (Shannon 1994, p. 2).

The methods

Critical ethnography can create a dialogue with research participants so that they can examine the personal, political, social, cultural, historical and economic aspects of their contexts to develop local knowledge of use to their own situations (Hammersley 1992; Jordan & Yeomans 1995; Street 1998). Therefore, critical ethnography is a reflexive research process that offers a means to reveal 'the complex micro politics of social relationships in the situation and the researcher's position within those politics' (Wellard & Street 1999, p. 133). In this way, critical ethnography goes beyond the surface features of social settings to uncover and examine the power relations and influences affecting and determining the nature and consequences of human behaviour.

Although there are no prescriptive rules to follow in planning and undertaking a critical ethnography, the methods used will be congruent with certain principles of critical inquiry. A critical ethnography will probably:

- focus on a setting in which specific day-to-day practices can be observed
- intend to bring about changes in the status quo by submitting the research area to constant and systematic political critique
- involve researcher–participant collaboration in open and honest communication and critical reflection
- attempt to acknowledge and deal with potential power differences and struggles between research participants
- generate a frank and critically aware discourse which allows participants to express their ideas, assumptions and concerns regarding the research process and the evolving aims of the research
- involve participants equally in actively engaging in problem-locating and strategy-solving within the agreed structures and processes of the research.

Given the nature of the principles of critical ethnographic research as listed previously, the methods to ensure that issues of power are addressed may include: group processes such as discussion and debate, participant observation, and reflective practice strategies such as keeping diaries, writing narratives and engaging in individual and group critiques.

Nursing research examples

Sally Wellard and Annette Street (1999, p. 132) used a critical ethnographic approach to explore 'the development of home-based care, in particular home-based dialysis, using a case-study approach ... to identify the issues of families involved in home care'. Data sources included interviews developed into case studies with the family of a person with end-stage renal disease (ESRD) and a focus group of nurses caring for people with ESRD. Three families were studied for the case studies, and their experiences of home-based care were explored through in-depth interviews, informal conversations, and observations of family interactions. Verbal interactions were audiotaped and transcribed where possible and a field work journal was used to record observation of family interactions and the chief researcher's own reflections. Emergent issues included the development of the home-based clinic, the role of women, social isolation, and the lack of effective support from general practitioners and their health services.

Each family allocated 'clinic' space in their home, and dialysis 'dominated the lives of the families studied, pervading their space and time and affecting every aspect of their living' (p. 133). For example, a 'strict use of time was evident in all three families and the timetabling of treatments demonstrated the control of activity that dialysis dictated' (p. 133). The inflexible routines affected negatively any social and leisure activities outside the home. Women accepted the role of caregivers or home-makers, increasing their work activities and demonstrating 'the normalising models that act as truth in our society, where it is assumed that a wife in any "normal" family will adopt the carer's role' (p. 134). As sole providers of their husbands' dialysis support, the women never had a day off and there was no respite available, leading to social isolation.

Families reported that general practitioners were often uninformed, unable to be of practical help in managing the complications of renal dialysis, and of limited availability in out-of-office hours. Therefore, families 'found themselves positioned in the health-care system as knowledgeable, yet not powerful', giving rise to ongoing tensions (p. 135). Accordingly, families learned to manipulate the system, while remaining

> captive to a system that fails to recognise their knowledge and understanding of their own bodies and treatment, or legitimate insight into the best management of their condition, based on their previous experience. Such encounters extended discomfort and produced great anxiety for patients and families (Wellard & Street 1999, p. 135–6).

The implications of the research included the need for acknowledgement that home-based clinics cause significant disruption to families, and extra work and social isolation for women carers. In cognisance of the constraints and issues in dealing with the health care system, nurses were urged to develop 'practices that are sensitive to patients and family needs' and for specialist nurses with the required skills to provide respite (p. 136). Also suggested were educative processes to accommodate home-based treatments, refresher courses to maximise safety and benefits, improved communication with families and patients that enables questioning from all members of the family, and further collaborative research 'for critical dialogue between all the stakeholders ... to determine the desired outcomes' (p. 136).

Potential nursing research questions

A critical ethnographic approach may be taken for any research interest that involves becoming familiar with the rituals and practices of nurses and nursing with the intention of being politically provocative in order to challenge the accepted understandings and established power sources in the culture. Because it has emancipatory potential, critical ethnography can be used in any setting that will inform nurses about the influences and constraints operating against nurses in their work. For example, nurses may work together to raise their awareness about work circumstances that may benefit from a critical appraisal in places such as wards, clinics, administrative offices, schools, universities and community settings.

If you want to consider possibilities for a critical ethnographic study, begin by thinking about your clinical setting and some of the rituals and practices that you may have noticed there. In what ways are these rituals and practices taken for granted? To what extent are nurses aware of the taken-for-grantedness of aspects of their work? Are there political struggles 'in the open' or on a hidden level? Is there any interest among colleagues in working together to set up systematic politically active research processes and methods to raise awareness, questions and critique about selected practices in the culture?

Key terms associated with postmodern thought

The following terms have been adapted from Rosenau (1992, pp. xi–xiv).

- An **agent** or **agency** is someone assumed to have authority and power. For example, in nursing practice, nurses are agents and have agency by virtue of their knowledge and skills as clinicians.
- An **author** is a person who creates a text, or is responsible for an outcome. For example, nurses researching their practice are authors who are responsible for their own practice and for research projects and articles that disseminate the results.
- **Deconstruction** is a postmodern method of analysis that tears a text apart to reveal its contradictions, but not with the intention of improving, revising, or offering a better text. For example, all of the projects presented in this book could be subjected to a postmodern deconstruction to reveal their contradictions in claiming (overtly or covertly) to offer 'truth'.
- **Discourse** is all that is written and spoken and invites dialogue or conversation. For example, many critical and postmodern approaches to epistemology invite active and open discussion in their processes.
- **Intertextuality** refers to infinitely complex and unending interwoven interrelationships that do not arrive at an end point or consensus. For example, no absolute claims are made about any area of interest or inquiry and the relationships of texts.
- **Narratives** are views or stories and postmodernists are opposed to grand/meta-narratives or world views based on claims to legitimise their 'truth'. However, mini/micro/local/traditional narratives as stories making no truth claims are acceptable to postmodernists.
- The **reader** is the observer, who is given the power of interpreting the text; thus postmodernists empower the reader over the author.
- **Reading** refers to understanding and interpretation that in postmodern terms may be 'my reading', 'your reading' or 'a reading' without judgement of adequacy or validity of the said reading. This means that researchers do not assume superior positions over the readers of projects in dictating meaning.
- **Text** refers to everything, so that all events and phenomena are texts.
- **Voice** is the modern conception of the author's perspective, but postmodernists question the attribution of privilege or special status to any voice. Thus, a 'public voice' is more acceptable, making discourse broadly understandable.

Nursing research discourse reflecting postmodern influences

This section deals with nursing research discourse reflecting postmodern influences, rather than 'postmodern research' per se, because my reading of various postmodern ideas leads me to suspect that to write and speak of the latter would constitute an oxymoron. An oxymoron is a contradiction in terms. It would be a contradiction in terms to claim that 'postmodern research' per se exists or could exist, because postmodernists agree on their rejection of grand narratives, and to construct a form called 'postmodern research' would be the same as constructing a grand narrative, which is antithetical to postmodernist claims for the plurality, diversity, relativity and multiplicity of truth.

All of the approaches described in this section, specifically action research, feminism, and critical ethnography, constitute grand narratives, as they are based on certain assumptions about how knowledge is gained and verified through research methods and processes. The discourse arguing the legitimacy of grand narratives creates various positions. For example, some feminist scholars believe that the emancipatory impulse of feminism is silenced by postmodernism (Farganis 1994; Benhabib 1995); therefore it has no value in advancing the interests of women as members of oppressed groups. In nursing, Kermode and Brown (1995) have argued that failure to recognise the grand narratives of capitalism and patriarchy have left uncontested these issues as sources of power. However, there are researchers who have held onto important aspects of a 'grand narrative' while integrating what they see as compatible aspects of postmodernism (Fahy 1997; Glass & Davis 1998; Hall 1999).

Kathleen Fahy (1997, p. 27) addressed the apparent oxymoron of postmodern feminist emancipatory research by arguing that 'postmodernism can be compatible with politically motivated, humanistically based inquiry'. Postmodernist feminist research might be considered an oxymoron because postmodernism rejects grand narratives, and as social theories on the oppression of women, feminisms are grand narratives. Also, postmodernisms are of various types, many of which reject research endeavours as being the work of 'authors', who try to influence others through their superior opinions. Therefore, to link feminism with postmodernism is tricky, on the basis that feminism is a grand narrative and it has a research agenda for women based on certain emancipatory intentions.

The postmodern critique of humanism is that its orientation towards autonomy, integrity, human rights and self-conscious rationality has led it into valuing the right of the individual over those 'of the community, other animals and the environment' (p. 28). Also, humanists have privileged reason over emotion and 'this has meant that decisions about the world and how we should live have been made and enacted without reference to emotions, values or relational attachments' (Johnson 1994 in Fahy 1997, p. 28). Humanists' inattention to women's ways of knowing has also created a humanist subject who 'turns out not to be a universal "human"'; rather the image is of one particular culturally constituted form of human subjectivity: the young, strong, white, elite male' (p. 28). Also, humanism 'is vulnerable to criticism because atrocities have been committed and oppressive social practices have been perfected in its name' (p. 29).

In the face of these and other critiques of humanism, Fahy (1997, p. 30) argued

> it is difficult, if not impossible to be both feminist and anti-humanist. Feminists value human freedom, autonomy and self-conscious reflexivity; these are humanistic

> values that imply an inner, authentic subject ... Present day feminists have rejected the notion of a set of universal essential human needs that define what it is to be human. I acknowledge that the individual's identity is, to a large extent, discursively and historically constituted, resulting in an identity that is both fragmented and dynamic. I reject, however, the postmodern notion that there is no true or authentic self ... It is this 'authentic self' who is vital to the emancipatory project. The goal of emancipatory feminism is to facilitate the emergence of the true self and the creative project of human becoming ... When we can link our feelings, emotions, intuitions and reason together then we are in the best position for deciding what to do and how to proceed in life. Embracing both humanistic and postmodern ideas creates a productive synergy from which to theorise.

In view of this argument, what are the implications for nursing research of Kathleen Fahy's discourse reflecting postmodern influences on her perception and practice of feminism? Kathleen recognises the risk that humanist and feminist research processes may place the researcher in the role of 'expert' and the researched in the role of 'normalised'. To overcome this possibility, she suggests that 'feminist researchers need to be continuously conscious of the power differential that exists between themselves and participants', (pp. 31–2) and find ways to balance it through reciprocity, negotiation, equality, sharing and friendship.

In concluding her argument for reconciling the apparent oxymoron of postmodern feminist emancipatory research, Kathleen Fahy (1997, p. 32) contends that

> Postmodern notions of power and subjectivity can strengthen the theoretical power of emancipatory studies ... some forms of postmodernism serve the purposes of researchers who want their practices and their theories to contribute to changing the present towards a better future ... These emancipatory theories should ... be based on a colligation of reason and emotion; on an embodied rationality. Ultimately, it is not reason, logic or intellectual analysis that controls human decisions or gives our lives their meaning and direction. One must feel, emotionally and biologically, a sense of active excitement about being alive in order to create and protect a life worth living. Helping research participants and/or nursing clients to achieve this state is far more challenging and far less arrogant than providing prescriptions about what research participants or nursing patients 'should' do in order to be happy and healthy.

Although Nel Glass and Kierrynn Davis (1998, p. 44) admit that 'the "merging" of feminism and postmodernism ... is contentious, offering a diversity of opinions that culminate for some scholars as binary opposing beliefs', they contend that both discourses are changing, making it 'timely to explore the contemporary debates by considering an integrated on-the-move feminist postmodern approach to nursing research'. While accepting as the main tenet of feminism that women are oppressed within patriarchal societies, Glass and Davis (1998, p. 45) disrupt modernist feminism by presenting views in what they term 'the dissatisfaction debate' and 'the fragmentation debate' to arrive at the solution of 'an integrated turning point' in nursing research. The disruption refers to the questions they raise about feminism in light of postmodern thinking.

'The dissatisfaction debate' relates to the postmodern 'dissatisfaction with monolithic theories and grand narratives' (p. 46), because of their inability to reflect the positions of individuals. For example, Nel Glass noticed that the 'oppression narrative' makes the generalisation 'that all women and nurses are oppressed equally' (p. 47) thus failing to take account of the needs of individuals within groups.

'The fragmentation debate' is linked with the dissatisfaction debate and relates to the multiplicity of views opposing grand narratives, resulting in the situation that the 'emphasis on local, contextual, and therefore multiple explanations of reality is viewed as fragmentary rather than cohesive' (p. 47). Even so, scholars such as Kierrynn Davis would not view this fragmentation negatively, but rather 'celebratory, because it concerns the subject in process, and it can be visionary, resisting, struggling and nonideological' (p. 48). Glass and Davis (1998, p. 48) contend that it is 'the failure to realize the different views, types, stances, turns, and constructs of the postmodernisms that has led many critics to maintain a negative view of postmodernism as fragmentary, chaotic, nonpolitical, and therefore without emancipatory intent' (p. 48). They also cite a tendency for critics to focus on skeptical postmodernism and its concentration on nihilism, negativity and hyper-reality as a reason for ignoring affirmative stances in which 'fragmentation is considered potentially liberating ... [with] concepts capable of producing a general social theory' (p. 48).

'An integrated turning point' in nursing research is suggested as a solution, for which Glass and Davis 'have taken an interdisciplinary approach and drawn on ideas from within the nursing literature, feminist postmodernism, and postmodern sociology' (p. 48). The researchers asked themselves a critical question in relation to difference: 'Can one's individualism be comprehensively explained, theorized, and ultimately "celebrated" by an integrated turn[ing point] in nursing research?' (p. 49). They agreed with Lather (1991) in Glass and Davis (1998) that links can be drawn between feminism and postmodernism, in that modern feminist theory encourages conflicting theories within itself, has an emphasis on praxis and self-reflexivity, 'recognizes the importance of subject and agency in the effort toward transforming society', and has 'begun to move from essentialism toward social construction of the subject and the questioning of difference' (p. 49). In other words, some of the concepts held as central and important within feminism and emphasised by postmodernism are present already and/or are being worked with 'on-the-move' by feminist scholars and researchers.

Another 'component of the integration involves the preservation of feminist notions of celebrating women's voices' consistent with the postmodern influences of validating socially constructed existence, blurring boundaries, acknowledging the need for dialogue or conversation 'rather than an authoritative voice', and giving women's voices 'new scripts, texts and discourses' (p. 49). Therefore, the shared aspects of feminism and postmodernism include 'a context that validates and celebrates difference and variety ... inclusive of "marginalised voices"', 'constantly changing phenomena', no 'fixed unique identity', no ideal decontextualised observers, and identity 'in a constant state of movement' (pp. 49–50).

In describing the research implications influenced by the integrated turning point of modernist feminism toward postmodernism, Glass and Davis (1998, p. 50) suggest the need to refocus to emphasise 'the contexts that create meaning combined with a revisioning to the extent that everything is open to interrogation', for example, by resituating 'perceptions of identity, subjectivity, agency, language, and power'. They expect that 'these research directions will potentially destabilize previously held assumptions concerning interpretive validity and concurrent emancipatory research', and would 'involve inscribing and subverting of those who speak rather than what is said', resulting in unease, nervousness and possibly resistance. Even so, they remain 'optimistic that we can accurately represent all individual women and nurse research participants', and that we can acknowledge diversity, retain our 'individual integrity ... of how we represent ourselves and others' while 'being true to oneself', being responsible to others while validating difference and, in turn, celebrating 'common humanity' (p. 50). Added to this, the integrated nursing research model redirects focus 'toward deference, partiality, and multiplicity', 'eliminates the search for a universal truth or the right answer', incorporates a conversational-style research method, represents 'a critical wariness regarding any generalizations', and allows feminists to read postmodernist 'writings critically to accept what [is] useful from a feminist perspective' (pp 50-51).

In a compelling argument for diversity of knowledge development in nursing, Hall (1999) revisits marginalisation using critical, postmodern and liberation perspectives. If you are interested in postmodern influences on nursing knowledge and potential research questions, this article can be downloaded in hard copy from the Internet or located in the serial section of your library.

The co-author's postscript to postmodernism

I have experienced a certain tension in writing about postmodernism, even when being careful to qualify it as *informing* nursing research, rather than being postmodern research per se. As a co-author of this book, I have given you my own reading of scholars' writing and I realise that this may be in direct opposition to your or someone else's interpretation as a reader of the text. My dilemma resides in putting myself in a position of legitimate authority as a co-author of this book, but as a teacher and researcher I put myself in a position of legitimate authority every day of my working life. My response to this dilemma of my authority as co-author is moderated by postmodernist ideas of offering multiple ideas, and highlighting possible contradictions, while providing paradigmatic maps for you that make sense of the vast terrain of nursing research. In this sense, I offer teaching as a form of guidance and hope that my explanations offer you choices for understanding complex and novel texts.

Summary
This chapter dealt with qualitative research methodologies that have political awareness and social change as their 'up-front agenda'. Critical research methodologies have an active intention to question the taken-for-granted aspects of a culture in order to change it positively. Critical approaches can address the power imbalances in nursing conditions, relationships and organisations, and question assumptions about the way things are and the way they need to be.

This chapter clarified some common qualitative theoretical assumptions about the importance of critical research approaches and defined key terms associated with critical methodologies, such as empowerment, emancipation, hegemony and praxis. Three forms of qualitative critical methodologies were described, specifically action research, feminisms, and critical ethnography in terms of their methodologies, methods and potential for raising and dealing with nursing research questions of a political nature. Critical social theory, poststructuralism and postmodernism were compared briefly, some key postmodern thought terms were described, and research and projects were presented that have used various postmodern ideas in their approaches.

Main points
- Critical research approaches address social and political issues in human life, and in nursing they can address the power imbalances in nursing conditions, relationships and organisations, and turn upside down some taken-for-granted assumptions about the way things are, and the way they need to be.
- Critical methodologies generate emancipatory knowledge that has the potential to free people from the oppressive conditions of their entrenched historical, social, political, cultural and economic circumstances, to something that can be better for them.
- Critical methodologies involve research methods that encourage people to come together to share collaboratively, to surface their personal and collective concerns and to attempt to own more equally their research problems, processes and outcomes as co-researchers.
- Even given the historical connections of qualitative interpretive and critical research methodologies to postmodernism, many postmodernists argue that these methodologies constitute in *varying degrees* grand or meta (master) narratives that assume some authority in addressing issues of justice, truth and theory, and thus run counter to some postmodern thinking.
- Empowerment is the process of giving and accepting power; in critical research the methods and processes are geared towards helping people to find their own power, to liberate them from their oppressive circumstances and self-understandings.
- Emancipation is freedom *from* something *to* something, and for nurses, critical research approaches can assist in experiencing freedom from the bonds of taken-for-granted expectations and roles, to more knowledgeable, skilful and creative practice.

- Hegemony means ascendancy or domination of one power over another, when social systems and people give the impression that they are unassailable, and that the conditions they have produced are not only good, but also appropriate for the people over whom they have control.
- Praxis is change through critical reflection on practice, and in qualitative critical research it is facilitated through participatory, collaborative methods and processes.
- Action research goes to the site of a concern or practice, and works with the people there as co-researchers, to generate solutions to problems (thematic concerns) with which they have agreed to deal, through action cycles of systematically and collectively planning, acting, observing and reflecting.
- Feminism is a social movement concerned with women's issues and lives and many kinds of feminisms such as liberal, Marxist/socialist, radical, poststructuralist, and postmodern representations, reflect transitions in defining and addressing women's concerns.
- Critical ethnography uses reflexive research processes that have exploratory, descriptive and emancipatory aims, to create a dialogue with research participants so they can go beyond the surface features of their social settings to uncover, examine and begin to deal with, the power relations and influences affecting them.
- 'Postmodern research' cannot exist per se, because postmodernists agree on their rejection of grand narratives, and to construct a representation called 'postmodern research' would be tantamount to constructing a grand narrative, which is antithetical to postmodernist deconstruction that supports the plurality, diversity, relativity and multiplicity of truth claims.
- As qualitative critical approaches constitute grand narratives, various responses to postmodernism from nursing researchers have been that the emancipatory impulse is silenced by postmodernism; grand narratives such as capitalism and patriarchy are left uncontested as sources of power; and that it is possible to retain important aspects of a 'grand narrative' while integrating compatible aspects of postmodernism.

Review Questions

1   Qualitative critical methodologies are derived from some key ideas in critical:
    a   psychology
    b   social science
    c   feminism
    d   philosophy

2   Qualitative critical methodologies all agree that the process of producing and verifying knowledge is essentially:
   a   empirical ✓
   b   conservative
   c   political ⓒ
   d   scientific

3   The ascendancy or domination of one group over another so that they give the impression they are unassailable is:
   a   oppression ✓
   b   emancipation
   c   praxis
   d   hegemony ⓓ

4   Qualitative critical methodologies attempt to redress social imbalances in:
   a   status ✓
   b   class
   c   power ⓒ
   d   ethnicity

5   Action research processes are:
   a   participatory and collaborative ✓ⓐ
   b   directed and controlled
   c   subjective and relativistic
   d   uniform and individualistic

6   The three forms of action research influenced by Habermas's 'knowledge-constitutive interests' are:
   a   empirical, interpretive and critical ✓
   b   absolute, relative and postmodern
   c   primary, secondary and tertiary
   d   technical, practical and emancipatory ⓓ

7   Feminisms are concerned with the issues and lives of:
   a   all people
   b   women ✓ⓑ
   c   families
   d   minority groups

8   The feminism which seeks equal rights within present social structures is: ✓
   a   Marxist
   b   radical
   c   liberal ⓒ
   d   socialist

9   For an ethnography to become critical it must be:
    a openly ideological, socially critical, overtly political and emancipatory
    b problem based, cyclical, participatory, collaborative and emancipatory
    c woman focused, process oriented, outcomes driven and emancipatory
    d ethnic oriented, culture based, covertly political and emancipatory

10 Given the nature of critical ethnographic research, the methods used will most probably include
    a surveys and questionnaires
    b structured interviews
    c primary sources
    d reflective practice strategies

Discussion Questions

1   What are the main differences between critical methodologies, poststructuralism and postmodernism?

2   Define empowerment, emancipation, hegemony and praxis, in relation to the intentions of qualitative critical research.

3   Describe the methodology and methods, and provide one nursing research example, of action research.

4   Describe the methodology and methods, and provide one nursing research example, of feminism.

5   Describe the methodology and methods, and provide one nursing research example, of critical ethnography.

References

Angus, L. 1986, 'Research traditions, ideology and critical ethnography', *Discourse*, vol. 7, no. 1, 59–77.

Baudrillard, J. 1983, *In the Shadow of the Silent Majorities*, Semiotext(e), New York.

Best, S. & Kellner, D. 1991, *Postmodern Theory: Critical Interrogations*, Macmillan, London.

Benhabib, S. 1995, 'Feminism and postmodernism', in *Feminist Contentions: A Philosophical Exchange*, eds S. Benhabib, J. Butler, D. Cornell & N. Fraser, Routledge, New York.

Bunting, S. & Campbell, J. C. 1990, 'Feminism and nursing: historical perspectives', *Advances in Nursing Science*, vol. 12, no. 4, 11–24.

Carr, W. & Kemmis, S. 1986, *Becoming Critical: Education, Knowledge and Action Research*, Falmer Press, Lewes.

Cheek, J. 2000, *Postmodern and Poststructural Approaches to Nursing Research*, Sage Publications, Thousand Oaks, California.

Cheek, J., Shoebridge, J., Willis, E. & Zadoroznyi, J. 1996, *Society and Health*, Longman Australia, Melbourne.

Chein, I., Cook, S. & Harding, J. 1948, 'The field of action research', *American Psychology*, vol. 3, 43–50.

Chenoweth, L. & Kilstoff, K. 1998, 'Facilitating positive changes in community dementia management through participatory action research', *International Journal of Nursing Practice*, vol. 4, 175–88.
Chinn, P. L. & Wheeler, C. E. 1985, 'Feminism and nursing', *Nursing Outlook*, vol. 33, no. 2, 74–7.
Culbertson, J. A. 1981, 'Three epistemologies and the study of educational administration', *Review, The University Council for Educational Administration*, vol. 22, no. 1, 1–6.
Davies, B. 1994, *Poststructural Theory and Classroom Practice*, Deakin University Press, Geelong.
Delmar, R. 1994, 'What is feminism?' in *Theorising Feminism: Parallel Trends in the Humanities and Social Sciences*, eds A. Herrmann & A. Stewart, Westview Press, Boulder, Colorado.
Dick, R. 1995, 'A beginner's guide to action research', *ARCS Newsletter*, vol. 1, no. 1, 5–9.
Doering, L. 1992, 'Power and knowledge in nursing: a feminist poststructuralist view', *Advances in Nursing Science*, vol. 14, no. 4, 24–33.
Dzurec, L. C. 1989, 'The necessity for and evolution of multiple paradigms for nursing research: a poststructuralist perspective', *Advances in Nursing Science*, vol. 11, no. 4, 69–77.
Evans, M. 1997, 'Introducing contemporary thought', in *Speaking Feminisms and Nursing*, ed. N. Glass, Polity Press, Cambridge, UK.
Fahy, K. 1997, 'Postmodern feminist emancipatory research: is it an oxymoron?' *Nursing Inquiry*, vol. 4, 27–33.
Farganis, S. 1994, 'Postmodernism and feminism' in *Postmodernism and Social Inquiry*, eds D. Dickens & A. Fontana, University College Press, London.
Fay, B. 1975, *Social Theory and Political Practice*, Allen & Unwin, London.
Fay, B. 1987, *Critical Social Science: Liberation and Its Limits*, Polity Press, Cambridge, UK.
Foucault, M. 1990, *The History of Sexuality. Volume 1: An Introduction*, Penguin Books, London.
Frey-Hoogwerf, L. 1996, 'A journey towards continence through emancipatory action research', *International Journal of Nursing Practice*, vol. 2, no. 2, 77–81.
Gatens, M. 1992, 'Power, bodies and difference', in *Destabilizing Theory: Contemporary Feminist Debates*, eds M. Barrett & A. Phillips, Polity Press, Cambridge, UK.
Giroux, H. A. 1983, *Theory and Resistance in Education*, Heinemann Educational Books, London.
Giroux, H. A. 1992, *Border Crossings: Cultural Workers and the Politics of Education*, Routledge, New York.
Gitlin, A., Siegal, M. & Boru, K. 1989, 'The politics of method: from leftist ethnography to educative research', *Qualitative Studies in Education*, vol. 2, no. 3, 237–53.
Glass, N. 1994, Breaking a social silence, women's emerging and disruptive voices: a feminist critique of post-registration nursing education in rural Australia. Unpublished PhD thesis, University of New South Wales.
Glass, N. 1997, 'Breaking a social silence: registered nurses share their stories about tertiary nursing education', *International Journal of Nursing Practice*, vol. 3, 173–7.
Glass, N. 1998, 'The contested work place: reactions to hospital based RNs doing degrees', *Collegian*, vol. 5, no. 1, 24–31.
Glass, N. 2000, 'Speaking feminisms and nursing', in *Nursing Theory in Australia: Development and Application*, ed. J. Greenwood, Pearson Education Australia, Frenchs Forest, NSW.
Glass, N. & Davis, K. 1998, 'An emancipatory impulse: a feminist postmodern integrated turning point in nursing research', *Advances in Nursing Science*, vol. 21, no. 1, 43–52.
Gore, J. 1992, 'What we can do for you! What can "we" do for "you"?: Struggling over empowerment in critical and feminist pedagogy', in *Feminisms and Critical Pedagogy*, eds C. Luke & J. Gore, Routledge, New York.
Habermas, J. 1972, *Knowledge and Human Interests*, Heinemann, London.
Habermas, J. 1973, *Theory and Practice*, Heinemann, London.

Hall, J. 1999, 'Marginalization revisited: critical, postmodern, and liberation perspectives', *Advances in Nursing Science*, vol. 22, no. 2, 88–102.

Hammersley, M. 1992, *What's Wrong with Ethnography?* Routledge, London.

Jackson, D. & Raftos, M. 1997, 'In uncharted waters: confronting the culture of silence in a residential care institution', *International Journal of Nursing Practice*, vol. 3, 34–9.

Jagger, A. 1983, 'Political philosophies of women's liberation', in *Feminist Frontiers*, eds L. Richardson & V. Taylor, Random House, New York.

Johnson, P. 1994, *Feminism as Radical Humanism*, Allen and Unwin, St Leonards, NSW.

Jordan, G. & Weedon, C. 1995, *Cultural Politics: Class, Gender, Race and the Postmodern World*, Blackwell, Oxford.

Jordan, S. & Yeomans, D. 1995, 'Critical ethnography: problems in contemporary theory and practice', *British Journal of Sociology of Education*, vol. 16, 389–408.

Keatinge, D., Scarfe, C., Bellchambers, H., McGee, J., Oakham, R., Probert, C., Stewart, L. & Stokes, J. 2000, 'The manifestation and nursing management of agitation in institutionalised residents with dementia', *International Journal of Nursing Practice*, vol. 6, 16–25.

Kemmis, S. & McTaggart, R., eds, 1988, *The Action Research Planner*, 3rd edn, Deakin University Press, Geelong, Australia.

Kermode, S. & Brown, C. 1995, 'Where have all the flowers gone: nursing's escape from the radical critique', *Contemporary Nurse*, vol. 4, no. 1, 8–15.

Koch, T., Kralik, D. & Kelly, S. 2000, 'We just don't talk about it: men living with urinary incontinence and multiple sclerosis', *International Journal of Nursing Practice*, vol. 6, 253–60.

Lather, P. 1991, *Getting Smart: Feminist Research and Pedagogy with/in the Postmodern*, Routledge, New York.

Lewin, K. 1946, 'Action research and minority issues', *Journal of Social Issues*, vol. 2, 34–46.

Lumby, J. 1997, 'Liver transplantation: the death/life paradox', *International Journal of Nursing Practice*, vol. 3, 231–8.

Manias, E. & Street, A. 2000, 'Possibilities for critical social theory and Foucault's work: a toolbox approach', *Nursing Inquiry*, vol. 7, 50–60.

McTaggart, R. 1991, 'Principles for participatory action research', *Adult Education Quarterly*, vol. 41, no. 3, 168–87.

Mohanty, C. T. 1994, 'On race and voice: challenges for liberal education in the 1990s', in Giroux, H. A. & McLaren, P. eds, *Between Borders: Pedagogy and the Politics of Cultural Studies*, Routledge, New York.

O'Brien, B. & Spry, J. 1995, 'Expanding the role of the clinical nurse consultant', *Australian Journal of Advanced Nursing*, vol. 12, no. 4, 26–32.

Poole, M. J. & Isaacs, D. 1995, 'Family vs career: nursing student discourses', *Nursing Inquiry*, vol. 2, no. 2, 100–5.

Ramudu, L., Bellet, B., Higgs, J., Latimer, C. & Smith, R. 1994, 'How effectively do we use double staff time?' *Australian Journal of Advanced Nursing*, vol. 11, no. 3, 5–10.

Ray, M. A. 1992, 'Critical theory as a framework to enhance nursing science', *Nursing Science Quarterly*, vol. 5, no. 3, 98–101.

Reinharz, S. 1992, *Feminist Methods in Social Research*, Oxford University Press, New York.

Retsas, A. 1994, 'Problematic telephone orders: empowering nurses through action research', *Australian Journal of Advanced Nursing*, vol. 11, no. 2, 19–27.

Rosenau, P. 1992, *Post-Modernism and the Social Sciences: Insights, Inroads and Intrusions*, Princeton University Press, New Jersey.

Seidman, S. 1994, *Contested Knowledge*, Blackwell Science, Oxford.

Shannon, S. J. 1994, Dilemmas of a feminist ethnography. Paper presented at the Discursive Construction of Knowledge Conference, Adelaide, South Australia.

Speedy, S. 1987, 'Feminism and the professionalization of nursing', *Australian Journal of Advanced Nursing*, vol. 4, no. 2, 20–8.

Stevens, P. E. 1989, 'A critical social reconceptualization of environment in nursing: implications for methodology', *Advances in Nursing Science*, vol. 11, no. 4, 56–68.

Street, A. 1995, *Nursing Replay: Researching Nursing Culture Together*, Churchill Livingstone, Melbourne.

Street, A. 1998, 'From soulmates to stakeholders: issues in creating quality postmodern participatory research relationships', *Social Sciences in Health*, vol. 4, 119–29.

Stringer, E. 1996, *Action Research: A Handbook for Practitioners*, Sage Publications, Thousand Oaks, California.

Tong, R. 1989, *Feminist Thought: A Comprehensive Introduction*, Unwin Hyman, Sydney.

Walter, R., Davis, K., & Glass, N. 1999, 'Discovery of self: exploring, interconnecting and integrating self (concept) and nursing', *Collegian*, vol. 6, no. 2, 12–5.

Weedon, C. 1991, *Feminist Practice and Poststructuralist Theory*, Basil Blackwell, London.

Wellard, S. & Street, A. F. 1999, 'Family issues in home-based care', *International Journal of Nursing Practice*, vol. 5, 132–6.

Wheeler, C. E. & Chinn, P. L. 1989, *Peace and Power: A Handbook of Feminist Process*, National League for Nursing, New York.

Wilkinson, J. M. 1992, *Nursing Process in Action: a Critical Thinking Approach*, Addison-Wesley Publishing, New York.

CHAPTER 14

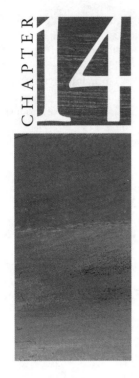

Qualitative methods

chapter objectives The material presented in this chapter will assist you to:

- discuss the rationale for choosing congruent methods in qualitative research
- describe the central importance of contexts and people in qualitative research
- discuss some data collection methods that may be used in qualitative research.

Introduction

There are many methodologies that underlie the generation of a variety of forms of knowledge, and there are many ways or methods in which information can be collected. In qualitative research, usually there are attempts to ensure that the methods by which new information is collected are 'in tune' with the particular theoretical assumptions that underlie the kinds of knowledge that are being generated in the project. Being 'in tune' is another way of saying that methods and forms of knowledge need to be congruent, and for many qualitative researchers, methodological congruency is an issue they face as they plan research projects.

This chapter begins by exploring some of the issues around methodological congruency. This is an issue you may need to face if you think that the research questions you have might be answered well by a qualitative approach. You will then discover the importance of research contexts and people, because all the circumstances of the setting and the people within them have a great bearing on how interpretations are made in qualitative research.

Following this, a list of methods that may be used in qualitative research will be described alphabetically. You will see that the methods are many and varied, and in some cases they may seem quite creative and fun to you. Given that all the examples of methods are discussed briefly by way of introduction, you would be well advised to read further than the descriptions given here, should you be thinking of using them in your research.

Choosing congruent methods

Methods are the ways or means by which new knowledge is collected and analysed, and they can include controlled trials, interviews, surveys, questionnaires, observation, field notes, historical documents, and so on. For example, empirico-analytical methodologies include an assumption that knowledge is real and trustworthy if it is found through objective means, so the researcher will need to use methods that involve strict observation, manipulation and measurement of variables to produce new knowledge of that type. For the quantitative researcher, a survey, questionnaire or controlled trial may be the appropriate data collection method.

Conversely, qualitative methodologies are based on the assumption that knowledge that is real and trustworthy is found through paying attention to what people say and do in specific circumstances; therefore, methods may be chosen that collect information that is language based and specific to people's particular experiences.

The word 'may' has been used deliberately to show that instances of matching methodologies to methods may not always be the case. Some researchers who have labelled their research 'qualitative' may use surveys and questionnaires, for example in an action research phase. Some 'quantitative' researchers may argue that they can 'qualify' quantitative data by using interviews and converting the findings into numbers. This is not stated to confuse you, rather to say that things may not be as clear cut as they seem at first, and you would do well to be alert to instances when these arbitrary distinctions become blurred.

For many researchers using qualitative approaches to their work, issues of congruency are important. The attention to choosing congruent methods is based on the assumption that if a methodology is a set of theoretical assumptions, and a method is a means for generating a certain type of knowledge, then it seems reasonable to assume that there needs to be a degree of fit between the type of knowledge that is to be generated and the means that are available to achieve it.

If a qualitative research project is based on the assumptions that people are interpreters of their own experiences and that matters of their context and relationships are important components of how they can make sense of their experiences, the types of methods that are selected to reflect these assumptions need to be appropriate. For example, a research project that seeks to explore the lived experiences of nurses and patients would need to select some methods through which those people would have the best chance to express their experiences. In such a case, participant observation and participant interviews would be consistent with the epistemological (knowledge-producing and proving) assumptions.

The reasons the methods for the previous example could be argued as being appropriate are that, through participant observation, the researcher has gone to the participants' own place of living and working to watch them on site and interact with them there. Through interviews, opportunities are given for people to express their experiences through language, experiences which may be different from those that could be represented in a prepared survey or questionnaire. In a forced-choice survey or questionnaire there may not be sufficient opportunity for a richer expression of variations in people's experiences. This is not to deny the likelihood that a very well-constructed, highly tested and amended questionnaire may not go some way in getting to the meaning of people's experiences, but most probably it would not allow for unique cases and unexpected responses that people may offer in a trusting conversation-like interview, that would give deeper insights into the area of interest.

Research contexts and participants

In its broadest sense, 'context' means the set of features specific to a particular setting, including the place, time and circumstances. Research contexts are those features of the research setting that need to be taken into account when deciding to undertake a research project. In qualitative research, it is important to acknowledge the features of the setting as having a bearing on how people might interact within them, so these features are described clearly as part of the project report.

A general principle of qualitative research would hold that people are placed in time and space, and therefore that they cannot help but be situated somewhere, and as such, they have some degree of involvement in their respective contexts. Benner and Wrubel (1989, p. 82) claim that 'there can be no situationless involvement'. In other words, where people are placed has a bearing on how they will interpret their situations, and this is an important point to bear in mind when asking them to speak of their experiences. Applying this principle to nursing practice, nurses and patients will make sense of their experiences in relation to the situations they find themselves in, such as the ward or unit they are in, the time of day and their unique set of circumstances, including for example the social, political, economic, physical, emotional and spiritual aspects of their lives.

People are central to qualitative research because they are the prime sources of information. People's experiences may seem insignificant to them because they may be regarded as simply part of living their lives, but qualitative research has an interest in commonplace experiences. It encourages people to delve into their experiences, and to realise that it is through their accounts that personal and practical knowledge may be generated for themselves and for others. For example, if we are to understand the meaning of illness and disease, it can be directly from the accounts of the experiencing people. If we are to understand and change the powerful constraints acting on nurses in health care organisations, we can work collaboratively with nurses in their practice settings. People are the key, because it is through the expression of their stories that we come to understand their experiences.

Subjectivity refers to personal experiences and personal truths that may or may not have some resonance with other people's subjective experiences and truths. The 'subjective' knowledge that is generated through qualitative research methods does not make a universal claim to be true for everyone and for all things in all times and places, nor does it rely on proving things to be true through the objectivity of human senses. Therefore, subjectivity in qualitative research is linked inextricably with the relative nature of knowledge and the possibilities of understanding the complexities of human phenomena from the standpoints of the experiencing individuals.

Qualitative research emphasises the central roles of the research context and people in generating knowledge that is personal and practical, and which comes from the perspective of people engaged actively in their lives. In contrast to research methods of an 'objective' nature, qualitative research values what people have to say about how they feel, what they believe and think, based on whatever information they have amassed as participants in experiencing life.

Rigour in qualitative research

In relation to research, 'rigour' means the strictness in judgement and conduct which must be used to ensure that the successive steps in a project have been set out clearly and undertaken with scrupulous attention to detail. This allows the project to be scrutinised by others for evidence of methodological accuracy and worthiness. In other words, the interest is in whether the project's findings can be relied on as reflecting 'the truth' of the matter. 'Truth' appears here in inverted commas to denote its relative and uncertain status, in that the generation and verification of absolute truth is a debatable point in terms of whether it is actually possible.

In quantitative research, rather than referring to rigour in a general sense, the more specific words 'validity and reliability' would most probably be used. Validity refers to the extent to which the means used in the research to collect and analyse data do what they are supposed to do. Reliability refers to the extent to which consistent results can be achieved on repeated undertaking of the research project. These checking processes ensure that the strict rules and steps of the scientific method have been followed and reflected in the project. If the processes are judged to be accurate, the likelihood is greater that the research findings are 'true'. The criteria for rigour are related directly to the underlying assumptions of what constitutes knowledge and truth and how these are best generated and proven. Another way of stating this, is that criteria for rigour are related directly to the underlying epistemological assumptions. If you refer to Chapter 12, you can review the differences between the assumptions underlying the use of quantitative and qualitative research approaches.

Qualitative research is no less rigorous than quantitative research, but it uses different words to demonstrate the ways of making explicit the overall processes and worthiness of a project, because it is based on different epistemological assumptions. As Emden and Sandelowski (1998) rightly point out, issues of 'rigour' in qualitative research have gone through many 'translations', and this is especially so in nursing research. Please note that I use inverted commas intentionally around the word 'rigour' in relation to qualitative research, to denote the transition in meaning it has traversed from quantitative into qualitative methods, and the difficulties it has had in throwing off quantitative epistemological assumptions.

Adjustments to imagining qualitative concerns about 'rigour' began with Guba and Lincoln (1981) who suggested the renaming of validity and reliability categories into trustworthiness to reflect the people-oriented nature of qualitative research. The reason for this is that the assumptions, methods and processes of qualitative and quantitative research differ. Sandelowski (1986) took up this suggestion and applied it well to nursing. The criteria of credibility, fittingness, auditability and confirmability will be discussed later in this section.

Qualitative researchers (Beck 1993; Sandelowski 1986; Yonge & Stewin 1988) argued that it is unreasonable to judge a qualitative research project against the criteria designed for a quantitative investigation. For example, qualitative research works on the assumption that 'truth' is relative and context-dependent. This means that what is seen to be true may change, and it may reflect the features of the time, places and circumstances in which people find themselves. Also, quantitative research uses objectivity in searching for objective knowledge, whereas many qualitative research approaches acknowledge and use the subjectivity of research participants and value the subjective knowledge they offer.

Determining 'rigour' in qualitative research

Various means of determining 'rigour' in qualitative research have been suggested (Sandelowski 1986; Denzin 1989; Hall & Stevens 1991; Beck 1993). There is not one accepted test of 'rigour' in qualitative research, just as there is not one way of doing qualitative research, although the 'translation' of criteria now extends to postmodern thinking and the concept of goodness (Emden & Sandelowski 1998, 1999). This means that researchers must use the most appropriate means of assessing 'rigour' in qualitative projects, to reflect the methodological assumptions of the project.

For example, in some feminist research approaches 'rigour' is judged by the extent to which the project reflects 'dependability' and 'adequacy' (Hall & Stevens 1991). Stability and similarity across data collection methods and findings are the degree of dependability, and this equates with reliability. Meaningful research outcomes reflect adequacy, which comprises aspects of reliability and validity.

According to Hall and Stevens (1991), areas contributing to 'rigour' are:

- reflexivity, by continually critiquing the research process
- credibility, by assessing the progress and outcomes through member checks
- rapport, experienced as open, trusting group dynamics
- coherence, by constantly confirming the research process
- acknowledging complexity in the research and its participants
- achieving consensus in decision-making
- addressing relevance to women's concerns
- attaining honesty and mutuality
- naming, using women's own terms and concepts, to denote the project's objectives, processes and outcomes
- achieving relationality, by forming collaborative interpersonal relationships to challenge ideas and respect differences.

Whereas these attempts to ensure 'rigour' are relevant for feminist research assumptions and processes, they may have little or no relevance for other qualitative researchers who do not place strong emphasis on collaborative relationships in research.

Burns and Grove (1993, p. 64) argued that 'rigour' in qualitative research is 'associated with openness, scrupulous adherence to a philosophical perspective, thoroughness in collecting data, and consideration of all the data in the subjective theory development phase'. They suggest that in order to be rigorous in qualitative research the researcher must be open to new ideas by being willing to let go of old ideas (deconstructing), and by examining many dimensions to form new ideas (reconstructing). Although deconstructing and reconstructing reflect the open, exploratory nature of qualitative research, these concepts do not provide potential qualitative researchers with actual steps in how to attain 'rigour'.

Denzin (1989) suggested using triangulation to create multiple references which converge to draw conclusions that may be claimed as the 'truth'. He identified data, investigator, theory and methodological triangulation.

Data triangulation uses multiple data sources, such as interviewing many participants about the same topic in a study. Investigator triangulation uses many individuals to collect and analyse a single set of data. Theory triangulation uses many theoretical perspectives to interpret data. Methodological triangulation uses multiple methods such as interviews, document analysis and observation. By using many triangulation sources as described, Denzin (1989) suggested that a data cross-checking system would ensure the 'rigour' of a project.

Sandelowski (1986) applied the ideas of Guba and Lincoln (1981) relating to 'rigour' in qualitative research in general, to nursing research in particular. The categories for determining 'rigour' are credibility, fittingness, auditability, and confirmability.

Credibility

Credibility means the extent to which participants and readers of the research recognise the lived experiences described in the research as similar to their own. If there is recognition of the phenomenon just from reading about it in the transcripts or research reports, credibility is achieved.

Fittingness

Fittingness refers to the extent to which a project's findings fit into other contexts outside the study setting. The term is also used to mean the extent to which the readers of the research find it has meaning and relevance for their own experiences.

Auditability

Auditability is the production of a decision trail which can be scrutinised by other researchers to determine the extent to which the project has achieved consistency in its methods and processes. A high degree of auditability would allow another researcher to use a similar approach and possibly arrive at similar or comparable conclusions.

Confirmability

Confirmability of a project is achieved when credibility, auditability and fittingness can be demonstrated. This relies on the confirmation of participants, whose subjectivity is valued as instructive in assessing the extent to which the project achieves neutrality from the researcher's stated biases.

These criteria for 'rigour' will appear quite different from those described in this book to ascertain reliability and validity in quantitative research. This is completely admissible, given that the two broad approaches have many differences in what constitutes truth and the best ways of finding it. Given the longer standing positive reputation of quantitative research, and the tendency to judge qualitative research against quantitative criteria, Yonge and Stewin (1988, p. 65) present some challenges for qualitative researchers to:

- develop and use rules, terms and procedures to describe qualitative research processes accurately
- ensure that participants are actively involved in all phases of the research project, including being present at dissemination of the findings through presentations, and are informed of publication
- understand the purposes and implications of using terms such as validity and reliability
- tolerate uncertainty and confusion (particularly when pitted against an articulate positivist!) as a new language to describe the relevance of qualitative inquiry emerges
- recall that there is an essential difference between qualitative and quantitative methods of inquiry and that if both are to be mixed, the researcher must provide a sound rationale.

Emden and Sandelowski (1998, 1999) have taken up Yonge and Stewin's (1988, p. 65) challenge to qualitative researchers, and have evolved their ideas for the 'conceptions of goodness in qualitative research'. In a thought-provoking, two-part paper, they review the transformations of criteria in qualitative research, noting the renaming of various approaches as more distance from quantitative criteria for 'rigour' has been accomplished. In the first part the authors 'trace efforts to define "goodness" in qualitative research within various fields, including nursing' noting that they 'continue to reflect a search for order' (Emden & Sandelowski 1998, p. 206). In the second part of the paper, the authors describe the problematic shortfalls in 'rigour' and 'criteria' by applying postmodern thinking. They point out that criteria attempt to define and limit reality in the assumption that 'truth' is out there, waiting to be discovered, harnessed, and applied to problems of explanation, prediction and control in the human world. Thus, 'criteria' *and* 'rigour' have an 'ancestry [that] can be similarly traced to positivism and its problems' (Emden & Sandelowski 1999, p. 3).

Emden and Sandelowski contemplate 'the demise of criteria' to show how authors have attempted to sever 'qualitative research from the tenets of positivism'. One approach has been of 'conceiving criteria not as definite rules but as ever evolving and open ended "lists"' (Smith 1990, cited in Emden & Sandelowski 1999, p. 3). Another approach has been to use enabling conditions 'to do with dialogue, a community of interpreters, rhetoric, conversation, and imagination' (Schwandt 1996, cited in Emden & Sandelowski 1999, p. 3). Even so, Emden and Sandelowski (1999, p. 4) cite Lincoln (1995) who wrote: 'We are not ready to close down the conversation or to say farewell to criteria quite yet'. Emden and Sandelowski remind readers of the practical realities of keeping qualitative research 'alive as a coherent whole' and satisfying criteria of goodness for 'those required to make speedy judgements about the quality of qualitative work, such as members of human research ethics committees, funding bodies, and editorial review boards, as well as consumers and designers of the research in the first place' (p. 4).

In responding to the conundrum of goodness in qualitative research in the postmodern era, Emden and Sandelowski (1999, p. 5) raise the possibility that 'uncertainty can be turned to advantage, and novel avenues of thought forged, whereby both the impracticability of the grand narrative is recognised, as well as the richness and value of local contexts and meanings appreciated'. This means that researchers can opt to integrate the best of the modern and postmodern worlds of research into ensuring goodness in their projects. Emden and Sandelowski also raise the courageous and baldly honest possibility of a 'criterion of uncertainty' not in terms of methodological weakness, but as an 'open acknowledgement that claims about our research outcomes are at best tentative and that there may indeed be no way of showing otherwise' (p. 5). However, they admit, that 'within all terms and usages, the criterion problem lurks' and that in a postmodern world that 'decries all such searches for order and meaning' it is 'never too late to ask … "Whose criteria?" "Criteria for what?" and "Why criteria at all?"' (Emden & Sandelowski 1999, p. 6).

Methods that may be used in qualitative research

In this next section you will be introduced to a variety of methods that may be used in qualitative research projects, in various combinations, according to the requirements of the research question or area. For ease of access, the methods are listed alphabetically. Bear in mind that methods are used to gather information considered most likely to be of assistance in fulfilling the aims and objectives of a research project. This means that they have been considered carefully and put into place and used with thoughtfulness in relation to what they may offer. Bear in mind also, that if we are informed by postmodern thought, we might hold only as tentative any knowledge that comes about, however carefully we undertake our methods.

Archival searches

Archival information consists of original hard copies of treasured documents such as logs, diaries, government agencies' agendas and minutes, reports, photographs, newspapers, books, private papers donated by families to the archives, and so on. Historians are well versed in archival searches with respect to what to seek and how to make the best of the information once it is gathered and copied.

This method involves going to archival repositories, such as purpose-built archival buildings and libraries, to seek specific research information of an historical nature. Archives are listed in telephone directories and/or contact details may be gained by phoning the information centres of country and city councils. There is usually a search fee to gain access to records, and photocopying charges apply. The cost of archival data collection should be itemised in project budgets, so that the cost does not become a problem for the overall management of the project. Remember also, that once you are in amongst the archives your enthusiasm for finding treasures may get the better of you, so for the sake of time, effort and expense, keep your research focus in mind, so that you do not become unduly sidetracked.

Categories of copied data can be sorted systematically into a favoured filing system, which can be accessed easily by yourself and other members of the research team. Boxes, hanging files, cupboards and shelves may store information in some practical order, such as by time, place, or main content. Labelling items with full reference details, dates, times, sources, and so on, makes for easier management of the data, when it is time for analysis.

For further information on how to do archival searches and manage literature, refer to Sorensen (1988) and Streubert and Carpenter (1995, pp. 201–3) and the relevant sections in this book.

Artistic expression

Sometimes it might be appropriate in the research design to collect data in the form of a direct and creative demonstration of the participant's experiences through artistic expression, such as painting, drawing, montage, photography, poetry, dance, music, symbols, singing and so on. At times, the data may be accompanied by the creator's interpretations of the piece, or the data may stand as they are, to be interpreted by other means, such as through group discussion and/or the researcher's methods of interpretation.

Data collected through artistic expression may be particularly useful in research aimed at finding the experience of certain conditions/states/perspectives from the unique viewpoint of individuals. Participants may be invited to use a variety of artistic expressions to represent themselves and issues in their lives through creative images. Alternatively, as the researcher, you may decide to express some of your observations through an artistic medium, such as poetry, to add further richness to the other sources of data.

Careful storage and sorting of artistic data are important, because symbolic representations are best interpreted in relation to the person representing them. Therefore, items and their interpretive accounts must be stored together, labelled clearly and fully for later analysis if necessary. Details such as the artist's name or pseudonym, date, time, intention of the artwork, preliminary interpretational remarks and so on, may be useful in making sense of the contribution of any form of creative expression when applied as a research method.

If this form of data collection sounds interesting to you, you might like to read Mary Ebbott's article: 'Integrating the arts into clinical care' (Ebbott 1996). The article deals with 'exploring the spiritual, intangible dimensions of the creative arts' and their integration into therapeutic nursing (Ebbott 1996, p. 105). As an application of the article, research methods for exploring the effectiveness of arts in nursing could be undertaken by the arts and artists themselves; that is, information could be collected and analysed using the artistic expression and interpretation of the participants.

In addition to using the artist's expression as a form of knowledge generation in itself, creative means may also be used when reflection is a part of a project. Taylor (2000a) lists many ways in which artistic expression can aid reflection, and by association, assist research. These include writing, audiotaping, creating music, dancing, drawings, montage, painting, poetry, pottery, quilting, singing and videotaping. Any of these methods may be used alone or in combination. In the area of artistic expression, you are limited only by your own imagination, but remember the unlocking of creative potential needs to be related to the aims and objectives of your project, otherwise it may eventuate to be fun without practical application.

Case studies

A case study can be considered as a method or a design. In other words, some researchers focus on the discrete analytical means along the way (methods), while others look to the broader stream of events in the research project (design). On the whole, authors tend to agree that a case study is a research strategy that comprises an all-encompassing, comprehensive method and set of strategies (Burns & Grove 1997; Woods 1997) that allow people, practices and phenomena to be described over time according to their contextual features (Stake 1994; Yin 1994; Fitzgerald 1999).

The case study method describes fully, selected foci of research interest, such as individuals, groups, or institutions. The researcher uses a case study method to try to understand over time as much as possible about the area in focus, so the method is characterised by intensive analysis of all the determinants involved.

As there is no clear-cut way of doing a case study, it is really up to the researcher to set up a practical and systematic approach to gathering, recording, analysing and presenting information. For example, Cowley et al. (2000) wanted to understand how community nurses in England carry out health education needs assessments with clients, so they used four 'cases' based on geographical locations to observe recently qualified practitioners during regular shifts over a total of 134 home visits. Semistructured interviews were carried out after the observation periods to explore with nurses their rationale for decisions and procedures during needs assessments. Assessment and curriculum documents were also analysed as a form of triangulation of data. Patterns of the data were compared repeatedly and explanations were developed, leading to analytical generalisations (not statistical generalisations).

In planning a case study you need to consider your research questions and how you might best answer them. This may mean that you will need a variety of strategies in sequence, that will ensure a comprehensive approach to the area of inquiry. As an illustrative case, consider a research student (whose project I am supervising) who wanted to explore the subjective experiences of people with moderate depression in relation to Healing Touch (Healing Touch International 2000). As she was not interested in proving that Healing Touch 'cures' depression, she was not required to undertake an experimental design in which she could show statistically that Healing Touch alone was the healing factor.

After exploring the literature around case study and methodologies, the research student realised that she could combine a case study approach with an overarching methodology of grounded theory, as the two are complementary in their intentions to explore an unknown area of inquiry inductively. Grounded theory also provides an analytical method and permits theory building, while a case study approach facilitates investigation and comparison over time of single (or collective) cases, using a variety of data collection methods. This being so, she designed a project including five weekly Healing Touch treatments of one hour's duration. The first session involved assessment with the Beck Depression Inventory (Foreman 1997) to identify moderate depression, and the completion of the Healing Energy And Life Through Holism (HEALTH) tool (Healing Touch International 2000) for a holistic health assessment. The participants and researcher kept a reflective journal to record their experiences and the researcher also made case notes of participants' pre- and post-treatment responses. The final session included a further Beck assessment, an interview about each participant's subjective experience, and review of the data entries. The data will be analysed by a constant comparative process with the aim of generating a theory (Strauss & Corbin 1990). From this case study, the researcher will make recommendations as to the use of a theory in the provision of Healing Touch for people with moderate depression.

Given the two examples above, you may be able to see that the case study approach you take will be entirely up to you, as long as you can show that the sequence of methods relate to exploring most directly and comprehensively the research questions and aims you have posed. You need also to consider issues of trustworthiness (see this chapter), appropriate methods of data analysis (see Chapter 16) and interpretation (see Chapter 17). Read as widely as you can and see how other researchers have organised their case studies and be prepared to critique those methods and designs that could have been more creative and/or comprehensive in their approaches. Some examples to get you started are Dale (1995), Sharp (1998), Byrar (1999), Pegram (1999) and Vallis and Tierney (1999).

As with all research involving human participants, a case study requires ethical approval and the consent of all participants in each and every part of the case study in which they are involved. For example, if you are interested in undertaking a single case study about an exemplary woman who has survived cancer, you would need to think through all the usual steps of a research project. For instance, what do you want to know, why, how, when, and for whose purposes? How will the case study be important to nursing and health? Having determined these ideas, you need to work with the person to set up a practical approach to recording her experiences. She might agree to having her stories audiotaped and transcribed. She might also agree to allowing you to spend some time with her in observation of her daily life, or she might have photographs and personal records that she will allow you to make public.

As you can see, the approach to a case study is open and creative, but this should not frustrate you if you have given the method sufficient thought and have planned it carefully with the people involved. The analysis and interpretation of the sections of the case study will depend on what is appropriate for the method used. For example, interviews and journal entries may require thematic analysis and the findings may be combined into a collective interpretation or retained as single case trajectories, depending on how the case study was set up. The people involved may want to offer their interpretations, some observational comment may be appropriate, and photographs and document analysis may add to the descriptive potential of the case study. The presentation of the case study may be as a journal article for publication, or it may be of sufficient depth and breadth to warrant publication in a book or monograph.

Fieldwork

Fieldwork occurs where the action is happening, out in the 'field' of inquiry. Fieldwork methods may vary according to the intentions of the research, but they usually consist of combinations of observation, participation, documentation and analysis. A common form of data collection in fieldwork is the documentation of field notes. These are notes made by the researchers to themselves, that will form part of the data when the entire project is drawn together. Field notes need to be made as soon as possible, so that the events are still fresh in the researcher's mind.

For instance, if you want to do an ethnographic study of the inside culture and activities of a community health centre, part of the data would be notes that are written whenever it becomes necessary and/or advisable to capture the thickest possible description of what is happening, to whom, when, why, how and where. To save the effort of having to transfer the information later, a portable computer can be used to record the notes, making copies readily accessible.

If paper and pen are used for making notes, a system of careful storage is necessary to maintain the chronological and contextual order of the information. If computers assist the process, files should be identified easily and checked periodically to ensure that the disk is still operable. When the analysis phase begins, the records should be complete and legible.

Another alternative for researchers who prefer oral rather than written accounts is to use a portable audiotape system. In this way observations can be recorded rapidly and with the relative spontaneity of spoken words. All tapes should be identified with the date, time and general content of the recording, so that they can be organised easily for later analysis.

Fieldwork and observation/participant observation are related methods, in that fieldwork can be taken to mean broader activities such as those undertaken in ecological studies. Here, the emphasis is on the methods of observation researchers use when they are undertaking qualitative projects. For further explanation, see this section: Observation/participant observation.

Group processes

Some research methodologies use group interaction processes, through which to collect and sort data. Group interaction processes are particularly suitable for collaborative research such as action research, feminist research or research that is informed by poststructural and/or postmodern ideas. In all of these cases, the underlying assumptions of the research are that people need to be empowered to find and use voice, multiple perspectives are valued, group members have agreed on the research problems and those members are the best ones to solve the problems through their own collective processes. It is advisable to think ahead about how to collect and sort this kind of data, to ensure that the group processes are of optimal value. In other words, you will invite a purposive sample of people to gather together, given that they have the experiences needed to offer insights into the research topic.

When people get together there needs to be some direction, otherwise they have a tendency to talk over the top of one another, to break into separate chatting sessions, and generally to lose direction. Facilitation of the group conversations is needed, and it can be by the researcher as a facilitator, or all of the group members may take a turn in facilitating by a 'rotating chair' process in which everyone takes responsibility for facilitation at some time. Shy or inexperienced members can be encouraged to apply the skills of group facilitation, learning at first by modelling their behaviours on those of an experienced group facilitator. Skills in group processes are many and varied and you are advised to read beyond this text for suggestions on how to do this effectively. For example, Beebe and Masterson (1994) wrote up a study that could be helpful if you are interested in bringing a group together for research purposes.

Collecting information within the group needs to be given some thought in order to capture how the group interacts together and what has been discussed and decided collectively. Some methods for collecting information may include note-taking, audiotaping, videotaping, or by collective review processes at the end of the session. A good idea is to have the group generate ideas and for them to be written clearly on a whiteboard as the meeting progresses, so that members can decide collectively on the main ideas, areas to be prioritised and areas for further action. It may be useful to create small groups and present the main ideas to the whole group at the conclusion, or group members may take responsibility for contributing to a brainstorming or ideas-collating exercise at the end of the session. Whatever occurs, it is important to gather in the most important ideas, so that the perspectives of the group can be represented adequately. It is also important that the group members validate their ideas by confirming that the interpretations that have been made reflect faithfully the meaning that was intended.

A focus group is a particular type of group, in that it has certain processes that distinguish it from a group convened for less specific reasons. A focus group is a collection of people working together on a particular research issue. The people who attend are research participants who have given their consent to be involved in the project, having been invited deliberately for their knowledge and/or skills in the area to which the research relates. The group is facilitated by the researcher or by a research assistant with the necessary skills to keep the group focused on its aims and objectives. In some cases, researchers may use their grant monies to pay an expert skilled in running focus groups to facilitate the meeting or series of meetings.

The process usually involves a brainstorming session, in which the focus group members respond to questions and comments made by the facilitator and/or in response to group discussion. Responses are recorded on an object visible to the group, such as a blackboard, whiteboard, overhead transparency or butchers' paper. The facilitator calls for all spontaneous responses with 'no holds barred', then the group works together to collate and prioritise ideas to remove duplications, 'off the wall' remarks, or responses that are judged by the group to be of minimal help or relevance to the research question/aim/context.

Focus groups help research by getting a number of people together to solicit their contributions. This means that many ideas are collated, it is less expensive than individual interviews and, in some cases, the group can collaborate on analysing and interpreting the data. The disadvantages of focus groups are that the less vocal members can be overlooked if they are not 'drawn out' carefully by the facilitator, the responses may not be as rich and full as they might be in the privacy of an interview and it is difficult to track an individual's perceptions in amongst the group's responses, leaving the interpretations broad and relevant only to the collective responses of the group.

If group processes are to be used sequentially, say, for one hour per week for six months, a great deal of data will be generated and many twists and turns in the life of the group will need to be documented to represent the processes and outcomes of the group. This may be the case in an action research project in which members are committed to regular meetings to work through action cycles. When groups meet regularly, it is a good idea to create some documenting processes. An idea is to have all group members keep a journal of events and their responses to them, and/or to maintain meeting agendas and minutes. I found both these processes to be very helpful in an action research and reflective practice project (Taylor 2000b; Taylor, in press), because the group confirmed the minutes each week as a form of data validation, and the information was present in the minutes when I came to the point of writing the final report and preparing a journal article.

Interviews

Qualitative interviews are more like conversations than interrogations. Unlike quantitative research, in which you might reasonably expect to find a structured interview format resembling a oral survey or questionnaire, the epistemological assumptions of qualitative research favour a less structured approach. The reasons for this are that a qualitative interview is designed to encourage participants to tell their stories and relate their experiences in the deepest and richest way possible, bearing in mind inevitable project constraints such as time, transcription costs, interviewee ability as conversationalist and storyteller, and so on.

You may locate many descriptors for qualitative interviews in the literature, such as 'in-depth focused' (Walker, Hall & Thomas 1995), 'in-depth semi-structured' (Nolan, Owens & Nolan 1995), and 'unstructured formal' (Hogston 1995). It is not really important that researchers are prescriptive about the 'labelling' of a qualitative interview, but it is essential to indicate as clearly as possible the processes that were used, especially in the part of the project report that describes methods and processes. For example, interviews may be focused or non-directive, depending on how the participant is invited to respond. Some guiding questions may be necessary to keep a clear direction in a focused interview, but it is very important that the questioning does not extend to a long list, as depth of responses may be sacrificed for breadth of coverage. If you have many questions to ask in rapid-fire sequence, consider a survey, as this can cover a lot of material, with many people, in a relatively short time.

When a research participant is interviewed with an invitation to tell a story, the researcher's directive may be as simple as 'Tell me about your experience of ...', or 'I understand that you have experienced ... Can you tell me about that please?' Some lead-up conversation may be necessary to settle the storyteller emotionally, and to ascertain that s/he is clear about the focus of the research and how the story can contribute. The plain language statement and the consent form handed out prior to the beginning of the research can indicate all of the necessary information about the project and the participant's involvement. Participants may also be given a list of guiding questions that will be asked to engage the interviewee in a storytelling and/or conversational process. When an interviewee requires prompts, simple encouraging words may help, such as: 'What happened then?', 'Where/when did that happen?' 'How were you involved?' 'How did that make you feel?' As with all good communication, being attentive and responding appropriately are important skills for unfolding effective conversations and stories.

In summary, qualitative interviews can be structured with a list of set questions to be asked, or they can be relatively unstructured with little more than an invitation being issued by the researcher for the participant to talk about an area of interest. In between both end points is a semistructured interview, a conversation in which the researcher invites the participant to talk, encouraging a free flow of words and ideas but at the same time keeping the person relatively on track in the conversation if s/he has a tendency to wander off the point. For example, you might say something like: 'Tell me more about that please?', and 'We seem to have got off track; you were saying ...'.

The best way to collect interview data is on audiotape, although video may be advisable in cases in which nonverbal cues are important. Buy reliable tapes to minimise the risk of data loss. To prevent loss of data you might also prefer to make backup copies of the tapes and store them in a different place from the originals. The audiotapes can be transcribed to form written text for analysis, or they may be replayed, to allow for the recognition of themes. If participants are shy of the audiotape machine, a time of general talking with the player on may be necessary in order for people to feel less conscious of it. If anxiety prevails about the use of the audiomachine, it may be necessary to take notes, although this method may take up your attention and energy, and you may miss important content details and voice inflections.

Interview transcripts generate lots and lots of data that must be managed systematically. If you are an organised sort of person, this will come easily to you. If you tend towards the haphazard end of the continuum, you might like to get the advice of a practical person who can set you straight on how to organise your sorting and filing system so that data are not misplaced or otherwise mistreated.

In the absence of an organised and practical person here are some clues that might help you. The transcripts are most easily managed on computer disk. Make a copy of each transcript, transfer it to a separate well-functioning computer disk and store it in a different place to prevent loss. Keep a main copy of the transcript either on a floppy disk or the hard disk of the computer, and ensure that any alterations made to the main document are also made to the copies. This will help you to keep all of the work current thereby preventing confusion as to which is the most recent working copy. It also means that if there is a computer glitch or the floppy you are using deteriorates, the information loss will only be as extensive as the last updated disk copy. Consider procuring a filing cabinet with hanging files for hard copies, foolscap folders, and a lockable computer disk container with plenty of disk labels. Some forethought in organising the storage of your data will prevent a lot of concern and chaos later.

If you do not have access to computer facilities, you may be using typed hard copies of transcripts. There is a similar need for caution in storing and filing these forms of data. Make multiple copies of the hard copies. Ensure they have all of the identifying details written on them. Keep a list of all the transcripts according to participants' actual names and pseudonyms and lock this away so that anonymity is maintained. Store the typed transcript copies in a paper filing system such as manilla folders, and keep a copy in a different location to minimise the risk of loss.

Journal keeping

The journal form of data collection is useful for research in which participants are conversant with, and willing to indulge in, reflective writing for the purposes of the research. It may be just like keeping a diary that sets out the events of the day and reactions to them, such as in a journal you keep about being a research student. A journal of this nature might record your impressions of your meetings with your research supervisor, joys and pains of being a researcher, and any thoughts, insights and inspirations you have along the way. You might also find it useful to record information about your role in the research and how you manage being a nurse researching some aspect of nursing or health. Thus, a journal used in this more focused way may help you to reflect on your experiences of having multiple roles and responsibilities, while noticing the issues in everyday practice from the perspective of an interested participant observer divorced temporarily from the busyness of work.

Another way of using a journal is to enlist the cooperation of participants in keeping one for information gathering. You may also keep a reflective journal of your experiences as a co-researcher sharing equally in group processes. If you choose to use this method of data collection, you need to ensure that participants are willing, able and eager to write reflectively. The literature is clear that people benefit from coaching in order to reflect effectively (Greenwood 1993; Conway 1994). You may need to build some time into your project to coach participants in the methods and processes of reflection and these skills can be acquired, especially if you want them to go beyond descriptive accounts of their personal stories to making sense of their experiences. I suggest that you refer to my book on reflection for nurses and midwives if you are serious about making the best use of having participants and co-researchers keep journals (Taylor 2000a).

In using a journal all participants need to be clear about the objectives of the activity, otherwise many words may be written that may have little hope of informing the research. So often, ideas can wander so far off the point of a project, that the richness of the information is compromised. This does not mean that there is no room for discussion and journalling tangential to the project's main interests, but you should be careful to ensure that precious time given so generously by the participants is used to its best advantage, as a sign of respect for their contributions.

Journals may be private or semi-private, and therefore, participants may decide on what they choose to divulge for the research data. Group processes or discussions with individuals can clarify expectations about the use of journal entries as data. Participants need to agree to disclosing material in the amount and level of privacy they choose. Indeed, there may be excerpts that are so deeply personal, that they are known only to the writer, who may use them as aids for working through personal and professional issues. Areas that can be shared publicly can be spoken about in meetings and/or photocopied for incorporation into research reports and papers using pseudonyms.

The amount of material that can be generated will depend on the objectives of the exercise and the amount of disclosure that is required, but journal keeping is likely to amass a substantial amount of information that needs to be sorted in some way, in order for it be useful. Photocopies of the 'public domain' journal entries can be made, after words and phrases are adapted as ethical safeguards to reduce the risk of identifying people and places. Interpretations will be most useful if they are made by the person doing the writing, in collaboration with another person, possibly the researcher, who acts as a critical friend, asking constructive questions to bring out the richness of the content.

For further information on keeping a journal for the purposes of using critical reflection on practice for yourself or prospective research participants, you might like to read Street (1995, pp. 147–71). This is a comprehensive step-by-step account of how to set up and maintain a journal so that it is useful for more than personal reflection. The method and process Annette Street describes can help nurses to make sense out of their practice and work in ways to change those parts of it that they would like to change. Alternatively, if you need a simple-to-follow 'recipe book' approach to when, why and how to keep a journal and do reflective practice, refer to my book as mentioned previously (Taylor 2000a).

Literature searches

Part or all of a research project may involve searching for literature. Literature features in applied research as data, when it is used to show how the findings relate to published accounts of the same area of interest. In pure research, the project may consist of literature entirely, such as in the scholarly critiques expected in philosophical projects. Literature is collected from all its likely sources and repositories, and collated in a succinct and focused analysis, to show the strengths, weaknesses, connections, and gaps in what is written and how each writer contrasts to and/or augments other writers in the area.

Some helpful questions to keep in mind, to ensure a thorough literature review are:

- What is the purpose of the literature review? In other words, what is the relationship between the literature review and the research questions?
- Who has written in the area? What social/occupational roles do they occupy?
- What has been written in the area? What key propositions have been made and do they fall into key areas? What has been seen as problematic and what solutions/strategies/actions have been proposed and/or tested in relation to the area of concern?
- How have other scholars received this material? Has this material been subsumed into existing paradigms? Has it challenged existing theories or does it reinforce present ideas?
- What research projects have been carried out in this area? What methods have been employed and were they appropriate for the research questions investigated?
- What are the major findings of the research projects?
- Are research findings across various studies consistent, conflicting or both?
- What debates have there been about the content (substantive) and approach (methodological) components of these projects?
- What have been the main issues in the debates?
- What important issues appear to be overlooked, and constitute gaps, silences and omissions?
- What are the common threads in the research issues, debates, findings and themes?
- How can these common threads guide an evaluation of the knowledge that has been gathered to date, and how they can be informative for further inquiry?

If your literature review is under the special scrutiny of a discourse analysis, you need to use an even deeper level of examination, by asking questions as listed in Chapter 16 in the section: Discourse analysis.

Literature may be collected in piles and bundles, but it is of little use if it is not managed well. It is a good idea to create a running bibliography on computer disk, which keeps a record of the referencing details of the literature and the main ideas within it. If lists and descriptions are kept on computer disks, they can be cut and pasted readily into the research document. If computer technology is not available, coloured cardboard cards can be used to store information in secure filing boxes.

For some further information on how to collect and analyse literature, consult relevant sections of this book and Parahoo (1997).

Member checks

A member check is a procedure used within qualitative research methods to ensure that participants validate their contributions to the overall project, as a source of determining the trustworthiness of the project. This might mean that researchers invite participants to check various parts of the project to see whether the researcher is reflecting and interpreting their contributions in the way the participants intended. On a practical level, this means that participants might be given transcripts of interviews to ensure that the information is complete and accurate, or comment may be sought on the way in which the researcher has interpreted various themes in the data.

Even though it is good practice to use member checks in qualitative research, be aware of some of the likely scenarios that may arise. For example, people have a tendency to speak in broken sentences, adding redundancies, such as 'ums', 'ahs' and 'you knows'. When they receive a transcripts full of these kinds of grammatical glitches, they may be embarrassed at best, and want to withdraw their contributions at worst. Be prepared for this eventuality, and if there are no methodological contradictions, tidy the transcript without changing the meaning of the words, or warn the reader to be forgiving of their use of spoken language, given that it is fairly typical of us all to speak in this way.

Also be clear about what the participant is checking. There are many reasons for giving a transcript back to participants, and some may need to be spelt out clearly. A transcript may be checked before or after analysis and the participant needs to be given directions in their part of the process. For example, you may ask them to check the content of the transcript to ensure that the conversation is as they remember. Alternatively, you may invite them to add or delete information they deem necessary, or to give their opinion on whether the outcomes of the analysis are 'in tune' with their reading of the transcript. If there are certain functions you do not expect the participant to perform in relation to member checking, make this clear, and ensure that all provisos have been communicated previously in the plain language statement that accompanied the consent form they signed before they became involved in the project.

Observation/participant observation

Types of observation vary according to the research approach. They can be structured, unstructured and participant observation. Structured observation, requiring strict attention to objectivity through checklists of events and behaviours, is inappropriate in qualitative research generally, because there is no intention to standardise data collection conditions as would be the case with empirico-analytical research. However, there may be some need for this type of observation as part of a larger issue-based participatory action research project, when the observation component of an action cycle has a particular intention to identify predetermined categories of events and behaviours (Keatinge et al. 2000). If you are interested in using structured observation refer to Chapter 8 in this book.

In unstructured observation, the researcher observes a context systematically and carefully, but with no predetermined categories in mind. The observation is done with open-mindedness as to what may occur, keeping in mind the central purposes for being there as stated in the research objectives. The researcher's attention is drawn to what is happening, where, when, how and why, without actual involvement in the setting as a participant. This means that the observation periods are flexible in relation to the place in which the observation of the people and events occurs, as well as the time of day, length of time, and expectations about the aspects to be observed. Observations are documented as field notes, that describe the broad features of the setting. This kind of observation is useful for an ethnographic project, in which the researcher is present in the setting as an unobtrusive observer (Fiveash 1998; Rossiter & Yam 1998; Josipovic 2000).

As it would seem, participant observation is about getting involved in the action in a setting, whilst observing the details within it. Sometimes it is necessary to spend some time in a particular setting to see what happens there. There may be different reasons for observing the area, including getting to know who and what comes and goes, finding out about the routines, seeing how people interact with one another, and so on. For example, observation phases would be needed to gather data in ethnographic research, or observation may form part of the data collection phases of research that is not necessarily ethnographic, for instance, in action research.

Observation usually involves watching and attending systematically to a setting, then retreating for some time to write up the impressions. If the data are written directly into a word processing system, it will save a lot of time in typing them up for later analysis. If there are no technological aids such as computers, impressions can be written into a logbook or some other permanent record system.

It is important to be fully aware of why you are acting in the role of a participant observer, so be familiar with the aims and objectives of the project in which the method is occurring. You need to be 'loitering with intent', so to speak, so that you can 'tune in' intentionally to those areas of the context most directly related to your project. You need to be aware of the people who have given their consent to be observed during interactions and to exclude anyone who has not consented. Attending to ethical issues means not only having informed consent to observe people, but also changing names and identities of people and places to pseudonyms to maintain privacy and anonymity.

Having gained consent it is important to 'blend in' as much as you can, so that people are unaware or become less aware of your presence, except in specific cases in which you need to make your presence known for ethical or methodological reasons. Done well, participant observation is not conspicuous and therefore has less chance of disrupting the usual features of the setting. It may take a little time to settle into the situation before the actual work of observation begins. This allows people a chance to get used to having you around in a researcher capacity. Even if you are researching your own work area, people may feel self-conscious if they know you are doing research (which they will, because you are ethically bound to tell them and to gain their consent to observe them).

You may be involved in the interaction to varying degrees, but you need to avoid being a central person in the interaction. For example, you may be assisting in making a bed or washing a patient, but as a researcher on a designated project, you will most probably not have responsibility for patient care. Exceptions to this will be when nurses decide to do action research projects and use their own practice as an area of inquiry and reflection.

You will need to develop a watchful approach to what is happening around you. Learn to 'tune in' and see as many details as possible in the situation. Use a systematic approach to watching and documenting what you see. For example, think carefully before you write field notes about:

- Who was involved?
- What was the nature of the interaction?
- What were the sights, sounds and smells?
- What happened?
- When did it happen?
- What were the outcomes (effects) of the interaction?

Write the field notes as soon as possible after the interaction. It is not advisable to write during the interaction as it important to be active, but not intrusive in the interaction. Also it gives an unconcerned and thoughtless image if you stand there writing on a clipboard or in a book while busy nursing activities happen around you. It is quite cumbersome and artificial to collect data notes and descriptions in the course of participating in the setting, so a better alternative is to retreat periodically to write up impressions before rejoining the action for further phases of participant observation.

The data are best written in a richly descriptive form, and they read easier if they are written in the present continuous tense, for example *'I walk to the office and I see a woman waiting to speak with me. She is looking apprehensive, and as I approach her she says she wants to talk to someone about her husband. Her face is serious and drawn and a little girl is tugging at her hem'*.

When you write notes, be as descriptive as you can. Don't worry about grammar or spelling, as these are minor glitches that can be fixed easily later. Concentrate on describing the situation as comprehensively as you can so you and others reading your account can understand what happened, why, when, to whom, and with what outcomes (effects).

Ensure that you have a selection of interactions occurring over time with the people involved; thus various people will be involved over many shifts or times of day. Participants need to be assured that you will not use their names on the accounts and that other identifiable information will be hidden. You can be careful in this respect as you write, by referring only to 'the nurse', 'the patient', 'the relative', the doctor' and so on.

In sorting the data it is important to gather the information in some kind of permanent storage system, such as a computer disk, and ensure that each description of the setting is labelled according to the date, time, and other important details that may have some bearing in the later analysis. In qualitative research, field notes may count as data to be analysed or process notes to document the research progress, so it is feasible and advisable to use them in the text of research reports, journal articles and conference presentations, when disseminating your results.

Photography

Photographs can be highly significant sources of data, assuming that you have permission to take and store them. In some health care settings, such as hospitals and private clinics, clients may want to have their identities hidden. Also, organisations may have strict rules about the use of cameras and videos, with respect to the anonymity of their clients and the workplace. Remember also, that certain groups of people such as Indigenous people, may have strong cultural taboos about having their images caught on camera. There may be potential for violating sacred beliefs by using photographs. Because of the risk of the researcher's unwitting insensitivity to certain people and/or institutions, always check thoroughly each and every time before you go ahead and assume that it is appropriate to use photography.

Photographs can be taken that represent the features of the research setting and/or participants. For example, if a project involved exploring the routines of a nursing home, other sources of data such as participants' observation and interviews could be augmented well by selected pictorial images. Photographs could be sorted into categories and labelled accordingly, and the best images, in terms of the most descriptive photos, are chosen for inclusion in the research report. Details of the photographs could also be analysed to contribute to informing the research questions.

A final reminder. Before any photographs are published you need to ensure that you have the permission from the humans who might feature in them. As you might be able to imagine, photographs as a research method can do a great deal to augment other methods you may have used in the overall project, and they will add lift and polish to the final work when it is presented for assessment and/or publication.

Storytelling

Researchers have tended to use the words 'story' and 'narrative' interchangeably. When Wiltshire (1995, p. 75) examined the use of the terms 'story', 'narrative' and 'voice' within health care, he pointed out that the words have been used synonymously in relation to telling stories and he claims that they all have therapeutic dimensions. Polkinghorne (1988) is more precise, differentiating a story as a single account reviewing life events in a true or imagined form, and a narrative as a scheme of multiple stories 'that organises events and human actions into a whole' (p. 18).

Whether as a single story or as in the organising scheme of a narrative, data for qualitative research can be gathered easily and effectively through having people relate accounts of their experiences relevant to the research. It is an effective way of involving people in research, because it is not unusual for people to think that they have little to offer research projects, and some people may feel intimidated by the thought of participating. However, people may respond to the invitation to tell a story.

For example, if you want to find out about how patients perceive nursing care, they can be encouraged to tell a story about it. The lead-in to encourage the story could be as simple as: 'Please tell me about a time in which you were happy with the nursing care you received here'. Alternatively, another story may be encouraged by the lead-in: 'Please tell me about a time in which you were not pleased with the nursing care you received here'.

The story can be recorded on audiotape for later analysis, but some audiotape-shy participants may feel happier about writing their stories and adding illustrations. In some cases, stories may be enacted in traditional ways – dance, rituals – and other creative means, such as poetry, music, singing and film. If creative means are used, it is important that the artist is the interpreter of her/his own story, the accounts of which are stored by a recordable means to which the artist agrees.

As with all effective communication, if a storyteller has optimal conditions for speaking, the likelihood of a rich and deeply thoughtful story is enhanced through listener silence and attention. Once the storyteller has clear parameters for the story, resist the impulse to interject, unless the narrator is wandering right off the track and looks like being lost in irrelevancies. Look back in this section to 'Interviews' for further comments on how to encourage participants to tell their stories.

I never cease to be amazed at how research participants weave their stories. I remember working with palliative care nurses (Taylor 1995) who were interested in exploring what they meant by a 'good death'. They remonstrated at the outset that they had not done and could not *do* research. I invited each nurse to tell me a story about a person they had nursed who, in the nurse's opinion, had had a good death. When they told their stories, they cast their nets wide over particular patients and their families, first setting the context in broad 'pencil' outlines and then 'colouring in' the detail of each person's experience with the skill and artistry of clinicians immersed in the daily scenarios of their practice. All I had to do was sit back, listen, pay attention, check occasionally that the audiotape was still working and reach for the tissue box each time the stories melted me to tears! The stories were rich and full and the analysis of the transcripts provided many insights into nurses' perceptions of a good death.

In storing and preparing data from transcribed stories, some considerations are noteworthy. It is important to label the tape containing the story according to the participant's pseudonym, and with the date, time, and other contextual features of note. If many stories are stored on a single audiotape, use a numerical code on the label and keep and prepare a list of corresponding names and pseudonyms on computer disk or hard copy files. This prevents data confusion and ensures that each participant's story is attributed to the experience of that person, even though particular identities remain hidden. Set up a filing system and lock audiotapes, floppy disks and hard copies of stories away securely, as required by ethical procedures. You need to make a hard copy of each story to return to participants to validate their accounts.

For further reading on storytelling and narrative inquiry refer to the following articles: Bailey (1996); Poirier and Ayres (1997); Emden (1998); and Koch (1998).

Videotaping

Moving pictures give even more scope than still photographs for data, so their value as sources of data is self-evident. The same precautions apply to videotaping as have been outlined for photography. It is imperative that ethical clearance is gained before videotaping begins.

Also, do not underestimate the amount of knowledge and practice that are needed to produce videos that look professional and which record sound and movement well. Even with care in the recording phase, the video may need considerable editing to extract the extraneous details associated with the production glitches. If you are considering this medium, check out some of the traps for beginners, by consulting someone conversant with videotaping. The videos need to be labelled clearly, or have specific identifying information recorded at the beginning of the taping, to ensure that the information is represented in its correct context.

Summary

This chapter explored some of the issues around methodological congruency, which is an issue researchers may need to face if they think that the research questions they have might be answered well by a qualitative approach. Research contexts and people in qualitative research were described as being important, because all the circumstances of the setting and the people within them have a great bearing on how interpretations are made in qualitative research.

A list of methods that may be used alone or in combination in qualitative research were described in alphabetical order. Some of the methods, such as artistic expression, photography and videotaping, are so creative that little has been written about them in the nursing research literature to date. It is hoped that this chapter has given you motivation to think about the kinds of methods that you might like to incorporate in a qualitative research project you might be planning.

Main points

- In qualitative research, usually there are attempts to ensure that the methods by which new information is collected are congruent with the particular theoretical assumptions that underlie the kinds of knowledge that are being generated in the project.
- There is not one accepted test of 'rigour' in qualitative research, just as there is not one way of doing qualitative research, although the 'translation' of criteria now extends from trustworthiness to postmodern thinking and the concept of goodness.
- Credibility means the extent to which participants and readers of the research recognise the lived experiences described in the research as similar to their own.
- Fittingness refers to the extent to which a project's findings fit into other contexts outside the study setting, and the extent to which the readers of the research find it has meaning and relevance for their own experiences.
- Auditability is the production of a decision trail which can be scrutinised by other researchers to determine the extent to which the project has achieved consistency in its methods and processes.
- Confirmability of a project is achieved when credibility, auditability and fittingness can be demonstrated, and this relies on the confirmation of participants, whose subjectivity is valued as instructive in assessing the extent to which the project achieves neutrality from the researcher's stated biases.
- In postmodern thinking, 'rigour' and 'criteria' are problematic, in that they follow on from positivism in attempting to define and limit reality in the assumption that 'truth' is out there, waiting to be discovered, harnessed, and applied to problems of explanation, prediction and control in the human world.
- Archival searches locate information consisting of original hard copies of treasured documents as historical data, such as logs, diaries, government agencies' agendas and minutes, reports, photographs, newspapers, books, and private papers donated by families to the archives.
- A research design may collect data in the form of a direct and creative demonstration of the participant's experiences through artistic expression, such as in painting, drawing, montage, photography, poetry, dance, music, symbols, and singing, accompanied by the creator's interpretations of the piece, or through group discussion and/or the researcher's methods of interpretation.
- A case study is a research strategy that comprises an all-encompassing, comprehensive method and set of strategies that allows people, practices and phenomena to be described over time according to their contextual features.
- Fieldwork occurs where the action is happening, out in the 'field' of inquiry, and it comprises combinations of observation, participation, documentation and analysis to study a culture or other phenomenon of interest 'on the inside' to capture the thickest possible description of what is happening, to whom, when, why, how and where.

- A focus group is a collection of people, who have been invited to work together purposefully, brainstorming, collating and prioritising ideas around a particular research issue focused on a project's aims and objectives.
- A qualitative interview is like a conversation designed to encourage participants to tell their stories and relate their experiences in the deepest and richest way possible, through clear guidance on what is required, a genuine invitation to speak, and communicative facilitation on the part of the researcher.
- Data derived from entries from journal keeping may include researchers' and participants' impressions of meetings, conversations, research settings, roles in the research (in light of having multiple roles and responsibilities), information gathering and personal reflection.
- Part or all of a research project may involve searching for literature from all its likely sources and repositories, and collating it in a succinct and focused analysis, to show the strengths, weaknesses, connections, and gaps in what is written and how each writer contrasts to and/or augments other writers in the area.
- A member check is a procedure within qualitative research methods that involves seeking participants' validation of their contributions to the overall project, as a source of determining the trustworthiness of the project.
- In unstructured observation, the researcher observes a context systematically and carefully, but with no predetermined categories, keeping in mind the central purposes for being there as stated in the research objectives, thereby attending to what is happening, where, when, how and why, without actual involvement in the setting as a participant; whereas participant observation is about getting involved in the action in a setting, whilst observing the details within it.
- Photographs can be highly significant sources of data, for their value in representing the features of the research setting and/or participants.
- Whether as a single story or as in the organising scheme of a narrative, data for qualitative research can be gathered easily and effectively through having people relate accounts of their experiences relevant to the research.
- Videotaping moving pictures has even more scope than still photographs as data, but ensure that ethical clearance has been gained before videotaping begins and do not underestimate the amount of knowledge and practice needed to produce videos that look professional and record sound and movement well.

Review Questions

1. In qualitative projects, researchers use alternative terms for 'rigour' because:
   a reflecting the 'truth' is not as important as it is in quantitative research
   b qualitative and quantitative assumptions about 'truth' differ
   c 'truth' is absolute, objective, generalisable and context independent
   d qualitative and quantitative research are not of an equal standard

2. The production of a decision trail which can be scrutinised by other researchers to determine the extent to which the project has achieved consistency in its methods and processes is:
   a credibility
   b fittingness
   c auditability
   d confirmability

3. Methods used in qualitative research:
   a may be in various combinations according to the requirements of the research question or area
   b need to be limited to one or two to ensure that the research question or area remains focused
   c attempt to gather data which are capable of being analysed numerically for predictive ability
   d always include interviews with participants because they provide rich research data

4. The method of accessing logs, diaries, government agencies' agendas and minutes, reports, photographs and private papers donated by families is referred to as:
   a an archival search
   b a literature review
   c a member check
   d a case study

5. Fieldwork involves:
   a observing, documenting and analysing secondary sources of information in various locations
   b taking notes of people's accounts of their experiences, when it is not appropriate to go where they are
   c being where the action is, using a variety of methods, to describe a specific area of research interest
   d doing experimental work in laboratories which simulates actual experiences in the field

6 Group processes may be used typically in collaborative research approaches such as:
   a action research
   b surveys
   c ethnographies
   d grounded theory

7 In qualitative research, interviews are:
   a carefully directed and strictly structured
   b used as preliminaries to questionnaires
   c used to maintain consistency across respondents
   d more like conversations than interrogations

8 A procedure used to ensure that participants validate their contributions to the overall project as a source of ensuring the trustworthiness of the research is:
   a triangulation
   b artistic expression
   c member checking
   d journal keeping

9 When storytelling is used as a method in qualitative research, it is important to:
   a protect the identities of the people and the places in each story
   b set a time limit so that participants do not ramble off the point
   c structure the story with a list of specific directions and questions
   d ensure that everything recorded can be measured numerically

10 When using videotaping as a method of data collection, it is important to note that participants' permission is:
   a unnecessary
   b always necessary
   c sometimes necessary
   d seldom necessary

Discussion Questions

1 What is methodological congruency and why it is considered important in qualitative research?
2 Discuss the rationale for choosing congruent methods in qualitative research.
3 In relation to epistemology, why are contexts and people important in qualitative research?
4 How do Emden and Sandelowski (1998, 1999) deal with the problem of trustworthiness of qualitative research in a postmodern age?
5 Discuss five methods of data collection in qualitative research.

References

Bailey, P. H. 1996, 'Assuring quality in narrative analysis', *Western Journal of Nursing Research*, vol. 18, no. 2, 186–94.

Beck, C. T. 1993, 'Qualitative research: the evaluation of its credibility, fittingness, and auditability', *Western Journal of Nursing Research*, vol. 15, no. 2, 263–6.

Beebe, S. A. & Masterson, J. T. 1994, *Communicating in Small Groups: Principles and Practices*, 4th edn, Harper Collins, New York.

Benner, P. & Wrubel, J. 1989, *The Primacy of Caring*, Addison-Wesley Publishing Co., Menlo Park, California.

Burns, S. & Grove, N. 1993, *The Practice of Nursing Research: Conduct, Critique and Utilization*, W. B. Saunders Company, Philadelphia.

Burns, S. & Grove, N. 1997, *The Practice of Nursing Research: Conduct, Critique and Utilization*, 3rd edn, W. B. Saunders, Philadelphia.

Byrar, R. 1999, 'An examination of case study research', *Nurse Researcher*, vol. 7, no. 2, 61–78.

Conway, J. 1994, 'Reflection, the art and science of nursing and the theory–practice gap', *British Journal of Nursing*, vol. 393, 114–18.

Cowley, S., Bergen, A., Young, K. & Kavanagh, A. 2000, 'A taxonomy of needs assessment, elicited from a multiple case study of community nursing education and practice', *Journal of Advanced Nursing*, vol. 31, no. 1, 126–34.

Dale, A. E. 1995, 'A research study exploring the patient's view of quality of life using the case study method', *Journal of Advanced Nursing*, vol. 22, no. 6, 1128–34.

Denzin, N. K. 1989, *The Research Act*, McGraw-Hill, New York.

Ebbott, M. 1996, 'Integrating arts into clinical care', *International Journal of Nursing Practice*, vol. 2, no. 2, 105–8.

Emden, C. 1998, 'Conducting a narrative analysis', *Collegian*, vol. 5, no. 3, 34–9.

Emden, C. & Sandelowski, M. 1998, 'The good, the bad and the relative: conceptions of goodness in qualitative research: part one', *International Journal of Nursing Practice*, vol. 4, no. 4, 206–12.

Emden, C. & Sandelowski, M. 1999, 'The good, the bad and the relative: conceptions of goodness in qualitative research: part two', *International Journal of Nursing Practice*, vol. 5, no. 1, 2–7.

Fitzgerald, L. 1999, 'Case studies as a research tool', *Quality in Health Care*, vol. 8, 75.

Fiveash, B. 1998, 'The experience of nursing home life', *International Journal of Nursing Practice*, vol. 4, no. 3, 166–74.

Foreman, M. 1997, 'Measuring cognitive states', in *Instruments for Clinical Health Care Research*, 2nd edn, eds M. Stromberg & S. Olsen, Jones and Bartlett Publishers, Boston.

Greenwood, J. 1993, 'Reflective practice: a critique of the work of Argyris & Schon', *Journal of Advanced Nursing*, vol. 18, 1183–7.

Guba, E. & Lincoln, Y. 1981, *Effective Evaluation*, Jossey-Bass, San Francisco.

Hall, J. M. & Stevens, P. E. 1991, 'Rigor in feminist research', *Advances in Nursing Science*, vol. 13, no. 3, 16–29.

Healing Touch International 2000, *Healing Touch Research Survey*, HTI, Denver.

Hogston, R. 1995, 'Quality nursing care: a qualitative enquiry', *Journal of Advanced Nursing*, vol. 21, 116–24.

Josipovic, P. 2000, 'Recommendations for culturally sensitive nursing care', *International Journal of Nursing Practice*, vol. 6, 146–52.

Keatinge, D., Scarfe, C., Bellchambers, H., McGee, J., Oakham, R., Probert, C., Stewart, L. & Stokes, J. 2000, 'The manifestation and nursing management of agitation in institutionalised residents with dementia', *International Journal of Nursing Practice*, vol. 6, 16–25.

Koch, T. 1998, 'Story telling: is it really research?' *Journal of Advanced Nursing*, vol. 28, no. 6, 1182–90.

Lincoln, Y. S. 1995, 'The making of a constructivist – a remembrance of transformations past', in *The Paradigm Dialogue*, ed. E. G. Guba, Sage Publications, Newbury Park.

Nolan, M., Owens, R. G. & Nolan, J. 1995, 'Continuing professional education: identifying the characteristics of an effective system', *Journal of Advanced Nursing*, vol. 21, 551–60.

Parahoo, K. 1997, *Nursing Research: Principles, Process and Issues*, Macmillan London.

Pegram, A. 1999, 'What is case study research?' *Nurse Researcher*, vol. 7, no. 2, 5–16.

Poirier, S. & Ayres, L. 1997, 'Endings, secrets, and silences: overreading in narrative inquiry', *Research in Nursing and Health*, vol. 20, 551–7.

Polkinghorne, D. E. 1988, *Narrative Knowing and the Human Sciences*, State University of New York, Albany.

Rossiter, J. & Yam, B. 1998, 'Promoting the nursing profession: the perceptions of non-English-speaking background high school students in Sydney, Australia,' *International Journal of Nursing Practice*, vol. 4, 213–19.

Sandelowski, M. 1986, 'The problem of rigour in qualitative research', *Advances in Nursing Science*, vol. 8, no. 3, 27–37.

Schwandt, T. A. 1996, 'Farewell to criteriology', *Qualitative Inquiry*, vol. 2, 58–72.

Sharp, K. 1998, 'The case for case studies in nursing research: the problem of generalization', *Journal of Advanced Nursing*, vol. 27, no. 4, 785–9.

Smith, J. K. 1990, 'Alternative research paradigms and the problem of criteria', cited in Emden, C. & Sandelowski, M. 1999, 'The good, the bad and the relative, part two', *International Journal of Nursing Practice* vol. 5, no. 1, 2–7.

Smith, J. K. 1990, 'Alternative research paradigms and the problem of criteria' in *The Paradigm Dialogue*, ed. E. G. Guba, Sage Publications, Newbury Park.

Sorensen, E. S. 1988, 'Archives as sources of treasure in historical research', *Western Journal of Nursing Research*, vol. 10, no. 5, 666–70.

Stake, R. E. 1994, 'Case studies', in *Handbook of Qualitative Research*, eds N. K. Denzin & Y. S. Lincoln, Sage Publications, Thousand Oaks, California.

Strauss, A. & Corbin, J. 1990, *Basics of Qualitative Research: Grounded Theory Procedures and Techniques*, Sage Publications, Newbury Park.

Street, A. 1995, *Nursing Replay: Researching Nursing Culture Together*, Churchill-Livingstone, Melbourne.

Streubert, H. J. & Carpenter, D. R. 1995, *Qualitative Nursing Research: Advancing the Humanistic Imperative*, J B Lippincott Co., Philadelphia.

Taylor, B. 1995, 'Promoting a good death: nurses' practice insights', in *Issues in Australian Nursing*, eds G. Gray & R. Pratt, Churchill-Livingstone, Melbourne.

Taylor, B. 2000a, *Reflective Practice: A Guide for Nurses and Midwives*, Allen and Unwin, Melbourne.

Taylor, B. 2000b, Improving the practice of hospital nursing through reflective practice and action research, unpublished research report, School of Nursing and Health Practices, Southern Cross University, Lismore, NSW.

Taylor, B. (in press), 'Identifying and transforming dysfunctional nurse–nurse relationships though reflective practice and action research', *International Journal of Nursing Practice*.

Vallis, J. & Tierney, A. 1999, 'Issues in case study analysis', *Nurse Researcher*, vol. 7, no. 2, 19–35.

Walker, J. M., Hall, S. & Thomas, M. 1995, 'The experience of labour: a perspective from those receiving care in a midwife-led unit', *Midwifery*, vol. 11, 120–9.

Wiltshire, J. 1995, 'Telling a story, writing a narrative: terminology in health care', *Nursing Inquiry*, vol. 2, no. 2, 75–82.

Woods, L. P. 1997, 'Designing and conducting case study research in nursing', *NT Research*, vol. 2, no. 1, 48–56.
Yin, R. K. 1994, *Case Study Research*, Sage Publications, New York.
Yonge, O. & Stewin, L. 1988, 'Reliability and validity: misnomers for qualitative research', *Canadian Journal of Nursing Research*, vol. 20, no. 2, 61–7.

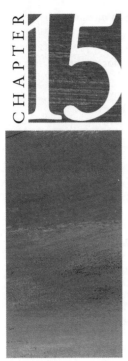

CHAPTER 15

Qualitative data collection and management

chapter objectives The material presented in this chapter will assist you to:

- recognise forms of qualitative data, such as words, images and numbers
- discuss the usefulness of qualitative data in relation to context, lived experience, subjectivity and potential for change
- prepare for data collection by deciding on data forms and combinations
- use strategies for collecting the data
- recognise people, place and equipment pitfalls to avoid
- use collection hints for storing main copies and coding the data
- discuss the use of computers in collecting and storing qualitative research data.

Introduction

Research is about searching again; literally, *re-searching*, or looking again. This means that there has to be some agreed ways of going out and looking for, gathering in, and then storing the information until it is time to do something with it. You could, of course, just go out and look and make up your collection and sorting processes as you go along, but in the tradition of all good 'hunters and gatherers' you would be wise to have a plan and some well-tried strategies before you set out.

This chapter is about being practical and systematic in collecting and managing qualitative data. Some hints have been given to you already, in Chapters 12 and 13, about how to collect and manage data gathered using certain qualitative methods, so this chapter will continue the 'how to' theme of managing assorted practicalities in preparation for analysing the data.

We begin by discussing the forms of qualitative data, such as words, images and, to a lesser extent, numbers, and the usefulness of qualitative data in relation to context, lived experience, subjectivity and potential for change. This is followed by some strategies for preparing for data collection, and deciding on data forms and combinations. Then there are hints on pitfalls to avoid in the process and ideas for storing main copies and coding the data. Finally, there is some introductory discussion on the use of computers in collecting and managing qualitative data.

Forms of qualitative data

Qualitative research can offer many things to research inquiry in general, but probably the best features of its contributions lie in its stories and accounts of living, and the richness of meanings within its words. Qualitative research assists people to tell their stories about what it is like to be a certain person, living in a particular time, place, and set of circumstances. This means that even the most ordinary people can do research, or be part of research, because if they can speak and tell stories about subjects they know best, such as their own life experiences, they can be part of qualitative research. The researcher invites them to share stories and from these stories, rich and useful data can be gleaned.

Words

The 'tools' or data for building new knowledge in qualitative research are mainly words, because they are the medium through which people express themselves and their relationships to other people and things, in and beyond their lives. As you discovered in Chapter 14, other data forms in qualitative research can include the demonstration and interpretation of artistic expression, such as painting, drawing, montage, poetry, dance, music, symbols and singing. Still photographs and videos may also be counted as data, but for the most part, qualitative research data are collected and stored in the form of words, whether they be from archival searches, case studies, field notes, group process outcomes, interview transcriptions, journal entries, literature searches, observation notes and/or written accounts of stories.

The usefulness of qualitative data

Qualitative data have a great deal to offer in the form of new and revised knowledge to researchers, through their deep and rich description of context, lived experience, subjectivity and potential for change.

Context

Qualitative data are bound to their particular context. As you may have read previously, 'context' means all of the features of the time and place in which people find themselves, and in which they locate their descriptions of things and people in their lives. People live their daily lives in the moment, yet they also remain connected to their past, and hopeful of their future. People cannot help but be placed in, and involved in, their particular time and place situations. In qualitative research, descriptions of contexts are useful in bringing forward new ideas about people's lives, their circumstances and the meaning they place on the events and phenomena around them. Qualitative data offer direct access to people's accounts of their experiences. Qualitative researchers consider participants' contextual appraisals as being worthy of inclusion as data in research projects.

Lived experience

Qualitative data can give researchers accounts of lived experience, which means how it is to live a life in regard to being someone or something unique. This implies that every human and every human situation is a lived experience. People live out their lives on a day-to-day basis in ways that are unique, and the level of conscious awareness of their existence may vary between people. Reflection is the key to making sense of human existence, because lived experiences accumulate and make sense as they are remembered. Thinking about what has happened and is happening to themselves and others, and of other phenomena of interest, gives people a sense of finding some meaning that is relevant to themselves and to others with whom it resonates. Therefore, qualitative data are gathered in word form to be available for analysis processes, which are congruent with the particular qualitative approach taken in the project.

Subjectivity

Qualitative data can take subjectivity into account. 'Subjectivity' means that which comes from the individual's sensing of inner and external things. Knowledge which comes from subjectivity does not make a universal claim to be true for everyone and for all things in all times and places; rather it refers to personal experiences and personal truths that may or may not be like other people's subjective experiences and truths. In the social world of daily life, humans take account of one another's sense of self and they share their experiences and truths through what is referred to as 'intersubjectivity.' When qualitative researchers are trying to understand the relationships between people, they take account of, and value, the intersubjectivity between people, as it is expressed to them in words as data.

Potential for change

Gathering and analysing qualitative data have the potential for change in two main ways. In the qualitative interpretive research approaches, such as historical research and grounded theory, change can occur when people raise their awareness of something and make adaptations in their perceptions and/or actions to accommodate the new insights. In qualitative critical research approaches, such as action research and feminisms, the intention to bring about change is stated at the outset of the research, so that the methods used in the research ensure that there is a high degree of possibility for change to occur as a result of the projects.

Postmodern possibilities

While repudiating the grand narratives of qualitative interpretive and critical research approaches, postmodern thinking searches for meaning by questioning taken-for-granted assumptions about 'truth' and 'being'. Disciples of extreme forms of skeptical postmodernism would see no reasons for, or ways of, doing research, because they claim authors use their authority as writers to control and censure readers; thus the 'death of the author' halts academic inquiry. In effect, all data are as dead as the author, because words, images, meanings and symbols constitute a 'fixed system of meaning', and, as representations, they are rejected by skeptical postmodernists because they do not allow for diversity (Rosenau 1992, p. 96).

While affirmative postmodernists reduce the author's authority to offering options for public debate, they do not abandon the author completely. This position allows researchers as the authors of projects to collect data and offer tentative insights for readers' interpretations and discussion. In some readings of postmodernism, representation is permissible, but in improved political forms that assist oppressed minorities and women to find voice (Fahy 1997; Glass & Davis 1998), leaving room for participatory and emancipatory research data that focus on the specific circumstances of participants and find multiple and contradictory personal and local solutions.

Preparing for data collection

Given the rich variety of qualitative data, it may seem difficult at first to decide what to gather and store for analysis. You need to remember that the data you collect and use will be related directly to the methods you use. This means that certain methods may produce words as data, while other methods may produce photographic images or some numbers. These are the forms of qualitative data described in the section above.

Deciding on data forms and combinations

How will you decide on the forms of data you want? Believe it or not, this can be a fun part of a project, in which you get to make some decisions about the best ways of doing things. It all gets back to some very simple, yet fundamental questions: 'What do I want to know?' 'Why?' 'How will I find out the information?' The answers to these questions give you the basis for deciding on forms of data that would serve best the aims and objectives of your project. Some examples may help you to grasp the point being made here.

For the sake of continuity, the distinctions will be used that were made in previous chapters of this book between interpretive and critical forms of qualitative research. For each methodology, some methods and forms of data will be suggested (see Table 15.1). This does not mean that these combinations are the best or only ways of looking at choosing forms of data; rather they are meant to be guidelines only, so that you can be as creative as you like when you are making decisions of this nature in your research.

From this exercise in setting out some of the possibilities for using qualitative data forms, you may see that data forms basically get down to combinations of words, images and numbers, which act as pieces of information that need to be analysed and interpreted, with the research questions, aims and objectives in mind. Therefore, your choice of data forms will depend on the nature and intentions of the research and your willingness to use combinations of methods, which will in turn produce certain combinations of data. You have to be very clear about what it is you want to explore and why, before you can be confident that the methods you choose will give you the data you need to find some insights and answers to the research questions you have raised.

Deciding on what data to collect will be determined by why you want it and how reasonable and sensible it is to access it. Therefore, it is important to think about what it is you want to know and why, before you decide on what data you will collect and how. For example, it would make a great deal of sense to arrange to talk with the actual people concerned if you want to know about their first-hand accounts of their experiences, rather than relying solely on secondary sources such as literature. Alternatively, if you are doing historical research and all of the primary people sources have 'passed over to the great majority' (died), secondary sources such as relatives, friends and documents of various kinds may be your only data sources (unless you can convince the sceptics that you have communication with 'the other side').

Some qualitative approaches allow for a mixture of people and paper sources. In an oral history, for instance, you might like to augment the person's story of their life with some personal and public domain documents and photographs. These data not only add strength to the oral account, but may also give

Table 15.1 Methodologies, methods and possible data forms

Methodology	Possible methods	Possible data forms
Interpretive research methodologies		
Grounded theory	Participant observation Interviews	Words, photographs Words
Phenomenology	Participant observation Interviews Creative writing	Words, photographs, video Words Words
Historical research	Archival searches Interviews Document analysis	Words, photographs Words Words
Ethnography	Participant observation Field notes	Words, photographs, video Words
Critical research methodologies		
Action research	Surveys Questionnaires Interviews Participant observation Group processes Reflective journal	Words, numbers Words, numbers Words Words, photographs, video Words Words, drawings
Feminist research	Group processes Interviews Reflective journal Surveys Questionnaires Creative expression	Words Words Words, drawings Words, numbers Words, numbers Words, painting, poetry, dance
Interpretive interactionism	Participant observation Interviews Group processes Reflective journal	Words, photographs, video Words Words Words, drawings
Critical ethnography	Participant observation Interviews Group processes Reflective journal	Words, photographs, video Words Words Words, drawings

validation to what has been said, and add visual interest to the person's life story.

Having decided on the data forms that would best serve your research questions, aims and objectives, you need to spend some time thinking about how each of the data forms will be analysed and how the various forms of analysis will be integrated into producing interpretations that best express the findings of the research. Analysis will be dealt with in detail in Chapter 16. You need to realise at this point that thinking about possible ways of analysing data should begin around the same time that you are deciding on what forms of data to collect. The reason for this is that there is little point in collecting data that you do not know how to use, or which may have little or no relevance in fulfilling the aims and objectives of the research.

Strategies for collecting the data

Once you have decided on what kinds of data are needed, you then need to give consideration to how you will go about collecting them. The method of data collection may vary according to what you want to achieve in the research, and it can include single or multiple data collection methods. A selection of data collection methods was described in Chapter 14. You might like to refer to these before you continue.

Pitfalls to avoid

People problems

One of the greatest problems in any research is lack of communication. Essentially, qualitative research is people-oriented, so the best advice you can be given is that you have respect for, and be inclusive of, all the people involved. This means that before you step out to collect the data, you have observed certain basic steps, such as: you have full ethical clearance from the institutions involved; consent forms and plain language statements are prepared ready to read and sign; and people know you are coming and they know who you are, what you are doing, and what you expect from them in terms of their degree of involvement.

Sometimes you may find that you need to make several phone calls or write letters to confirm the details of the research and all of the arrangements. Even then, you may find that people do not show up, or you arrive and they have little or no idea of who you are and why you are there to talk with them. That is all right because contingency plans can be negotiated on the spot, and you can learn from those experiences to make your initial approach better the next time. As the researcher, you have the responsibility to be as clear and concise as you can be and to be prepared for any contingencies that may arise.

Place problems

Find a place to collect data that is conducive to the methods you are using. For instance, if you are undertaking interviews, encourage participants to meet you in a quiet and private place so that they can speak freely and what they say can be heard clearly on the recording equipment. As a general rule, avoid busy places that have high traffic flows, banging doors and ringing phones, because they are not conducive to collecting data, unless, of course, it is the specific setting in which you intend to take field notes.

Make sure that the people in the setting who are not involved in the project know who you are and why you are there. It would be extremely unpleasant to be frogmarched out of a high security or 'closed to the public' area which you had not gained permission to enter. If you cannot gain admission to restricted areas, negotiate another place in which to meet participants, or think of creative means by which data may be gathered. For example, once they understand what it is they are to do, and how and why, research participants may be willing to take active roles in collecting data. You may find they are willing to be involved in reflective practitioner methods which allow them to develop critically aware means of assessing their workplaces and work practices. For instance, they may be interested in keeping their own reflective journals and attending group meetings for regular discussion with you and the other participants.

Equipment problems
If you are working with equipment such as audiotape recorders, tapes, videotape recorders and the like, make sure they work before you take them to your research setting. Many embarrassing and frustrating moments can be avoided by checking the energy levels of batteries, or having spares, or by buying good-quality recording tapes that do not get chewed up in the machine. When you arrive at your meeting place, set up the equipment and check that it works. If one power point does not work, try another. It is not always the case that the actual equipment is trying to sabotage your efforts. Other forces could be at work!

Collection hints
There is so much variety in qualitative data that it is difficult to speak in generalities about collecting it, but for the sake of avoiding undue repetition, we will try. One way to think of it is to remember that forms of qualitative data may be words mainly, images sometimes, and numbers occasionally or whenever mixed methods are used.

Have confidence in participants' contributions
I would like to make a personal observation about collecting qualitative data. Through experience, I have found that research participants in qualitative projects will do the best they can to give you their wholehearted accounts of their experiences, as long as they know what it is they have been asked to talk about and why. I have come to have confidence in participants' attention to the process, and I am astounded constantly by the generosity of their contributions. The researcher's part in this process is to be clear about the aims and objectives of the research (even if they are stated broadly). It is also important to be open to people, nonjudgemental of their idiosyncrasies and life choices, and attentive to the basic rules and conventions of effective interpersonal communication.

Know if you are collecting words, images and numbers, alone or in combinations
As noted previously, you are aiming to collect data in the forms of words, images and numbers, alone or in combinations. The kinds of methods that may produce words as data are participant observation, interviews, creative writing, archival searches, document analysis, open-ended responses in surveys and questionnaires, group processes and some forms of creative expression. Data as images may be produced through participant observation, archival searches and creative expression of artistic forms such dance, painting and poetry. Qualitative research

which uses mixed methods as part of the information-seeking processes may produce numbers as data through surveys and questionnaires.

Choose the appropriate method
When using methods to collect words, images and numbers, you need to begin with some degree of confidence that the methods you are using to collect them will gather what it is you want. Going out with the inappropriate method is like going to fish for a shark with a tiddler line. It simply will not work, or if you do manage to 'land' something, it may be more trouble than it is worth.

Check the usefulness of the method
All you need to do at this stage is to check, and possibly test, the validity of the method you are choosing. Ask a few friends to check over the way in which you intend to collect the data. For example, they may be willing to read through the questions you intend to ask or they may allow you to interview them. This trial run will not only allow you to see how you are coming across as a facilitator of the method, but it may also show you whether you are getting the information you want from the methods you are using. Use a checklist before collecting data.

You could also ask yourself some questions to check the ability of the method to gather the data you hope to gather. The reason you would be wise to ask yourself these questions is that they may help to ensure that the research will do what it intends to do, by means that are open and transparent to all of the people concerned. Questions may be:

- 'What am I exploring in this project?' 'Why?'
- 'What are my intentions for using this method?'
- 'What kinds of data will it produce?'
- 'Is the method likely to produce data that will contribute towards insights and answers to the research questions or general area of interest?
- 'Have I been as clear as I possibly can in telling the research participants who I am, why I'm requesting their involvement and how I would like them to contribute?'
- 'Will I collect the information I actually want to collect; that is, will it be relevant to the project?'
- 'What are my plans for analysis; that is, what do I intend to do to make sense of the data when I collect them?'

Having decided that you are ready to go and collect the data, you need to be prepared on the day, being aware of possible people, place and equipment pitfalls to avoid.

Other practical hints
Some other practical hints to consider during the information-gathering sessions are to:

- introduce yourself and reiterate your gratitude for the participant's involvement

- spend some time in general talk, if necessary, to create a relaxed and open setting for the data collection
- label the data with the participant's name, time, date and setting for the collection
- keep to time – if you have told the participant that you will be taking a certain amount of time for the process, you must be aware of that, and negotiate with her/him if more time is needed
- maintain clear and open communication during the data collection
- check during the collection on the working order of any equipment you are using, to ensure that it is still doing what it is meant to do
- keep on track – this means that you need to keep focused on what it is you are doing, so the data you collect are what you want
- inform the participant when the end of the collection has come, and tell him/her what will happen next in the project, and how s/he is involved
- say 'Thank you!' and mean it, because participants' contributions to your research are an act of generosity on their part and you should acknowledge that sincerely.

Storing main copies: maintaining security and integrity

Data in the form of words, images and numbers may be stored as paper, computer disks or items of artistic expressions, such as paintings, poetry and so on. It is no exaggeration to say that the data you collect are tantamount to a rich, raw resource; therefore, you need to treat them well to maintain their security and integrity. If you doubt this, ask some people with a PhD what they did in relation to the storage of their data. Some of the stories could be interpreted as the result of extreme anxiety related to the fear of loss of this precious information. Some researchers store paper and computer disks in the fridge, or the lining of curtains, or at a friend's house. These actions are rationalised in terms of the likelihood of theft, loss or destruction of data by fires, floods and all imaginable natural disasters. It is entirely up to you to decide what is appropriate for you in storing data.

Regardless of where you store data, they should be kept in locked storage. Security relates to ensuring that data are stored according to agreed guidelines. The NHMRC regulations for the storage of data dictate that they be stored in a locked area under the supervision of the researcher for five years after collection. Any copies of the data should be stored likewise.

Integrity refers to keeping data stored in such a way that they are maintained in their best state for use and possible review. Main copies are the 'heart' of the research; therefore, they need to be treated carefully. Transcripts, documents, photographs, computer disks, hard copies of items of artistic expression and other forms of data need to be stored in a safe place, away from potential threats, such as dogs, cats, kids, sun, rain and so on. Treat the data as you would things of value to you, and their integrity should be assured. Check on their integrity from time to time and take steps to amend your storage plans if the data are not keeping as well as you intend.

Coding the data

Ethical requirements demand that data maintain the anonymity and privacy of the research participants and places. There are several ways you can do this.

Pseudonyms

You can ask the participants to suggest a pseudonym by which they would like to be known, and to select code names for organisations mentioned in the data. If they are hesitant to do this, you get the chance to make up names, and this can be fun, using the first names of friends and relatives. When the data are ready to be analysed, they can be organised according to the order in which they were collected, or according to the alphabetical ordering of the pseudonyms.

Numbering

A more impersonal way of coding the data for anonymity and privacy is to use a numbering system and to eradicate proper nouns, in relation to places. For example, the text could read: *'Participant 1 referred to her experience at the local hospital'*. Manual and computer codes may be used to hide the identities of participants and places. The researcher decides on the construction of the code, and then stores the main key to the code with the data in the locked area. Manual and computer codes can use letters, words or numbers, alone or in combination. It does not really matter what system is used, so long as it is logical and consistent throughout, and it has the potential to represent the data in their entirety.

Use of computers in qualitative data collection and management

Computers are incredibly useful in qualitative research, because one of their main areas of expertise is in handling words through word processing functions. Words can be written, amended, added and re-arranged with ease, by word processors in computers. As you may have read already, words are the most common data in qualitative research, and they need to be collected, stored, analysed and interpreted carefully. Computers can be useful in all of these activities.

Direct collection and storage system

Computers can be used as a direct collection and storage system, such as in field research for note-taking. It may be much simpler and more efficient to create field notes directly onto a disk, than onto paper for later transfer to disk. Computer disks can be copied to ensure that there are backup versions of the data, and these can be accessed with relative ease at all stages in the research.

A means of smooth, creative thinking

Another interesting 'plus' about using computers in qualitative research is that they may soon allow researchers to take on smooth thinking processes while working with them. That is, if you are a person who imagines that you think best by using paper and pencil, you might be surprised to find out how quickly you get over your first efforts at two-finger typing on the computer keyboard, to becoming 'at one' with the computer. From my experience, I can attest to the usefulness of having research data on disk that can be arranged and re-arranged and later 'cut and pasted' into a document. I was also impressed by the way I soon learned to think 'through' the computer as well, and even better than I had done before with my pencil in hand, poring over reams of paper. Try it. I hope you find it to be the case also.

Examples of computer systems

Any of the Apple and/or IBM-compatible computer word processing systems is useful for qualitative research, because of their ability to store and manage words. Some of the more sophisticated and expensive computers may also allow you to collect and store still or moving images, because they can be connected to audiovisual recording equipment.

Disks

Computer disks are sold by different companies for various prices. Be careful when buying computer disks that they are of good quality and that they suit the computer you use. Check to see what symbol appears on the screen when you insert the disk, because some may be formatted for one computer system only. For example, if you are a Macintosh user, some IBM-compatible disks may need to be formatted to Macintosh before you store data on them, without worries about opening the documents safely. Have a person who knows how, 'step you through' converting the disk to a compatible form. Checking to ensure that the format is correct may prevent problems related to storing, reading and working with the material at a later date.

Qualitative data analysis systems

Although there are many ways in which qualitative data can be analysed, there is a growing tendency to use computer systems solely, or as an adjunct to manual analysis techniques. Specific computer systems that have been used for analysis include the Macintosh word processing system Hypercard, Ethnograph (Siedel 1992) and NUD*IST (Qualitative Solutions and Research 1995). The strengths and weaknesses in using these systems will be discussed in detail in Chapter 16.

Data are usually entered into qualitative analysis systems in the form of transcripts containing sections of text prepared from the interviews, group discussions, researcher's notes and so on. The ways in which the various kinds of transcripts are prepared are specific to the requirements of the particular qualitative analysis system. Always check the instructions accompanying the system, or if that is not available, seek advice from a person who has used or created the system. You may prefer to attend a training course made available by the manufacturers/designers of the system, as this will give you a comprehensive overview of the operation of the complete package and provide you with a 'hotline' if problems arise.

Summary

This chapter intended to give you some practical and systematic strategies and hints for collecting and managing qualitative data. We discussed the forms of qualitative data, such as words mainly, some images, and the occasional use of numbers in mixed methods. Knowledge about human context, lived experience, subjectivity and potential for change were listed as the benefits in using qualitative data. These were followed by strategies for preparing for data collection, and deciding on data forms and combinations. Some hints were suggested on person, place and equipment pitfalls to avoid in collecting data and you were introduced to processes for storing main copies and coding data. Finally, there was some introductory discussion on the usefulness of computers in collecting and managing qualitative data. All of these areas may assist you in making the most sense out of the qualitative data analysis which follows in Chapter 16.

Main points

- Research is about searching again, literally *re-searching*, or looking again, implying the need for some agreed ways of looking for, gathering in, and then storing the information until it is time to do something with it.
- Qualitative research can offer many things to research inquiry in general, but probably the best features of its contributions lie in its stories and accounts of living, and the richness of meanings within its words, which assist people to tell their stories about what it is like to be a certain person, living in a particular time, place and set of circumstances.
- The 'tools' or data for building new knowledge in qualitative research are mainly words, because they are the medium through which people express themselves and their relationships to other people and things, in and beyond their lives.
- Qualitative data can offer new and revised knowledge through their deep and rich description of context, lived experience, subjectivity and potential for change.
- Descriptions of contexts are useful in bringing forward new ideas about people's lives, their circumstances and the meaning they place on the events and phenomena around them; qualitative data offer direct access to people's contextual accounts of their experiences.
- Thinking about what has happened and is happening to themselves and others, and of other phenomena of interest, gives people a sense of finding some meaning that is relevant to their lived experience and to others with whom it resonates.
- Knowledge which comes from subjectivity does not make a universal claim to be true for everyone and for all things in all times and places; rather it refers

to personal experiences and personal truths, and the way humans take account of one another's sense of self and share experiences and truths through 'intersubjectivity'.
- Gathering and analysing qualitative data causes change by raising awareness and creating and maintaining an intentional change agenda.
- Extreme forms of skeptical postmodernism would see no reasons for, or ways of, doing research, because they claim authors use their authority as writers to control and censure readers; thus the 'death of the author' halts academic inquiry.
- Affirmative postmodernists do not abandon the author completely, but they reduce the author's authority to offering options for public debate, thereby allowing researchers as the authors of projects to collect data and offer tentative insights for readers' interpretations and discussion.
- Qualitative data forms consist of combinations of words, images and sometimes numbers, which act as pieces of information that need to be analysed and interpreted with the research questions, aims and objectives in mind; therefore, be clear about what is to be explored and why, so the methods chosen will give relevant and appropriate data.
- Pitfalls to avoid in data collection include being aware of potential people, place and equipment problems that can be minimised by adequate foresight and planning.
- When collecting data have confidence in participants' contributions; know if you are collecting words, images and numbers, alone or in combinations; choose the appropriate method; check the usefulness of the method; and maintain effective and gracious communication throughout the interpersonal encounter.
- Data are rich, raw resources; therefore, treat them well to maintain their security and integrity.
- Code data with useful and uncomplicated pseudonyms and numbering systems.
- Computers can be used in qualitative data collection and management as direct collection and storage systems and to facilitate smooth, creative thinking.
- Specific computer systems for qualitative data analysis can manage large amounts of data tagged to participants' identities and dialogue, but they may not be able to find the finer nuances of meaning possible through manual methods.

Review Questions

1. The main 'tools' or data for building new knowledge in qualitative research are:

    a numbers
    b words
    c images
    d statistics

2. In qualitative research, all the features of time and place in which people find, describe and analyse themselves, are referred to as their:

    a context
    b lived experience
    c subjectivity
    d world

3. Qualitative interpretive approaches have the potential for change because they:

    a have a stated change agenda of mobilising direct political action
    b demonstrate the relationship between cause and effect variables
    c can allow change agents to predict and generalise future cases
    d can raise people's awareness of areas that need to be different

4. In relation to pitfalls to avoid in qualitative research, people problems can be avoided by better:

    a funding
    b organisation
    c transport
    d communication

5. When deciding on data forms and combinations in qualitative research, some simple yet fundamental questions to ask are:

    a What do I want to prove? How? Where will I find the information?
    b What do I want to predict? When? How will I find the information?
    c What do I want to know? Why? How will I find the information?
    d What do I want to show? Why? When will I find the information?

6. When you are collecting data from participants in qualitative research, it is a good hint to:

    a assume they are out to trick you
    b have confidence in their contributions
    c create and use foolproof methods
    d remain objective and detached

7 What does integrity mean when used in relation to storing qualitative data? It refers to:
   a checking that the data are truthful and trustworthy
   b keeping the data locked away securely for five years
   c replacing real names and places with pseudonyms
   d storing data in their best state for use and possible review

8 Qualitative data are coded because:
   a ethical requirements demand that data maintain the anonymity and privacy of the research participants and places
   b medical and nursing jargon is misleading and needs to be stated in plain language
   c the process transforms them into items which can be more readily analysed and interpreted
   d the information is a secret which must be kept by the researchers until it is ready to be divulged

9 Computers are incredibly useful in qualitative research because of their ability to:
   a convert data collection items into statistics and graphs
   b collate words, images and numbers into numerical categories
   c handle words through word processing functions
   d run software packages that ensure mathematical accuracy

10 An example of a qualitative data analysis system is:
   a Anovar
   b SPSS
   c CINAHL
   d NUD*IST

Discussion Questions

1 Why are words the main forms of qualitative data?
2 Discuss the usefulness of qualitative data in relation to context, lived experience, subjectivity and potential for change.
3 How will you decide upon which data forms to use in your qualitative research project?
4 List the main people, place and equipment pitfalls to avoid when collecting qualitative data.
5 Discuss the use of computers in collecting and storing qualitative research data.

References

Fahy, K. 1997, 'Postmodern feminist emancipatory research: is it an oxymoron?' *Nursing Inquiry*, vol. 4, 27–33.

Glass, N. & Davis, K. 1998, 'An emancipatory impulse: a feminist postmodern integrated turning point in nursing research', *Advances in Nursing Science*, vol. 21, no. 1, 43–52.

Qualitative Solutions and Research 1995, *NUD*IST (Non-Numerical Unstructured Data: Indexing Searching & Theorising)*, application software package, QSR, Melbourne.

Rosenau, P. 1992, *Post-Modernism and the Social Sciences: Insights, Inroads and Intrusions*, Princeton University Press, New Jersey.

Siedel, J.V. 1992, Ethnograph, Version 4.0, Qualis Research Associates, Corvallis, Oregon.

CHAPTER 16

Qualitative data analysis

chapter objectives The material presented in this chapter will assist you to:

- consider some approaches for getting started in analysing qualitative data
- describe and use manual and computer-assisted methods of thematic analysis
- find explicit and implicit themes within the text
- be aware of benefits and constraints in using qualitative data computer analysis systems
- locate examples of completed qualitative analyses
- describe the analysis of images as qualitative data.

Introduction

The main data derived from qualitative research methods are words. In Chapter 15 you may have noticed that much reliance is placed on the trustworthiness of language. This is because language is the main way in which qualitative researchers make sense of the answers to the questions they pose in their projects about human phenomena. This reliance on language is in contrast to the main approach of quantitative research methods, which tend to trust the value of numbers as tools for analysis.

However, you may remember that things are not so 'black and white' as to assume that 'words equal qualitative' and 'numbers equal quantitative'. In keeping with the tendency to maintain caution in categorising research approaches too quickly into insulated methods, you need to remember that qualitative researchers may also use a mixture of methods, and place their trust in words and numbers, to produce new or amended knowledge about a thing of interest to them.

In this chapter, we will deal with some 'how tos' of qualitative analysis. It will be assumed that words are the main data for analysis, and the chapter will deal most comprehensively with their analysis. A small part of the text will be devoted to the analysis of images as data. For help in how to analyse numbers as data, please refer to Chapter 10, where it is dealt with most comprehensively.

You may find that research books and researchers seldom are useful in telling potential researchers how to undertake a method of qualitative analysis so, for the most part, much of what follows is a compilation of hints and strategies that have worked for me over the years. I hope that you will find them helpful.

Approaches to analysing qualitative data

Good news! The cringe has gone from nursing scholarship and research about whether qualitative research is 'good enough'. It was swept away by the debates of the 1960s and 1970s (Henderson 1964; Kratz 1978) and the bold new assertiveness of the 1980s and 1990s (Winstead-Fry 1980; Goodwin & Goodwin 1984; Allen 1985; Chinn 1985; Kermode & Brown 1995) into the postmodern age of valuing multiple discourses (Glass & Davis 1998). If you doubt this, look over items of nursing scholarship of these decades that are now historical documents and you will see that changes to wider views of research have been happening for some time.

The coming of age of qualitative research

Qualitative research in nursing has 'come of age'. It is assured of a secure and respected place at the start of the new millennium. These assurances are given to you because you need to realise at the outset that your approach to analysing qualitative data should be a confident one. The findings of your research should be judged by qualitative criteria and deemed of value by readers who understand and value the knowledge-producing and verifying assumptions of qualitative research.

However, although qualitative research has come of age, it does not mean that the research will not be open to critique. It is a positive measure of scholarship to welcome critique. Qualitative research will continue to be criticised and even invalidated by other researchers. Some researchers may not know about the philosophical debates that questioned the use of the scientific method as the only way of generating knowledge in human inquiry. This might mean these researchers continue to use quantitative criteria for judging the worthiness of a qualitative project. For example, some human research ethics committees may be composed solely or mainly of members who are schooled in quantitative research approaches and nothing else.

Other researchers who use qualitative approaches may judge a project against the particular assumptions of their favoured theoretical orientation. For example, a researcher using a critical approach such as action research or critical ethnography may criticise an interpretive approach for failing to deal with issues of power and domination.

The orientation of the qualitative researcher

It is suggested that you make a personal approach to qualitative research analysis with an orientation of respect for people, their experiences and words, and have confidence in finding meaning in them. Your orientation may not have these features when you first approach the task of analysis, but it is entirely possible that you may develop them over time. As was suggested previously, if you have chosen your methods wisely, and the research participants know what it is you want to know and why, the data you collect are likely to have some insights and answers to your questions.

Being ready physically and emotionally

Qualitative analysis requires that you read, look and listen to language with wakeful alertness. This means that you need to be feeling physically and emotionally fresh before you try to do the analysis, so choose a time of day when you know you are feeling the best. It might also help to use some sort of centring technique to get you into a mood that allows you to be fully present. For instance, if you meditate, spend some time relaxing with your particular technique.

If you are not conversant with meditation or other forms of relaxation, try this simple visualisation. Stand upright with your feet flat on the ground. Imagine that you are a tree. Feel your roots going deep into the ground. Feel the gentle wind in your branches. Allow yourself to experience this sense of stability for a few minutes of silence, and then, when you are ready, begin your work.

Getting started

The words you have collected may be stored in hard copies or on computer disks. How to take care of them has been discussed in the previous chapter. The time has now come to organise the data ready for analysis.

Make copies

Begin by making copies of all of the data, in whatever forms they are stored. Ensure that you keep the original copy to one side and stored carefully, with identifying details and the date written clearly on it. The duplicated copy can be labelled: 'Working Copy', to differentiate it as the copy on which the analysis will be done. Be sure to update and label copies as your work progresses, so that you do not become confused by differing versions of the same electronic document.

Decide on an organising system

Decide on a system for organising the paper or computer files. You may need to buy some manilla folders to store paper files in their respective bundles, or you might need to code and name each computer file according to the content of data stored therein. The principle to keep in mind is the need to be practical and careful in getting the data ready for analysis.

Have confidence in words as data

If you have been careful in the choice and implementation of the research methods, you can be fairly confident that within the words collected as data are the answers to the questions you have posed. If you have spoken with research participants who have responded well to the invitation to speak of their experiences and you have been careful to ask the sort of questions that will give them a chance to supply the answers you need to fulfil your research objectives, then you will probably be amazed and somewhat humbled at the magnitude and the richness of the textual information which people will offer.

Methods of thematic analysis

One overarching approach to identifying the answers to research questions embedded in the data is a method called thematic analysis. As you might guess, thematic analysis simply means a method for identifying themes, essences or patterns within the text. In this case, text refers to the selection of words with which you are working. An interesting observation is that many researchers may talk about thematic analysis, but when it comes down to it, very few of them are able or willing to communicate to you just what it is they do to find the themes, essences or patterns within the text. Even when they tell you that they used a specific method, for example, Spradley (1979), Leininger (1985), Strauss (1987) or Sarnecky (1990) and you go to the source and read about it, more often than not, you may be still none the wiser as to how to actually go about doing the analysis. This chapter hopes to remedy that situation to some extent.

Methods appropriate to intentions

Qualitative analysis of words may be by either manual or computer-assisted means. The intentions of the analysis will determine what is done with the words. For example, researchers with exploratory and descriptive intentions may use analysis methods that produce groups of themes and sub-themes. Although there is no strict prescription, these methods are helpful because they allow a descriptive interpretation of human experiences. Practical guides for manual and computer-assisted methods of data analysis are described in this chapter.

Researchers with intentions to bring about changes may prefer critical analyses of discourses and the other economic, political, cultural, social and historical determinants. These analyses may involve thematic approaches, but with extra scrutiny to bring into awareness silences and gaps in the discourse as well as issues of power and domination. Methods that provide analysis for qualitative critical research approaches based on critical social science, and for research influenced by poststructural and postmodern thinking, are described in this chapter.

Finding explicit and implicit themes within the text

It is one thing to tell you to find themes; it is yet another thing for you to feel confident that you can. The following hints on how to find themes may help you, regardless of whether you use a manual or a computer-assisted method of thematic analysis.

Know what you are looking for

The first 'rule' when looking for themes is to know what you are looking for! It sounds so obvious, but it can be so difficult to remember. Before you start looking for themes, review your research proposal. What are the research project's aims and objectives? Keep those ideas firmly in your mind as you go about finding themes. Why? So that you will recognise a theme when you see one! It is so easy to become sidetracked once you get in amongst the thick undergrowth of the data. Keep your aims and objectives in mind so you find what you set out to find!

Locate specific words for explicit themes

If you are searching for specific words or combinations of words, it is a relatively simple task to look for their appearance within sections of the text. The word 'health' for instance, will figure keenly in a discussion about health promotion. This is an explicit theme, in that it may float with relative ease to the top of a well of words when doing an analysis. Explicit themes are apparent because they provide direct answers to direct research questions, so they speak out loudly when you are reading and unless you are becoming tired or otherwise uninterested, it is difficult to miss them.

Look closely for implicit themes

It is important to recognise that a theme will not always be stated as a direct word or words, or even as an easily recognisable concept. Take the example of health, for instance. People might talk about feeling 'good', 'well', 'happy', 'energised', 'bountiful' and so on. There may be no mention at all of health-like words, but rather a story, an innuendo, a hint or a fine wisp of language that portrays a health-related situation.

So how will you recognise an implicit theme? You will recognise it because of the way it fits into the total context of what has been said. By now, you may be very familiar with the transcript, so you will be ever watchful for what it can tell you. An implicit theme may lie like a fine weave in the tapestry of the conversation. When you locate it you know that you have it, because its fine threads will be connected with other parts of the text and you will see where they began and where they finished. It will be a joyful discovery and it will fire you up to look for more.

Be sure it is a theme

How can you be absolutely sure that you have located an explicit and/or implicit theme? Well, how do you know it is a fish on the line when you go fishing? It is a similar problem. You will know you have located a theme because it bears resemblance to what you thought you might find; that is, it appears to have within it some features of the thing for which you are looking. It might not look exactly like the whole thing for which you are looking, but you will know that it is related because it comes up in front of your awareness in answer to the questions you have been posing as you analyse the text for signs of it. It is part of the pattern of answers you are intending to find within the text, and you know it is relevant because its identity is connected directly and sometimes indirectly to the stated research aims and objectives. Yes, you have found a theme! Congratulations!

Now that you have some idea of how to recognise a theme when you see one, we will switch back to discuss two main ways of approaching thematic analysis; that is, through manual and computer-assisted methods.

Manual approaches

Even in this age of technology, it is still reasonable to choose to analyse qualitative data by manual methods. It is entirely a matter of what you prefer and what is the best way for you to handle the data carefully and effectively. Qualitative research tends to produce a great many words stored on a lot of paper, so if you choose a manual method of analysis, you need to be sure that you are systematic about the way in which you handle the data. As mentioned previously, to chart a course through these data, you will need to document your analytical progress by a tagging system called thematic identification. It will show the pathway through which you made sense of the words and put them into some order for interpretation.

Review the research aims and objectives

The first thing is to remember why you have researched what you have researched. This is not only to give you a renewed sense of commitment to the project, but also to revive for you the main purposes of the research. What did you say you would do in the research; why and how? Revisit the words you wrote in your proposal and centre on the key ideas to make sure you are clear about what it is that needs to emerge from the information you have amassed from the research participants. This means you will need to look again at the statements you made about the aims and objectives of the research, and keep these in mind while you are doing the analysis.

Read and re-read
Having gained a refreshed and re-focused view of the research objectives and strategies, begin by reading and re-reading the text. As you may suspect, there is likely to be a lot of information in the transcripts, some of which is useful directly, and some of which may need to be stored away for another time. There are many ways to proceed at this point and these are some of them. Feel free to be creative in adjusting the following suggestions to suit yourself. Remember that there is no one way to do this, and that as long as you are clear about the research aims and objectives you can adjust the analysis methods to fit the unique requirements of the project and its participants.

Make multiple copies
Number the pages of your transcript either sequentially from '1' onwards or using a number number (1-1, 1-2 etc.) or letter number (A-1, A-2 etc.) combination to number each transcript or each group of transcripts. Make multiple copies of the page-numbered transcripts. Ensure one copy is kept untouched as a guide. It is a good idea to put a large column on the left of the page in which to write notes about ideas that come to mind. You might like to have the audiotape of the interview playing as you read the transcripts, so that you can capture the intonations and emphases of the speakers' words.

Know the text thoroughly
Read the transcripts one by one. Be ready to pick up the nuances in the text. Endear yourself to the text so that you come to know it on an almost intimate basis. You may have to read it many times over to get to this stage of familiarity. As you attend to the text, remember the research question and/or objectives, so that your attention falls on the relevant words, phrases, sections of dialogue, and gross and fine connections between parts of the document.

Allow time for it to come together
Do not try to catch the whole of the meaning in an instant, or even in the first protracted sitting. Let the information percolate and incubate in your mind for a while. When you relax from reading, you may watch with interest as the connections start to pop into your mind, sometimes at the most inopportune moments – you may be at home involved in your family life and find your mind drifting to the research.

The 'pile on the kitchen table' method

What you do next will depend on what you like to do when you 'play'. You can do the 'pile on the kitchen table' method, in which you cut out any sections of text that appear to be connected to a theme and arrange them in mounds. After you have amassed various groupings, try to reduce them into fewer groups, so that the essential themes that remain are those that cannot be subsumed into other categories without losing some of their meaning. Do not attempt this method near children, pets, or open windows because accidents can happen at this point!

The 'colour coding' method

You might prefer the 'colour coding' method, in which you collect a wide range of coloured pens and go through the text marking in colour codes those words, ideas, sections and/or nuances that appear to be connected.

Finding the right word

When you have the kitchen table covered in piles or you have completed the colouring, go back to place a card containing a word or words on top of each pile or write a word or words in the column beside each colour to capture the main idea represented by that colour. List the words and review then reduce the list so that similar ideas merge into groups. You have reached the limits of the reduction when you can no longer move ideas without losing some of their specialness in relation to the research. What remains (because they defy further movement into groupings) are the distinct themes.

The concise version of the manual thematic method

In point form, here is 'how to do' a manual thematic identification of research themes.

- Read and re-read the text.
- Make multiple copies of the page-numbered transcripts.
- Ensure one copy is kept as a guide.
- Keep in mind the research question and/or objectives.
- *Either* cut out any sections of text that appear to be connected to a theme and arrange the cut-out bits in mounds, then
- try to reduce them into groupings that cannot be subsumed into other categories without losing some of their meaning
- *or* use the 'colour coding' method, marking in colour codes those words, ideas, sections, and/or nuances that appear to be connected.
- Find a word or words to capture the ideas in each pile or to represent each colour.
- List all the words and review them.
- Reduce the list so that like ideas merge into respective groupings.
- You have reached the limits of the reduction when you can no longer move ideas without losing some of their specialness in relation to the research. These are your themes.

Computer-assisted approaches

If you are not into paper cut-outs or colouring in, you might like to try some computer-assisted and hard copy strategies for finding themes. Computers are wonderful inventions. They are helpful particularly to the qualitative researcher, because they have the ability to move mountains of words around documents with the greatest of ease.

Make a disk copy

Start by making a disk copy of the main text to be analysed. (If you have developed research neurosis, the chances are that you will have multiple disk copies stored all over your home or office!) Remember, if you have been clear with your participants about what you wanted to know from them, the chances are that they will have given you the information you need. It will be all there in the transcripts. All you have to do is to locate these ideas in the participants' language.

Tidy the transcript

If you are working with a transcript of an interview, drop off any extraneous details from the copy, such as side conversations or comments not central to the research, and also 'ums', 'ahs', and 'ohs'. I realise that some people are loath to drop these linguistic hesitations, but unless the research is looking at these things directly, say in a study of the lived experience of hesitation (this is a joke), they serve no purpose except to make the participant sound awkward, to impinge on the flow of language and to thicken the text with irrelevancies. If you feel nervous about dropping extraneous details, even on a copy, listen to your intuition, because it is probably trying to tell you that something lurks there that is far from extraneous.

Read and section

Start from the beginning of the sequence to be analysed and read through the text as it scrolls on the computer screen. You may have become very conversant with the information already through reading and re-reading, so this is another chance for extra insight. As parts of the text relating to the research interests appear, section them off under a subheading that is relatively descriptive. As you progress through the document, you may find that 'sectioning' the document through the use of headings and subheadings can help you to organise the text and create connections between themes that are raised in one part of the text and reiterated in another part. In a practical sense, 'sectioning' is as simple as pressing the 'return' key several times to push a chunk of text several lines down to isolate it for separate consideration. This will provide some direction through the document and chart the course of ideas as they emerge from the information. Use your spontaneity to use creative subheadings, but keep the meaning as direct as possible to what appears underneath the subheading. The subheadings and general labels may contain some actual words that appear in the text or a short phrase that reflects most closely the explicit content and implicit meaning of the sectioned text.

Look for themes

As you work slowly and systematically through the scrolling document, look for explicit and implicit themes, as described previously. Explicit themes may pop up conspicuously, while implicit themes may hide away for a time. As you read sections of the text, ask yourself: 'What is this saying?' 'Is there anything here that relates to my research aims and objectives?' 'Is there anything here connected implicitly to what I have read before?'

It may be possible to locate themes straight away, as you proceed through the analysis or you may find sub-themes as you continue looking for explicit and implicit ideas. Sub-themes are related to main themes, and they are like subsections, or further elaborations on a theme. Do not become overly concerned at the first 'run through' about trying to find all there is to find, because some of the sub-themes and implicit themes may remain hidden until later. At this stage, do not even worry about whether they are themes or sub-themes, because you can sort that out later.

Be aware of your feelings

As you go through the analysis, be aware of any emotions you may be feeling as the researcher. Analysis can be a fairly taxing and tiring experience, so be sensitive to how you are feeling, and why that might be. For instance, do not become too disheartened if you think you are not finding enough. Sometimes one or two themes may be hidden in a mountain of data. Remember it is quality you are after, not quantity! If the analysis process seems to be getting 'all too much' for you, it might be a good idea to take a rest from analysis for a while, and go outside for a walk, or create some space from the task until you feel fresh and ready again.

Review after a break

When you return to the analysis, begin at the start of the document again, so that you can remind yourself of where you are and how you got there. It is a way of refreshing yourself about the context of the analysis before you go on to make further progress, or to finish a particular part of the analysis overall. Work through the document as described before, looking carefully for themes and 'sectioning' text into serviceable and practical chunks, until you come to the point at which you consider that you have analysed the document.

Be patient with the first run through

What you will have at this stage is a copy of the working document, which may have some headings, subheadings, themes and sub-themes, alone or in various combinations. In other words, it still looks a bit messy! At this stage your working document would be tantamount to one of Leonardo's sketches, before he tackled the finished artwork. (How's that for an ambitious analogy!) In other words, it is the essence and basis of the final analysis. Now you need to tidy the working document and collate the actual themes.

Collate the themes

This is where a computer is so useful, because you can copy all of the working document so easily, ready for its transformation. In order to collate the themes within the text you can copy the entire analysis of what you have just done (with its headings, subheadings, themes and sub-themes, alone or in various combinations). Paste that copy of the document into the end of the working document, so that you have the same document twice on one file. Alternatively, you might prefer to create a new file. This now means that you have the working document duplicated, so that you can make the next refinements.

Now, go through and drop off everything in the second, or duplicated copy of the analysis to date, except the subheadings, themes and sub-themes that you generated previously. Review the list and concentrate on the research interest again by asking yourself: 'What does this say about the research interest?' The answers to this question, or others phrased in a similar vein, will give you the themes for the research. As you ask this question, look for connections between the words and phrases you see listed there. Do some of them look similar? Are they similar enough to be merged together, without losing their essential identity? If yes, put them together. If no, leave them separate.

You keep going through this thinking, shifting and collating process until everything settles into the place it fits best, in relation to the original questions you posed in your project, and the aims and objectives you had in relation to them. When it has all come to its steady state, you have your themes.

Name the themes

You can name the themes whatever you want. You have gone through the 'labour and delivery' of your analysis, so you get the honour of 'naming your children'. Spare a thought, however, for the readers of your research, by not making the theme names too obscure or exotic. Humour and/or simplicity are permissible in naming themes, so feel free to think creatively. Remember, though, to allow the name of the theme to reflect its nature, otherwise you could end up in the silly situation of naming the theme inappropriately, and this will be of little use to anyone trying to make sense of your project.

Combine to form common themes

The method of analysis thus far is useful for a single text analysis; however, if you have interviewed a number of people, you may want to analyse each transcript separately and then combine the group accounts together to find common themes. This is just a simple matter of attending to each transcript as described above and making a document for each participant. Go through each document and attend to the analysis as described previously. When all of the documents have been analysed separately, if you want to combine them to find common themes, do this by duplicating the final versions of the separate analyses on a computer and putting them together in one file.

The aim of the collective analysis is to find the ideas that are different enough to remain in their own categories. If themes are similar, merge them. For instance, if women say that they are happy, sad, confused and so on, these are all emotions. Incorporate these ideas under one heading of 'emotions' and be sure to include in your description of the theme, what the term means and what elements are included. In other words, you make your own definition of the theme based on what you have incorporated within it and what it has come to mean through the analysis process.

A good idea when naming common themes is to write a short phrase consisting of a verb and noun, that reflects the participant's experience and is consistent with the project's focus. For example, when I asked people with arthritis how they managed their lives (Taylor 2001), they gave accounts that had within them themes that were indeed their daily strategies, such as managing mornings, ensuring personal comfort, keeping a positive attitude, doing housework, cooking meals, getting exercise, existing in day-to-day life and so on.

The concise version of the computer-assisted method

The words taken to describe some ways of doing computer-assisted analyses are many, so to reiterate in point form:

- Make a disk copy of the main text to be analysed.
- Drop off any extraneous details from the copy, such as 'ums' and so on.
- Read through the text as it scrolls on the computer screen.
- Section the text off under subheadings that are relatively descriptive.
- As you progress through the document, make connections between themes that are raised in one part of the text and reiterated in another part.
- Collate the themes.
- Review the list while asking yourself: 'What does this say about my research interest?'
- Name the themes meaningfully.
- For multiple interviews analyse each transcript separately and then combine the accounts to find common themes.
- Define the themes and describe their components.

Other methods of text analysis

In qualitative research, words make up the texts, language and discourses that carry the meaning of human experience. Qualitative data analysis seeks to scrutinise and organise words in light of the research objectives and the particular methodological assumptions about the approach taken. Methods of data collection and analysis are not bound by methodologies; that is, a qualitative approach such as ethnography does not 'own' participant observation, and action research does not 'own' participatory group processes. Even though these two examples are known to use selected methods often, they do not use them always, nor do they exclude other possible methods. With this in mind, there are other analytic methods that can be used in a variety of approaches stretching across and beyond methodologies and research paradigms, such as narrative analysis and discourse analysis.

Narrative analysis

Storytelling is a popular method of qualitative data collection for all of the reasons cited in Chapter 14. Making sense of the stories can be through a variety of methods, including thematic analysis as described in this chapter. An interview can be converted to a story through amending the text to make the participant's words paramount. If you are considering creating stories from interview transcripts, a useful method of 'core story creation' is described by Emden (1998, p. 35), who suggests the following steps:

1 Read the full interview text several times within an extended time frame (several weeks) to grasp its content.
2 Delete all interviewer questions and comments from the full interview text.
3 Delete all words that detract from the key idea of each sentence or group of sentences uttered by the respondent.
4 Read the remaining text for sense.
5 Repeat steps 3 and 4 several times until you are satisfied that all key areas are retained and all extraneous content is eliminated. Return to the full text as often as necessary to recheck.
6 Identify fragments of constituent themes (subplots) from the ideas within the text.
7 Move fragments of themes together to create one coherent core story, or series of core stories.
8 Return the core story to the respondent and ask: 'Does it ring true?' and 'Do you wish to correct/develop/delete any part?'

Having created a core story, the next analysis task is emplotment, which is

> a process of working with one or more plots of a story in such a way that the significance of the story is disclosed; that is, emplotment ascribes some sense to a story – at potentially different levels of complexity (Emden 1998, p 36)

At the practical level of how to manage emplotment, Emden (1998, p. 37) explains that she tracked the plots

> aided by pencil and paper as I sought to keep track of the best fit possibilities between events as described by the participants and the emergent plot ... identified by me. This moving back and forth helped ensure that a preconceived plot structure was not imposed on events.

In tracking plots, you could use pencil and paper, or you might prefer to mark the text with highlighter pens so that each story line through the transcript appears in a particular colour. Alternatively, if you are adept at reading from a computer screen, you may be able to convert sections of text in the same plot into a different font type and size, thereby indicating different tracks of various plots.

Searching carefully through text in this way will eventually locate sets of events that are common to all stories, that 'grasp together as one story' (Polkinghorne 1988) in Emden (1998, p. 37). Thus, the events as related by participants (storytellers) constitute the contexts of the stories, and the task of narrative researchers is to undertake an analysis that will 'make sense of all the events as one story' (Emden 1998, p. 37). To see how narrative analysis translates to a research report, I suggest you locate a copy of Carolyn Emden's 1995 research.

Discourse analysis

In a general sense, discourse means a series of written or spoken utterances with a formal and organised connotation, such as in a dissertation, lecture, sermon, conversation or text on a certain subject. In effect, discourses as systems of statements can be on any topic. In nursing there are multiple discourses on the knowledge and skills nurses need to practise effectively, such as evidence-based practice, primary nursing, team nursing, and nursing diagnosis approaches. In a specific philosophical sense, discourse can be defined as a 'group of ideas or patterned way of thinking which can be identified in textual and verbal communications, and can also be located in wider social structures' (Lupton 1992, p. 145). Therefore, many epistemological (knowledge-producing and validating) and ontological (meaning of human existence) discourses underlie research approaches (defined in this book as methodologies). It is possible to speak of reflexivity in the form of discourse analysis in a variety of disciplines such as 'socio-linguistics, sociology, anthropology and philosophy ... [and in] a range of theoretical frameworks, including phenomenology, structuralism, Marxism and feminism' (Heslop 1996, p. 53). However, it is reasonable to assume that if you locate a research article or report in the present nursing literature, then it will most probably be referring to a critical social science or poststructuralist form of discourse analysis (Heslop 1996; Powers 1996; Crowe 1997; Cheek 2000; Manias & Street 2000).

Bearing in mind that there is no prescription for *doing* discourse analysis, I'm now going to describe some interpretations of Foucauldian thought before suggesting a 'poststructural process'.

Although opinions vary on the constitution of discourse analysis, a name appearing almost routinely in nursing literature is that of Michel Foucault, a philosopher whose work has had a profound influence on Australian nurse-researchers since the 1980s (see more about Foucault in Chapter 13). The method of discourse analysis used in this section is influenced by my 'reading' of the work of Foucault (1980).

Interpretations of some Foucauldian thought

The rules of discursive practices form and maintain discourses that in turn constitute power and knowledge relationships. For example, ethical requirements in research projects maintain the power bases of people on committees, who may favour particular design approaches and methodologies and thus obstruct the passage of those projects that do not fit the discourse judged by them to be important and 'true'.

Knowledge that counts as 'truth' is that which has won recognition in a culture as being successful and thus has gained and exercised power. For example, biomedical technology has been so highly successful in treating diseases that the powerful discourse of medicos has influenced other members of the health team to the extent that biomedical discourse is the benchmark by which effective patient management is judged. The power-knowledge of biomedical discourse is immersed in the culture of health care settings, especially those organised around hierarchies and bureaucracies that exercise the power of 'ownership' of human health care by experts.

Power can operate in many directions in micro-levels of a culture and people, through their knowledge, can change their subject positions to disrupt and challenge power relations. Therefore, power-knowledge not only maintains existing 'truth', but it can also shift, circulate, spread and change. For example, nurses are not necessarily bound by biomedical discourses as they too can exercise their power-knowledge by changing their subject positions in the health care team, as individuals capable of resistance against injustice.

A 'poststructural process'

A Foucauldian-style discourse analysis is a complex undertaking because it requires 'careful reading of entire bodies of text and other organising systems (such as taxonomies, commentaries and conference transcriptions) in relation to one another in order to interpret patterns, rules, assumptions, contradictions, silences, consequences, implications, and inconsistencies' (Powers 1996, p. 211). If you are intending to use a Foucauldian-style discourse analysis you would be well advised to read widely in Foucault's writing (for example, Foucault 1972, 1975, 1978, 1979) and authors who have interpreted his writing (for example, Dreyfus (1987); Foss and Gill (1987); Rawlinson (1987); Kusch (1991) and Bouchard (1997). If you are considering a postgraduate research project at master's degree or PhD level, you need to immerse yourself in these and other references, especially in relation to how Foucauldian thought has influenced nursing and health research. These suggestions are given in light of the idea that there is no particular way of doing a discourse analysis and if you are attempting to undertake a thorough process reflecting Foucauldian thought, you will need a comprehensive understanding of his discourse on knowledge and power.

Essentially, a discourse analysis asks questions about the knowledge and power inherent in all kinds of spoken- and written-life texts. Julianne Cheek (2000) offers a method of *'doing'* discourse analysis, so this will be used to highlight how you might go about doing something similar. She uses Parker's (2000) key features of research using discourse analysis, noting his contention that there is 'no set "recipe"' (Cheek 2000, p. 51) for analysing texts. Bear in mind that 'texts' may be interview transcripts, all kinds of academic and general publications, professional and public documents, and media sources such as films and videos.

According to Parker (in Cheek 2000), the first feature (phase, stage) of discourse analysis is the *introduction*, in which a literature review is done to position the project in relation to other research. Then, 'the types of questions/issues driving the research are discussed in order to contextualise the research' (Cheek 2000, p. 52). The second phase is *methodology*, describing the texts to be analysed, why these and not others were selected and how the selected texts will be obtained. For example, how will the interview be conducted and what type of articles will be collected? In the third phase, *analysis* occurs using 'a degree of intuition' and no set 'discursive frames' (p. 52); that is, using questions such as: 'What ways of speaking and thinking about the reality in question are not present and why might that be so?' (p. 52). In the last phase, *discussion*, 'analyses are linked to other material in the area in order to draw out points of discussion about the substantive area under scrutiny' (p. 52) and there is reflection by the researcher on her/his position on the issues raised.

You should note that in the third phase other questions could be raised to facilitate further discourse analysis of the textual comparisons, such as:

- What patterns and rules are present?
- How have the patterns and rules been constructed?
- What are the assumptions?
- What are the possible sources of these assumptions?
- What contradictions are apparent?
- What discourses are silent?
- What discourses are dominant?
- What are the consequences of the silenced discourses?
- What are the consequences of the dominant discourses?
- What are the implications of the discourse?
- What are the inconsistencies in the discourse?

Cheek (2000) presents Parker's (2000) features of discourse analysis in a synoptic version. For excellent examples to give you ideas about how you can do a discourse analysis, read Cheek's (1997a) article in which she analysed how four selected Australian print media represented toxic shock syndrome from the use of tampons. In another project (Cheek 1997b), Cheek analysed a conversation between a client and a health care professional to show that assumptions affect positions when communicating about health and health care.

Computer systems that manage qualitative data

Sometimes you may find that you can use manual methods of analysis in conjunction with a word search function on your computer. For Macintosh computers Hypercard is a program that can be used to organise data in the analysis processes. There is no prescription as to what must be done, so feel free to do whatever you need to do to obtain the most comprehensive and thorough analysis that you can, so that the richest meanings can emerge.

Another avenue you might like to explore is the use of a computer almost exclusively to locate the themes for you through the use of qualitative data analysis systems. *NUD*IST* (Qualitative Solutions and Research 1995) and *Ethnograph* (Siedel 1992) are systems that can group and order conceptual categories which have been decided progressively by the researcher. These are examples of computer systems that manage the qualitative data, with greater and lesser degrees of success depending on the aim of the researcher who is using them.

Benefits in qualitative data computer analysis systems

The main benefits of using qualitative data computer analysis systems are that they can manage large amounts of data and they are relatively easy to use.

Managing large amounts of data

Qualitative data computer analysis systems allow for whole transcripts and groups of transcripts to be merged and matched. This means that you have the potential to mix together all of the text and to do a collective analysis with ease. The added value of the systems is that they allow you to retrieve words and phrases from all of the combined transcripts that are connected to the context of the information. This means that sentences and phrases can be moved around the disk and located later, with their contextual features intact, which helps you to remember what words were said by whom, when and where. This is a very handy function for qualitative researchers who are making sense of large masses of words contained within the transcripts of high numbers of lengthy open-ended interviews.

Relatively easy to use

Systems are becoming easier to use as new versions appear on the market. They come complete with their own operating manuals for IBM-compatible or Macintosh computers. You may be able to access these systems through a site licence in an institution, or you can buy them directly from the manufacturers. Workshops run by the developers on how to use the systems are available, and it is advisable to avail yourself of them, and/or be assisted by someone who is proficient in using the particular system you have chosen.

Constraints in using qualitative data computer analysis systems

The main cautionary note in using qualitative data computer analysis systems is that the fullest interpretation may be missed because of the system's inability to locate implicit themes.

Inability to locate finer nuances
When using any computer system for qualitative analysis, a cautionary note is that the resultant analysis and interpretation of the data are only as rich as the meaning that is tagged to the words, through a thorough analysis of the text. This means that the finer nuances of the text may be missed if the researcher relies entirely on the sophisticated word search ability of the system, and does not look between the words to find the implicit meanings within words, phrases and sections of text. In qualitative research, the richest and finest meanings may be hiding within the total context of the words, so that it is only through protracted and clear-minded attention to the text that these connections are made. It's a bit like relying on the spell checker on your computer. It won't pick up words that are spelt correctly but used incorrectly. You (or some critical friend) must read all documents for errors that are beyond the 'ability' of the computer.

Examples of completed qualitative analyses
Before you embark on a qualitative analysis method, it may help you to look at completed forms that have been published. The main publication sources are books, journal articles, theses and published conference presentations.

Books about qualitative research
An example of completed qualitative analysis informed by phenomenology can be found in my book *Being Human* (Taylor 1994, 2000). In Chapters 3–8, you will see the detail of how I created sub-themes and if you refer to Chapter 14 you will see how they came together in the overall research themes.

In brief, this method of computer-assisted thematic analysis was created at the time of my research, because I could find no real guidance in how to do 'a phenomenological analysis' and I needed to try to get to the nature of the phenomenon of ordinariness. After a period of reading and re-reading, and through the computer-assisted thematic analysis I had devised, I located sub-themes I called aspects. The eight major aspects were: facilitation; fair play; familiarity; family; favouring; feelings; fun and friendship. Each of these aspects was defined according to its component parts. For example, facilitation refers to the enabling qualities and activities of both nurses and patients, whereby certain challenges being experienced by one person are made easier to face by the other person. Some qualities and activities (component parts) of facilitation include: appreciating skilful nursing care; appreciating help; facilitating independence; facilitating learning; facilitating coping; facilitating comfort; facilitating acceptance of body image changes; facilitating changes; calming fears; building trust; giving confidence; and allowing the experience to unfold.

However, because in this project I was trying to illuminate the ontological nature of ordinariness in nursing, I realised during the analysis that I needed to go deeper into the nature of each aspect illuminating the phenomenon. In other words, I went beyond the common themes to what I imagined was a phenomenological level of analysis, to what I termed actualities. Informed by some philosophical ideas, I moved from analysis to interpretation, and found that within facilitation there was 'allowingness'; within fair play there was 'straightforwardness'; within familiarity there was 'self-likeness'; within family there was 'homeliness'; within favouring there was 'favourableness'; within feelings there was 'intuneness'; within fun there was 'lightheartedness'; and within friendship there was 'connectedness'.

At this point of a project, it becomes very difficult, sometimes, to say just what one actually does when doing a qualitative analysis, especially at the interface of analysis and interpretation. In this project I remember feeling that the analysis was incomplete, and a philosopher confirmed this when I posed the question to him: 'How do I know that this project is phenomenological and not just qualitative?' He replied that the main feature of phenomenology is an attempt to explicate Being (existence, ontology). So I returned to an important methodological assumption of phenomenology, which asserts that in order to know the nature of the thing of interest, one goes to the thing itself. If one goes to the phenomenon and searches out its nature, and if one can assume that one indeed has illuminated the thing intended, the effects of its nature can only be the effects of the thing itself; it cannot be anything other than itself. This path of reasoning is in line with Heidegger (1962), who was unable to explicate Being through a temporal analysis, but he referred to Being as 'Es' (Itself). Therefore, if Being is Itself, it can be nothing else.

Using this reasoning, I remembered that I had moved from the place and people features of the research context to find the nature of the phenomenon, so I decided that it was now necessary to move 'backwards' from the phenomenon towards the research context in order to locate the effects. I imagined Being as residing within context, and context as residing within Being. To me, they became one and the same and they could not be something different from each other; therefore, I supposed that the nature of the phenomenon reflected its effects. I conceptualised the move from context to phenomenon, to find the nature of the thing, and the move from phenomenon to context, to find the effects of the thing, as a mirror image. The nature of the phenomenon within the actualities of the phenomenon reflected back towards the qualities and activities as effects that emerged out of the context. This logic being reasonable, it then followed that the effects of the phenomenon of ordinariness in nursing were those very qualities and activities (component parts) that comprised the aspects of the phenomenon.

A helpful book for seeing how an author has managed qualitative data analysis using a poststructural approach has been written by Julianne Cheek (2000). I suggest you borrow or buy this book, as Cheek answers in the affirmative the question of whether postmodern thinking is of any use for nurse-researchers, and she provides practical assistance on how projects can be undertaken. She also demonstrates how she was informed by Foucauldian ideas to use discourse analysis in a project examining media texts relating to toxic shock syndrome in adolescent females.

Examples of research and thesis documents

You would be well advised to procure examples of research and thesis documents to give you a wide appreciation of the types of approaches that are possible. If you scan refereed nursing journals that feature nursing research, you may find examples of qualitative nursing research that set out clearly the methods of data collection and analysis. Some of the journal articles cited in the qualitative part of this book may give you some guidance as to how the researchers managed data analysis. However, journal articles are constrained by word limits and you may have to resort to the original report or thesis document to glean practical assistance on how to go about the actual process of data analysis.

Often libraries keep holdings of research theses for honours and master's degrees and PhD awards. Sometimes these theses have been copied on microfiche or the full-text, hardbound copies are available for reading in the library. Locate theses whose titles and abstracts suggest adherence to a particular approach, such as an interpretive or critical methodology, or suggest postmodern influences. The methods of analysis contained within these theses have been judged by examiners to be of a quality sufficient to warrant the academic award, so you can place a certain amount of trust in them as guiding documents. Realise, however, that there is no one best method of qualitative analysis and it is permissible to amend and re-create some methods, as long as you are consistent with the methodological assumptions of the research approach and describe your analysis method fully and clearly.

Research project presentations

Oral accounts of qualitative analyses may be given by nurses presenting their projects at professional conferences. In this case, you would be well advised to attend the presentation then seek the presenters out afterwards to request elaboration on how they managed the analysis component of their research design. Conference presentations may be published in a book of proceedings and these may be a good source of worked examples of research analysis. Even so, do not be afraid to use the contact details offered publicly to communicate with researchers who have worked through the vagaries of data analysis. Depending upon their interest and cooperation, you may learn a great deal from successful researchers willing to share their techniques and strategies for data analysis.

Adjust analytic methods with a rationale

Be energetic and thorough in seeking out examples of analytic methods, but remember that no one qualitative method is sacrosanct. Do not be afraid to adjust an analytic method. As a standard procedure for report writing, you need to explain what you did in the analytic stage as part of your rationale for the research methods. The main aim is to ensure that what you have done is defensible in respect of the methodological assumptions that you used to structure the research methods in the first place.

The analysis of images as qualitative data

As words are the main tools of qualitative research, the analysis of them has taken up the largest part of this chapter. However, a discussion of qualitative analysis would not be complete without the acknowledgement of images as sources of qualitative data. You may remember that previously it was noted that some artistic expression, such as photographs, video and/or dance, may be admissible as data for qualitative analysis.

For the purposes of this chapter, the whole area of aesthetic judgement will be left to one side, as that is a highly specialised field in the arts which cannot be represented adequately here. Instead, the discussion will centre on the analysis of images that are generated by research participants as descriptive forms to augment or represent their personal expression of a phenomenon of research interest.

Analysis by the creator of the image

Images may be created by the researcher as photographs or videos, or they may be created by research participants as forms of expression to describe their experiences. This being so, it follows that the images would be analysed most accurately by the people who created them. This would mean that participants analyse and describe the images they created according to their intentions for creating them in relation to the research. Researchers would discuss with participants their analysis of the content of images and create a dialogue with them in making connections to the research aims and objectives. Therefore, the analyses of images as data are made in relation to the aims and objectives of the research and the intentions of the researcher and/or participant. The interpretations that result from the analysis of the images are what the person creating them says they are. These analyses and interpretations are admissible as they are relevant to the person involved; thus they add to the richness of the research findings. The research project report will need to show clearly that these analyses and interpretations are acknowledged as being those of the respective participants.

Summary

This chapter dealt with some 'how tos' of qualitative analysis. It was assumed that words are the main data for analysis, and the chapter dealt most comprehensively with their analysis. A small part of the text was devoted to the analysis of images as data. As I have found that most research books and researchers are seldom useful in telling potential researchers *how* to undertake a method of qualitative analysis, the chapter contained a compilation of hints and strategies that have worked from personal experience. I hope that you found them informative and that they continue to be helpful when you need to refresh your memory of them and put them into action in your own research.

Main points

- The orientation of a qualitative researcher undertaking the intellectual task of data analysis needs to include being ready physically and emotionally.
- Getting started in data analysis includes making copies, deciding on an organising system and having confidence in words as data.
- Qualitative analysis of words may be by either manual or computer-assisted means and the intentions of the analysis will determine what is done with the words.
- To find explicit and implicit themes within the text, know what you are looking for, locate specific words for explicit themes and look closely for the nuances of implicit themes.
- A theme bears resemblance to what you thought you might find, and it appears to have within it some features of the thing for which you are looking; that is, it is part of the pattern of answers you are intending to find within the text, and you know it is relevant because its identity is connected directly and sometimes indirectly to the stated research aims and objectives.
- A manual thematic analysis method is to read and re-read the text; make multiple copies of the page-numbered transcripts (ensuring one copy is kept as a guide); keep in mind the research question and/or objectives; isolate (by cutting out or colour coding) any sections of text that appear to be connected to a theme; reduce the 'themes' to a word or two each and list them; and, finally, collect them into groupings until they cannot be subsumed into other categories/groupings without losing their specialness in relation to the research aims and objectives.
- A computer-assisted data analysis method is to make a disk copy of the main text to be analysed, drop off any extraneous details from the copy, read through the text as it scrolls on the computer screen, section the text off under a subheading that is relatively descriptive, make connections between themes that are raised in one part of the text and reiterated in another part, collate the themes, review the list while asking yourself: 'What does this say about the research interest?', name and define the themes and describe their components.
- Caroline Emden suggests creating a core story by: reading the full interview text several times within an extended time frame (several weeks) to grasp its content; deleting all interviewer questions and comments from the full interview text; deleting all words that detract from the key idea of each sentence or group of sentences uttered by the respondent; reading the remaining text for sense; repeating the previous two processes several times until you are satisfied that all key areas are retained and all extraneous content has been eliminated; returning to the full text as often as necessary for rechecking; identifying fragments of constituent themes (subplots) from the ideas within the text; moving fragments of themes together to create one coherent core story, or series of core stories; and returning the core story to the respondent for checking.

- Emplotment involves the researcher going carefully through text to track plots and locate sets of events that are common to all stories, then undertaking an analysis that will make sense of all the events as one story.
- Discourses are groups of ideas or patterned ways of thinking, writing and speaking immersed in social structures that constitute power and knowledge relationships.
- A discourse analysis asks questions systematically and thoroughly about the knowledge and power inherent in all kinds of spoken and written life texts, in relation to the nature and construction patterns and rules present, the kinds of assumptions and their possible sources, and the contradictions, silences, dominance and inconsistencies in the discourse.
- The main benefits of using qualitative data computer analysis systems are that they can manage large amounts of data and they are relatively easy to use, whereas the main cautionary note is that the fullest interpretation may be missed because of the system's inability to locate implicit themes.
- Examples of completed qualitative analyses can be located in books, journal articles, theses, and published conference presentations.

Review Questions

1. Getting started in qualitative data analysis includes:
   a making copies
   b deciding on an organising system
   c having confidence in words as data
   d all of the above

2. Qualitative analysis of words may be by:
   a manual or computer-assisted means
   b manual means only
   c computer-assisted means only
   d intuitive or manual means

3. To find implicit themes within the text:
   a locate specific words
   b look closely for the nuances
   c connect key words
   d disregard irrelevancies

4. You know you have found a theme because it:
   a bears no resemblance to what you thought you might find
   b appears to have within it some features of the thing for which you are looking
   c is not part of the pattern of answers you are intending to find within the text
   d is not connected to the stated research aims and objectives

5. A theme has reached its full identity when:
   a. the total number of themes is consistent with the aims and objectives of the research project
   b. it is represented by the idea that you imagined it would be from the start of the research
   c. it cannot be subsumed into other categories/groupings without losing its specialness
   d. it is no longer possible to think up new terms to name the emerging phenomena

6. Caroline Emden's method of transforming interview transcripts into concise and informative documents is termed creating ... stories.
   a. essential
   b. short
   c. key
   d. core

7. The process of going carefully through text to track plots and locate sets of events that are common to all stories, then undertaking an analysis that will make sense of all the events as one story, is termed:
   a. emplotment
   b. encasement
   c. encoding
   d. emancipating

8. Groups of ideas or patterned ways of thinking, writing and speaking immersed in social structures that constitute power and knowledge relationships are:
   a. dialogues
   b. discourses
   c. debates
   d. dissertations

9. The main benefit of using qualitative data computer analysis systems is that they:
   a. are completely subjective
   b. are readily available
   c. can manage large amounts of data
   d. require no training

10. The main limitation of using qualitative data computer analysis systems is that they:
    a. are difficult and cumbersome to use
    b. are dependent on a knowledge of mathematics
    c. are expensive
    d. may miss implicit themes

Discussion Questions

1. Describe some approaches for getting started in analysing qualitative data.
2. Describe two manual methods of thematic analysis.
3. What processes are used to find explicit and implicit themes within the text?
4. Describe computer-assisted methods of thematic analysis.
5. Compare the benefits and limitations of using manual and computer-assisted methods of thematic analysis.

References

Allen, D. G. 1985, 'Nursing research and social control: alternative models of science that emphasise understanding and emancipation', *Image: Journal of Nursing Scholarship*, vol. 17, no. 2, 58–64.

Bouchard, D. E. (ed.) 1997, *Knowledge, Counter-Memory, and Practice: Selected Essays and Interviews of Michel Foucault*, Cornell Press, Ithaca, New York.

Cheek, J. 1997a, 'Contextualizing toxic shock syndrome: selected media representations of an emergent health phenomenon 1979–95', *Health*, vol. 1, no. 2, 183–203.

Cheek, J. 1997b, 'Negotiating delicately: conversations about health', *Health and Social Care in the Community*, vol. 5, no. 1, 23–7.

Cheek, J. 2000, *Postmodern and Poststructural Approaches to Nursing Research*, Sage Publications, Thousand Oaks, California.

Chinn, P. L. 1985, 'Debunking myths in nursing theory and research', *Image: Journal of Nursing Scholarship*, vol. 17, no. 2, 45–9.

Crowe, M. 1997, 'The power of the word: some post-structural considerations of qualitative approaches in nursing research', *Journal of Advanced Nursing*, vol. 28, no. 2, 339–44.

Dreyfus, H. 1987, 'Foucault's critique of psychiatric medicine', *Journal of Medicine and Philosophy*, vol. 12, 311–33.

Emden, C. 1995, 'Scholars in dialogue', in *Scholarship in the Discipline of Nursing*, eds G. Gray & R. Pratt, Churchill-Livingstone, Melbourne.

Emden, C. 1998, 'Conducting a narrative analysis', *Collegian*, vol. 5, no. 3, 34–9.

Foss, S. K. & Gill, A. 1987, 'Michel Foucault's theory of rhetoric as epistemic', *Western Journal of Speech Communication*, vol. 51, 384–401.

Foucault, M. 1972, *The Archaeology of Knowledge*, Tavistock, London.

Foucault, M. 1975, *The Birth of the Clinic*, trans. A. M. Sheridan-Smith, Vintage/Random House, New York (original work published 1973).

Foucault, M. 1978, *The History of Sexuality*, vol. 1: An Introduction, trans. R. Hurley, Vintage/Random House, New York (original work published 1976).

Foucault, M. 1979, *Discipline and Punish*, trans. A. M. Sheridan-Smith, Vintage/Random House, New York (original work published 1975).

Foucault, M. 1980, *Michel Foucault. Power/Knowledge: Selected Interviews and Other Writings*, Harvester Press, Brighton, England.

Glass, N. & Davis, K. 1998, 'An emancipatory impulse: a feminist postmodern integrated turning point in nursing research', *Advances in Nursing Science*, 21, no. 1, 43–52.

Goodwin, L. D. & Goodwin, W. L. 1984, 'Qualitative vs quantitative research or qualitative and quantitative research?' *Nursing Research*, vol. 33, no. 6, 378–80.

Heidegger, M. 1962, *Being and Time*, Harper & Row, New York.
Henderson, V. 1964, 'The nature of nursing', *American Journal of Nursing*, vol. 64, no. 8, 62–8.
Heslop, L. 1996, 'The (im)possibilities of poststructuralist and critical social science nursing inquiry', *Nursing Inquiry*, vol. 4, 48–56.
Kermode, S. & Brown, C. 1995, 'Where have all the flowers gone: nursing's escape from the radical critique', *Contemporary Nurse*, vol. 4, no. 1, 8–15.
Kratz, C. R. 1978, *Care of the Long Term Sick in the Community*, Churchill-Livingstone, Edinburgh.
Kusch, M. 1991, *Foucault's Strata and Fields: an Investigation into Archaeological and Genealogical Science Studies*, Kluwer Academic Publishers, Dordrecht, The Netherlands.
Leininger, M. 1985, *Qualitative Research Methods in Nursing*, Grune and Stratton, New York.
Lupton, D. 1992, 'Discourse analysis: a new methodology for understanding the ideologies of health and illness', *Australian Journal of Public Health*, vol. 16, 145–50.
Manias, E. & Street, A. 2000, 'Possibilities for critical social theory and Foucault's work: a toolbox approach', *Nursing Inquiry*, vol. 7, 50–60.
Parker, I. 2000, 'Discourse dynamics: critical analysis for social and individual psychology', in *Postmodern and Poststructural Approaches to Nursing Research*, ed. J. Cheek, Sage Publications, Thousand Oaks, California.
Polkinghorne, D. E. 1988, *Narrative Knowing and the Human Sciences*, State University of New York, Albany, New York.
Powers, P. 1996, 'Discourse analysis as a methodology for nursing inquiry', *Nursing Inquiry*, vol. 3, 207–17.
Qualitative Solutions and Research 1995, *NUD*IST (Non-Numerical Unstructured Data: Indexing Searching & Theorising)*, application software package, QSR, Melbourne.
Rawlinson, M. 1987, 'Foucault's strategy: knowledge, power and the specificity of truth', *Journal of Medicine and Philosophy*, vol. 12, 372–95.
Sarnecky, M. T. 1990, 'Historiography: a legitimate research methodology for nursing', *Advances in Nursing Science*, vol. 12, no. 4, 1–10.
Siedel, J. V. 1992, *Ethnograph*, version 4.0, Qualis Research Associates, Corvallis, Oregon.
Spradley, J. P. 1979, *The Ethnographic Interview*, Holt, Rinehart & Winston, New York.
Strauss, A. L. 1987, *Qualitative Analysis for Social Scientists*, Cambridge University Press, New York.
Taylor, B. 1994, *Being Human: Ordinariness in Nursing*, Churchill-Livingstone, Melbourne.
Taylor, B. 2000, *Being Human: Ordinariness in Nursing* (adapted), Southern Cross University Press, Lismore, NSW.
Taylor, B. 2001, 'Promoting self-help strategies by sharing the lived experience of arthritis', *Contemporary Nurse*, vol. 10, no. 1–2, 117–25.
Winstead–Fry, P. 1980, 'The scientific method and its impact on holistic health', *Advances in Nursing Science* (Jan.), 1–7.

CHAPTER 17

Interpreting qualitative findings

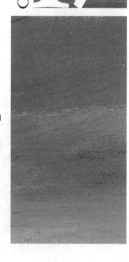

chapter objectives The material presented in this chapter will assist you to:

- differentiate between analysis and interpretation
- acknowledge the relative nature of qualitative research interpretations
- relate varieties of findings to specific methodological approaches
- use qualitative interpretive and critical categories to make general statements about interpretive processes
- describe processes for synthesising qualitative interpretive and critical results
- identify postmodern influences on interpretation as another perspective for nursing research.

Introduction

To some extent in qualitative research, analysis and interpretation appear to overlap, but they are not the same. There is a transition from a systematic review and analysis of the words, images and/or numbers (alone or in combination) to interpretive statements that can be made, revealing insights and relative answers to the areas being researched. In some cases, the transition is marked by step-by-step development of theory, for example the structured approach of grounded theory (Strauss 1975). In other cases, such as phenomenological research, the transition from analysis to interpretation is not as structured, yet readers can locate analytic steps in the research process (Colaizzi 1978). Towards the postmodern end of the continuum, transitions may be relatively imperceptible, as analysis and interpretation blend as relative explanations are located, based on the multifaceted nature of human discourse and the tentativeness of the research questions.

There are many kinds of qualitative research; therefore, there are many means of analysing and interpreting the meaning which emerges from them. This chapter will introduce you to some of the ways in which the analysis phase of qualitative research leads to interpretation and theories/results/findings/insights/recommendations/implications. The reason for presenting all these words in this way is that language is important. In this part of a qualitative research project, language indicates the differences in various kinds of qualitative research and the assumptions that underlie them. As has been shown in other chapters of this book, it is very difficult to represent qualitative research approaches as a general group. Differentiation is required between different methods and processes of interpretation that are used, with basic assumptions about the nature of human knowledge in mind.

Although processes for interpreting analysed information vary according to research methodologies, for ease of reference and the sake of continuity, this chapter will distinguish between them under the categories of interpretive qualitative research and critical qualitative research. This approach for categorising qualitative research was introduced in Chapter 12. The explanation was given then, that even though the categories of qualitative interpretive and qualitative critical research are very broad, they nonetheless simplify what could be a very complex issue for new researchers. It is hoped that the qualitative interpretive and qualitative critical categories will allow you to make general statements about the various processes of interpretation that you may read about, or choose to use in your own projects. In addition, some discussion on postmodern influences on interpretation is offered, as another perspective for nursing research.

Differentiation between analysis and interpretation

It is important to draw a distinction between analysis and interpretation, as they are separate processes. In order to be able to make interpretations, data must be analysed thoroughly. Although some writers promise information on interpreting qualitative research (Knaff & Howard 1984) and other writers get closer to the nub of the problem by discussing the problems of doing qualitative interpretation (Ammon-Gaberson & Piantanida 1988), overall there is very little direction in the nursing literature as to how to go about qualitative research interpretation. There is also minimal guidance on how interpretation relates to and differs from analytic research processes.

As far as possible, qualitative researchers must attempt to set out the analytic and interpretive phases of the project for readers of the research. This may be a difficult task, because qualitative analysis and interpretation is not always clear cut. This contrasts with quantitative approaches, in which instruments are considered valid and reliable and interpretations stem directly from discussing relationships between discrete variables.

Defining analysis and interpretation

Qualitative analysis and interpretation are related, yet they are different.

Analysis

Analysis involves reviewing research data systematically with the intention of sorting and classifying them into representational groups and patterns. To describe analysis, Ammon-Gaberson and Piantanida (1988) use the analogy of stacking pebbles into piles. After analysis, the data have been organised from their raw state as words, numbers and images (alone or in combination) into groupings and symbolic forms that require explanation to ensure that the meaning is clear.

Interpretation

Interpretation involves working with the forms of analysed information so that statements can be made about what they mean in light of the intentions, methods and processes of the research. The analogy of the pebbles is extended here to the point at which an artist puts them into configurations to depict their central purpose and elaborate their meaning (Ammon-Gaberson & Piantanida 1988). In qualitative research, if the interpretations and explanations of the analysed data are not given, readers will be left to infer their own conclusions. This raises issues around interpretations from various perspectives.

Just as a work of art can be left open to multiple interpretations, so also can qualitative research findings. This is in line with the context-dependent and relative features of qualitative research approaches. For example, qualitative researchers and participants will place their unique interpretations on the data, having been involved actively in the project. Readers of the research may not necessarily agree with the researchers' and participants' interpretations or they may posit other possible conclusions about the findings. Readers of the research should be able to trace the processes that were used in a project, so that they have a sound rationale for their differing interpretations.

Analysis generally precedes interpretation

Generally speaking, analysis precedes interpretation, although some qualitative researchers, such as those using phenomenological writing, describe an intuitive grasp of the data, having focused on it so closely and thoroughly. Also, some qualitative researchers who use participatory research methods and processes with participants as co-researchers may experience spiralling and integrative processes in which analysis and interpretation blend and seem to become indivisible. Bearing in mind these and other possible exceptions to the rule, the approach taken here will to be to assume that interpretation occurs after a period of analysis, however protracted and by whatever means.

Interpretation requires immersion in the text

Language is the basis of qualitative research. Although images and numbers can also be part of qualitative analysis and interpretation, words are the main symbols from which meaning is derived. Because words are the main source of interpretation, many approaches require a high degree of familiarity with the text. Text was defined previously as the transcript and/or record of words. Text may be interview transcripts, field notes, historical documents, journal entries, summaries, audio recordings of group discussions and so on. Essentially, text can mean any sources of words that contribute to finding meaning in the research interest.

Invariably, qualitative interpretations of words and language require protracted time with the text to ensure that meaning is located and that it is as clear as possible to convey to other people. Therefore, qualitative interpretation is generally not a matter of putting data through a computer system to come up with statistical relationships for interpretation. Rather, analysis is usually through reading and re-reading text, with manual or computer-assisted means. Interpretation follows after further reflection and validation by people such as other researchers, co-researchers, participants and peers.

Qualitative research findings as relative interpretations

The findings of research projects will be disseminated to readers as information which can be relied on as trustworthy. This is another way of saying that, to the best of their abilities, the researchers claim to share truthful findings. In Chapter 12 there is a discussion on what constitutes truth according to the major distinctions of quantitative (empirico-analytical) and qualitative (interpretive and critical) research traditions. The methods for knowledge generation, analysis, interpretation and validation differ according to assumptions about what constitutes new and/or amended truth and worthwhile knowledge. If you are unclear about these distinctions you may like to refer to this section in the early part of Chapter 12.

Interpretations as relative truth

Qualitative researchers agree that there is no way of guaranteeing absolute truth, because truth is relative and elusive. This means that truth can change according to all kinds of context-dependent determinants associated with people, places, times and conditions in which it resides and emerges. Therefore qualitative researchers interested in human phenomena attempt to explore the changing nature of knowledge, assuming that truth is tentative and unpredictable.

The idea that truth is relative may appear to leave open the whole issue of whether qualitative interpretations can be relied on as having some foundation for adding to knowledge. Even though truth is regarded as being relative, it is considered important to reveal it in its various forms. The main difference between qualitative and quantitative assumptions about knowledge in this regard is that the former do not seek to generate absolute, indisputable truths and facts. This is because they agree that the changing and complex nature of human existence does not permit research approaches to guarantee this kind of knowledge. Even so, qualitative researchers use various means of demonstrating the worthiness of their projects. For example, measures for ensuring validity may involve asking the participants to confirm that the interpretations are truthful for them. These issues are discussed in the section dealing with rigour in Chapter 14.

Interpretations by other names

Various words are used synonymously to mean interpretations. Qualitative research reports may use words such as theories, findings, results, insights, strategies, implications, examples of reflective awareness and changed practice, and so on. The words used may have been selected specifically to reflect the assumptions and intentions of the research methodology. That is because qualitative research is set up in different ways to fulfil different purposes. For example:

- a grounded theory approach may put forward interpretations as theories (Wilson 1993)
- a phenomenological approach may document insights (Walters 1996)
- a feminist approach may describe competing discourses (Glass 1994)
- an action research approach or a critical ethnography may report examples of reflective awareness and changed practice (Street 1998; Wellard & Street 1999; Koch, Kralik & Kelly 2000)
- a project influenced by postmodern ideas may document the presence of multiple and contradictory voices (Cheek 2000).

The scope of interpretation

Most qualitative research approaches do not claim to generate interpretations that can be considered to be generalisable to the wider population. An exception to this is grounded theory, which sets out to make general statements in the form of theories about what might be expected in similar circumstances.

Phenomenological approaches that provide insights might typically expect that interpretations will be useful for those people with whom they resonate. In other words, if readers of the research find it is relevant for them, then it has scope in being informative to them.

Action research approaches reporting examples of reflective awareness and changed practice have scope for local theories of practice. This means that the people who have participated in the project have realised local, personal truths that are relevant for them. The scope of the interpretations is broader when the people involved in the research influence other people, policies and practices in the wider setting.

Research using postmodern thought may not deem to offer anything concrete, but to leave all ideas open as tentative, or make multiple interpretations and give authority to readers to make their own interpretations (Cheek 2000). In some cases, key postmodern ideas, such as difference and voice, may be retained as the central core and integrity of a grand narrative (Glass & Davis 1998).

Qualitative findings in relation to methodological approaches

Qualitative findings will differ according to the underlying theoretical assumptions of the approach and the intentions of the research. There are many ways of categorising methodological approaches in qualitative research; however they invariably lead to a great deal of detail and confusion. For this reason, the approach taken here will be to use the categories explained previously in Chapters 12 and 13 of this book.

A very simple and comprehensive way of thinking about kinds of qualitative research is to categorise them according to interpretive and critical forms and differences. Although categorisations of this kind have their shortcomings, they are useful for students who are trying to plot their way through a wide and deep range of ideas about research. As an important postscript, some possibilities will be considered of the diverse thought that postmodernisms offer.

Qualitative interpretive methodologies

Qualitative interpretive research methodologies intend mainly to generate meaning, by exploring, explaining and describing things of interest in order to make sense out of them. Examples of these methodologies are historical research, grounded theory, ethnography and phenomenology. These methodologies have been described previously in Chapter 12.

Qualitative critical methodologies

Qualitative critical methodologies aim to bring about change in the status quo by questioning aspects that are taken for granted. Through systematic political critique, these methodologies attempt to expose factors of control, oppression, power and domination and cause raised awareness and change activities.

Examples of these methodologies are critical ethnography, feminisms, interpretive interactionism and action research. These methodologies have been described previously in Chapter 13.

Similarities and differences

In doing what they intend to do as their first priority, qualitative interpretive and critical research methodologies also manage to do other things. For example, they both generate meaning by looking closely at a phenomenon of interest. Also, they can both bring about change.

The major difference between interpretive and critical qualitative research is in the main intention of what they hope to achieve through the research process. Interpretive forms are involved mainly with generating meaning. Critical forms concern themselves with change. Even though they both can bring about change, they differ in the intensity of their intentions and their choice of methods to do this. Critical methodologies are most intense in bringing about change. This is because they have an 'up-front' change agenda and they tend to use participatory research processes to realise their change intentions.

Qualitative interpretive and critical categories of interpretive processes

Processes for interpretation may differ according to what kind of qualitative research it can be considered to be; that is, whether it is essentially an interpretive (concerned mainly with meaning) or critical (concerned mainly with change) project. Some researchers may argue that they have combined methodologies across the interpretive and critical categories. In this case, they may need to use a combination of interpretive processes, appropriate to the assumptions, aims, objectives, methods and processes of the project.

Clarifying some preconditions for qualitative interpretation

A researcher may have made a clear decision as to the placement of a project in either the interpretive or critical methodology categories. Alternatively, the project may be placed in a combination of methodologies. In some cases a project may defy categorisation altogether into methodological groupings, for example, postmodern research. Regardless of the nature of the project, there are some general necessary preconditions for interpretation of which qualitative researchers are advised to be aware.

The need for congruency

Congruency is correspondence or agreement. In qualitative research, it means the fit or correspondence between foundational ideas and the activity phases of the research. Even though the phases of a project may be planned carefully at the outset, parts of the overall project may change over the course of the research. Therefore, before embarking on making sense of the analysed data it may be useful to take some time to re-orient to the overall project. This will involve you asking yourself some questions to check on the congruency of the project's assumptions, aims, objectives, methods and processes.

Some questions which may be posed are:

Assumptions
- What ideas underlie this project about the nature of knowledge and how it is verified?
- What choices were made about selecting a paradigm in which the project would fit most appropriately?
- If no paradigm category was chosen then, does it matter now?

Aims and objectives
- What did I intend to research?
- Why did I want to research these things?
- At this stage, to what extent has the project fulfilled its stated purposes?

Methods
- What methods were chosen to gather the information?
- To what extent do the methods appear to be a good fit with the assumptions, aims and objectives of the research?
- To what extent did the methods gather the information required?

Processes
- How was the research undertaken in terms of the researcher–participant relationships?
- How was the research undertaken in terms of the overall management of the project?
- To what extent did the processes appear to be a good fit with the assumptions, aims, objectives and methods of the research?

Reasons for asking questions between analysis and interpretation

The reasons for asking certain questions at the transition from analysis to interpretation are to re-orient to the overall project; to check on the degree of congruency between the assumptions, aims, objectives, methods and processes; and to prepare for the process of interpretation.

Re-orienting to the overall project

In re-orienting to the overall project, the researcher's memory is refreshed and an assessment can be made as to the whether the project has progressed generally as anticipated to this point. If it has not gone as expected, it might be helpful to look at ways in which it has differed and locate the reasons why. It may be necessary to have this in mind when beginning the interpretation as this will help to sort out twists and turns in the data that otherwise may be confusing.

Checking on the degree of congruency

Congruency may not be an issue for some qualitative researchers. Some researchers may argue that they are using certain methods which make their project qualitative in nature (Gething 1992; Semmens & Peric 1995–6). They might contend that there does not need to be any justification of theoretical underpinnings of methodologies. Therefore, it would follow that they would see no need to find agreement between the project's methodology and its aims, objectives, methods and processes.

However, it is worth bearing in mind that most qualitative research provides a theoretical basis for its choice of methodological approach, methods and processes (LoBiondo-Wood & Haber 1994; Bunkers et al. 1996), but because there are many qualitative approaches from which to choose, they do not all have the same assumptions about what constitutes knowledge and how to go about finding and verifying it. Supporters of having a theoretical basis might argue that researchers need to be clear about the degree of congruency within and between all the research phases because it helps them prepare for interpretation and because it will provide a strong rationale for readers of the research as to what has been done, and why and how it has been done.

Preparing for the process of interpretation

When it comes time to move from analysis to interpretation, using the questioning exercise listed in this chapter may help you to determine the degree of congruency in the research to date. It will help you to focus thoroughly on the data. This intense focusing may help you to extract meaning that is congruent with the assumptions, aims, objectives, methods and processes of the research. It will also mean that some time will elapse between the analysis and interpretation phases of the research. This will not only give you time for thinking, but it will also permit time for reading and re-reading so that there is deeper and deeper immersion in the data, in preparation for making sense out of it.

Processes for synthesising qualitative interpretive and critical results

In the strictest dictionary sense, processes are series of actions that produce changes or developments (*Collins English Dictionary* 1998). In qualitative research involving humans, however, the interest is not so much in the actions themselves but in how the actions are done through interpersonal processes. The processes for synthesising qualitative interpretive and critical interpretations happen as cognitive activities within the researcher. This interpretation process must happen for the researcher to make sense of the analysed data.

From analysis to interpretation

Being able to describe interpretation is tantamount to being able to describe cognitive processes such as making intellectual leaps, connections, intuitive grasps and so on. This makes interpretation a very difficult thing to describe on a biochemical and psychological level. Philosophers have taken different approaches to tackling the vexed problem of what it is inquirers do when they interpret, by addressing various forms of hermeneutics (Gadamer 1975 trans.; Habermas 1981). (Hermeneutics is taken here broadly to mean processes of interpretation.)

Hans-Georg Gadamer is a philosopher in the phenomenological tradition. Gadamer (1975 trans.) decided that all understanding is hermeneutical, because hermeneutics is the 'basic being-in-motion of There-being, which constitutes its finiteness and historicity and hence includes the whole experience of the world' (Gadamer 1975 trans., p. 323). This means that Gadamer reasoned that interpretations were available to humans as beings in the world. He argued that things can be made apparent through understanding the nature of human existence. For him, the key to understanding existence is through language.

Gadamer contended that it is the task of hermeneutics to make distinctions between true and false prejudices, by a process of effective historical consciousness. Gadamer suggested that effective historical consciousness was analogous to the I–Thou relationship in which openness to the other and willingness to be modified creates a dialogical relationship (Gadamer 1975 trans., p. 323). By this he was advocating the need to be open to and surprised by what may emerge through interpretation.

For Jürgen Habermas, interpretation is more a matter of realising that knowledge is socially constructed through human interaction and that interpretation involves social, cultural, economic and political and personal dimensions. He proposed a kind of critical hermeneutics that:

> focuses on the communicative conditions under which meaning is produced and on power/justice dimensions of intended and unintended social consequences of interpretations. Critical hermeneutics has a commitment to both understanding and exposing how power imbalances and misunderstandings constrain and distort interpretations (Allen 1995, p. 180).

Habermas linked truthful interpretation to the idea of rational consensus gained through discourse. This means that people have the potential to create their own interpretations through non-coercive and non-manipulative rationality. He considered that people orient towards finding truth through daily communicative acts or speaking, and that ideal speech situations involve comprehensibility of the utterance, truth of the content, rightness of the performative content, and veracity of the speaker. This kind of rationality has been criticised by Bernstein (1978) who says that Habermas's idea of ideal speech is not real, because it has not paid attention to people's choice and will, cultural diversity and language differences.

For the postmodernists the whole idea of interpretation is open for debate. As Rosenau (1992) explains:

> Post-modernists recognise an infinite number of interpretations (meanings) of any text are possible because, for the skeptical post-modernists, one can never say what

one intends with language, ultimately all textual meaning, all interpretation, is undecidable. Because there is no final meaning for any particular sign, no notion of a unitary sense of text, these post-modernists argue that no interpretation can be regarded as superior to any other. In its world of plural constructions, diverse realities, an absence of certainty, and a multiplicity of readings, post-modernism refuses to privilege one statement over another; all interpretations are of equal interest.

Postmodern definitions of interpretation are influenced by *deconstruction*, which 'involves demystifying a text, tearing it apart to reveal its internal, arbitrary hierarchies and its presuppositions' (Rosenau 1992, p. 120). Deconstruction involves looking at the 'margins' of a text, to its contradictions, inconsistencies, and what is excluded, unnamed and concealed, not to unmask errors (as this would imply a search for truth) but to transform and redefine it. In this way, postmodernist deconstruction discloses tensions, but does not seek to resolve them, as this would give authority to the most correct interpretation. The consequence of postmodern deconstruction, therefore, is a never-ending critique of text to reveal its contradictions and to question the authority of the author.

Where does postmodern deconstruction leave nurse-researchers? If we are to take a skeptical view of postmodernism, we would be caught up 'in an infinite regress of deconstruction, where nothing is better than anything else' (Richardson 1992, in Rosenau 1992, p. 122). On a practical level, no research meanings would be viewed as defensible interpretations, providing no definite answers or even tentative guidance, reasonable for the moment. However, nursing needs guidance in practice, education and management, and in this postmodern world, trends towards evidence-based practice are paramount, and these favour quantitative measures and prioritise qualitative measures last as indicators of useful, 'truthful' interpretations.

So, is postmodernism interesting, but of no practical use for nurse-researchers? Debates have argued both cases. Kermode and Brown (1995) would argue that postmodernism is not only of no practical use for nursing, but also that it can deaden our sensitivities towards capitalism and patriarchy, which may be left uncontested as sources of power and domination in postmodern times because of an 'anything goes' relativism inherent in postmodernism. In response, nurse-scholars and researchers argue that a narrow view of postmodernism takes account only of the skeptical literature and does not allow postmodernism to create wider and deeper possibilities for conceptualising and practising nursing (Glass & Davis 1998; Cheek 2000). On an optimistic note, a postmodern 'interpretation' leaves the reader in authority as the interpreter of any life text, and in nursing, that means making choices about what constitutes nursing, while heeding caution about accepting unquestioningly all kinds of dominant discourses in grand narratives.

All in all, what is written about interpretation may provide cold comfort to a nurse-researcher who knows very little about philosophy and who simply wants to know how to go about interpreting qualitative data. The next section will attempt to break through the lack of direction to give clues to ways in which interpretation might be done. It will be done by raising some questions and suggesting some tentative answers. Examples of research will be given to demonstrate differences that will be noted in qualitative interpretive and critical research interpretations.

The assumptions underlying the listing of these suggested processes relate to differences in research relationships between researchers and participants. Qualitative interpretive methodologies involve participants by working with them in research processes, rather than doing research 'to' subjects. However, qualitative interpretive methodologies are not as mindful of participatory group processes and co-researcher status for participants as qualitative critical methodologies.

How do I go about the process of interpretation when I have used a qualitative interpretive methodology?

- Go through the exercise of asking yourself the questions listed in this chapter as preconditions for qualitative interpretation.
- Take some time away from the project. Take a walk, go on a holiday – in whatever way you prefer, give yourself some space. (This will depend on the time you have available to complete the project, of course!) 'Time out' will let the analysed data percolate through your mind.
- Although you are taking a rest from the project, notice any ideas that come up in your mind. Write them down, even if they seem insignificant.
- Remember that interpretation subsumes all the phases in the research that have gone before.
- Remember that the products of the analysis are incomplete in themselves. They only have fullest meaning when they have been described and explained through interpretation.
- Resume your work and re-read the analysed data. Review how you came to make the themes/essences.
- If you have already named any of the themes/essences in the analysis phase, why did you choose those words? Are they still relevant? Would other words represent them more effectively?
- Clarify in your mind what the themes/essences mean. Try writing down words and sentences that explain them to other people.
- If you are not a rapid writer and your thoughts are moving too fast, speak into an audiotape recorder and rephrase your thoughts over and over until you are sure you are saying what you mean to be saying. Commit the final version to writing.
- If you prefer vocalising your interpretations as they happen, ask a valued friend or colleague who is aware of the intentions of the research, to listen to you as you speak spontaneously about what you think the analysed data mean in light of the overall project. After you have finished the clearest possible explication of what you want to say, invite the person to ask questions and to be frank about any parts of your interpretations that did not seem to ring true to the overall intentions and phases of the project.

- Create definitions and explanations that represent most faithfully the clearest and truest meaning that you can extract from the analysed data.
- Ensure that you have created and explained links between definitions and explanations, that are congruent with the assumptions, aims, objectives, methods and processes of the research.
- Links between definitions and explanations need to be clear and your reasons for making them should be able to be traced by readers.

For excellent examples of interpretation of nursing research using interpretive methodologies, refer to the following projects:

- Fiveash, B. 1998, 'The experience of nursing home life', *International Journal of Nursing Practice*, vol. 4, 166–74.
- Hemsley, S. & Glass, N. 1999, 'Nurse healers: exploring their lived experience as nurses', *Australian Journal of Holistic Nursing*, vol. 6 (2), 28–34.
- Irurita, V. 1999a, 'Factors affecting the quality of nursing care: the patient's perspective', *International Journal of Nursing Practice*, vol. 5, 86–94.
- Irurita, V. 1999b, 'The problem of patient vulnerability', *Collegian*, vol. 6 (1), 10–15.
- Johnstone, M-J. 1999, 'Reflective topical autobiography: an underutilised interpretive research method in nursing', *Collegian*, vol. 6 (1), 24–9.
- Zeitz, K. 1999, 'Nurses as patients: the voyage of discovery', *International Journal of Nursing Practice*, vol. 5, 64–71.
- Jones, C. & Chapman, Y.B. 2000, 'The lived experience of seven people treated with autologous bone marrow/peripheral blood stem cell transplant', *International Journal of Nursing Practice*, vol. 6, 153–9.

How do I go about the process of interpretation when I have used a qualitative critical methodology?

Given that critical methodologies have an emancipatory intent for groups of oppressed people, the interpretive processes may often be shared by the people involved.

- Go through the exercise as a group, asking each other the questions listed in this chapter as preconditions for qualitative interpretation.
- Acknowledge the potential of group members to make a collective interpretation of the information, based on their active involvement in the collaborative project.
- Give the group the option of taking some time away from the intensity of the project. The time can be negotiated. This will depend on the time you have available to complete the project and on other factors the members may raise as being important.
- If the members decide to take time away from the project, suggest that during the time away they notice any ideas that come to mind. Ask them to write them down, even if they seem insignificant, so that they can be shared with others in the whole group.

- Resume or continue group meetings and decide on a way of reviewing the analysed data. Review how you came to make the decisions you made at the time of analysis.
- Remember that multiple interpretations of competing discourses are possible. There may be no easy answers to complex socio-political questions that have been raised by the research; rather the group may be able to identify some tentative connections and interpretations related to interpersonal and institutional power relationships.
- Remember that the interpretations subsume all the phases in the research that have gone before.
- Remember that the products of the analysis are incomplete in themselves. They only have fullest meaning when they have been described and explained through critical appraisal and interpretation.
- If the group has already named any of the issues/themes/ideas/action cycles that were generated in the analysis phase, why did they choose them? Are they still relevant? Would other issues/themes/ideas/action cycles represent them more effectively now, in the light of further critique and new information?
- In an open group discussion clarify what the issues/themes/ideas/action cycles mean. Ask group members to write down words and sentences and explain them to other people. Invite them to share them with the other group members.
- It may be useful to have an audiotape recorder during the sharing of interpretations. Expose the interpretations to critique. Try to reach consensus on a shared and agreed set of statements about the interpretations. Note any possible alternate interpretations in light of the unique social, historical, economic, political, cultural and personal determinants of the research setting, intentions, processes and methods. Commit the final version to writing.
- You could also suggest that group members work in pairs to discuss individual interpretations. Suggest that they speak spontaneously about what the analysed data might mean in light of the overall project. Encourage members to make the clearest possible explication of what they want to say. Suggest that they raise questions about interpretations and seek other possible explanations and conclusions. These are then shared with the whole group.
- As a group, create statements and explanations that represent most faithfully the multiple discourses that can be extracted from the analysed data.
- Ensure that you have created and explained links between the multiple discourses, that are congruent with the assumptions, aims, objectives, methods and processes of the research.
- Links between the multiple discourses need to be clear as possible and the linking should be argued carefully for the benefit of the participants and the readers of the research.
- Ensure that the final version of the overall interpretations represents all the group intend them to mean after full discussion and critical appraisal of the social, historical, economic, political, cultural and personal determinants operating in the research.

For excellent examples of interpretation of nursing research using critical methodologies, refer to the following projects:

- Glass, N. 1997, 'Breaking a social silence: registered nurses share their stories about tertiary nursing education', *International Journal of Nursing Practice*, vol. 3, 173–7.
- Jackson, D. & Raftos, M. 1997, 'In uncharted waters: confronting the culture of silence in a residential care institution', *International Journal of Nursing Practice*, vol. 3, 34–9.
- Lumby, J. 1997, 'Liver transplantation: the death/life paradox', *International Journal of Nursing Practice*, vol. 3, 231–8.
- Chenoweth, L. & Kilstoff, K. 1998, 'Facilitating positive changes in community dementia management through participatory action research', *International Journal of Nursing Practice*, vol. 4, 175–88.
- Glass, N. 1998, 'The contested work place: reactions to hospital based RNs doing degrees', *Collegian*, vol. 5, no. 1, 24–31.
- Walter, R., Davis, K. & Glass, N. 1999, 'Discovery of self: exploring, interconnecting and integrating self (concept) and nursing', *Collegian*, vol. 6, no. 2, 12–15.
- Wellard, S. & Street, A. F. 1999, 'Family issues in home-based care', *International Journal of Nursing Practice*, vol. 5: 132–6.
- Keatinge, D., Scarfe, C., Bellchambers, H., McGee, J., Oakham, R., Probert, C., Stewart, L. & Stokes, J. 2000, 'The manifestation and nursing management of agitation in institutionalised residents with dementia', *International Journal of Nursing Practice*, vol. 6, 16–25.
- Koch, T., Kralik, D. & Kelly, S. 2000, 'We just don't talk about it: men living with urinary incontinence and multiple sclerosis', *International Journal of Nursing Practice*, vol. 6, 253–60.

What will the interpretations look like?

- Interpretations will not look alike. They will differ according to the ways in which they were extracted from the data.
- Interpretations will bear a resemblance to the language of the methodologies that guided them.
- Interpretations may be represented as diversely as words, phrases, sentences, models, theories, action strategies, group summaries and so on.
- Interpretations may be put forward to readers of the research as theoretical propositions, findings, results, insights, strategies, implications, and examples of reflective awareness, changed practice, multiple discourses and so on.

How will I know that the interpretations are relevant?

- Interpretations will have a high chance of being relevant if they can demonstrate methodological congruency. This means that they show that they are related directly to the analysed data, which in turn is related to the assumptions, methods and processes of the research.

- Interpretations have meaning only in terms of the research, because they are specific to the research. Interpretations are context-dependent; that is, they are relative to the total set of circumstances that make up the research.
- Ways of checking relevance differ according to the methodological approach.
- The tests of relevance that are applied are particular to the approach taken.
- For further information on relevance refer to the section on rigour in Chapter 14.

Interpreting the text in light of the literature

The need to do a research project may be based on a review of the literature review that confirms knowledge gaps or conflicting results. In contrast, if a researcher is interested in taking an inductive approach, such as that taken in grounded theory, the literature review may be delayed until during or after the data collection. Even so, at some point, qualitative researchers will go to the literature to see what it contains on an area of interest.

Interpretations may compare to or contrast with the results of other studies. Research reports may include a section in which the connections are spelt out clearly. If connections are found between the newly interpreted data and those already in the literature, qualitative researchers would not necessarily use this discovery to make a claim for the truthfulness of the interpretations. Rather, the similarities would be documented in the research report as a point of interest.

The other reason for consulting the literature is to provide a firm grounding for the interpretations in the methodological tradition of choice. For example, a phenomenological project may use certain concepts to show readers that the assumptions underlying the choice of methods and processes relate to the project; a feminist project will be guided by the literature relating to feminisms and feminist research processes; and a critical ethnography may cite references derived from critical social science to augment its questioning approach to the research interest. In each of these cases, the aim is to present key ideas of the methodology to show the kind of knowledge it is capable of generating in research projects. Research reflecting postmodern influences may stand outside methodological categorisation on the basis that they represent grand narratives. Even so, nurse-researchers reflecting postmodern influences may appeal to literature that affirms key ideas, such as multiple voices, difference, fragmentation and deconstruction. For methods of narrative and discourse analyses, see the relevant sections in Chapter 16.

Summary

This chapter alerted you to the need to differentiate between analysis and interpretation in qualitative research. The relative nature of qualitative research interpretations was acknowledged, given that there is agreement in the methodologies that due to the complex nature of human relationships, there is no absolute and unchanging truth.

Interpretations differ according to specific methodological approaches. For example, qualitative interpretive methodologies tend to highlight context-dependent meanings and qualitative critical methodologies will tend to expose multiple interpretations associated with power relationships in socio-political settings. Postmodernism questions the whole idea of interpretation and definitions of interpretation are influenced by deconstruction, which involves looking at contradictions and inconsistencies at the 'margins' of a text.

As a practical guide for new researchers, processes were outlined for making qualitative interpretive and critical interpretations and some postmodern influences on interpretation were identified.

Main points

- Interpretation involves working with the forms of analysed information so that statements can be made about what they mean in light of the intentions, methods and processes of the research.
- Generally speaking, analysis precedes interpretation, although some qualitative researchers describe an intuitive grasp of the data, while others may experience spiralling and integrative processes in which analysis and interpretation blend and seem to become indivisible.
- Invariably, qualitative interpretations of words and language require protracted time with the text to ensure that meaning is located and that it is as clear as possible to convey to other people and it may also be validated by other researchers, co-researchers, participants and peers.
- Qualitative researchers agree that there is no way of guaranteeing absolute truth, because truth is relative and elusive; therefore, truth can change according to all kinds of context-dependent determinants associated with people, places, times and conditions in which it resides and from which it emerges.
- Various words are used synonymously to mean interpretations, such as theories, findings, results, insights, strategies, implications, examples of reflective awareness and changed practice, and so on, according to the assumptions and intentions of the research methodology.
- Most qualitative research approaches do not claim to generate interpretations that can be considered to be generalisable to the wider population, with the exception of grounded theory, which sets out to make general statements in the form of theories about what might be expected in similar circumstances.
- Research using postmodern thought may not deem to offer anything concrete, but to leave all ideas open as tentative, or make multiple interpretations and give authority to readers to make their own interpretations.
- Processes for interpretation may differ according to what kind of qualitative research it can be considered to be, that is, whether it is essentially an interpretive (concerned mainly with meaning) or critical (concerned mainly with change) project, although some researchers use a combination of interpretive and critical processes, appropriate to the assumptions, aims, objectives, methods and processes of the project.

- In qualitative research, congruency means the fit, or correspondence, between foundational ideas and the activity phases of the research.
- The reasons for asking certain questions at the transition from analysis to interpretation are to re-orient to the overall project, to check on the degree of congruency between the assumptions, aims, objectives, methods and processes, and to prepare for the process of interpretation.
- For the postmodernists the whole idea of interpretation is open for debate, because postmodern definitions of interpretation are influenced by deconstruction, which involves looking at the 'margins' of a text, to its contradictions, inconsistencies, and what is excluded, unnamed and concealed, not to unmask errors (as this would imply a search for truth), but to transform and redefine it.
- On an optimistic note, an affirmative postmodern 'interpretation' leaves the reader in authority as the interpreter of any life text, and in nursing, that means making choices about what constitutes nursing, while heeding caution about accepting unquestioningly all kinds of dominant discourses in grand narratives.
- The process of interpretation in qualitative interpretive methodologies involves protracted reading and reflecting on the data to create definitions and explanations that represent most faithfully the clearest meaning that can be extracted from the analysed data in light of the descriptive intentions of the project.
- The process of interpretation in qualitative critical methodologies often includes collaborative group processes to sift through multiple interpretations of competing discourses to find tentative answers to complex socio-political questions involving social, historical, economic, political, cultural and personal determinants, in light of the descriptive intentions of the project.
- Interpretations will not look alike, as they will bear a resemblance to the language of the methodologies that guided them and they may be represented as diversely as words, phrases, sentences, models, theories, action strategies, group summaries, theoretical propositions, findings, results, insights, strategies, implications, and examples of reflective awareness, changed practice, multiple discourses and so on.
- Interpretations have a high chance of being relevant if they can demonstrate methodological congruency; that is, they show that they are related directly to the analysed data, which are in turn related to the methodological assumptions, methods and processes of the research.
- Research projects reflecting postmodern influences may stand outside methodological categorisation on the basis that they represent grand narratives; however, nurse-researchers reflecting postmodern influences may appeal to literature that affirms key ideas, such as multiple voices, difference, fragmentation and deconstruction.

Review Questions

1. Analysis precedes interpretation:
   a generally
   b never
   c always
   d seldom

2. Invariably, the time needed for qualitative interpretations of words and language is:
   a lengthy
   b short
   c truncated
   d brief

3. Qualitative researchers agree that there is no way of guaranteeing truth, because truth:
   a is relative and elusive
   b can change according to context
   c is absolute and measurable
   d is both a and b

4. Words used synonymously to mean interpretations are:
   a theories, findings and results
   b insights, strategies and implications
   c examples of reflective awareness and changed practice
   d all of the above

5. A qualitative research approach which sets out to make general interpretive statements in the form of theories about what might be expected in similar circumstances is:
   a phenomenology
   b grounded theory
   c action research
   d ethnography

6. Research using postmodern thought:
   a offers concrete interpretations
   b leaves all ideas open as tentative
   c forms singular interpretations
   d gives interpretive authority to researchers

7 The fit, or correspondence, between foundational ideas and the activity phases of the research is methodological:
   a correlation
   b comparison
   c congruency
   d contradiction

8 The reasons for asking certain questions at the transition from analysis to interpretation are to:
   a re-orient to the overall project
   b check on the degree of congruency
   c prepare for the process of interpretation
   d do all of the above

9 The process involving looking at the 'margins' of a text, to its contradictions, inconsistencies, and what is excluded, unnamed and concealed is:
   a deconstruction
   b construction
   c reconstruction
   d preconstruction

10 Interpretations have a high chance of being relevant if they can demonstrate methodological:
   a congruency
   b trustworthiness
   c reliability
   d coherence

Discussion Questions

1 Differentiate between qualitative analysis and interpretation.
2 Discuss why findings differ in their language according to specific methodological approaches.
3 Describe the processes for synthesising qualitative interpretive results.
4 Describe the processes for synthesising qualitative critical results.
5 Describe postmodern influences on interpretation as another perspective for nursing research.

References

Allen, D. G. 1995, 'Hermeneutics: philosophical traditions and nursing practice research', *Nursing Science Quarterly*, vol. 8, no. 4, 174–82.

Ammon-Gaberson, K. B. & Piantanida, M. 1988, 'Generating results from qualitative data', *Image: Journal of Nursing Scholarship*, vol. 20, no. 3, 159–61.

Bernstein, R. 1978, *The Restructuring of Social and Political Theory*, University of Pennsylvania Press, Philadelphia.

Bunkers, S. S., Petardi, L. A., Pilkington, F. B. & Walls, P. A. 1996, 'Challenging the myths surrounding qualitative research in nursing', *Nursing Science Quarterly*, vol. 9, no. 1, 33–7.

Cheek, J. 2000, *Postmodern and Poststructural Approaches to Nursing Research*, Sage Publications, Thousand Oaks, California.

Colaizzi, P. 1978, 'Psychological research as the phenomenologist views it', in *Existential Phenomenological Alternatives for Psychology*, eds R. S. Valle & M. King, Oxford University Press, New York.

Collins English Dictionary 1998, 4th Australian edn, HarperCollins Publishers, Glasgow.

Gadamer, H.-G. 1975 trans., in *Truth and Method*, eds G. Barden & J. Cumming, Seabury, New York.

Gething, L. 1992, 'Nurse practitioners' and students' attitudes towards people with disabilities', *Australian Journal of Advanced Nursing*, vol. 9, no. 3, 25–30.

Glass, N. 1994, Breaking a social silence, women's emerging and disruptive voices: a feminist critique of post-registration nursing education in rural Australia, unpublished PhD thesis, University of New South Wales.

Glass, N. & Davis, K. 1998, 'An emancipatory impulse: a feminist postmodern integrated turning point in nursing research', *Advances in Nursing Science*, vol. 21, no. 1, 43–52.

Habermas, J. 1981, *The Theory of Communicative Action: Reason and the Rationalization of Society*, Beacon, Boston.

Kermode, S. & Brown, C. 1995, 'Where have all the flowers gone: nursing's escape from the radical critique', *Contemporary Nurse*, vol. 4, no. 1, 8–15.

Knaff, K. A. & Howard, M. J. 1984, 'Interpreting and reporting qualitative research', *Research in Nursing and Health*, vol. 17, 17–24.

Koch, T., Kralik, D. & Kelly, S. 2000, 'We just don't talk about it: men living with urinary incontinence and multiple sclerosis', *International Journal of Nursing Practice*, vol. 6, 253–60.

LoBiondo-Wood, G. & Haber, J. 1994, *Nursing Research: Methods, Critical Appraisal, and Utilisation*, Mosby, St Louis.

Richardson, L. 1992, 'The collective story: postmodernism and the writing of sociology', in *Post-Modernism and the Social Sciences: Insights, Inroads and Intrusions*, ed. P. Rosenau, Princeton University Press, New Jersey.

Rosenau, P. 1992, *Post-Modernism and the Social Sciences: Insights, Inroads and Intrusions*, Princeton University Press, New Jersey.

Semmens, J. & Peric, J. 1995–6, 'Children's experiences of a parent's chronic illness and death', *Australian Journal of Advanced Nursing*, vol. 13, no. 2, 30–8.

Strauss, A. L. 1975, *Chronic Illness and Quality of Life*, C.V. Mosby Co., St Louis.

Street, A. 1998, 'From soulmates to stakeholders: issues in creating quality postmodern participatory research relationships', *Social Sciences in Health*, vol. 4, 119–29.

Walters, J. 1996, 'Being a nurse consultant: a hermeneutic phenomenological reflection', *International Journal of Nursing Practice*, vol. 2, no. 1, 2–10.

Wellard, S. & Street, A. 1999, 'Family issues in home-based care', *International Journal of Nursing Practice*, vol. 5, 132–6.

Wilson, H. S. 1993, *Introducing Research in Nursing*, Addison-Wesley Nursing, Menlo Park, California.

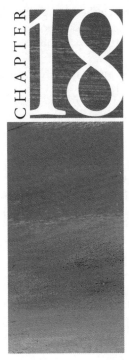

CHAPTER 18

Disseminating the findings

chapter objectives The material presented in this chapter will assist you to:

- understand the reasons for preparing a research report
- identify the intended recipients of the research report
- write a research report
- identify the elements of a quantitative and a qualitative report
- submit a research report
- give a conference or seminar presentation
- prepare and present a poster
- prepare a journal article
- prepare a monograph.

Introduction

The research report is a formal account of the research project. It is the major means by which you disseminate essential information about your research project. It can be either in written form, in which case it becomes a permanent record, or it can be an oral report to a group of colleagues at a seminar or conference.

Students who are taking units at either the undergraduate level or graduate diploma level, in which they are required to write a research report as a part of learning about the research process, will find the material in this chapter useful. In Australia, most undergraduate nursing courses have a unit on nursing research. Some of these focus mainly on proposal writing and the consumption of research, while others take students through the whole research process, including writing a report. In addition, many postgraduate diploma courses have a research component. Honours students and higher degree students will find the material in this chapter useful as a starting point for writing their theses. Students who are studying units for which there is no written research report will still find this chapter useful for learning to assess other research reports.

The emphasis in this chapter is on student research reports because they are a common student exercise, and part of the process of learning about research. Students may also present seminars, reports at conferences, and posters. Few students will publish a research report in journals; student assignments in their original form are seldom suitable for publication because their content, length and organisation are normally unlike the type of copy that journal editors want (Robertson 1994). If reworked, student research reports may be able to become journal articles. Therefore, some mention is made of journal writing in this chapter. There are publications that specialise in teaching about writing for journals, for example Wiltshire (1995), Greenwood (1998) and Plawecki and Plawecki (1998). Anyone doing a thesis should find the rudiments of report writing in this book helpful, but should obtain specialist books in thesis writing such as Anderson and Poole (1998) and Walters (1999).

If carrying out nursing research comprises a part of your employment, you have a responsibility to share the findings of your research with colleagues. There are a number of reasons for this. First, a report is essential because research that is not reported is meaningless and does not contribute to building a body of knowledge that is useful to nursing. Secondly, the findings may be useful to colleagues to help them make their practice more effective. Thirdly, the findings may be useful in helping others to plan their research more effectively. Finally, a research report allows your peers to evaluate the quality of your research. In return for fulfilling your responsibility, you will have the reward of helping other people, recognition by your colleagues and assistance with your career development.

The research report

The most important purpose of a research report is to communicate key aspects of the project to the research consumer. Readers will probably be reading your report so that they can replicate your study, to do their own literature review, to plan a new study or to help find a solution for a clinical practice problem. In all of these situations, readers will be evaluating your study for validity and usefulness. To do this they need to be able to determine how your study was conducted.

Research reports are presented in different media, have different lengths and serve different purposes. First, there are written reports such as classroom project reports, journal articles and theses or dissertations. These are intended to be read. Secondly, research findings may be presented as oral reports such as seminar reports and conference papers. These convey information spoken to an audience, and are therefore an auditory or audiovisual experience.

A classroom research report is usually submitted as an assignment of about 2000–3000 words. It follows a standard format for a research report, as detailed below.

A journal article will normally be between 3000 and 5000 words long. The main purpose of a journal article is to disseminate the results of the research to a large target audience. Journal articles often take a year between submission and publication. There is very little opportunity for direct comments to the researcher after publication; however there is feedback built into the review process that precedes publication. Journal articles have the potential to reach the whole profession or specialty group. If you are involved in writing up a paper either for a classroom assignment or a journal article, there are numerous writings on the topic to help you. Examples are an article by Greenwood (1998) and books by Day (1998) and Dees (1999).

A dissertation is a long, detailed discourse, and need not be a research report. A thesis is a research dissertation submitted for an honours degree or a higher degree such as a master's degree or a doctorate. The words 'thesis' and 'dissertation' tend to be used interchangeably, with the word 'thesis' preferred in Australia. The purpose of a thesis is to test the student's ability to demonstrate proficiency in the research process. A thesis for a master's degree will usually be at least 25 000 words long. A doctoral thesis will be much longer, up to 100 000 words. A thesis may only ever be read by a limited number of people who have an interest in the topic. If you are writing a thesis, you should obtain at least one specialist book in thesis writing. Examples are: *How to Write a Better Thesis or Report* (Evans 1995), *Assignment and Thesis Writing* (Anderson & Poole 1998) and *How to Write Health Sciences Papers, Dissertations and Theses* (Thomas 2000).

The purpose of conference and seminar papers is to communicate work in progress or completed results to a specific target group of interested persons. Papers allow personal communication with colleagues about your work, and allow for critical feedback. Conference papers are normally distributed to the conference delegates, and others who may be interested in purchasing them. Seminar papers may be distributed to those attending the seminar.

A poster is a presentation on poster board, usually at a conference, with the researcher in attendance to answer questions. You can prepare the poster yourself from stencilled letters or other printing. If you can afford it you can have almost any stage of the poster prepared professionally. The text can be prepared from a computer program such as PowerPoint. The poster can be screen-printed in very large font on the board by a printery. The final product can be professionally laminated. You can compose the poster from a series of A4 pages linked by arrows, which are far more portable than a full-sized poster.

A poster presentation is strongly visual; however, the visual information is supplemented by discussion between the presenter and the viewer. With the proliferation of nursing research there has been an increasing tendency to use the poster as a medium for presenting research since many can be presented in one session. Posters also allow nurse-researchers to present work in progress or completed work. They are a good way to begin presenting research because they are a lot less intimidating than presenting a paper before a class or a conference. Posters are very small in comparison to any other medium. Posters are usually kept by the presenter. You can learn more about poster preparation in articles by Maltby and Serrell (1998), McCann and colleagues (1999), Cantrell and Bracher (1999) and Jackson and Sheldon (2000). There is even a whole book on poster presentation (Gosling 1999).

In the future, it is to be expected that the limited dissemination of conference papers and minor reports will change because of the ability to post many communications on the World Wide Web. Even theses are becoming available electronically. However, the large volume of a thesis will ultimately restrict the audience for it.

The written report

The target audience

Before beginning to write the report, consider the target audience. Whether you are writing for a lecturer, a thesis examiner or a journal editor, there will be expectations on their part as to the structure and content of the report. A lecturer will probably be most interested in whether or not the student has shown a comprehension of the research process. A thesis examiner will be interested in whether the student has demonstrated proficiency in the subject and in planning and executing research and interpreting the findings in their scientific context. A journal editor will be looking for evidence that the content of the report is suited to the journal's readership. For example, a clinical nursing research journal will want clinical implications.

If a journal readership is your target, it is first necessary to select a journal that is aimed at that group. You can find out about the journals in a database such as CINAHL. In deciding which journal to target, consider its style, its readership and the type of article it publishes. For example, if your report is very specialised in content, you should aim at a journal that specialises in that content so that the information you have to present reaches an appropriate audience. You may also want to consider the demographics of the readership – if your article is heavily Australian context-dependent, you will do better to target an Australian journal. Depending on the quality of the report, you may choose to target a refereed (peer-reviewed) or a non-refereed journal.

Guidelines

Whatever the target readership of your research report, you must obtain and follow any guidelines for the preparation of research reports. If you are writing for a classroom project, you should follow any guidelines that you have been given, as marks may be allocated for presentation and referencing. Many universities have guidelines for thesis presentation, which you should obtain if you are doing a thesis or research project as part of a graduate diploma, honours degree or higher degree. Most university calendars state the rules for presentation of theses for a research degree. They address type of paper, margins, line spacing, binding, number of copies and so forth. These should be followed exactly. If you are writing for a journal, make sure you acquire a copy of their guidelines for authors and follow them exactly. These will concern referencing and presentation of the article. It is also worth photocopying several articles and analysing the approach that successful authors have used.

Planning and writing your report

When you have assembled the guidelines, you should plan your writing approach. It is wise to make an outline, as detailed as possible. The outline can include the major topics and subtopics. Then write the sections of the report according to the format below, or whatever variation is specified by the guidelines. You will probably need to revise the report several times, polishing it as you go. If possible, have someone critique the report.

The style of writing for a research report is generally the same as for a research proposal. This can be read in more detail in Chapter 6; however the major points will be reviewed here. The style should be concise, clear and coherent. One of the greatest scientific discoveries of all time, that of the molecular structure of deoxyribonucleic acid (DNA) was reported in an elegantly written one-page letter to the journal *Nature* (Watson & Crick 1953). Your style should suit your target audience. A report of quantitative research is usually written in the formal scientific style to convey objectivity. A report of qualitative research may be written in the personal style. Use good English that is appropriate for your audience, and avoid jargon and sexist language. Avoid the passive voice wherever possible. The tense is less of a problem in a research report than in the proposal because the report will mainly be in the past tense. The exception is statements of everyday knowledge, which are written in the present tense.

Structure of the report

In this chapter, we are giving you material on how to write both quantitative and qualitative research reports, with examples of both.

Common initial elements of quantitative and qualitative reports

The research report has three major components: the preliminaries, the body and the supporting materials, presented in that order. The preliminaries introduce the report; the body contains the main information and the supporting materials contain the references and appendices.

A sample format for a research report is as follows:

Sample format of a research report

Preliminaries
    Title page
    Required forms*
    Acknowledgements*
    Abstract
    Table of contents*
    List of tables*
    List of figures*
    Executive summary†
Body of report
    Introduction
    Literature review
    Methodology
    Results
    Discussion
Supporting materials
    References
    Appendixes

Key: * denotes applicable only to thesis or long report
      † denotes applicable only to long report

Figure 18.1 Sample format of a research report

For a student research assignment, it is not necessary to use the components marked in Figure 18.1 with the symbol *. It is also not necessary to divide the content into chapters; the body of the report can be all one section. Begin each section on a new page. For a thesis or longer report, it is customary to use separate chapters for the introduction, methodology, results and discussion. If the literature review is long, it may merit a chapter on its own.

Headings and subheadings should be used within the document as shown in Chapter 6. Headings for tables and figures should also follow a system. Usually tables and figures are numbered from 1. If using the chapter system and there are many tables and figures in various chapters, the number of the chapter can be used as a prefix. For example, tables in Chapter 1 would be labelled Table 1.1 etc., while those in Chapter 3 would be labelled 3.1 etc. The headings are usually indented in the table of contents and they may be indented in the text.

Components of the report

Preliminaries

The first part of the report is the 'preliminaries' or pages that precede the body of the report. A short report will need only a title page and an abstract. Great care and attention should be given to the title and abstract. In this day of electronic databases, the title will appear in lists of documents in many searches and the abstract will be accessed by many of those generating the search. It becomes the showcase for your work since it will be what determines whether researchers access the full paper. A longer report will require additional preliminaries such as a table of contents including a list of tables and a list of figures, both with page numbers to help the reader locate the tables and figures easily. A thesis will require additional papers to be inserted, such as a statement that the thesis is entirely the work of the candidate and a list of acknowledgements.

The title page
The title page should be similar to a title page of a research proposal, which was discussed in Chapter 6. The title page gives the title of the proposal as well as the author's name, position and qualifications. The author's postal and email addresses should be given, as well as telephone and fax contact numbers. The date should be placed somewhere on the page; this can be done easily as a footer if you are using a word processor.

We are now going to give you extracts from a quantitative report on the kangaroo mother care study (Roberts, McEwan & Paynter 2000) for which you read the proposal in Chapter 6. This report is published with permission from *Neonatal Network*.

Elements of a quantitative report
Preliminaries
The title
The title of the report should be a mini report, or thumbnail sketch, of the work, conveying the essence of the report while stimulating interest in the study. The title can be either a statement or a question and should reflect the major theme of the report and the type of investigation, which can be achieved by using key words. Students often err on the side of excessive length when developing titles for theses, as they try to convey everything about the project, but a good title will be a concise statement or question of no more than 15–20 words. Sometimes the agency for which you are writing will have restrictions on the length of the title. For a journal article, it is important to use key words that can be indexed so that the article can be retrieved by researchers. It is best to avoid expressions such as 'An investigation of …' or words similar to those. That is self-evident and simply takes up space. 'The influence of …' or 'The effect of …' in a short report are both unexciting and are therefore unlikely to catch the interest of the reader. Strangely enough, it is often best to compose the title last, because it must reflect the most up-to-date material in the report. An example of a title that piques the interest of the reader is 'Gender bias in cardiology: are women missing out on PCTA?' (Hildon 1994).

An example of a title is as follows: *A comparison of kangaroo mother care and conventional cuddling care.*

The abstract
The abstract is a succinct and accurate description of the project you have conducted, an introduction to your research report which gives the reader a

summary of the project, highlighting its major themes. A well-written abstract will give a potential reader a good thumbnail sketch of the project. The abstract is one of the most important parts of the report because, essentially, it is a marketing device. It is the 'hook' that entices readers to select your research (Evans 1994). The abstract helps the person doing a literature search to make a decision about acquiring your article.

Abstracts are sometimes submitted for consideration of the presentation of a paper at a research meeting or conference. Abstracts may be published in conference programs to help delegates decide what part of the conference to attend. In fact the abstracts may be the only part of the conference proceedings that is published.

As with the title, the abstract can also be written near the end, or last. It should summarise the objectives, methodology, major findings, and implications of the project. It should be concise, with a word limit of 250–300 words; in other words, no more than one page. Its major purpose is to help readers decide whether or not to read the entire report. The abstract is usually located between the title and the actual report. In writing an abstract, consider what you as the reader would want to know about this project. The abstract should not require the reader to refer to other supporting materials to understand it.

The content of the abstract starts with a brief introductory sentence that tells the reader what the study was about – this is the problem statement. If you used a theoretical framework, identify it. Then put in a sentence or two to explain the design and methodology of the study, including the sample and data collection methods. The next sentence or two should be the longest part of the abstract, giving the major findings and any conclusions. Finally, you conclude with any recommendations.

An example of an abstract is:

> In this study, kangaroo mother care (KMC) and conventional cuddling care (CCC) were compared in two neonatal nurseries in Darwin, NT, Australia. Thirty mother–infant dyads were randomly assigned to the Kangaroo Mother Care Group or the Conventional Cuddling Care Group. Both groups of mothers cuddled their babies for a minimum of two hours per day, five days a week while in the study, with the KMC group having skin-to-skin contact while the CCC group had contact through normal clothing. The results showed no difference between groups on the Parental Stress Scale (NICU) or the Parental Expectations Survey. Infants in both groups experienced equivalent maintenance or rise of temperature while out of the incubators, equal weight gain, equal length of stay in hospital and equal duration of breastfeeding. It was concluded that KMC was equivalent but not superior to CCC although further research is recommended.

You can see that the abstract is very similar to the abstract for the proposal in Chapter 6, but with the addition of the results.

Body of report

The body of your report should be a straightforward description of the problem, the methodology and the findings plus the interpretation of those findings. There should also be an assessment of the significance and the adequacy of the study design, and recommendations for further research. There are four major sections in the body of the research report: the introduction, or 'why I did it'; the methodology, or 'what I did'; the results – 'what I found'; and the discussion – 'what it means' (Tornquist 1986). The introduction and methodology sections in the body of the research report are similar to the sections of the research proposal with the same titles. There may be minor variations in format required for different purposes, but these sections are fairly standard.

The introduction

The purpose of the introduction section is to acquaint the reader with the problem, background and purposes of the study. The introduction goes from the general to the specific, and sets the scene for your research question or problem. In fact it includes your problem statement/research question and it should answer the questions 'What problem was investigated?' and 'Why was it done?' The introduction to your research report is similar to the introduction section of your research proposal, except that the significance of the study is discussed in the discussion section. The introduction emphasises the study's importance and sets it in a context of previous work in the area. If it is a quantitative project, the introduction section contains a review of theoretical and empirical literature and the hypotheses. In a thesis, the review of the literature may occupy a separate chapter.

An example of an introduction is:

> This study compared the use of kangaroo mother care (KMC) with standard or conventional cuddling care (CCC) in premature and small-for-gestational-age (SGA) infants in Darwin, Australia. Kangaroo mother care is the positioning of a near-naked infant at or between the mother's breasts so that there is skin-to-skin contact. KMC was initiated at Bogota, Colombia, in South America, in order to overcome the lack of staff and equipment to care for premature infants and small infants.[1-3] KMC has been reported in the literature since the mid-1980s as having been in use in Scandinavia, and California.[2,4] It has also been implemented safely with intubated infants of over 700 gm who are physiologically stable.[5] The reported advantages of KMC for the infant are maintenance of skin temperature, reduced incidence of apnea and bradycardia, stable transcutaneous oxygen level, longer quiet sleep periods and shorter hospital stay.[4] Increased quiet sleep frequency and reduced activity level have also been reported.[6] Some of these benefits could lead to a shorter hospital stay and therefore have potential for considerable savings on the total cost of special care nursery (SCN) care.

Note how the introduction sets the scene for the report and justifies the study. It recaps a bit of the history of KMC.

The literature review

A good quantitative research report will contain in its introduction an adequate review of the literature. As in the research proposal, the review of the literature comprises the review of both theoretical and empirical literature and it is normally constructed in much the same way as the review for the proposal.

However, you will probably prune the literature review now to be congruent with what findings you wish to report. For example, if one part of your findings turned out to be unusable for some reason, and you decide to eliminate it from the report, you would delete the literature now redundant. When writing for a journal, you need to prune the literature review to include only the few most relevant studies, because of space restrictions. It should emphasise the findings and include a critique only where it was relevant to your methodology Even more drastic reductions may be necessary for a conference paper or a poster. For these purposes, the aim is not to demonstrate your ability to review the literature, but to provide a brief summary of the relevant findings so that the reader can place your work in the context of previous work and so that you can interpret how your findings fit into the overall work on the subject.

An example of a literature review is:

The literature contains reports of several studies of KMC, some of which dealt with maternal outcomes, and some with infant outcomes. In terms of infant outcomes, various researchers have found that KMC is equal or superior to conventional incubator care. Ludington-Hoe and colleagues and Smith found that infants' average temperature rose significantly after KMC and that average oxygen saturation was not decreased significantly.[7,8] In terms of infant activity and sleep state, Ludington-Hoe and colleagues found that the amount of time in quiet regular sleep increased and activity states significantly decreased after KMC.[7] However, Whitelaw and colleagues found that by six months of age there was no difference between KMC and control groups in the duration of sleeping, feeding, being held and playing but that the KMC group spent significantly less time crying.[9] Several researchers have found that KMC decreased the length of stay in the incubator and the hospital.[9-11] Wahlberg and colleagues found both a decrease in stay and an increase in weight gain in KMC infants.[10]

KMC has also been found to have better outcomes for breastfeeding. Wahlberg and colleagues and Affonso and colleagues found considerably higher participation rates of breastfeeding in KMC than among CCC mothers, while Whitelaw and colleagues found that the mean duration of lactation was considerably longer in the KMC group than the normal-contact group.[9-11]

Finally, KMC has been found to result in improved maternal confidence. Affonso and colleagues and Smith found that mothers who had given KMC bonded better to the infant and had increased maternal confidence.[8,11] Curry, however, found that the control group and KMC did not have significant differences in attachment behaviours or self-concept scores.[12]

In summary, the previous research demonstrated that KMC may result in positive maternal and infant outcomes. However, these findings have been produced by research that was exploratory and sometimes characterised by lack of a control group.

The researchers' hypotheses in the study were the following:

1 KMC infants would have gained more weight on average by the date of discharge from hospital, then at six weeks and at three months compared with CCC infants
2 KMC infants would have equal or better temperature maintenance during KMC than CCC infants would have during CCC
3 KMC infants would have a shorter hospital stay than CCC infants.

It was also hypothesised that KMC mothers would:

4 breastfeed for longer than CCC mothers
5 report less stress than CCC mothers
6 feel more confident of their parenting skills than CCC mothers.

Note that the literature review has been integrated around the dependent variables and succinctly summarises the literature on the subject. You can see that the hypotheses arise from the literature.

The methodology

The methodology section describes in detail the methodology that was used in the study. Again, the methodology section of the report will be very similar to that of the proposal, assuming that there have not been many changes, but, of course, it will be written in the past tense.

The principle of this section is that it should describe your methods and processes in enough detail to allow another researcher to replicate your study – to conduct another study using the same methodology – so the methodology must include the design, setting, participants, sampling, instruments, and procedures for the study and it should answer the questions: 'On whom was the research carried out?', 'How?', 'When?' and 'Where?' It is important to report the methodology accurately and completely because it helps the reader to evaluate its validity and the researcher's interpretation of the findings. It also facilitates comparison with other studies on the subject (Gething 1995).

When writing the methodology section, you should make a brief statement about the design of the study, explaining why that design was appropriate to the research question. Quantitative designs were discussed in Chapter 7, and qualitative designs in Chapters 12 and 13.

The hypothesis should be stated as a description of what the anticipated outcomes were. It should show the relationships between the variables, stated in measurable terms. The independent and dependent variables should be identified and stated in measurable terms.

Next, the setting for the research should be given, showing where it took place. In a report it is not appropriate to give the names of agencies in which you carried out the research, unless they have given their permission to be identified.

The participants should be described next. State the characteristics of the group from which the participants were selected and where they were found, and give your rationale for selecting this particular group of participants. You should give the ideal size of sample, how you arrived at this figure, and the size you ended up with.

State the type of sample that you used, as discussed in Chapter 8. If it is a convenience sample, there will not be much to say except the basis of the convenience; for example, they were the patients on a ward. If it is a random or a stratified random sample, say how the sample was drawn from the population. Indicate any steps that you took to prevent bias in the sample. Describe the criteria for participant selection and give the rationale for the criteria. You should give the details of how the participants were recruited – by letter, by telephone or through personal contact.

Once you have described your sampling procedures, you should state the number of groups and the number of participants in each group, and how they were allocated to the groups. Any special procedures, such as matching participants on criteria, should be addressed.

In the instruments and materials section, you should describe the instruments or materials that you used, including any questionnaire or tool. It is not necessary to explain any standard tests, but you should explain any unconventional techniques, tests, or instruments. If an instrument is new, you should include details of how it was developed and tested before use. If it has been used before, you should give the details of its origin, how much it has been used before, and its reliability and validity. You should describe any questionnaire that you used or state its name if it is well known. If your report is a thesis or a student research project, include a copy of the questionnaire in an appendix, but this is not necessary for a journal article.

If you used a physical instrument, it should be named if it is well-known, or described if it is unusual or new. You should say how the instrument is scored or measured, for example, on a Likert scale. You can use diagrams or photographs of an instrument to avoid long descriptions and to stimulate interest. You should say why the instrument was suitable for the acquisition of reliable, valid data. These concepts were discussed in Chapter 8.

In the procedures section, you describe the procedures that were used in the study. If it was an experiment, you describe how an experimental treatment was applied. You state how, when, and where you collected the data, in enough detail to allow someone to replicate your procedures, including such procedures as participant observation, questionnaire administration, and application of an instrument or experimental treatment. Describe any calibration of the instruments or any training given to data collectors. For questionnaire administration, describe how you distributed the questionnaires, how they were returned to you, and whether the respondents were anonymous or identified.

You should say when you carried out your data collection procedures and how long they took. Any relevant particulars concerning the exact time the procedures were carried out should be included if they were important to the design of the study.

In the data analysis section, you should describe briefly how you recorded your data and your procedures for managing them. These include coordination of data management if a multiple site is involved, and data entry into the computer, including coding of data.

Next, you should describe your data analysis in relation to your research question or hypotheses. You should say whether you analysed the data by hand or computer, and if the latter, you should name the data analysis package and which procedures you used. You should state which statistical tests you carried out to test each hypothesis.

It is not necessary in a research report to go into a great deal of detail about the ethical considerations. However, you should state that permission was given by the relevant ethics committees and name them. The reader will thus be assured that reasonable ethical procedures were in place. You should discuss briefly any procedures that were in place to protect participants from harm. In a short report this can be integrated with the appropriate parts of the report, such as the procedures section.

If you did a pilot study, give a brief description here. You should describe any changes in the methodology that resulted from the pilot study, and justify them.

An example of a methodology section is:

The settings for this study were the Special Care Nursery at the Royal Darwin Hospital and the nursery at the Darwin Private Hospital. The study was approved by the university and hospital human research ethics committees and written consent was obtained from parents.

The participants in the study were 30 mother–infant dyads in which the infants were premature or SGA and needed special care. There were 13 female (7 CCC and 6 KMC) and 17 male (7 CCC and 10 KMC) infants of whom three-quarters (77 per cent) were delivered by Caesarean section because their mothers were high-risk clients. Four dyads were from Darwin Private Hospital, with the rest from Royal Darwin Hospital. Table 1 shows other characteristics of the sample.

Table 1 Characteristics of study group and total sample

Variable	KMC Group (n=16)		CCC Group (n=14)		Total Group (n=30)	
	$\overline{X}$	SD	$\overline{X}$	SD	$\overline{X}$	SD
Mother's age (yrs)	26	6	28	6	27	6·8
Gravidity	2	1	2	2	2·4	1·9
Parity	1·6	0·9	1·5	0·9	1·6	0·9
Birth age (weeks)	31·7	3·1	31·2	2·4	31·5	2·7
Apgar 1 minute	5·9	2·8	6	2·4	6	2·6
Apgar 5 minutes	7·8	2	8·4	2	8	2
Birthweight (gm)	1562	465	1481	409	1524	434
Enrolment weight (gm)	1687	418	1693	212	1690	332·5
Infant days in hospital	48	28	46	19	47	23·7
KMC/CCC per day (hrs)	1·6	0·9	1·8	0·9	1·7	0·9

To be enrolled in the study, the infants had to meet criteria similar to those of Ludington-Hoe and colleagues.[7] They had to have been born at 30 or more weeks' gestation or corrected age, with a 5-minute Apgar of 5. They had to be medically stable with clearance from the unit specialist and have no congenital abnormalities or central nervous system impairment. The infants had to have had a stable temperature for 24 hours, to have been extubated for more than 48 hours, and to have ceased cot or headbox oxygen for at least 24 hours. Nasogastric or oral feedings were to be 1 to 4 hourly. Infants could have nasal continuous positive airway pressure in place or a nasal cannula delivering oxygen at less than 0·2 L/min. At the time of entry into the study, infants had to be being cared for in an open crib or an incubator; could have an intravenous infusion in progress; and may have been on a course of antibiotics, theophylline, dexamethasone or other drugs that did not maintain systemic function (that is, no inotropes). They could not have had phototherapy within the last 24 hours. Any episodes of mild apnoea or bradycardia would have required mild stimulation only; infants who had been resuscitated were excluded.

Parents had to have a good understanding of the English language, be resident in the Darwin area and be prepared to spend a minimum of 2 hours a day for 5 days a week over a maximum of 4 weeks. Mothers who had a history of drug use were excluded from the study.

The study used an experimental design in which 30 dyads were assigned randomly to either the experimental KMC Group (n=16) or the control CCC group (n=14). This was done by means of envelopes that contained the random group assignment, stratified by gender to ensure equivalent numbers of male and female infants in each group. The only difference in the treatment of the groups was that the KMC group had skin-to-skin contact with the mother while the control group had contact through the clothing.

The revised Parental Stressor Scale–NICU (PSS–NICU) of Miles, Funk and Kasper[13] was used to measure the maternal stress levels. This questionnaire comprised 46 items measuring parents' reactions to the NICU. The items were grouped into four scales: 'Sights and Sounds', 'Baby's Looks and Behaviour', 'Relationship with Baby' and 'Staff Behaviours and Communication'. Miles et al. reported internal consistency coefficients for these scales ranging from 0·74 to 0·87. Each item was rated on a scale of 1 to 5 where 1 was 'not at all stressful', 2 was 'a little stressful', 3 was 'moderately stressful', 4 was 'very stressful' and 5 was 'extremely stressful'.

Mothers' perceptions of their maternal competence were measured by the Parental Expectations Survey (PES) developed and validated by Reece.[14] This survey is based on social learning theory. This questionnaire contains 25 items of parents' perceptions of their ability to take care of their baby. The items were rated from 0 'cannot do' through 5–6 'moderately certain can do' to 10 'certain can do'. Reece reported the reliability coefficient (Cronbach's alpha) for this scale at over 0·9.

Clinicians in both hospitals were briefed by the researchers on the protocols of the study to ensure equivalent performance of the procedures. On enrolment, the parent(s) were instructed by the SCN researchers about the care of the infants during the study. The amount of KMC/CCC was recorded on a KMC/CCC chart (Table 1). KMC/CCC was done in privacy, in a comfortable cane armchair that was able to be rocked. KMC infants were dressed only in a diaper, with the addition of a bonnet for smaller babies, to decrease heat loss via the scalp. The babies were then placed on the mother's skin and covered with a light blanket to ensure privacy. The CCC infants were swaddled in infant clothing and a light blanket. The temperature was measured by axilla for three minutes, before and after the KMC/CCC episode, by the clinician caring for the infant. The ambient temperature of the nurseries is controlled by air conditioning at 79·7°F (26·5°C) at all times of the year, and the control is separate from that for the rest of the hospital. Any monitors were left in place on the infant during the period of care. Breastfeeding was permitted as desired.

Infants were normally weighed naked by the clinicians, according to the usual hospital procedure, twice a week at approximately the same time of day on an electronic scale.

Data on the infants' gestational age, gender, birthweight, Apgar at 1 and 5 minutes, weight at discharge, and length of stay in the hospital were collected by chart audit. Data on weight gain were averaged across the length of stay in the hospital. Data on enrolled mothers were also collected from the chart: age, parity, mode of delivery and duration of breastfeeding while in the hospital. Data at six months was by mother's report. Infant weights were measured at the well baby clinic and were reported by mothers; mothers also reported whether they were still breastfeeding at that time.

Toward the end of the infants' stay in the Special Care Nursery, the mothers were given the PSS–NICU questionnaire on stress, which they returned by mail. Six weeks after discharge, or three months after birth, whichever was the later, the mothers were contacted by telephone to determine whether they were still breastfeeding, and were given the PES questionnaire. Six months after birth, the mothers were contacted to determine whether they were still breastfeeding.

Data were analysed using two-tailed independent t-tests to establish initial equivalence of the groups, one-tailed t-tests, Mann-Whitney U-tests and chi squares to compare the two groups on outcomes, and paired t-tests to compare pre- and post-KMC/CCC temperatures. A level of significance of $p = 0.05$ was set.

Note that the methodology section describes the setting, the sample, the instruments, ethical aspects, procedures and data collection procedures.

The results

The results section is very exciting to write because here you present your findings, the 'nitty gritty' of all of your hard work. This section presents an account of the findings of your investigation, which should be derived from your data analysis. The results comprise the text and supporting illustrations, such as tables, graphs, charts, photographs and models derived from the data.

The researcher has the responsibility of deciding which results should be reported. In a student report or thesis, it is customary to present all findings, whether important or not, significant or not. However, for other reports, pruning to key findings will be necessary to meet criteria for presentation time or journal space. It is never appropriate to elect to present only findings that support your hypotheses or beliefs.

Researchers often err on the side of over-reporting. They do this for three reasons – because they believe that every finding is equally important, because they think that if they have gone to the trouble of doing the procedure it must be reported, and because of their inability to sort the wheat from the chaff (Brown 1995). A report that is full of irrelevant detail can obscure the important findings. The aim is to make the key findings stand out.

The results tell a story, but should be presented in order of their importance, since people tend to read the first bit of a section more carefully and may skip over the following parts (Brown 1995). In a quantitative report, the results can be structured around the hypotheses. If your report is of a qualitative project, you present the findings as a narrative, focusing on the themes that have emerged. It is customary to interpose quotations from the interviews or journals to embellish or clarify the themes.

The results should be presented in such a way as to address the research question. You never present the raw data or your analysis of them in the results section; you present your analysis of the findings and the statistical significance, if it is a quantitative project.

If you have many results on several subtopics, use appropriate headings and present all the results on each subtopic together, even mixing qualitative and quantitative if you are using both approaches. You will have to decide whether to present the quantitative or the qualitative data first.

For quantitative results, the statistical tests should be reported with the appropriate result, giving the test, the result of the test, and the probability value. Some journals or bodies require that the degrees of freedom are also presented. The statistical test is usually presented in brackets after the result has been reported. Note that the letters that represent the statistical test, for example, 't' and the probability 'p' should be given in italics. In the past, the p value used to be expressed in terms of greater or less than the level of significance, which was usually 0·05. Thus, $p = <0·05$ meant that the result was significant, while $p = >0·05$ meant that it was not. Today, the exact p values should be given since computers can now generate them. The exact reporting of the p value allows the reader to see how close to significance the results were. If the computer gives a p value of 0·0136, the number should be rounded off to two decimal places, i.e. 0·01.

In quantitative research reports, include a statement of whether or not an hypothesis was supported with each result. This will include a statement about the null hypothesis and the research hypothesis. The possibilities are: (1) that the null hypothesis was rejected, in which case the research hypothesis was supported; (2) the null hypothesis was not rejected, in which case the research hypothesis was not supported; and (3) the null hypothesis was rejected but the findings were in the opposite direction from that predicted by the research hypothesis, which was not supported.

Supporting illustrations

Various devices can be used to present results in ways other than using words. Photographs, diagrams, models, flow charts, graphs and tables are all alternative ways of presenting information. Tables are called tables; all the rest are collectively called figures. Tables and figures are called illustrations. Judicious use of illustrations will provide variety and enhance clarity. Illustrations are also concise and, therefore, economical methods of presenting information in ways that are reader-friendly. However, it is important not to over-use these devices. Never use a table or figure when you can say the same thing in one or two sentences. Reserve illustrations for the presentation of more complex data. The old saying that a picture is worth a thousand words is certainly true for figures and graphs: they should be used instead of a thousand words, but not instead of ten or twenty.

Illustrative devices should be introduced in the text before they are presented. Give each illustrative device a caption and a number. Put the caption of a table at the top of it, and the caption of a figure below it. The caption should inform the reader about the findings in the table or figure, but should not include the name of the statistical test. For short reports, the figures and tables may be numbered consecutively throughout, but for reports and theses that have chapters, it is useful to use the number of each chapter as part of the numbering system.

Tables have been discussed already in Chapter 10. When using tables, avoid giving too much detail; keep in mind what information you want your reader to extract and build the table to make the extraction as easy as possible (Brown 1995). Many researchers make the mistake of expecting the numbers to speak for themselves. They also make the mistake of falling in love with the numbers in their data and forgetting that they are a means to an end rather than an end in themselves (Brown 1995). Round the numbers off to the level of their significance. There is no virtue in using three decimal places if your data are not accurate to three decimal places. For example, if your number is 572 out of 1000, or 57.2%, but the standard deviation is 10%, your figure is accurate only to 57% at best and 60% is really close enough. All numbers should be rounded off to the same number of decimal places, and the decimal points should be under each other in a column. This is easy to do by using the centring tab function on the word processor, or the table function. Make sure that your columns and rows have top and side headings. If inferential statistics were used, the results of these tests should be presented at the bottom of the table. You can see an example of a table in the 'Results' section of our sample report.

A figure is a pictorial representation instead of a numerical one. It may be a photograph, model, flow chart or graph. Most journals have requirements concerning the presentation of photographs. Graphs are the most commonly used figures in a research report, and they may be hand-drawn, but these days most computers come equipped with a program that will generate graphs from your data. When preparing graphs, it pays to frame the graph, use visually prominent symbols, place labels for the values outside the graph and choose a scale that is appropriate for the data.

A graph will usually compare findings for groups, or within a group. For example, it may compare the results of two groups on the dependent variable. Most modern statistical computer programs will generate graphs, but graphs can also be made using graph paper, or pen and ink drawings on plain paper. When preparing graphs, the dependent variable is usually on the X or horizontal axis and the independent variable on the Y or vertical axis. The axes should be labelled. You can see examples of different types of graphs in Chapter 10. Different types of graphs are useful for different purposes, and the results that you want to show should be considered when you are selecting a type of graph. Tests of significance can be reported at the bottom of the figure, or in the text.

The simplest graph is a line graph. Line graphs will have a connecting line between points, as is used in a temperature, pulse and blood pressure chart. Only a few lines or curves should be shown on a line graph.

A histogram, or bar graph, is commonly used. This demonstrates the manner in which the number or percentage of instances of the dependent variable occurs in different groups. The bars can go either from side to side, or from top to bottom. It is helpful to give numerical labels to the bars if your computer program will generate them. Pie graphs are used to show a percentage breakdown, and are useful for describing a group on a variable. A regression graph will show the scattergram with a line drawn to show the relationship between **X** and **Y**.

The information in figures and tables should not just be repeated in the text. The narrative should concentrate on interpreting the table or figure. However, the reader should be able to interpret the figure or table without the text.

The tests of significance and other data analysis particulars are included in the results section, along with the actual result. Some people prefer to put the data analysis only in the results section, but wherever it is put, it should be comprehensive, giving the reader enough detail to understand exactly what you did.

The results section is purely for the presentation of the findings. It is inappropriate to discuss your opinions of the meaning of the data here. These comments should be saved for the discussion section.

An example of a results section is:

> KMC and CCC groups were not significantly different on mother's age, parity, gravidity, gestation age, type of delivery, Apgar ratings, gender of baby, baby's birthweight, weight at the beginning of the study or time in KMC/CCC. Thus, the groups were considered initially to be equivalent.
>
> In comparing the two infant groups, the researchers found no statistically significant difference on any of the outcome variables for the KMC and CCC groups. With respect to hypothesis 1, both groups gained an average of 23+/−7 grams per day while in hospital. There was no significant difference in weight gain at six weeks, three months or six months. Infants in the KMC group had gained 52+/−24 gm/day at six weeks, 39+/−12 gm/day at three months and 30+/−6 gm/day by six months; infants in the CCC group had gained 55+/−15 gm/day at six weeks, 42+/−10 gm/day at three months and 30+/−6 gm/day by six months.
>
> For hypothesis 2, the temperatures were analysed for the first 11 episodes of KMC/CCC. At that point, there were only 20 dyads left in the study, not enough to analyse statistically. For all episodes, temperatures remained stable or rose by 0·2°–0·4°F (0·1°–0·2°C) for both groups. However, when the KMC and CCC groups were compared, there was no significant difference in temperature gain for any episode. The group mean temperature before KMC/CCC for both groups was 98·1°+/−0·2°F (36·7°+/−0·1°C) and after KMC/CCC it was 98·4°+/−0·4°F (36·9°+/−0·15°C). Concerning hospital stay (hypothesis 3), the KMC group spent an average of 48+/−28 days in hospital; the CCC group spent an average of 46+/−19 days.
>
> For the duration of breastfeeding (hypothesis 4), 10 KMC and 11 CCC babies were breastfeeding at discharge, with 9 KMC and 6 CCC babies breastfeeding at six weeks, 7 KMC and 5 CCC babies breastfeeding at three months and 4 from each group breastfeeding at six months.
>
> The Parental Stress Scale (NICU) scores were not significantly different in the KMC and CCC groups (hypothesis 5). The mothers in the sample expressed moderate to very stressful responses to all four subscales, i.e. nursery environment, infant appearance, relationship with the infant, and staff behaviour and communication (Table 2 overleaf).

Table 2: Parental Stress Scale: KMC and CCC						
Scale	KMC $\bar{X}^1$	Group SD	CCC $\bar{X}$	Group SD	Whole $\bar{X}$	Group SD
Sights and sounds of nursery	3·3	0·88	3·2	0·82	3·3	0·84
Looks and behaviour of baby	4·0	0·84	4·0	0·88	4·0	0·84
Relationship with baby	4·4	0·46	3·4	1·16	4·0	0·95
Staff behaviours and communication	4·4	1·3	4·3	1·6	4·35	1·4

For the Parental Expectations Survey, which was administered after the clients had been discharged, the total sample's mean score on the scale was 8·6+/−0·71, with all items having a mean score of 7·5 or higher, indicating a high level of confidence in their parenting abilities. There was no significant difference in the KMC and CCC groups' scores (hypothesis 6): the mean score of the KMC group was 8·4+/−0·75 and that of the CCC group was 8·8+/−0·62.

Note that the report gives only the findings and does not attempt to discuss their importance. The statistical significance of the findings should be reported. In the example above, the main findings are reported in a table to allow ease of access.

The discussion

The discussion section is the last section of the body of the report, and should explain the importance and relevance of your findings. This is where you get a chance to demonstrate your ability to interpret the meaning of the findings. In this section, you highlight the most important findings, interpret them in relation to issues raised in the introduction section and place the results in the context of the theory and research on the topic (Gething 1995).

In quantitative studies, you discuss the meaning of the findings for the support or non-support of the research hypotheses. You will have given in the results section the actual statement about whether or not the null hypotheses have been rejected, and research hypotheses have been supported. You now reiterate briefly the result and interpret its meaning for the reader. If your research hypothesis is supported, this is quite easy. However, if it is not supported, you are left with the task of explaining why not. This is usually either because of flaws in your methodology or because the prediction was not valid. When this happens, the temptation to throw it all in the bin can be strong, but do not despair. Sometimes negative findings are just as important as positive findings and can have just as significant an impact on practice. Borderline findings can stimulate further research, as can reports with a methodological flaw; which can prevent other researchers from making the same mistakes. In any case, as a student, your job is to learn to report the results, and the process of writing the report is more important than the product. It is how you interpret the results that counts, not the actual findings. You will not be marked down for insignificant results, but you will be failed for not submitting a report at all.

When interpreting the findings of your study, be sure to distinguish between statistical significance and clinical significance. Results cannot be clinically significant if they are not statistically significant. However, results are sometimes statistically significant but not clinically significant. This happens when the 'p' values are less than 0·05 (or whatever level of significance has been set) but the difference between the means of the two groups is low. This can occur because, as the sample size increases, the difference required for statistical significance decreases. In other words, with large numbers of participants, the difference required to reach statistical significance is small. In order to reach clinical significance, a difference should be at least 10% and preferably 20%. For example, suppose that you compared the dependent variable of the tidal volumes of two groups on two different types of pillows. A normal tidal volume is 500 ml. Unless you got a difference of more than 50 ml between the mean tidal volumes of each group, the result would not be clinically significant, although with a large enough sample it may have been statistically significant.

You must relate your results to the research that you have discussed in your literature review. This means that you will compare what you found to what was found by previous researchers. Your findings may agree or disagree with theirs, or they may agree with some and not with others. This does not need to be done as a separate section; it can be integrated with your interpretation of the findings. This is one of the hardest parts of the research report to write, and the one that most students do least well.

You should also relate your research to the theoretical or conceptual framework. If you were testing a theory, you should state whether your findings support, modify or refute the theory. If, however, a theoretical framework was used as a conceptual framework without testing the theory, you should describe how your findings are related to the theory.

The statement on the significance of the study follows. It should show why this study was worth doing. It should answer the question: 'So what?' It should show how the results of this study advance knowledge or practice in nursing and/or health. If there are possible applications of the results of this study, state them. At the end of the discussion section you can present conclusions and make recommendations for further research and/or clinical implementation of the findings.

An example of a discussion section is as follows:

This study was designed to investigate whether any difference in the KMC and CCC groups' outcomes for both infants and mothers was due to skin-to-skin contact alone. Skin-to-skin contact produced outcomes equivalent to those of CCC. Both groups of infants had similar lengths of stay in hospital and gained equal amounts of weight per day, with equivalent weight gains at six weeks, three months and six months. Because the pre- and post-treatment temperatures were the same or slightly higher on all occasions, the results suggest that both groups were able to be removed from the incubator for KMC/CCC without temperature control problems. Although KMC was not superior to CCC in reducing length of hospital stay or promoting temperature maintenance and breastfeeding, it was not inferior either. Perhaps the explanation for the positive effects for both groups may be the self-selected nature of the sample: the criteria for study enrolment required parents who were very committed to putting the time into caring for their infants in the neonatal intensive care unit. Furthermore, the infants were relatively older and healthier than those reported in previous studies. In any case, CCC may provide a useful alternative for women who do not feel comfortable with KMC.

This study's findings for temperature stability with KMC and CCC were similar to those of Ludington-Hoe and Smith for KMC. [7,8] The shorter hospital stay for KMC groups found by Whitelaw and colleagues, Wahlberg and colleagues, and Affonso and colleagues [9-11] cannot be equated to our findings because these three research groups used a control group with normal contact whereas our study compared two contact interventions.

In this study, the rates of breastfeeding declined steadily with the age of the baby. The results of this study did not confirm the results of Affonso and colleagues' sample for differences in breastfeeding; however, our study did not use an untreated control group.[11] Our findings also cannot be equated with the difference in duration of breastfeeding found by Whitelaw and colleagues, which those researchers presumed to be due to an increase in prolactin secretion induced by the baby's rooting for the breast.[9] The equivalence of breastfeeding duration for women in our study might be explained by an increase in prolactin secretion caused by both KMC and CCC.

In terms of maternal outcomes, there was no significant difference in the two groups' perceptions of stress and parental expectations. The PSS–NICU scores reflected moderate to high stress, but the PES scores were also high, indicating that the experience of the NICU did not interfere with the development of these mothers' confidence. The results of our study support the high maternal confidence levels found by Smith.[8]

A limitation of this study was the reliance on data obtained by clinicians for temperatures and weights. Clinical data on temperature and weight may include error because of the variations in the procedures for weighing and temperature-taking among nurses, and because of the lack of systematic calibration of scales and thermometers. The results of this study should also be interpreted with caution because of the small sample size. Later in the study, some mothers were requesting to do KMC and refused to enter the study because they did not want to take a chance of being in the CCC group, although one refused because she found the idea of KMC unappealing. In addition, some staff who were aware of the postulated benefits of KMC initiated it with the parents before the researchers were able to discuss the study with them, thus rendering them ineligible to participate.

In conclusion, this study has indicated that both KMC and CCC result in infant temperature maintenance while out of the incubator. Both interventions appear to be equivalent in terms of their effect on infant weight gain and hospital stay, duration of breastfeeding, parental stress and expectations.

In Chapter 6 we covered the rudiments of referencing, but you should follow the referencing system recommended by your institution. Whatever system is used, it is important to be accurate, particularly in a report that is going to be disseminated. Sloppiness in referencing will give the reader the impression that the research was sloppy, too. Even worse, errors in the journal name, volume number or issue number may prevent the reader from locating the reference, which negates a major reason for giving references. In a study of the accuracy of references in nursing journals, the researchers found minor errors in one-fifth to one-third of references, and major errors that prevented location of the article in 2.5% of references (Foreman & Kirchhoff 1987). The use of a reference manager such as EndNote will help to prevent mismatches between the in-text citations and the reference list. The references section of the article we have been following as an example was composed using Neonatal Network's version of the Vancouver system. This system is used by many nursing and medical journals – it numbers each reference and uses the same number every time the article is cited. The references from the article are:

1. Whitelaw A, Sleath K. Myth of the marsupial mother: home care of very low birth weight babies in Bogota, Colombia. Lancet 1985; 1 (8439):1206–8.
2. Anderson G. Skin-to-skin: kangaroo care in Western Europe. American Journal of Nursing 1989; 89(5):662–6.
3. deLeeuw R, Colin E, Dunnebier E, Mirmiran M. Physiologic effects of kangaroo care in very small premature infants. Biology of the Neonate 1991; 59:149–55.
4. Drosten-Brooks F. Kangaroo care: skin-to-skin contact in the NICU. MCN: American Journal of Maternal Child Nursing 1993;18(5):250–3.
5. Gale G, Franck L, Lund C. Skin-to-skin (kangaroo) holding of the intubated premature infant. Neonatal Network 1993;12(6):49–57.
6. Ludington S. Energy conservation during skin-to-skin contact between premature infants and their mothers. Heart and Lung 1990;19(5):445–51.
7. Ludington-Hoe SM, Thompson C, Swinth J, Hadeed A, Anderson G. Kangaroo care: research results and practice implications and guidelines. Neonatal Network 1994;13(1):19–27
8. Smith K. Skin-to-skin contact for premature and sick infants and their mothers. In: Biley F, Maggs C, eds. Contemporary Issues in Nursing. Edinburgh: Churchill Livingstone, 1996:31–78.
9. Whitelaw A, Heisterkamp G, Sleath K, Acolet D, Richards, A. Skin-to-skin contact for very low birth weight infants and their mothers: a randomized trial of kangaroo care. Archives of Disease in Childhood 1988;63:1377–82.
10. Wahlberg V, Affonso D, Perssons B. A retrospective, comparative study using the kangaroo method as a complement to standard incubator care. European Journal of Public Health 1992;2(1):34–7.
11. Affonso D, Wahlberg B, Persson B. Exploration of mothers' reactions to kangaroo method of prematurity care. Neonatal Network 1989;7(6):43–51.
12. Curry M. Maternal attachment behavior and the mother's self-concept: the effect of early skin-to-skin contact. Nursing Research 1982;31(2):73–8.
13. Miles M, Funk S, Kasper M. Neonatal Intensive Care Unit: Sources of Stress for Parents. AACN Clinical Issues 1993;2(2):346–54.
14. Reece S. The Parent Expectations Survey. Clinical Nursing Research 1992;1(4):336–46.

If you are writing a report for an organisation that demands a particular referencing style, be sure to follow it. If you are free to choose, you can decide whether the space and lack of interruption of flow of the document that the Vancouver system provides is more important than the reader-friendliness of the Harvard system.

Appendixes are used to include material that is too cumbersome for the main text, for example, questionnaires. Use appendixes wisely to avoid filling the report with unnecessary detail and interrupting the flow of the main text but ly material that supports or expands on the information in the body xt. Examples of things that are best put in an appendix are questionnaires, tools or tests, diagrams of instruments, consent forms and letters of support. Some disciplines may require, for a thesis, that the actual raw data be included in an appendix. Start each appendix on a new page, and index them alphabetically.

Putting it together

The mechanics of assembling the report are the same as for a proposal, which can be found in Chapter 6. It is important to use an appropriate heading system, which can also be found in that chapter. You will also need to construct a table of contents and for a long report the table of contents should include a list of tables and a list of figures. The table of contents should use the same system as the headings in the text. Make sure that all parts of the report are included and that you submit the required number of copies.

The presentation of a research report is similar to that of a proposal, using A4-size, good-quality, white bond paper. If possible, use a word processor with a legible 12-point font. Use double-spacing, particularly for class assignments, so that the lecturer can write between the lines. Make sure the pages are numbered correctly. If it is a longer report, some form of temporary or permanent binding will be required. Check again with your guidelines to make sure that you have conformed to them.

Before submitting the report, you should check it thoroughly for errors. It is vital to check the grammar and spelling, using the spellchecker and grammar checker on the word processor, if you have one. Particularly check that the numbers in the tables and figures are accurate and that your numbering of pages and captions is correct. This is especially important if you have been moving tables and figures around in the document. It is essential to check that your references are correct. It is crucial to proofread the document before submitting it in order to catch other errors, including word errors that the spellchecker will not pick up.

Writing the report of a qualitative project

A good qualitative report will contain all of the features of a good quantitative report, in terms of attention to the preliminaries, such as the title page, and the research summary or abstract. It will also pay the same amount of attention to clarity of presentation and thoroughness in setting out carefully all of the history and outcomes of the project.

To keep the accounts of how to write a quantitative report and how to write a qualitative report consistent, the structure of a qualitative proposal outlined in Chapter 6 (Taylor in press) will be used as a basis for making a report. In each of the sections questions will be raised, the written answers to which will form the draft of the report. Exceptions to the norm and other hints and ideas will be also included, so that you can see that qualitative reports not only differ from quantitative reports, they may also differ from other qualitative reports.

In the example which follows, the preliminaries of the report will not be reiterated. To refresh your memory of these ideas refer to the section in this chapter on common initial elements of quantitative and qualitative reports.

Preliminaries
The title
Improving the quality of hospital ward nursing care through reflective practice and action research with Registered Nurses

The aims and objectives
These are the same as those written for a proposal (see Chapter 6), but with the sentences converted to the past tense. Therefore, they read:

Aims
This project aimed to facilitate reflective practice processes in experienced Registered Nurses, in order to raise critical awareness of practice problems they face every day, to work systematically through problem-solving processes to uncover constraints against effective nursing care, and to improve the quality of care given by hospital nurses in light of the identified constraints and possibilities.

The literature review
The literature review for the report will be an amalgam of the literature presented in the proposal, plus that which has come to light since the project began. In the project being illustrated here, I added literature on dysfunctional nurse–nurse behaviours, such as horizontal violence and bullying, because this issue was raised by the action research group as a thematic concern. The extra literature appeared in full in the report (Taylor 2000b) and in a synoptic version in the journal article (Taylor in press). As the literature review for the report of the project is similar to the proposal, with addition of literature on dysfunctional nurse–nurse relationships, it will not be reiterated here. In your report writing, it is important to check that the literature review contains all of the elements of a good literature review as described in this chapter and in Chapter 3 of this book. Ensure that your literature review has these features, but be assured that it takes a lot of practice to write a comprehensive and strongly argued literature review.

Body of report
The research plan, including methodology, methods and processes
The body of a qualitative report contains sections on the methodology, methods and processes. The definitions for each of these sections, as they apply specifically to qualitative research, were given in Chapter 6.

Some questions to answer when writing the methodology section of the report are:

- What theoretical assumptions about the way knowledge is generated underlie the methods?
- What is the basic nature and intent of the chosen methodology?

- How did the methodology relate to this project?
- What were the main references to the methodological literature?

For example, a methodological section may read thus:

Methodology

In the context of this research approach, methodology means the theoretical assumptions of how knowledge is generated and validated, and these theoretical assumptions underlie the choice of methods. Given the collaborative nature of the project, a qualitative approach was chosen, informed by reflective practitioner concepts and the technical, practical and emancipatory intentions of action research.

The methods and processes used were appropriate for reflective practice strategies and action research. For the reflective practice component, methods included becoming familiar with some reflective practitioner literature and with the activities outlined in the project materials (Taylor, King & Stewart 1995; Taylor 2000a). Processes to enable effective reflection included coaching and practice in writing and in speaking descriptively in confidential and facilitative group meetings. Confidence was bolstered in undertaking reflection in practice (during practice) and reflection on practice (after practice) through individual and collective storytelling, journalling, critical analysis and discussion.

The methods of action research involved a four-phases problem-solving approach of collectively planning, acting, observing and reflecting. Each phase led to another cycle of action, in which the plan was revised, and further acting, observing and reflecting was undertaken systematically, to work towards solutions to problems of a technical, practical or emancipatory nature (Kemmis & McTaggart 1988). The planning and acting phases included appropriate methods of gathering and analysing data, such as participant observation, reflection and journalling. Cycles of action research led to further foci and members kept an action research approach to their work for as long as they chose, given that, typically, clinical nursing practice is fraught with many challenges on a daily basis.

If you have already read the proposal for this project in Chapter 6 of this book, you will notice that this section has been managed by changing the tenses to the past form. However, in a report of a project which is a thesis, the methodology may take part or all of a chapter. This is important to remember when using examples such as this to structure your own report. The research report must be appropriate to the audience.

At this point, you may also choose to insert a small section which outlines some key assumptions of qualitative research approaches. This will depend on the needs of the audience reading the report. If you think that there is a chance that they will be relatively uninformed about qualitative research, it might be advisable. For example:

Approaches to qualitative research

Knowledge derived from qualitative research is relative to the local and specific understandings people have of their realities. Action research and reflective practice are qualitative approaches that value people's experiences and the potential they have to make sense out of their own lives. This fits with the reliance of qualitative research on participants' context-dependent descriptions and the relative truths that emerge from their experiences.

Ethical requirements

It is important to report on the ways in which the ethical rights of the participants were safeguarded throughout the project. The report should address the following questions about ethical requirements.

- From which committees was ethical clearance obtained?
- What were the ethical considerations?
- How were informed consent, privacy and anonymity honoured?

For example:

Ethical requirements

Full ethical clearance processes through Southern Cross University and the Northern Rivers Areas Health Service preceded the commencement of the project. Research participants had the right to consent freely and without coercion. They were offered the right to refuse to participate, or to withdraw at any time, without penalty or coercion of any kind.

The first measure taken to ensure that research participants had the capacity to understand the research project was to ascertain that participants comprehended English. They could have been provided with the services of an interpreter, but this was not necessary. The forms given to participants were relative to their comprehension. Participants received detailed explanations, orally and in writing, of what the research involved, the aims and the processes of the research, and participants' commitments in it. Nurses were the main participants in this research, so the plain language statement and the consent form were written relative to their comprehension, bearing in mind that nurses are professionals conversant with language used in higher education institutions and health care settings. Even so, any words and sentences which may have caused confusion would have been paraphrased into simple English so that the meaning was clear and unambiguous, had this been necessary. The project was also explained orally, in plain language, by the researcher. Participants had opportunities to ask questions, make comments and voice any concerns that they may have had concerning the project at the outset and throughout its duration.

As this research encouraged nurses to share their practice stories, possible risks were that the privacy and confidentiality of patients may have been breached and that nurses may have felt vulnerable in sharing their experiences, leading to embarrassment or possible emotional catharsis such as tearfulness or anger. Nurses are educated in the need for patient confidentiality and they practise this daily in their work. Even so the researcher ensured that privacy and confidentiality measures were instituted and maintained. Stories written in journals and shared in group meetings were devoid of information that could have identified patients, relatives and staff. Pseudonyms were used and identifying material was omitted or renamed to protect the identities of people within any written transcripts. Reflective journals remained the personal property of participants and they were not read or sighted by the researcher, unless the participants consented. Reports and published material described the participants' stories and interpretations according to the issues they raised and the practice improvements they caused, rather than identifying specific people, places and situations. All data collected in the course of the research are secured in a locked storage compartment for five years and the responsibility for the safety and security of it resides with the researcher.

With respect to risks associated with emotional catharsis, the group offered support to its members and the researcher was an experienced nurse with 30 years of group management and support. No member became emotionally upset beyond the ability of the group to provide support, but an option of professional counselling was available. The risks of the project of breaches of confidentiality and emotional catharsis were communicated to participants at the outset of the project and repeated as often as necessary so that participants remembered the need for patient confidentiality and the availability of group and professional support. Benefits to participants included knowledge and practice of reflection and the improvement of nursing care.

Participants were informed orally and in writing that they were at liberty to withdraw from the project at any time, without penalty or coercion of any kind. As this project involved nurses who are healthy, consciously aware adults, they were able to consent for themselves. The issue of special cases did not apply to patients in this research, because verbal consent from legally competent adults was sufficient for the simple surveys which were used as part of the data collection phases in action research.

Methods and processes

The actual methods and processes used in the project must be reported. If these varied from those proposed, this should be noted. Some questions that may guide the writing of this section are:

- How were participants enlisted into the project?
- How were their rights honoured?
- What was the sequence of the research methods?
- What interpersonal processes were involved in undertaking the methods?

If there was no variation from the research intentions, parts of this section may be inserted by changing the sentences to the past tense. For example:

Number of participants and access arrangements

Experienced Registered Nurses (RNs) working in a large local rural hospital were invited by the researcher to participate and 12 RNs agreed to become involved on a one-hour-per-week basis for 16 weeks. Ethical processes were maintained throughout the project to protect participants' privacy and anonymity, and as this action research project involved collaborative group work, attention was paid to maintaining open and trusting processes within the group.

The nurses met weekly for one hour to discuss clinical problems raised by them in their journal writing and discussion. The researcher acted as group facilitator, and as a guide in the research processes, keeping meeting notes, writing up minutes, preparing agendas and contributing as appropriate. For the reflective practice component, methods included becoming familiar with some reflective practitioner literature and with the activities outlined in the project materials. Processes to enable effective reflection included coaching and practice in writing and in speaking descriptively, in confidential and facilitative group meetings. Confidence was bolstered in undertaking reflection in practice (during practice) and reflection on practice (after practice) through individual and collective storytelling, journalling, critical analysis and discussion.

The research processes began with nurses getting involved in locating in their practice issues and constraints that they wanted to change. It was important that the nurses 'owned' the research questions they generated and the intervention strategies, so time was taken initially to deal with some issues in the group and in their own practice. Such issues included power relationships in the group, which included relatively senior nurses who may have had a potential 'silencing' effect on other members of the group.

Common concerns were identified and reconnaissance was conducted, which means that an initial investigation of specific situations was undertaken to get an overall idea of what was happening. Members then focused on a specific concern of interest to them all. They wrote down their stories about the focus of concern and shared these accounts in the weekly meeting of the group.

The first action cycle occurred after the reconnaissance and a literature review, and it addressed itself to questions about the situation. The questions were: 'What is happening here?' 'Why is it happening?' 'What do we want to change about the situation?' Data collection strategies depended on what was needed and what would best serve the purposes of the research. The findings were pooled and discussed and the appropriate action was taken. Observation of the effects followed, before further reflection led to further action. In this way, the nurses evolved a collaborative working process for managing clinical issues of concern to them.

The planning and acting phases included keeping a journal as a method of gathering and analysing data. The non-confidential parts of journals were shared in the weekly group meeting. Participant observation occurred during practice in clinical areas. Notes and/or journal entries were made during or after the nursing activities, although, given the immediacy of clinical situations, it usually occurred afterwards.

The data analysis method included an analysis of journal experiences by individual and group critical reflection and problem-solving strategies. Group discussion also identified the specific nature and determinants of problems, the most appropriate methods to investigate problems further and the most practical and useful plan of action. Successive observation of the effects followed, before further reflection led to further action and analysis.

In the 16 weeks of the reflective practice and action research project, group members shared their experiences of nursing. After several meetings, a thematic concern of nurse–nurse relationships was identified. Over further meetings, an action plan was negotiated.

Analysis and interpretation

The report provides a description of how the analysis and interpretation of data was done. This is the part of the report that may differ from other qualitative projects. The reader must be able to see how you went about organising and making sense of the data, so be sure to set this section out carefully and clearly.

The report should also make the analysis and interpretation phases transparent by documenting them in the report. This means that the report should reflect faithfully the roles and contributions of all the people in the research to analysis and interpretation. The report should also provide excerpts of actual dialogue between researchers/co-researchers/participants, as sources of data to assist in validating interpretations and to act as a decision trail for readers.

Some questions which may guide you in writing up the analysis and interpretation phase of the project are:

- Whose writing informed the choice of analysis?
- What were the steps in the analysis?
- Who did the analysis; that is, was it done by an individual or by a group?
- How did the individual/group go about doing the analysis?
- How were the data organised when they reached analysed form?
- What were the sub-themes/collective themes/competing discourses?
- Who made the interpretations?
- How were the interpretations made?
- What interpretations were made?
- How were the interpretations validated?

Responses to these questions will differ considerably, depending on whether the report is describing a qualitative interpretive or qualitative critical project. However, as a practical guide, this section may contain statements such as these:

Analysis and interpretation

Analysis of journal experiences was managed by individual and group critical-reflection and problem-solving strategies. Group discussion was also used to identify the specific nature and determinants of problems as well as the most appropriate methods to investigate problems further and the most practical and useful plan of action. Descriptions of participant observation were analysed individually and collectively by manual thematic analysis techniques (Roberts & Taylor 1998). In each action research phase the findings were pooled and discussed and the appropriate action was planned and taken. Successive observation of the effects followed, before further reflection led to further action and analysis.

Action research involves a four-phases problem-solving approach of collectively planning, acting, observing and reflecting (PAOR). Each phase leads to another cycle of action, in which the plan is revised, and further acting, observing and reflecting was undertaken systematically, to work towards solutions to problems of a technical, practical or emancipatory nature (Kemmis & McTaggart 1988). Action research cycles represent aggregates of group activity over time in which key issues are addressed, during which the PAOR processes continue at the most effective rate and sequence relative to the issue being addressed.

In this project there were three discernible action research cycles. The activities within the three action research cycles were documented in the group's minutes, written by the researcher as facilitator and confirmed as faithful accounts weekly by the group members. These minutes represented the analysis and interpretation processes of individuals and the collective. The first cycle (Weeks 1–3) involved the development of group processes, and familiarisation with the research aims and action research and reflective processes. The second cycle (Weeks 4–7) involved using reflective processes to locate individual and collective practice issues. Individual reflections were about relationship difficulties, for example, in nurse–doctor and nurse–nurse communication. The third cycle (Weeks 8–16) involved working together on a common practice issue to generate and act and reflect on an action plan. The group analytic processes further identified the common thematic concern of dysfunctional nurse–nurse relationships, for which the group generated an action plan.

The report should be organised into sections or chapters in which the analysis and interpretation can be demonstrated. This action research in the report being used as an example required group discussion and collaboration; therefore, the documented group processes were sources of data from which interpretations were drawn. In the report (Taylor 2000b) the minutes of the meeting appeared in the relevant action research cycles to document the group's interpretive and action processes. For example, in the report, the table of contents was sequenced thus:

CHAPTER TWO: ANALYSIS AND INTERPRETATION

Action Cycles

The first action research cycle: meetings 1–3

The second action research cycle: meetings 4–7

The third action research cycle: meetings 8–16

Working together on a common practice issue

Generating and acting and reflecting on an action plan.

The report should demonstrate how individuals' accounts relate to those of other participants and, if it is appropriate to the methodology chosen, the report should discuss common themes that emerged from the data analysis and interpretation phases. In this research, the aim was to locate a thematic concern and to work on it collaboratively using action research. The theme of nurse–nurse relationships was established as part of the group processes, and following on from that an action plan was generated. For example, the negotiated action plan included:

Action plan

- Start a culture of 'positive strokes' and acknowledgement.
- Deal with the nurse directly and immediately and through recourse to policies and procedure.
- Provide strong leadership ourselves.
- Look carefully at the determinants of situations and try to 'turn them around'.
- Engage in conflict resolution.
- Raise the possibility that maybe this nurse is in need of recognition, acknowledgement and involvement in creating practice policies.
- Encourage the 'victims' to support one another; use evidence and documentation such as professional journals, incident forms, annual reviews and occupational health and safety procedures; use the line of command.
- Build skills to deal with situations directly, and/or ask for facilitation as soon as possible.
- Use 'people power' and a 'united front' to senior staff in the line of command.

This list of strategies led to the question: 'How?' For example, 'How can we handle issues directly, provide strong leadership and deal with conflict resolution?' Suggestions were by:

- remembering that all of the co-researchers in the group have experience and varying degrees of training in interpersonal communication skills
- approaching situations directly with a tentative and gentle attitude, seeking to clarify the situations
- listening reflectively
- organising face-to-face meetings between the key people in the situation
- paying strict attention to confidentiality
- employing specific skills such as stating one's own feelings and paraphrasing as necessary
- knowing the difference between aggression and assertiveness, so that direct approaches in conflict resolution use the attitude and skills discussed in such a way that all parties feel they are being heard and fair and reasonable solutions to nurse–nurse relationship problems can be negotiated.

Discussion and insights/recommendations/suggestions/conclusions

This part of a qualitative report can be labelled variously, depending on what the project has aimed to achieve through its methods and processes. Some qualitative reports will offer suggestions, while others will offer recommendations. It all depends on the justification they have for offering them.

The final stage of the report documents any pertinent discussions of the findings and offers suggestions and/or recommendations for nurses and nursing practice. Projects may conclude the research by offering suggestions for nursing practice, education and research. At times, however, and in line with the lack of certainty in qualitative research related to the relativity of 'truth', tentative statements are made, for example:

Discussion

> The earlier parts of the project (the first two action cycles) required plenty of time for learning about the research approaches and reflecting on nursing practice. The research was useful in introducing nurses to action research and reflective practice, but the varying degrees of success reflect the complexity of the thematic concern. As the literature suggests dysfunctional nurse–nurse relationships have a complex pathology and they may be difficult to eradicate. Even so, this project confirmed the necessity for reflective practice and continued collaborative research processes in the workplace to bring about a cultural change within nurses' collectives and in the places where they work to remove impediments to mutual respect and cooperation in nurse–nurse relationships. The action plan was put into place in the last three weeks of the project and members reported varying degrees of success in attempting to improve nurse–nurse relationships.

Qualitative reports will differ in their concluding parts, depending on the particular approaches they have taken. The report should demonstrate that the final discussion and conclusions are congruent with the overall plan, methods and processes of the research.

Remember that you can use this outline for forming drafts of the research report. You will need to go back over the drafts to correct grammar, to reword ideas, and to undertake other editorial tasks that ensure a high-quality report. It is a good idea to locate and study research reports so that you can see how they have been prepared. Do not hesitate to borrow from other researchers ideas that appear to work well, but only after verifying that they are appropriate for your research.

Presenting a report at professional meetings
Oral presentations

From time to time, a student may need to present an oral presentation of the report to an audience, for example the whole class, a seminar, or a student conference. A nurse-researcher may have to present a paper at a conference or seminar. Consider the audience. The oral report should be dynamic and interesting. The audience will not normally have access to the written paper at the time of the presentation, so clarity is essential. A good presentation seldom results from just reading a written paper, as the ways of conveying information by writing and speaking are different. It is boring to have to listen to a speaker read from a paper.

Visual aids can be useful to add interest to oral presentations. Use overhead transparencies, or if you are going to a conference, it is worth having professional slides made. If you have access to the software program PowerPoint or its equivalent, you can design professional-looking slides and transparencies. These are written using the Outline View (see Figure 18.2).

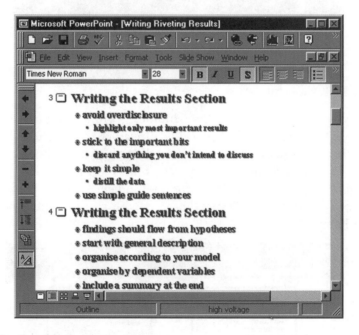

Figure 18.2 PowerPoint: Outline View

The Outline View is then converted to slides (see Figure 18.3 overleaf). You can also use PowerPoint to give a slide show using your computer in conjunction with a data beam that projects the presentation from the computer onto a big screen. A laptop computer is particularly useful for this purpose because of its portability. These slide shows are very effective because they use professionally designed layouts with dramatic colour schemes and allow for gradual introduction of points on the slide. PowerPoint presentations are becoming the norm at professional conferences.

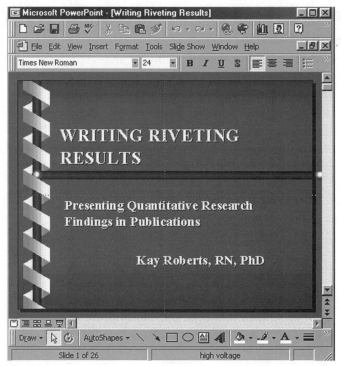

Figure 18.3 A PowerPoint slide

The presenter controls the presentation with a mouse. PowerPoint presentations can be embellished with special effects, including interesting transitions between slides and separate introduction of individual points. You can even introduce musical effects and hypertext links to Internet sites.

You can also generate handouts for the audience that reproduce varying numbers of your transparencies to the page, with space for note-taking if you wish. See Figure 18.4.

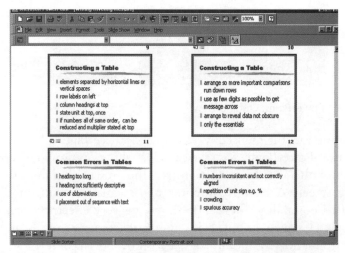

Figure 18.4 Handouts for the audience generated from PowerPoint slides

Finally, you can generate a set of notes for yourself that have one panel to the page that takes up only half of the page. On the other half, you can type brief notes in a large bold font that will help you to remember supporting information during your presentation of the paper. See Figure 18.5.

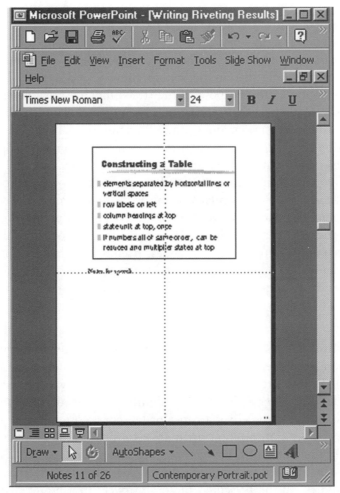

Figure 18.5 Speaker's notes generated from PowerPoint slides

The major errors made with these media are having too much information on the slide or transparency and having the printing too small. The latter is usually a consequence of the former. The printing should be in a large font. PowerPoint resists these errors. The material on slides should be oriented horizontally rather than vertically since the screen is wider than it is high (Day 1998). Consider the size of the room when composing your overheads or slides. If possible, check out the readability of the print from the back of the room. Make sure that your slides and transparencies are numbered and are in the correct order and the correct orientation (no upside-down slides!).

For most oral presentations, there will be some sort of time restriction: most presentations will not exceed 30–45 minutes, and may be as short as 10 minutes. Therefore you will need to be selective about what to include and you will need to plan the allocation of the time, including an allowance for questions. You can always also give a handout and just do the highlights. Handouts give the person something to take away and can include graphics to support the written report. Sometimes people give the abstract as a handout.

The presentation should be organised and logical, following a similar format to that of a written report. However, the audience will be far more interested in the results and implications than in the literature review and methodology, so give a brief introduction to the purpose of the study and any previous findings, then focus on the results and the implications. Do not include a lengthy account of the methods or extensive citations of the literature (Day 1998).

Preparation is essential for an oral presentation. You will need a copy of the full report, preferably double-spaced in larger print to allow easy and unobtrusive reading. If you are confident and know the topic well, a good method is to write the main headings on cards in large print or use PowerPoint speaker notes and speak to them. This allows you to make more eye contact with the audience. You can keep the written paper handy in case you get stuck. It is also useful to practise giving your paper to colleagues, friends or relatives. This gives you feedback and allows you to gauge the timing, and to practise using any equipment. Try to anticipate any questions or criticisms and have a reply ready.

Posters

A poster is usually presented at a poster session of a conference. Originally, poster sessions were developed to meet a need for catering for more presentations than could be accommodated on a conference program. The way the system works is that people offer (or are asked to submit) abstracts of presentations, then invitations are issued to deliver a paper or present a poster. At one time posters were seen as a type of rejection of an abstract (Day 1998). However, now they are an important part of a conference program, with large areas set aside for poster presentations. Some types of material, for example the results of complex research studies, can be presented more effectively in a poster than in an oral presentation (Day 1998).

The purpose of the poster presentation is to communicate the major points of the research project to a number of people who then have the opportunity to talk to the researcher about it. Usually there is a group of posters, with the presenters in attendance by their posters. The delegates walk around the room, looking at the posters, and stopping to talk to the researchers whose posters interest them. The researchers can then discuss the finer details of their projects with the delegates.

It is important to have a poster that will attract the attention of the delegates. Posters can result in publicity for the research and also in the presenter acquiring valuable ideas from colleagues. Guidelines for the presentation of posters can be obtained from the conference presenters. You should adhere strictly to these guidelines when developing your poster.

You can prepare a poster yourself using large sheets of cardboard. Printing can be done either by hand, using felt-tipped pens or paint, or you can print the text on the computer printer and attach it to the cardboard. If you are not constrained by financial considerations, you can do the poster on a computer program and have it printed professionally by a graphics company.

The poster should contain the title of the project, the name of the researcher, the purpose of the study, the research question, the method, the results, the conclusions and the implications.

The poster should have visual appeal and impact. It should get across the main points without being wordy. If it is too heavy with words, you might as well give delegates a copy of your research report. Remember, 'less is more'. The most common mistake is to have too much information on the poster. There should be very little text in a poster, with much of the space occupied by illustrations (Day 1998).

The poster should be able to be read easily at a distance of about 1.5 metres and should attract people to stop at your display. Letters should be at least 2.5 cm high, or 24-point font. Information using bullet points is easier to read than paragraphs. Be sure to lay the poster out carefully and proofread it. You may want to use arrows to direct the reader to read the poster in a logical sequence. Remember that any material below knee level will not be readable. The contrast of colours should be pleasing, but avoid too many colours as it may overwhelm the viewer. Creative presentation is important – try attaching a three-dimensional visual aid.

Care should be taken with transporting a poster to a conference: you should pack it in a tube and carry it with you during the journey. If you check it in with your luggage when you are travelling by air, it may become lost. Store it in the overhead compartment and remember to retrieve it at your journey's end.

If you are invited to present a poster at a conference, you can find more detail about the content and format of poster construction in the following publications: Russell, Gregory and Gates (1996), Maltby and Serrell (1998), Cantrell and Bracher (1999), Gosling (1999), McCann, Sramac and Rudy (1999) and Jackson and Sheldon (2000).

Writing for a wider audience

One of the most lamentable situations that can happen to research findings is that they are not communicated adequately to the wider audience beyond the span of the research report. Research is intended for public consumption, so that it can be scrutinised and have beneficial effects. An important feature of scholarship is in inviting open discussion and critique of original work, to verify the usefulness or otherwise of the new information. Whereas nursing research is open to anyone who shows interest in it, it makes the most sense to target nurses and people associated with nursing. Effective ways of doing this are through journal articles and monographs.

Writing a journal article

If you have not written a journal article before, you may be thinking that it is beyond your ability. If this is what you are thinking, please reconsider. Journals are media for communication. In nursing, there are many opportunities to choose a journal which is best able to communicate the results of your research. Wander into the nursing journal section of your library and take some time to browse. You will find many journals representing different areas of nursing. One of them is sure to suit you as a means of disseminating your research.

While you are looking through the journals that seem to suit you best, notice the format and style of the journal. Locate the section about notes for contributors. It may be on the inside front or back cover. This is a practical guide by the editor of the journal as to what is expected of you in preparing a manuscript for submission. Make a photocopy so that you can study it carefully and use it to guide you in writing your article.

The original research report that documents the whole of the research will need to be adjusted to suit the requirements of the journal. You will notice that there are word limits for the categories of articles. As you will be putting your research forward, you would be best advised to prepare your research as a feature article, which will undergo a review process. Do not let this concern you too much. You have managed to do the research and to present the report, so this is just another step in your evolution as a researcher.

Prepare the manuscript according to what it is you want to put forward in the article. For example, you may want to present a synopsis of the entire project or you may want to extract certain themes or sections from the project and elaborate on them. If you want to present a synopsis of the entire project, your challenge will be to represent the project overall faithfully, while keeping to the word limit. This will mean that you will have to make decisions about what you will leave out of the manuscript. Make sure that the essential features of the project remain intact according to the particular approach you have taken. If you are unsure what these features are, consult a reference on critique of research, for example, Polit and Hungler (1995). This will tell you what other people will be looking for when they read your research.

If you choose to extract certain parts of the project for further elaboration, you need to spend some time deciding on how you will do this. Be clear about the focus of the article you want to write. Ensure that it fits the content of the journal in which you are intending to publish. When you extract the section from the research report, read it carefully. It will most probably need a new introduction, a certain amount of extra work in the body of the text, and an appropriate conclusion.

When the writing phase is over, it is important to check the manuscript for spelling and grammatical errors. Check to see that it follows the referencing conventions of the journal and that it is set out clearly with headings and subheadings. Ideas should flow between sections, and the discussion and conclusions section should be well substantiated. When you think that you have the manuscript ready, give it to some colleagues to read for content, grammar, flow of ideas, fit for the selected journal and so on. You will then adjust the manuscript according to their feedback. Make sure you have added the other details as specified such as a title page, contact details and so on. Ensure that you have complied with the journal's requirements for content and format.

Always print your article in a large, easy-to-read font, for example 12-point Times Roman, and in double line spacing. Photocopy the required number of copies, including one for your files. Send them with a covering letter to the editor and then wait for feedback. It is a good idea to date the copy and note to which journal you sent it before filing it.

When the letter arrives from the journal editor, it may suggest some changes. Feedback from reviewers will be supplied to assist you in adjusting the manuscript. Alternatively it may be flawless and ready to publish as is, but this seldom happens, even to very experienced writers. The journal will then probably ask you for a copy of your article on disk, or to be submitted by email. The worst case is that the letter may inform you that the manuscript is not suitable for publication in that particular journal. If so, do not despair. Life is like that. You can't always get it right the first time. Consider resubmitting the manuscript to a more suitable journal. With a few changes you may find it fits another journal's requirements – but ensure you meet the next journal's specifications. If you want to publish, the trick is not to take rejections too much to heart. Above all, don't give up!

Another means of submitting a journal article is to write for an online journal, such as the *Australian Electronic Journal of Nursing Education (AEJNE)*. To access *AEJNE* get into the Internet, go to the home page for Southern Cross University, Australia, select Schools, select Nursing, and there you will find the journal link. The journal provides instructions for how you are to proceed in submitting a contribution.

If you want to learn more about publishing in journals, an excellent starting point for further reading is an article by Greenwood (1998). Another article you may care to access was written by journal editors (Plawecki & Plawecki 1998).

Writing a monograph

Definitions for a monograph differ, but there is usually agreement that a monograph is smaller than a book. It is usually presented as a soft-cover A5-size (half A4) document containing approximately 50 pages. It is usual for academic organisations to have their own printing facilities, and to publish their own monographs.

If you are thinking that you would like to try to have your work published in a monograph, your first port of call might be to an academic in the university or other tertiary institution. Ask this person whether the university has a monograph series for researchers. If the answer is yes, the rest of the inquiries will be up to you as to how you go about securing approval to submit a manuscript.

Do not put a lot of work in on a monograph unless you know it is appropriate for the publication series and that it will be reviewed for publication.

Preparing a monograph appears to be a larger task than preparing for submitting a journal article. In some it ways it may be, but on the other hand, it could be easier. For instance, the word limit will be larger, so there will be less challenge in presenting the research intact. Check with someone who understands copyright to ensure that you can cut and paste large sections of your thesis or research reports. You may find that much of the work you have already done can be transferred to the monograph manuscript. It will then be a matter of setting out a table of contents that gives the manuscript a good flow of ideas. Having done this, you will know where the areas for further elaboration lie, and these will be your main foci for writing.

As in any case of writing for publication, ensure that you follow the requirements of the publisher. Present the manuscript in its best possible version, after it has been thoroughly checked and re-checked by you and other willing readers. Send it to the publisher with a covering letter and wait for feedback.

Be prepared to make adjustments as directed by the publisher. If the manuscript is not appropriate for publication by that publisher, try working on the draft again and submitting it elsewhere. Remember, a rejection is not a comment about you as a person; it is a comment about a piece of written work and what the publisher wants.

Summary

In this chapter we have discussed the importance of a research report as a vehicle for disseminating the findings of the project and demonstrating professional accountability. We have also shown how to construct a research report. The mechanisms were outlined for presenting a research report orally and by poster to professional meetings. Ideas were also given about how to prepare a manuscript for submission for publication as a journal article or a monograph.

Main points

- A research report is a formal account of a research project and the major means of disseminating essential information about it. The report can be formal or informal, oral or written.
- Researchers have a responsibility to share findings so as to help build a useful body of knowledge, to help their colleagues practise more effectively, to help others plan research more effectively and to allow peer review.
- The purpose of a research report is to communicate key aspects of the project to research consumers so they can: replicate your study, do their own literature review, plan a new study or help find a solution for a clinical practice problem.
- When writing a report, consider your target audience and write to it after obtaining guidelines for content and presentation.
- In planning and writing the report, make an outline, write a draft and revise it, have someone critique it and rewrite it until it is the best you can do.

- The writing style generally is the same as for a research proposal – concise, clear and coherent, with good English usage and written in the past tense.
- The structure of the report is the same as for the proposal, with preliminaries, introduction, methodology and methods, but with the addition of results, discussion and conclusions.
- The results section should present the results concisely, with the judicious use of illustrations such as graphs and tables.
- The discussion section highlights the most important findings, explains their significance and relevance, interprets them in relation to issues raised in the introduction section and places them in the context of theory and previous research.
- The conclusions section draws conclusions derived from the findings, and includes recommendations for implementing the findings, for further research and for theory development.
- Supporting materials include references and appendixes.
- A qualitative report has many similarities with a quantitative report, including a research plan that covers methodology, methods and processes. The findings tell a story, using themes and sub-themes, with quoted material as appropriate. The discussion section presents insights, recommendations, suggestions and conclusions.
- In developing oral presentations, consider the audience, be dynamic and interesting, use visual aids, prepare and practise, and keep to time during the presentation.
- Posters communicate the major points of the research project to colleagues who have an opportunity to talk to the researcher. In preparing a poster, adhere strictly to the guidelines, and pay attention to creating visual appeal and impact.
- When writing a journal article, select the target journal, obtain and follow its author guidelines, prepare the manuscript, send it with a covering letter to the editor and wait for feedback.

Review Questions

1. The main difference between a good qualitative report and a good quantitative report, is that a qualitative report will:
   a be written better and be far more interesting
   b lack certainty in conclusions
   c be sure of 'truth' and predictions
   d feature numbers and graphs

2. A dissertation is:
   a a detailed report
   b not necessarily a research report
   c the same as a thesis
   d always 100 000 words long

3. Which of the following is in a research report but not a proposal?
   a. title page
   b. abstract
   c. findings
   d. supporting materials

4. Which of the following is part of the preliminaries of a research report?
   a. abstract
   b. introduction
   c. literature review
   d. methodology

5. Which of the following answers the question 'when?'?
   a. introduction
   b. findings
   c. preliminaries
   d. methodology

6. The important results should be presented first in a quantitative research report because:
   a. important things should be said first
   b. the reader will be less likely to skip them
   c. they are more likely to have graphics, which interest the reader
   d. all of the above

7. A graphic that shows the percentages of subgroups in a group is a:
   a. pie chart
   b. bar graph
   c. histogram
   d. polygraph

8. In a qualitative research report the findings are usually ordered in which way?
   a. with the important findings first
   b. as a story
   c. with the important findings last
   d. any of the above – it doesn't matter

9. Which of these will be read by the most people?
   a. findings
   b. discussion
   c. abstract
   d. introduction

10. The literature review in a research report will be related to that of the proposal in that:
    a. literature not relevant to the findings will be pruned
    b. literature later found to be relevant to the results will be added
    c. original literature that remains relevant will stay
    d. all of the above

Discussion Questions

1. Discuss the reasons for writing a research report.
2. Describe five ways in which a qualitative and quantitative report would differ.
3. Discuss how you would prepare a poster to illustrate a research paper.
4. Distinguish between a monograph, a thesis and a research article.
5. Discuss how you would prepare the presentation of your research report.

References

Anderson, D. & Poole, M. 1998, *Assignment and Thesis Writing*, 3rd edn, John Wiley & Sons, Brisbane.

Brown, R. 1995, *Key Skills for Writing and Publishing Research*, Write Way Consulting, Brisbane.

Cantrell, J. & Bracher, L. 1999, 'How to design and present a poster', *Advancing Clinical Nursing*, vol. 3, no. 2, 91–2.

Day, R. 1998, *How to Write and Publish a Scientific Paper*, 5th edn, Cambridge University Press, Cambridge.

Dees, R. 1999, *Writing the Modern Research Paper*, Allyn & Bacon Inc., Needham Heights.

Evans, D. 1995, *How to Write a Better Thesis or Report*, Melbourne University Press, Melbourne.

Evans, J. 1994, The art of writing successful research abstracts', *Neonatal Network*, vol. 13, no. 5, 49–52.

Foreman, M. & Kirchhoff, K. 1987, 'Accuracy of references in nursing journals', *Research in Nursing and Health*, vol. 10, 177–83.

Gething, L. 1995, *How to Manage Research Effectively*, The Sydney Nursing Research Centre, The Faculty of Nursing, The University of Sydney, Sydney.

Gosling, P. 1999, *Scientist's Guide to Poster Presentations*, Kluwer Academic/Plenum Publishers, New York.

Greenwood, J. 1998, 'The "write advice" or "how to get a journal article published"', *Contemporary Nurse*, vol. 7, no. 2, 84–90.

Hildon, A. 1994, 'Gender bias in cardiology: are women missing out on PCTA?', *Australian Journal of Advanced Nursing*, vol. 12, no. 1, 6–11.

Jackson, K. & Sheldon, L. 2000, 'Demystifying the academic aura: preparing a poster', *Nurse Researcher*, vol. 7, no. 3, 70–3.

Kemmis, S. & McTaggart, R. (eds) 1988, *The Action Research Planner*, 3rd edn, Deakin University Press, Geelong, Australia.

Maltby, H. & Serrell, M. 1998, 'The art of poster presentation', *Collegian*, vol. 5, no. 2, 36–7.

McCann, S., Sramac, R. & Rudy, S. 1999, 'The poster exhibit: guidelines for planning, development, and presentation', *Dermatology Nursing*, vol. 11, no. 5, 373–9.

Plawecki, H. & Plawecki, J. 1998, 'Writing for publication: understanding the process', *Journal of Holistic Nursing*, vol. 16, no. 1, 23–32.

Polit, D. & Hungler, B. 1995, *Nursing Research, Principles and Methods*, 5th edn, Lippincott, Philadelphia.

Roberts, K., McEwan, B. & Paynter, C. 2000, 'A comparison of kangaroo mother care and conventional cuddling', *Neonatal Network*, vol. 19, no. 4, 31–5.

Roberts, K. & Taylor, B. 1998, *Nursing Research Processes: an Australian Perspective*, Nelson ITP, Melbourne.

Robertson, J. 1994, 'Disseminating findings', in *Handbook of Clinical Nursing Research*, ed. J. Robertson, Churchill Livingstone, Melbourne.

Russell, C., Gregory, D. & Gates, M. 1996, 'Aesthetics and substance in qualitative research posters', *Qualitative Health Research*, vol. 6, no. 4, 542–52.

Taylor, B. 2000a, *Reflective Practice: A Guide for Nurses and Midwives*, Allen and Unwin, Melbourne.

Taylor, B. 2000b, Improving the practice of hospital nursing through reflective practice and action research, unpublished research report, School of Nursing and Health Practices, Southern Cross University, Lismore, NSW.

Taylor, B. (in press), 'Identifying and transforming dysfunctional nurse–nurse relationships though reflective practice and action research', *International Journal of Nursing Practice*.

Taylor, B., King, V. & Stewart, J. 1995, 'Reflective midwifery practice: facilitating midwives' practice insights into using a distance education reflective practitioner model', *International Journal of Nursing Practice*, vol. 1, 26–31.

Thomas, S. 2000, *How to Write Health Sciences Papers, Dissertations and Theses*, Churchill-Livingstone, Edinburgh.

Tornquist, E. 1986, *From Proposal to Publication*, Addison-Wesley, Menlo Park, California.

Walters, D. 1999, *The Readable Thesis: Clear & Effective Writing*, Avocus Publishing, Inc., Gilsum.

Watson, J. & Crick, F. 1953, 'Molecular structure of nucleic acids: a structure for deoxyribose nucleic acid', *Nature*, vol. 171, 773–8.

Wiltshire, J. 1995, 'Telling a story, writing a narrative: terminology in health care', *Nursing Inquiry*, vol. 2, no. 2, 75–82.

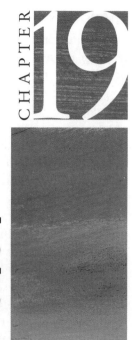

CHAPTER 19

Using nursing research

chapter objectives The material presented in this chapter will assist you to:

- discuss the status of utilisation of nursing research in clinical practice
- discuss barriers to the use of nursing research
- suggest strategies to overcome the barriers
- discuss evidence-based practice.

Introduction

In the final analysis, research must be useful in order to be of value. Nursing research is useful when it adds to nursing knowledge that nurses can apply to practice. In Chapter 1 we discussed the characteristics of nursing knowledge, so you may like to refresh your ideas about what constitutes nursing knowledge.

Nurses can enhance their practice by using nursing and health research as well as relevant research from other disciplines. For example, the health belief model (Becker 1974) explains why clients institute health-protective behaviours, and the body of research that has built up around the Self-Care Deficit Theory of Nursing (Orem 2001) explains why and how people perform self-care, what influences their self-care, and how to measure people's ability to do self-care.

Nurse–client interaction is a vital part of nursing practice. It is therefore important for us to incorporate into our practice research findings that enhance that interaction. This is particularly important in areas of nursing that deal with the emotional problems of the client, such as psychiatric nursing.

Nurses can use research evidence at any point of the nursing process. For example, in the assessment phase, we can use a protocol based on nursing research findings. In planning the care, we can make choices based on research findings. In implementing the care plan, we can choose research-based ways of giving expert care. Finally, we can use a research process in evaluating that care.

The Australian Nursing Council's Competencies for Beginning Practice have encouraged the use of nursing research in practice by including the recognition of the value of research as a nursing competency (Australian Nursing Council Inc. 2000). The Draft Competency Standards for the Advanced Nurse (Australian Nursing Federation/Department of Employment, Training and Youth Affairs 1996) include using nursing research to inform practice as a competency. The Code of Ethics for Australian Nurses incorporates a statement about nursing research (ANCI 1993).

In Chapter 1, we suggested that nursing is still in the process of developing a research culture. A research culture assumes not only the conduct of research but also its utilisation. In this chapter we want to establish that nurses do not routinely use research, explore the barriers and discuss strategies for encouraging the development of a research utilisation culture.

Applying nursing research to practice

Nurses can participate in the development of a scientific base for practice by utilising research findings and evaluating the effectiveness of specific changes in practice (Lindsey 1991). They can do this alone, but group efforts may be more productive. Mateo and Schira (1991) have proposed a model for utilising research findings in solving clinical problems, as has Kirchhoff (1991). The ideas of these writers form the basis for what follows here.

The Mateo Schira Model comprises two major phases of the process: 'delineating the problem' and 'exploring the solution'. In this model, the first step in delineating the problem is for nurses to become aware that there is a problem, such as an unsatisfactory clinical outcome or an inconsistency in practice. The next step is for the nurses to clarify the existence of the problem by discussing it with colleagues and carrying out a preliminary review of the literature. If they decide that there is a problem, the third step is the problem definition phase. The nurses now determine what is known about the problem, define which clients and/or nurses are affected by the problem and when they are affected, and identify personal and environmental factors that precipitate the problem. The next step is to define the characteristics of the intervention. Next is the resolution phase in which nurses determine whether the problem can and should be solved and how it can be solved.

The first step in the 'exploring the solution' phase is to determine how others have tried to solve the problem, including considering suggestions from colleagues. The second step is when research findings are used. Nurses locate the relevant literature and read, critique, and evaluate findings for utility in solving the problem. The research findings are evaluated to see if they are consistent. Other considerations are the applicability of the research findings to the actual situation; that is, how comparable with the setting in question are the characteristics of the settings of the research papers. The papers should also be significant and of scientific merit. Possible solutions should not be implemented if they are based only on one set of findings; that is, they should be supported by more than one study.

Next is a decision-making phase in which the clinicians evaluate the best potential solutions for applicability, feasibility and safety, including ethical aspects. Some considerations are: the compatibility of the proposed solution with institutional policies, the availability of human and financial resources, the level of administrative support, the possible effect of the timing of the proposed change, and the cost-benefit ratio. The risk of implementing the change must be compared with the risk of not implementing the change. The clinicians then select the best potential solution for implementation.

The nurses then draw up a plan for the implementation of change. It is important to secure the approval of the nursing administration and other gatekeepers and the cooperation of colleagues who will be involved in implementing the plan. It is crucial to secure the commitment of the clinical nurse consultant or nursing unit manager to implementing the change in practice.

The next step is for the nurses to communicate the plan to anyone who will be affected by the proposed change, using contact persons, fliers, organisational newsletters and other applicable media. A pilot study must be done in one unit in order to trial the implementation. They then analyse the results of the pilot study in terms of the initial patient care outcomes, the reaction of clients and staff, and the organisational considerations. They then revise the implementation plan if necessary.

After the trial and evaluation, the nurses implement the change on a wider basis throughout relevant parts of the organisation. During the implementation of the plan, it is important to encourage staff to support the project. Small incentives such as thank you notes and morning teas can be given. The contact person for the project will give ongoing formal and informal feedback to the staff involved.

Finally, the clinicians evaluate the effects of the implementation. The evaluation should determine whether or not the intervention was implemented as intended, and if not, why not (Goode 1995); and whether the proposed outcomes were achieved and whether the change was beneficial. If the change worked, it can be incorporated into the policies and procedures of the institution.

Even when the clinicians have successfully implemented the change, they must guard against becoming complacent. It is critical to continue to monitor research findings to see whether even better solutions present themselves.

Do nurses actually use nursing research?

Ideally, when confronted with a nursing practice problem, nurses would look up and utilise the research findings on that problem. Pearson and his colleagues (1997, p. 3) state that contemporary nursing is 'characterised by a large variability in practice and a serious lack of research utilisation'. They suggest that Australian nursing practice is seldom based on the best available evidence, that there is a lack of research synthesis, and that there is no evidence of systematic reviews carried out by Australian nurses. This low rate of usage is consistent with findings in the overseas literature (Capra, Houghton & Hattie 1992). However, nurses think that they do use research findings. In a study by Wright, Brown and Sloman (1996), the majority of their sample said they applied research findings to their client care, but there was no indication of how frequently this happens.

Another study in the Australian literature (Capra, Houghton & Hattie 1992) suggested that nurses are more likely to use research findings if it is easy to do so. Research findings concerning optimum pre-operative fasting periods were more likely to be applied on a ward on which nurses were given a summary of research findings to read than on a ward on which they were given the whole research report. Research findings are apparently more digestible in summary form.

Barriers to using nursing research utilisation

There are several reasons that nurses do not use nursing research in their practice. Twenty years ago, a UK researcher succinctly summarised the reasons that nurses did not use nursing research findings: they did not know about them, understand them, believe them or know how to apply them, and they were not allowed to use them (Hunt 1981). More recently in Australia, Wright, Brown and Sloman (1996) summarised the literature on nurses' stated reasons for not undertaking research or applying research findings as:

- a lack of understanding of research methodology
- the research–practice gap

- perceived irrelevance of research to practice
- primacy of the care mission
- lack of reward for application of research findings to practice
- lack of time and resources
- incompatible policies
- inflexible hospital structures.

A more recent study by Retsas and Nolan (1999) of 149 hospital nurses working in Australia found that the three most frequently cited barriers to using research were: insufficient time on the job to implement findings, insufficient time to read research and a lack of awareness of research findings.

Some of the factors that hinder research implementation are personal, some are professional, and some are institutional. In the USA, characteristics of the institution were perceived as greater barriers to research implementation than the presentability and accessibility of the research, the characteristics of the nurses or the quality of the research (Funk, Tornquist & Champagne 1991). Other papers commenting on the barriers to nursing research are Street (1995), Cavenagh and Tross (1996), Johnson (1996), McSkimming (1996), Wright, Brown and Sloman (1996) and Carroll et al. (1997).

A fundamental reason for nurses not applying research findings is that they are not aware of them because they do not read research articles. Two research studies of journal-reading habits of Australian nurses in New South Wales suggest that nurses do not read research articles very often (Nagy, Crisp & Brodie 1992; Wright, Brown & Sloman 1996). They found that few nurses read research journals and of those, few read them often. The reasons given for not reading journals were lack of easy access, insufficient time, lack of usefulness of the material and a lack of interest in research.

Another barrier to research utilisation is that nurses generally resist change. They can find all sorts of reasons that changing routines would not work in practice. A nurse at the Royal Children's Hospital in Melbourne tells of the attempt to implement the findings of the study by Birks and colleagues (1993) showing that water was as effective as gel in doing electrocardiograms. She stated 'We tried to change practice (wrote it into procedures and removed gel from ECG trolleys) ... but both nurses and doctors were resistant' (Spicer 1997).

One barrier to implementing research is that nursing research is only in its infancy in Australia. This slow development of nursing research can be attributed partly to a lack of interest in research and not having enough nurses trained in research techniques. It is also a result of a historical nursing research focus on education and the social sciences, which were the training ground for nurse-researchers prior to the relatively recent entry of nursing into the universities.

Nurses frequently lack confidence in their ability to complete research. Even those nurses who do research do not always complete their projects. Johnson (1996) reported that only three-quarters of the 68 clinical projects that had been initiated at the South Western Sydney Centre for Applied Nursing Research were completed.

Even if a study is completed, there is no guarantee that it will be published. It is widely recognised that there is not enough published clinical nursing research. Hicks (1995) found that while a majority of her sample had carried out some research, only 10 per cent had submitted it for publication. The greatest reasons for this were concern about the methodology, lack of confidence and lack of time. Few nurse-researchers who complete a project get it published in a journal (Johnson 1996).

There is a set of factors that comprise the research–practice gap. Nursing research is taught in the education system but does not make the transition to practice. There has been a historical separation of nursing education from nursing practice, which has not helped this problem. With research seen as something to be done only in the ideal world, practising clinicians have not implemented it. Clinicians think that the researchers do not address relevant problems. Researchers think that the clinicians are not asking the right questions, and even if they were, they do not understand the research process well enough to help the researchers to tackle the problems effectively (MacGuire 1990).

Another reason for the research–practice gap is the distrust of nurse clinicians for more abstract areas of knowledge, which includes nursing research. Clinicians tend to see research as an activity that fails to address their clinical problems. Since they see it as irrelevant, they do not implement it.

Clinicians may also see researchers as different from themselves. With reference to midwives, and therefore by extension to nurses, Hicks (1996, p vii) has stated that:

> Professional ideologies which promote the midwife as caring, nurturing, reactive and intuitive are not only deeply entrenched but are diametrically opposed to the stereotypic perceptions of the detached, objective, hard-nosed researcher. Consequently, for midwives to accept research as a routine part of their role means that they have to abandon, at least in part, their traditional professional persona.

Another barrier is that researchers normally write research for other researchers, and clinicians have difficulty in reading it. The emulation of scientists in a drive for professional status, and the resultant use of the scientific method by nursing researchers, has led to a tendency for researchers to express everything using research jargon. This tends to render research difficult to read if you are not a researcher. Fortunately, clinical nursing journals are now trying to improve their readers' access to research results by insisting on less emphasis on methodology and more emphasis on clinical implications. Researchers writing for clinicians can make their reports more user-friendly. They can explain the meaning of the results, identify previous studies that have contributed to their findings, and clarify the applications to practice.

Another reason for the failure to apply nursing research is that the system in which clinicians work may not encourage it. A bureaucratic system such as a hospital or other health service does not respond quickly to demands for change and promotes consistency and conformity to routine. Nurses feel powerless to change traditional practices. Furthermore, the emphasis on getting tasks done, rather than on considerations of best practice, can inhibit implementation of research findings.

Lack of time is a major barrier to implementation of research findings. Furthermore, lack of convenient access to libraries during work time does not encourage nurses to read research. The latter may change when nurses can access from computer terminals on their wards databases containing abstracted and full articles from research journals.

Strategies for encouraging research utilisation

Encouraging nurses to participate in research activities could develop a familiarity with research that might lead to more research utilisation. At the institutional level, nursing administration could offer research scholarships to apprentice a ward staff member to a researcher for one day a week as recommended by Street (1995). Time release could be provided for nurses to take part in research activities, and resources such as journal subscriptions would be a positive step.

The Australian nursing profession needs to implement some action project to encourage research utilisation in the clinical setting. There have been three major research utilisation projects in the United States in the last 25 years, aimed at teaching nurses how to use research (Lindsey 1991). One of these involved a group of nurses in developing and implementing research-based protocols concerning temperature measurement, teaching breastfeeding and pre-operative teaching. The nurses were helped to identify, read and critique relevant research findings; transfer the findings into clinical protocols; and determine if the desired outcomes occurred. One area in which nurses implemented changes successfully was temperature-taking, with the introduction of oral temperature-taking in patients with oxygen being administered by nasal prongs. The nurses involved reported increased research skills and an increase in their perception of themselves as professionals.

One of the strategies for increasing research conduct and utilisation is the setting up of professorial chairs of nursing based in, and funded by, the clinical area. Closely related is the appointment of other clinical nurse-researchers. Such appointees have the potential to provide powerful role models for increasing the utilisation of research in nursing. The actual presence of the researcher in the clinical area and resultant dialogue with clinicians is a key factor for making nursing research relevant. The clinical chairs have the responsibility for conducting clinical research that is relevant to the area and for promoting research utilisation as a part of improving clinical practice. They can also give seminars, inservice programs and workshops. They can involve the clinicians at every stage of the research projects and the clinicians can feel some ownership of the findings.

Before it is possible to implement research findings nurses must learn to read and critique research. Clinical nurse consultants or nurse-managers could promote research literacy by:

- encouraging nurses at the ward level to read research, for example by taking out a ward subscription to a relevant journal or prompting staff to go to the library during less busy periods on the ward
- encouraging nurses to attend conferences where research is presented
- encouraging research to be done on their ward or clinical area
- encouraging presentation of research results at ward inservice sessions.

However, applying strategies at the individual, ward and institutional level is not enough. We need to build encouragement of research utilisation into the system level. If we incorporated research activity and utilisation into promotion criteria, there would be some tangible reward for carrying out research, which would remove one of the most significant barriers.

Incentives at the system level are also important in promoting research utilisation. Nurses are going to have to demonstrate that they base their practice on evidence, that is, on research findings. Research findings applied to practice have had an influence on professional misconduct hearings. An expert witness giving evidence at a hearing of the New South Wales Nurses Tribunal based his evidence on sound research findings, which had an influence on the case (Shorten & Wallace 1997).

Evidence-based practice

Perhaps the most powerful influence in promoting the utilisation of research in clinical practice will be the introduction of evidence-based practice. Evidence-based practice is 'the conduct of health care according to the principle that all interventions should be based on the best currently available scientific evidence' (Shorten & Wallace 1997, p. 22). Evidence-based practice uses evidence from research, particularly experimental research, to establish sound clinical practices. Nurses must have a good grasp of the efficacy of nursing care strategies and the underpinning evidence to support them. This means adopting effective practices, questioning practices for which no evidence exists and eliminating those which have been shown to do harm. Examples of nursing practices that have been discarded when research proved them to be at best useless and at worst harmful include giving enemas during preparation for labour, some wound care practices and using soap and water massage to prevent pressure sores (Shorten & Wallace 1997).

The American medical profession began to develop evidence-based medicine 20 years ago, after a study reported that few current medical procedures had been shown by clinical trials to be effective. The evidence-based medicine movement was also stimulated by evidence of substantial variation in clinical practice patterns, increased financial pressure and the difficulty that clinicians have in incorporating rapidly evolving evidence into their practice. Evidence-based medicine has grown rapidly in the UK, Canada and the USA. It is a growth industry that has almost become a medical specialty on its own. It even has its own journal, *Evidence-Based Medicine*. However some notes of caution have been sounded. Naylor (1995) suggests that the culture of the clinician influences decisions about the value of the evidence and that there is a large area of practice for which current data are insufficient. What evidence there is may be skewed since researchers are more likely to publish positive than negative results.

However, evidence-based practice does not mean that every clinician must know every research finding to provide good care. That would be impossible, given even the inadequate amount of research that is published and the difficulty in accessing much of it. What has happened overseas and will no doubt happen here, is that committees of health professionals will review studies on certain aspects of care and develop integrated reviews of evidence.

The medical profession has set up an international initiative to facilitate the retrieval and synthesis of literature relevant to evidence-based practice. The Cochrane Collaboration is based in Oxford, England, and comprises specialised databases of systematic reviews to promote evidence-based practice. These reviews are disseminated through medical journals, CD-ROM, and the Internet (Robinson 1995). There are Cochrane Centres in various countries, including Canada, the UK, the USA and Australia. The Australasian Cochrane Centre is the result of a consortium formed between The University of Adelaide and Flinders University in Adelaide.

Nursing has been arguing for many years that it is a profession. In recent times it has used that argument to secure reasonable rates of pay. Professional status requires professional accountability. In this day of more highly informed consumers demanding the best health care, and of more legal accountability for professional practice, nurses must be able to give a rationale for their practice. This means being informed about effectiveness that has been demonstrated through research. In both clinical practice and medical education, professors of medicine now emphasise research findings as a basis for selecting the best treatment for the patient. One would expect professors of nursing to follow suit.

An important step in the foundation of evidence-based practice in nursing in Australia has been the establishment of the Joanna Briggs Institute for Evidence Based Nursing and Midwifery. It has headquarters at the Royal Adelaide Hospital and was spearheaded by Professor Alan Pearson of La Trobe University, formerly of The University of Adelaide. The Institute 'conducts primary research on the effectiveness of nursing practice; carries out systematic reviews; disseminates practice information sheets and condensed reviews; evaluates the effects of practice information on practice variability and costs; and conducts workshops on evidence based nursing in all states and territories' (Pearson, Borbasi, Fitzgerald, Kowanko, & Walsh 1997, p. 1). Every state and territory has a branch that is a consortium of universities and health care agencies. The Joanna Briggs Institute has done much to address the lack of systematic reviews identified by Pearson in the mid-1990s by producing a number of reviews. The process of systematically searching and reviewing the literature is described by Hek, Langton and Blunden (2000) for a study in England in the area of cancer nursing education.

Clinical practice guidelines

It is at the level of basic clinical practice that evidence-based practice needs to be fostered. Clinicians have problems in applying research – lack of evidence, lack of time to acquire the evidence, and a lack of research skills and experience to evaluate the evidence critically. Even if clinicians can acquire and appraise evidence, they may have difficulty in recalling it at the time it is required. This situation has led to the development of clinical practice guidelines or evidence-based protocols. They normally comprise a set of statements related to a specific condition or patient problem. Clinical practice guidelines are prepared by a committee of experts who translate the evidence into formulas for practice. Clinicians then implement the guidelines rather than distilling the research findings and making decisions based on the evidence. The latter half of the 1990s saw the development of hundreds of sets of clinical guidelines.

In Australia, the National Health and Medical Research Council has set up a preferred process for clinical practice guideline development (NHMRC 1995) and has also published clinical practice guidelines on the management of coronary heart disease (NHMRC 1996). The Joanna Briggs Institute issues regular clinical practice guidelines in the form of Best Practice Sheets. Practice matters covered so far include pressure sores, falls in hospitals and management of peripheral intravascular devices. The Joanna Briggs Institute has a website at http://www.joannabriggs.edu.au.

The criteria for prioritising and selecting a topic for development of clinical practice guidelines are:

- the condition is prevalent
- it places a burden of illness on the client
- it has potential for significant health benefits or risks
- it has relevance to local practice patterns
- there is a degree of variation in health care practice patterns
- guidelines are likely to influence change in clinical practice
- it affects costs of health care practices
- there is available sufficient high-quality evidence to support the guidelines (Browman, Levine, Mohide, Hayward, Pritchard, Gafni & Laupacis 1995).

Gyorkos and colleagues (1994) describe a model for developing clinical practice guidelines. First, the problem is formulated, including a description of the interventions to be evaluated, the process and outcome measures and the target population. The literature is then reviewed for published and unpublished studies; a process that includes the collecting of studies, the appraisal of each study, the analysis of similar studies, and the weighing-up of the overall level of evidence. Other sources of information are tapped such as routinely collected data, indirect or more peripheral evidence and expert opinion. A practice survey may be done to document current practice and its variability across settings. The evidence is evaluated and synthesised. Guidelines are then formulated, taking into account benefits, harms, costs and professional judgement of committee members. Recommendations are made as to whether an intervention should be included in practice or not.

However, when non-nursing groups impose guidelines on nursing it can be problematic. They encourage nurses to practise using a non-nursing framework and rate randomised clinical trials (RCTs) as the highest form of evidence and expert opinion as the lowest form. Enshrining clinical trials as the highest form of evidence excludes qualitative research, which is very important in answering nursing questions. Clearly, nurses should develop their own clinical practice guidelines and decide what evidence they deem is appropriate for sound practice. This requires nurses to break down the barriers preventing the implementation of research in the clinical setting, upgrading their skills concerning the consumption and practice of research, and identifying research priorities.

One problem with clinical guidelines is that they address only discrete parts of care and may be inappropriate for complex problems. It is also evident that nurses need to set up some criteria for judging the quality of nursing clinical practice guidelines. Guidelines can also provide the basis for negligence litigation and for insurance companies to refuse reimbursement for unproven treatments (Dracup 1996).

Another issue surrounding clinical practice guidelines is whether they will have the expected impact. After all, practitioners are slow to adopt other research, why would they adopt clinical practice guidelines? A study of medical practitioners' attitudes to clinical practice guidelines (Gupta, Ward & Hayward, 1997) showed that most general practitioners had positive views about the concept of clinical practice guidelines developed from evidence. However, most considered that guidelines were developed by experts who did not understand general practice. Fewer than half thought that they would improve client outcomes, and only half indicated that the guidelines had changed their practice.

Clinical guidelines have important legal implications because they can be used as a test of negligence. However, they should not be used as a recipe and carers should not suspend their clinical judgement (Tingle 1998). Tingle points out that tests for negligence are beginning to include research evidence and experts will have to include research evidence in their legal testimony. Evidence-based nursing is becoming a part of the clinical litigation process and lawyers and judges are becoming more specialist and sophisticated in the area (Tingle 1998).

Teaching nurses to be research consumers

As has been previously noted, nurses are not yet at a stage of professional development in which they naturally incorporate research findings into practice. This suggests that they have to be taught how to use research. Education is a powerful tool for teaching both students and practising clinicians about reading and using research. Students can be taught to read nursing research critically, to evaluate nursing research reports and to assess the applicability of research to practice. Nursing research is taught in most baccalaureate and graduate nursing programs in Australia. But how many go beyond the research process to address issues of using nursing research in practice? According to Horsley (1985, p. 138), some issues are:

- Who is responsible for using research in practice?
- What factors influence the use of research in practice?
- What constitutes successful utilisation of research in practice?
- Does using nursing research make a difference in practice, and if so, what difference does it make?

University educators can teach the nurse in the basic program to be aware of and to use nursing research. Nurse-lecturers can also give prominence to using research in postgraduate education aimed at producing clinicians. It is at the level of advanced practice that role modelling can have a strong influence on the behaviour of nurses.

Nurse-academics at all levels of nursing education have a responsibility to incorporate research findings into the actual material taught in the classroom, the nursing laboratory and the clinical area. Student must be required to include research findings in assignments such as care plans and case studies, as well as more theoretical assignments. Lecturers can encourage students to get in the habit of reading research material by assigning articles to read rather than books, as most research material is in journals rather than in books. However, basic nursing textbooks are now including some research findings to support their material and to give examples of relevant nursing research. For example, Crisp and Taylor's 2001 Australian adaptation of Potter and Perry's *Fundamentals of Nursing* includes numerous research highlights that incorporate implications for practice.

Unfortunately, teaching research utilisation in the classroom alone will not achieve the objective of turning nurses into research consumers. What happens in the actual practice situation is a far more powerful influence on behaviour than what happens in the classroom. Nurses tend to follow the practice of their colleagues in the wards. Since many of these colleagues have never been interested in research, they have socialised other nurses into ignoring research findings. Strategies for increasing nurses' awareness about research findings include: performing computer literature searches to identify relevant material; sharing of research abstracts, articles, and literature reviews; and the formation of journal clubs – discussion groups that meet to talk about research articles.

Summary

We have discussed in this chapter the reality that Australian nurses, like their overseas counterparts, do not read research and do not implement research findings in practice. The reasons for this vary, but they comprise such factors as: lack of interest, the difficulty in changing established routines in institutions, and the absence of professional rewards for the effort involved. In the future, the demand for evidence-based practice may provide a powerful stimulus for encouraging nurses to use research in practice.

Main points

- Health research must be useful in order to be of value. It should add to nursing knowledge that nurses can apply in practice. It may be supplemented by relevant research from other disciplines.
- In its current state, nursing practice is seldom based on the best available research evidence; there is a lack of research synthesis and there are few systematic reviews carried out by Australian nurses.
- Nurses think that they do use research findings and they are more likely to use research findings if it is easy to do so.
- Nurses who do not use research do not do so because they do not understand research methods; they see research as irrelevant to practice; they lack time, resources, and incentives; and they are restricted by hospital policies and structures.
- Evidence-based practice is 'the conduct of health care according to the principle that all interventions should be based on the best currently available scientific evidence' (Shorten & Wallace 1997).
- Evidence-based nursing is promoted by the Joanna Briggs Institute for Evidence-based Nursing and Midwifery, located in Adelaide. JBI conducts reviews and develops Best Practice Sheets, or clinical guidelines.
- Clinical practice guidelines are policies, protocols and clinical standards that provide guidance for good practice, where possible based on research evidence, but which may also take account of current practice and expert opinion (Duff, Kitson, Seers & Humphris 1996).
- The value and need to apply research is recognised by Australian nursing organisations including the Australian Nursing Council Inc., the Australian Nursing Federation and the Royal College of Nursing, Australia.
- Research findings can be used at any point of the nursing process.
- The Mateo Schira Model describes the process of utilising research findings in clinical practice.
- Health care institutions can encourage evidence-based practice by building it into job descriptions and criteria for job promotion, offering research scholarships and providing time release and resources for nurses to take part in research activities
- Clinical nurse consultants can encourage nurses to read research, provide reading material on the ward, encourage their staff to go to the library during less busy periods, encourage nurses to attend conferences where research is presented, encourage research to be done on the ward and facilitate presentation of research results at ward inservice sessions.
- Universities need to establish more chairs of clinical research, increase the number of nurses with research degrees, provide research training for clinicians and teach undergraduate students about evidence-based practice and how to 'do' it.
- To promote research utilisation, the profession needs to gain control of nursing research funding and use it to develop a larger research base with more clinical researcher positions and more joint clinical/research appointments.

Review Questions

1. Nurses can apply research to practice:
   a at every stage of the nursing process
   b only if it is nursing research
   c only in a limited number of settings
   d in all of the above cases

2. Barriers to research utilisation include:
   a realising that they do not use nursing research
   b lack of time
   c belief that it is irrelevant
   d b and c

3. The completion rate for clinical nursing research projects was shown at one hospital to be:
   a one-quarter
   b one-half
   c two-thirds
   d three-quarters

4. The proportion of completed nursing research submitted for publication has been estimated at:
   a 10%
   b 25%
   c 50%
   d 66%

5. Evidence-based practice:
   a was begun by the medical profession
   b applies to nursing and other allied health professions
   c fosters application of research to practice
   d incorporates all of the above

6. Reviews of evidence:
   a consider qualitative studies as the highest form of evidence
   b gather evidence from all published works on the topic
   c are conducted by centres for evidence-based practice
   d b and c

7. The evidence-based nursing and midwifery centre in Australia is the:
   a Florence Nightingale Centre
   b Lucy Osborne Centre
   c Joanna Briggs Institute
   d Alan Pearson Centre

8   Criteria for prioritising and selecting a topic for development of clinical practice guidelines include:
    a   the condition is rare but important
    b   practice patterns are uniform
    c   it must be universally applicable
    d   it has potential for significant financial benefits
9   Clinical guidelines:
    a   apply to all clients
    b   may be inappropriate for complex problems
    c   always encourage use of a nursing framework
    d   are unbiased
10 Factors comprising the research–practice gap include:
    a   historical separation of research and education
    b   clinicians believing researchers do not address relevant problems
    c   researchers believing clinicians are not asking the right questions
    d   all of the above

Discussion Questions

1   Is nursing a research-based profession? Discuss.
2   Describe the process of applying research to practice.
3   Discuss strategies for encouraging research utilisation.
4   Discuss the criteria for clinical practice guidelines.
5   How can nurses be encouraged to be research consumers?

References

Australian Nursing Council, Inc. 1993, *Code of Ethics for Nurses in Australia*, ANCI Canberra.
Australian Nursing Council, Inc. 2000, *National Competencies for the Registered and Enrolled Nurse*, ANCI, Canberra.
Australian Nursing Federation and the Department of Employment, Education, Training and Youth Affairs 1996, *Draft Competency Standards for the Advanced Practice Nurse*, ANF/DEETYA, Canberra.
Becker, M. 1974, 'The health belief model and sick role behavior', *Health Education Monographs*, vol. 2, 409.
Birks, M., Santamaria, N., Thompson, S. & Amerena, J. 1993, 'A clinical trial of the effectiveness of water as a conductive medium in electrocardiography', *Australian Journal of Advanced Nursing*, vol. 10, no. 2, 10–13.
Browman, G., Levine, M., Mohide, E., Hayward, R., Pritchard, K., Gafni, A. & Laupacis, A. 1995, 'The practice guidelines development cycle: a conceptual tool for practice guidelines development and implementation', *Journal of Clinical Oncology*, vol. 13, no. 2, 502–12.
Capra, M., Houghton, S. & Hattie, J. 1992, 'RNs' utilisation of research findings', *Australian Journal of Advanced Nursing*, vol. 10, no. 1, 21–5.

Carroll, D., Greenwood, R., Lynch, K., Sullivan, J., Ready, C. & Fitzmaurice, J. 1997, 'Barriers and facilitators to the utilisation of nursing research', *Clinical Nurse Specialist*, vol. 11, no. 5, 207–12.

Cavenagh, S. & Tross, G. 1996, 'Utilizing research findings in nursing: policy and practice considerations', *Journal of Advanced Nursing*, vol. 24, 1083–8.

Crisp, J. & Taylor, C. 2001, *Potter and Perry's Fundamentals of Nursing*, Harcourt, Sydney.

Dracup, K. 1996, 'Clinical practice guidelines', *Nursing*, 96, 41–6.

Duff, L., Kitson, A., Seers, K. & Humphris, D. 1996, 'Clinical guidelines: an introduction to their development and implementation', *Journal of Advanced Nursing*, vol. 23, no. 5, 887–95.

Funk, S., Tornquist, E. & Champagne, M. 1991, 'Barriers and facilitators of research utilization', *Nursing Clinics of North America*, vol. 30, no. 3, 395–407.

Goode, C. 1995, 'Evaluation of research-based nursing practice', *Nursing Clinics of North America*, vol. 30, no. 3, 421–8.

Gupta, L., Ward, J. & Hayward, R. 1997, 'Clinical practice guidelines in general practice: a national survey of recall, attitudes and impact', *Medical Journal of Australia*, vol. 166 (20 January), 69–72.

Gyorkos, T., Tannenbaum, T., Abrahamowicz, M., Oxman, A., Scott, E., Millson, M., Rasooly, I., Frank, J., Riben, P., Mathias, R. & Best, A. 1994, 'An approach to the development of practice guidelines for community health interventions', *Canadian Journal of Public Health*, vol. 85 (Supplement 1), S8–S13.

Hek, G., Langton, J. & Blunden, G. 2000, 'Systematically searching and reviewing the literature', *Nurse Researcher*, vol. 7, no. 3, 40–57.

Hicks, C. 1995, 'The shortfall in published research: a study of nurses' research and publication activities', *Journal of Advanced Nursing*, vol. 21, 594–604.

Hicks, C. 1996, U*ndertaking Midwifery Research*. Edinburgh: Churchill-Livingstone.

Horsley, J. 1985, 'Using nursing research in practice: the current context', *Western Journal of Nursing Research*, vol. 7, no. 1, 135–9.

Hunt, J. 1981, 'Indicators for nursing practice, the use of research findings', *Journal of Advanced Nursing*, vol. 6, 189–94.

Johnson, M. 1996, 'Australian clinical nursing research, where is it all?' *Australian Journal of Advanced Nursing*, vol. 13, no. 4, 4.

Kirchhoff, K. 1991, 'Strategies in research utilization', in *Conducting and Using Nursing Research in the Clinical Setting*, eds M. Mateo & K. Kirchhoff, Williams & Wilkins, Baltimore.

Lindsey, A. 1991, 'Integrating research and practice', in *Conducting and Using Nursing Research in the Clinical Setting*, eds M. Mateo & K. Kirchhoff, Williams & Wilkins, Baltimore.

MacGuire, J. 1990, 'Putting nursing research findings into practice: research utilization as an aspect of the management of change', *Journal of Advanced Nursing*, vol. 15, 614–20.

Mateo, M. & Schira, M. 1991, 'Exploring innovative ways in giving nursing care', in *Conducting and Using Nursing Research in the Clinical Setting*, eds M. Mateo & K. Kirchhoff, Williams & Wilkins, Baltimore.

McSkimming, S. 1996, 'Creating a cultural norm for research and research utilization in a clinical agency', *Western Journal of Nursing Research*, vol. 18, no. 5, 606–10.

Nagy, S., Crisp, J. & Brodie, L. 1992, 'Journal reading practices of RNs in NSW public hospitals', *Australian Journal of Advanced Nursing*, vol. 9, no. 2, 29–33.

Naylor, C. 1995, 'Grey zones of clinical practice: some limits to evidence-based medicine', *Lancet*, vol. 345 (1 April 1995), 840–2.

National Health & Medical Research Council 1995, *Guidelines for the Development and Implementation of Clinical Practice Guidelines*, Australian Government Publishing Service, Canberra.

National Health & Medical Research Council 1996, *Clinical Practice Guidelines for the Procedural and Surgical Management of Coronary Heart Disease*, Australian Government Publishing Service, Canberra.

Orem, D. 2001, *Nursing: Concepts of Practice*, 6th edn, CV Mosby, St Louis.

Pearson, A., Borbasi, S., Fitzgerald, M., Kowanko, I. & Walsh, K. 1997, Evidence-based nursing: an examination of nursing within the international evidence based health care practice movement. Discussion Paper No. 1, Royal College of Nursing Australia, supplement to *Nursing Review*, February.

Retsas, A. & Nolan, M. 1999, 'Barriers to nurses' use of research: an Australian hospital study', *International Journal of Nursing Studies*, vol. 36, no. 4, 335–43.

Robinson, A. 1995, 'Research, practice and the Cochrane Collaboration', *Canadian Medical Association Journal*, vol. 152, no. 6, 882–9.

Shorten, A. & Wallace, M. 1997, 'Evidence based practice: the future is clear', *Australian Nursing Journal*, vol. 4, no. 6, 22–4.

Spicer, M. 26 February 1997, Re: ECG. *NURSRES: Discussion list for nurse researchers*. (*NURSRES* is an on-line email list of nurses. This information was emailed to the author.)

Street, A. 1995, *Nursing Replay: Researching Nursing Culture Together*, Churchill-Livingstone, Melbourne.

Tingle, J. 1998, 'Developing clinical guidelines: present and future legal aspects', *British Journal of Nursing*, vol. 7, no. 11, 672–4.

Wright, A., Brown, P. & Sloman, R. 1996, 'Nurses' perceptions of the value of nursing research for practice', *Australian Journal of Advanced Nursing*, vol. 13, no. 4, 15–18.

Glossary

abstract A concise summary of a research report, preceding the report.

action research A qualitative critical research methodology that involves action cycles of collectively planning, acting, observing and reflecting.

affirmative postmodernism While agreeing with the critique of modernity, affirmative postmodernists have a more hopeful, optimistic view of the postmodern age in that they do not abandon the author completely, but they reduce the author's authority, offer options for public debate and allow researchers as the authors of projects to offer tentative insights for readers' interpretations and discussion.

agent or **agency** In postmodernism, someone assumed to have authority and power.

aims Overall intentions for the research.

analysis A method that involves reviewing research data systematically with the intention of sorting and classifying them into representational groups and patterns.

analysis of variance A statistical test that determines whether there is a significant difference in the mean scores of different groups on a dependent variable.

anonymity Concealment or obscuring of the identity of participants in a study.

applied research Research that concerns the application of knowledge to specific situations.

archival information Data for historical research which consists of original hard copies of treasured documents such as logs, diaries, government agencies' agendas and minutes, reports, photo-graphs, newspapers, books, and private papers donated by families to the archives.

artistic expression In qualitative research this is direct and creative demonstration of the participant's experiences through artistic expression, such as painting, drawing, montage, photography, poetry, dance, music, symbols, and singing, which may be collected as data.

assumptions of feminisms Certain key ideas that underlie feminisms, specifically that women are dominated and oppressed by masculinist structures and processes, and that women have the potential for being free from these constraints.

auditability A means of ensuring rigour in qualitative research, which involves the production of a decision trail that can be scrutinised by other researchers to determine the extent to which the project has achieved consistency in its methods and processes.

author In postmodernism, a person who creates a text, or is responsible for an outcome.

basic research Research that develops fundamental knowledge and tests theory.

bibliographic referencing system A computer program that allows the compilation of a library of references and the insertion of citations automatically in the text, with automatic referencing at the end of the document.

case study A research method that focuses on describing fully selected phenomena of interest over time, such as individuals in groups or institutions.

CD-ROM A compact disk with read-only memory on which a large amount of information is stored, for use in a computer.

cell The intersection of a row and a column in a table.

chi square A statistical test that determines within-group relationships on nominal variables.

CINAHL Cumulative Index of Nursing and Allied Health Literature – a database of published articles in the nursing and health field.

citation Reference in a text to another work.

clinical practice guidelines Evidence-based protocols for practice, comprising a set of statements related to a specific condition or patient problem.

code book Document containing a record of the codes used, and/or the placement of the data in a database.

coding Process that usually renders the data into numbers that can be entered into a database in a form in which they can be readily analysed.

coercion Obtaining of research participants through their fear that harm will befall them if they do not enter the study.

colour coding method of analysis In qualitative research, this is a method whereby words, ideas, sections, and/or nuances that appear to be connected ideas and themes are marked in colour codes for organisation into discrete categories.

comparative descriptive design Design in which two or more groups are being compared on particular variables.

computer-assisted analyses In qualitative research, this refers to using a computer solely, or in conjunction with a manual thematic method of analysis.

concept Abstract generalised idea that describes a phenomenon or a group of related phenomena.

conceptual framework Structure that forms a framework for a study, using concepts.

confirmability A means of ensuring rigour in qualitative research, whereby a project demonstrates that it has achieved credibility, auditability and fittingness.

congruency In qualitative research this means the correspondence, agreement or fit between foundational ideas and the activity phases of the research.

content analysis In quantitative research, content analysis means a numerical description of the appearance of specific ideas or expressions in a body of communications that use language.

context In qualitative research this means the set of features specific to a particular setting – including the place, time and circumstances – which need to be taken into account when undertaking research.

control group Group in an experiment that is exposed to everything that the experimental group is exposed to, except the treatment being tested.

convenience sample Sample that uses any available elements of the population that meet the criteria to enter the study.

core story creation A process of creating the essential features of a story ready for emplotment.

correlational design Design that examines the relationship of variables within one group without aiming to determine cause and effect.

counterbalanced design Design that attempts to achieve control by entering all subjects into all treatments.

covert observation Observation in which the person is not aware of being observed.

confidentiality Protection of the identity of research participants.

correlation coefficient Number that indicates the direction and strength of a relationship between two numerical variables.

credibility Means of ensuring rigour in qualitative research, whereby participants and readers of the research recognise the lived experiences described in the research as similar to their own.

critical discourse analyses In qualitative critical methodologies, these are the methods whereby language is submitted to a systematic critique of the personal, economic, political, cultural, social and historical determinants that shaped it.

critical ethnography A qualitative critical methodology which has the exploratory and descriptive mission of an ethnography, and the emancipatory aims of critical research approaches.

critical hermeneutics A qualitative critical methodology which has a commitment to understanding and exposing how power imbalances and misunderstandings constrain and distort interpretations.

critical research Qualitative critical methodologies which aim to bring about change through socio-political critique of the status quo.

critique Balanced assessment of both the positive and negative qualities of a research report, developed through a process of critical appraisal.

deconstruction A postmodern method of analysis that tears a text apart to reveal its contradictions, but not with the intention of improving, revising, or offering a better text.

Delphi technique Special questionnaire survey method of obtaining and analysing a range of expert opinions on a topic or issue without having a face-to-face meeting of the group, usually involving several rounds of the questionnaire.

dependent variable The variable that is hypothesised to be affected by the independent variable; the outcome variable.

descriptive design A research design that results in the portrayal of a phenomenon, person or group.

Dewey decimal classification A numbering reference system for locating books in libraries, using a three-number prefix, a decimal point and a multi-number suffix.

directional hypothesis An hypothesis that speculates about the direction that the findings will take.

discipline The status assigned to those areas of inquiry which can demonstrate that their knowledge constitutes something unique from other areas of knowledge interests.

discourse analysis Systematic and thorough questioning about the knowledge and power inherent in all kinds of spoken and written life texts, in relation to one another, in order to interpret patterns, rules, assumptions, contradictions, silences, consequences, implications and inconsistencies in the discourse.

discourses In postmodernism, groups of ideas or patterned ways of thinking, writing and speaking immersed in social structures that constitute power and knowledge relationships.

domain concepts These are the main ideas that form the basis of a complex construct; for example, the domain concepts of nursing are person, health, environment and nursing.

electronic journal Journal published only on the Internet.

electronic scanner Computer attachment that will scan or read text and print it into an electronic format.

emancipation In qualitative critical methodologies aiming for freedom, emancipatory research processes assist in freeing participants from their present conditions to something better.

emancipatory action research A form of action research that involves a group of practitioners taking responsibility for freeing themselves from the constraints of their practice through understanding and transforming the political, social and economic conditions that constrain them.

embodiment Humans living a life in a body, thereby having the capacity for embodied knowledge.

empirico-analytical research Research that is interested in observation and analysis using the principles of the scientific method.

empirics The science of nursing derived from empirico-analytical means.

emplotment A form of narrative analysis involving searching carefully through text in tracking plots, eventually to locate sets of events that are common to all stories.

empowerment A process of giving and accepting power.

epistemology The study of knowledge and how it is judged to be 'true'; whenever nurses raise questions about what they know, and how they know it is trustworthy, they are asking epistemological questions.

equivalent control group pre-test/post-test design A design that features random allocation of subjects to the control and experimental groups, pre-testing both groups on the dependent variable, giving the treatment to the experimental group but not the control group, and measurement of the dependent variable on a post-test.

ethnography A research approach that provides a 'portrait of people' by describing and raising awareness of a group of people's cultural characteristics, such as their shared symbols, beliefs, values, rituals and patterns of behaviour.

evidence-based practice The use of research findings, particularly experimental research, to establish sound clinical practices.

experiment A research design in which subjects are exposed to some event, or treatment, and their response to that treatment is measured to gauge the effect of the treatment on the subjects; a design that attempts to show whether one thing causes another.

experimenter effect An effect caused by the experimenter consciously or unconsciously affecting the results by a behaviour.

external validity The extent to which the findings of a study can be generalised, or applied, to the population.

extraneous variable A variable that may affect the outcome but is not central to the research question.

factorial design A design involving the measuring of two or more independent variables on a dependent variable.

feminisms Research methodologies that are concerned with women's issues and lives.

fieldwork Data collection where the action is happening out in the 'field' of inquiry, comprising combinations of observation, participation, documentation and analysis to study a culture or other phenomenon of interest 'on the inside', with the intention of capturing the thickest possible description of what is happening, to whom, when, why, how and where.

fittingness A means of ensuring rigour in qualitative research, whereby a determination is made of the extent to which a project's findings fit into other contexts outside the study setting.

flaming Destructive personal criticism sent on the Internet.

focus group A group of people who combine to work systematically on specific objectives, allowing each member to have a voice in the process and the outcomes.

frequency distribution A description of the distribution of the components in a group, giving sums and percentages.

gatekeeper A person in the research setting who can control access to participants.

'goodness' In postmodern terms, a process beyond trustworthiness that attempts to avoid definitions of rigour, based on the assumption that 'truth' is out there, waiting to be discovered, harnessed, and applied to problems of explanation, prediction and control in the human world.

grand theories (narratives) Grand theories and paradigms that are rejected by postmodernists as statements claiming universal truth that can be applied in all like cases.

grounded theory A research approach starting from the 'ground' of an area of human interest and working up in an inductive fashion to make sense of what people say about their experiences, then converting these statements into theoretical propositions.

Hawthorne effect The effect on the results when people behave differently if they know they are being watched.

hegemony In critical social science this means ascendancy or domination of one power over another in some social systems, which gives the people oppressed within those systems the impression that the dominant force is unassailable.

hermeneutics Processes of interpretation.

histogram Graphic representation of components in a group, showing size of components by length of bars.

historical research Qualitative research which seeks to discover new knowledge about what has happened in times past, in relation to specific portions of time and foci of interest. In nursing literature the term 'historiography' is synonymous with historical research.

history Events that happen during the course of the study that may affect the study results.

human research ethics committee A committee that deals with ethical matters pertaining to research on human participants.

hypothesis A statement of what the researcher thinks is going to be the outcome of the investigation.

IMRAD system A way of organising a research report that uses the sections Introduction, Method, Results, and Discussion.

in vitro **measurement** A measurement that is done on a sample taken from the participant, but analysed after it has been removed from the participant.

in vivo **measurement** A measurement taken directly on the participant, the value being obtained at the time of measurement.

independent groups *t*-test A statistical test that determines whether there is a significant difference in two different groups' means on the same variable.

independent variable A variable that can be manipulated by the researcher.

integrity In relation to data storage, this refers to safe means for keeping data stored in such a way that they are maintained in their best state for use and possible review.

internal validity The extent to which a study measures what it is supposed to be measuring and the effects measured are therefore attributable to the manipulation of the independent variable.

interpretation In qualitative research this involves working with forms of analysed information to make sense out of them so that statements can be made about what they mean in light of the intentions, methods and processes of the research.

interpretations In qualitative research these are the meanings made out of the research which may be referred to as theories, findings, results, insights, strategies, implications, examples of reflective awareness, changed practice, and so on, depending on the methodology used.

interpretive research Qualitative research methodologies which aim mainly to generate meaning; that is, they try to explore, explain and describe, in order to make sense out of things of interest.

intertextuality In postmodernism, this refers to infinitely complex and unending interwoven interrelation-ships that do not arrive at an end-point or consensus.

interval scale A scale in which the elements are constructed in equal intervals.

interviews In qualitative research these are more like conversations than interrogations and they can be based on questioning which is structured, unstructured or semi-structured.

journalling A form of data collection using reflective writing.

keyword A term that is used to describe an article and that is used in computerised database searching for references.

knowledge Knowing or familiarity gained by the senses.

language In qualitative research words are the main symbols from which meaning is derived.

level of confidence The degree to which the researcher is confident that the results are statistically significant and that the findings could not have occurred by chance alone.

Library of Congress system A referencing system for locating material in libraries, using a combination of letters and numbers.

Likert scale A scale on which respondents rank their attitudes or opinions on a continuum of response from strongly agree to strongly disagree.

literature The total body of writing that deals with the topic being researched.

lived experience The knowledge humans have of how it is to live a life in regard to being someone or something unique in everyday situations.

logbook A written record of the processes and/or products of the research project.

longitudinal design A design in which data are collected at intervals over a long period to see whether a phenomenon changes over time.

manual method of thematic analysis In qualitative research analysis, this is a systematic non-computer means of organising data that allows researchers to locate the finer nuances and themes not conveyed in verbally explicit ways.

maturation Growth or change of participants during a study in such a way as to affect the results.

'maxi' ethnography An ethnography with a large focus, for example, for comparisons between nursing practices in different countries or clinical settings, or nursing care of specific cultural groups.

mean The average score of a group of scores.

measurement The determination of the size or range of an object, characteristic or phenomenon.

median The middle score in a group of scores.

member check A procedure used within qualitative research methods to ensure that participants validate their contributions to the overall project, as a source of determining the trustworthiness of the project.

meta-analysis The analysis of multiple research reports to integrate and synthesise the findings on a particular topic.

metaparadigm The fundamental ideas of a discipline on which its knowledge is founded. In nursing the domain concepts are person, health, environment and nursing.

methods The ways by which new knowledge is collected and analysed, which can include controlled trials, interviews, surveys, questionnaires, observation, field notes, historical documents and so on.

microfiche A transparent plastic card with a large amount of information printed on it that you can read using a special magnifier.

'mini' ethnography An ethnography with small and local focus, for example, for framing questions about people and their practices.

mode The most frequently occurring score in a group of scores.

model A structure that represents objects, phenomena or concepts.

monograph A small book, which is usually a soft-cover, A5-size document containing approximately 50 pages.

mortality The dropping out of participants from the study in sufficient numbers to affect the results.

narrative In narrative methodology, a scheme of multiple stories that organises events and human actions into a whole.

narratives In postmodernism, views or stories. Postmodernists are opposed to grand/meta-narratives or world views based on claims to legitimise their 'truth'; however, mini/micro/local/traditional narratives as stories making no truth claims are more acceptable.

naturalistic setting A place in which people carry out naturally whatever phenomenon is under investigation.

netiquette A set of guidelines for behaviour when on the Internet.

nominal scale A scale comprising named categories.

non-equivalent control group design A quasi-experimental design that uses a control group but uses groups that either have already been established or are going to be established but not randomly.

non-probability sampling Sampling in which subjective judgements contribute to the selection of the sample.

normal curve A bilaterally symmetric curve that shows the distribution of data.

NUD*IST (Non-Numerical Unstructured Data: Indexing Searching & Theorising) A qualitative research computer package that provides a sophisticated word search to locate and analyse contextually specific text.

null hypothesis An hypothesis that does not predict a direction for the findings.

NURSRES An Internet list of nurses interested in research who communicate with each other by email.

objectives These are specific statements that are subsets of the overall intentions of the research.

one group – pre-test post-test design A design in which a pre-test and post-test are both done but the measurements are made on one group only.

one-shot case study A design in which the effect of an event, a phenomenon, administration of a substance, or other treatment is tested on a group after it has occurred.

ontology The study of existence itself; whenever nurses are asking about the nature of the existence of something or someone in nursing, they are asking ontological questions.

optical character recognition (OCR) A technology that enables the scanning of a document into a word processing file on the computer.

oral history A form of qualitative research in which oral evidence is gathered from a primary source whose accounts act as raw historical data that can stand alone or be synthesised with other sources to provide a picture of the past in people's own words.

ordinal scale A scale in which the elements are ranked numerically or on some criterion.

overt observation Observation of a participant who is aware of the observation.

paired (one-group) *t*-test A statistical test that compares two readings for each participant on the same variable.

paradigm A broad view or perspective of something, which may be referred to as a 'world view'.

participant observation Being involved in the action in a setting, whilst observing the details within it.

phenomenology ('phenomen-ology') The 'study of things' within human existence, by discovering, exploring and describing the essence of phenomena through attending towards them directly.

phenomenon Something that happens that can be perceived directly by the senses.

pie chart A figure showing the proportions of sub-groups in a group by showing a circle divided into 'pieces of pie' that are proportional to the sizes of the sub-groups.

'pile on the kitchen table' method A form of qualitative manual analysis in which sections of text are cut from a working text document and moved and organised into groupings until the essential features of themes are located.

pilot study A miniature replica of the planned research strategy, a trial run or a dress rehearsal for the main study, incorporating all aspects of the procedures of the main study.

placebo A substance that has no physical effect but mimics the experimental treatment.

placebo effect The effect on a person's mind or body from a belief that a treatment works, resulting in artificially high ratings of the effectiveness of the treatment.

population A group whose members have specific common characteristics of interest.

poststructuralism A methodology between critical social science and postmodernism, which focuses on discourses and discursive practices constituting power relations and knowledge.

post-test only, control group design A design using two groups, a control and experimental group, with a post-test given to both groups.

practical action research A form of action research that aims to improve existing practices and to develop new ones, by reflecting on taking deliberate strategic action.

practice discipline A specific label attached to those disciplines that are concerned with the development of professional knowledge and skills.

praxis Change through deliberate and systematic critical reflection on practice.

pre-experimental design A design that does not use a control group.

primary sources References to papers that are written by the author, as opposed to papers that are cited.

privacy The right of participants to decide which information they wish to disclose.

probability The likelihood that a finding could have occurred by chance.

probability sample A sample that attempts to portray the population in miniature.

process In qualitative research this refers to the 'how' of research, especially in relation to how the people in the research relate to one another.

pseudonym A false name by which a research participant is known to hide her or his identity.

Q-sort A method in which the researcher gives a participant a deck of cards containing items, and asks the participant to sort the cards according to pre-determined criteria.

qualitative data Information as words and language which can offer new and revised knowledge to researchers, through deep and rich descriptions of context, lived experience, subjectivity and potential for change.

qualitative interview A conversation designed to encourage participants to tell their stories and relate their experiences in the deepest and richest way possible, through clear guidance on what is required, a genuine invitation to speak, and communicative facilitation on the part of the researcher.

qualitative research A research paradigm that is interested in questions which involve human consciousness and subjectivity and value humans and their experiences in the research process.

quantitative research A process that attempts to find out scientific knowledge by measurement of elements.

quasi-experimental design An experimental design that does not have random allocation to control and experimental groups.

questionnaire A document containing questions to which a participant responds.

random sample A sample drawn at random from the target population.

range A number that reflects how spread out the scores are in a group of scores.

rating scale A scale on which respondents are asked to rate how often they carry out a behaviour, with responses ranging from never to always.

ratio scale An interval scale in which there is a true zero that is an absence of the element.

reader In postmodernism, the observer, who is given the power of interpreting the text; thus postmodernists empower the reader over the author.

reading In postmodernism, this refers to understanding and interpretation and it may be 'my reading', 'your reading' or 'a reading' without judgement of adequacy or validity of the said reading.

re-coding The process of altering data by changing the values, applying a weighting or executing a mathematical formula.

refereed journal A journal that requires its articles to have been refereed or critiqued by peers before publishing them.

refereed journal article An article that has been sent out for peer review before being accepted for publication.

relativity In relation to truth, this means that truth is elusive and can change according to all kinds of context-dependent determinants associated with the people, places, times and conditions with whom and in which it resides and from which it emerges.

replication Repeating a study using the same methodology.

research A careful search or inquiry, a course of critical investigation.

research design An account of the details of the methodology to be used in the study to answer the research question.

research plan In qualitative research this includes information about the study setting, participants and methods, and it also involves a description of the underlying methodological assumptions guiding the project.

research proposal A written account of the plan for the research project, presenting an argument as to why a particular problem should be investigated and what the appropriate methodology is to investigate it.

research question An explicit query about a problem or issue that can be challenged, examined and analysed and that will yield useful new information.

research summary See **abstract**.

review of the literature Reading, sorting and analysing the body of literature, then critiquing it and putting it into some kind of order.

rigour Strictness in judgement and conduct which must be used to ensure that the successive steps in a project have been set out clearly and undertaken with scrupulous attention to detail.

sample A part of the population that is studied, having been selected on some criterion.

scale A method that asks a respondent to rate an item on a numerical basis.

scientific method A set of rules for how to do research that can be considered to be rigorous.

scientific misconduct An act of deception or misrepresentation of one's own scientific work.

search engine A tool that will search the Internet for websites.

secondary sources Papers to which an author refers.

security In relation to data storage this means that data are stored according to agreed guidelines.

selection effect An effect resulting from non-random selection of participants from the comparison groups.

self-report A method of obtaining data directly from the participants in the study, using them as informants.

semantic differential scale A scale that asks the respondents to rate their response to an item using a bipolar pair of adjectives.

serendipitous finding A result that is unexpected, usually positive.

setting A place in which the researcher carries out the study and in which the phenomenon of interest can be observed.

simple descriptive design A design that measures known variables in a population or portrays the characteristics of participants.

skeptical postmodernism A pessimistic, negative, gloomy assessment which argues that the postmodern age is one of fragmentation, disintegration, malaise, meaninglessness, a vagueness or even absence of moral parameters and societal chaos, in which authors use their authority as writers to control and censure readers.

skew The distortion in a data curve resulting from unbalanced data.

Solomon four-groups design A special type of experimental design using two control groups and two experimental groups. One control and one experimental group are given the pre-test and the other two are not.

special participants Persons who have a diminished ability to give informed consent and are therefore at risk of exploitation.

standard deviation A number that is calculated from the data to show the amount of dispersion in the data.

static group comparison design A design in which a group that has experienced the event is compared with a group that has not in order to determine the effect of the event.

story A single account reviewing life events in a true or imagined form.

stratified sampling The selection of elements from a population that has previously been divided into groups called strata.

subjectivity Personal experiences and personal truths that may or may not have some resonance with other people's subjective experiences and truths.

table A meaningful presentation of numbers in rows and columns, the intersection of a row and column being a cell.

technical action research A form of action research which aims to improve techniques and procedures by having practitioners work collaboratively to test the applicability of results generated elsewhere.

text A selection of words with which the qualitative researcher is working.

texts In postmodernism, text refers to everything, so that all events and phenomena are texts.

thematic analysis A method for identifying themes, essences, or patterns within the text.

theme In qualitative research, this is an essential idea that is informative if it makes a unique contribution to the total description of the experience.

theory An attempt to describe, organise or explain a phenomenon or group of phenomena of a discipline.

time-series design A design in which the experimenter makes several measurements, both before and after the treatment.

triangulation Multiple references which converge to draw conclusions from data, investigator, theory and methodological sources.

true experimental design An experimental design that has three major features: use of an equivalent control group to control for extraneous variables, random assignment to experimental and control groups, and the ability to control the independent variable.

trustworthiness A process to determine the usefulness of qualitative research including the criteria of credibility, fittingness, auditability and confirmability.

type I error Rejecting the null hypothesis when it is true; that is, concluding that there are significant differences between the groups when there are not.

type II error Failing to reject the null hypothesis when it is false, concluding that there is no difference between groups when there actually is.

unfair inducement The offering of undue material gains for the purposes of recruiting research participants.

unobtrusive observation Observation in which the observer is either not visible or keeps a low profile.

unstructured observation The qualitative researcher observes a context systematically and carefully, but with no predetermined categories, keeping in mind the central purposes for being there as stated in the research objectives, thereby attending to what is happening, where, when, how and why, without actual involvement in the setting as a participant.

variable Something that varies or can be manipulated.

visual analogue scale A scale on which respondents are asked to indicate the quality of an experience on a linear, ruler-like indicator.

voice The modern conception of the author's perspective, but postmodernists question the attribution of privilege or special status to any voice; thus, a 'public voice' is more acceptable, making discourse broadly understandable.

voice-recognition program A computer program that translates the human voice into word processing files.

World Wide Web The network of Internet sites.

Answers to review questions

Chapter 1
1b, 2a, 3d, 4d, 5a, 6a, 7a, 8d, 9c, 10c

Chapter 2
1a, 2d, 3d, 4c, 5b, 6a, 7a, 8c, 9b, 10d

Chapter 3
1b, 2a, 3c, 4b, 5d, 6a, 7d, 8d, 9d, 10c

Chapter 4
1d, 2c, 3b, 4a, 5b, 6a, 7b, 8c, 9a, 10d

Chapter 5
1b, 2c, 3d, 4b, 5c, 6a, 7d, 8b, 9d, 10c

Chapter 6
1a, 2c, 3d, 4a, 5a, 6b, 7d, 8a, 9b, 10d

Chapter 7
1a, 2c, 3b, 4d, 5a, 6b, 7d, 8c, 9b, 10c

Chapter 8
1b, 2d, 3a, 4c, 5b, 6d, 7a, 8b, 9b, 10c

Chapter 9
1b, 2b, 3d, 4a, 5b, 6c, 7d, 8b, 9d, 10c

Chapter 10
1b, 2d, 3c, 4a, 5c, 6d, 7a, 8b, 9d, 10c

Chapter 11
1c, 2a, 3c, 4d, 5d, 6d, 7c, 8c, 9d, 10d

Chapter 12
1b, 2c, 3a, 4b, 5b, 6a, 7b, 8d, 9a, 10d

Chapter 13
1b, 2c, 3d, 4c, 5a, 6d, 7b, 8c, 9a, 10d

Chapter 14
1b, 2c, 3a, 4a, 5c, 6a, 7d, 8c, 9a, 10b

Chapter 15
1b, 2a, 3d, 4d, 5c, 6b, 7d, 8a, 9c, 10d

Chapter 16
1d, 2a, 3b, 4b, 5c, 6d, 7a, 8b, 9c, 10d

Chapter 17
1a, 2a, 3d, 4d, 5b, 6b, 7c, 8d, 9a, 10a

Chapter 18
1b, 2b, 3c, 4a, 5d, 6a, 7a, 8d, 9c, 10d

Chapter 19
1a, 2d, 3d, 4a, 5d, 6c, 7c, 8d, 9b, 10d

Index

Aborigines and Torres Strait Islanders, ethics of research 113–15
abstract
   in proposal 132, 147
   in report 61, 476–7
accessible population 202
action research 151–2, 347–51, 368, 454, 455
affirmative postmodernism 18, 22–3
agent/agency 362
aim of study 37–8, 41, 147, 428–9, 493
analysis of data 142–3, 158
   changing data 258
   computer assisted 266, 417, 426, 431–4, 438–40, 444, 445
   critiquing 70–1
   different from interpretation 450–2
   discourse 362–6, 436–8, 445
   discriminant 288
   image 443
   log-linear 287–8
   manual 428–30
   meta-analysis 217
   narrative 435–6, 444
   qualitative research 417–18, 424–45
   quantitative research 266–89
   thematic 426–8, 432, 433–4, 444
   in written report 497–500
analysis of variance 285, 287, 288
anonymity 109–10, 416
appendixes 162, 491–2
applied research 12, 513–23
approval 127, 128, 129, 130, 166–7, 168
archival information 382–3
artistic expression as data source 383–4
auditability 380

bar graphs 269, 270, 486
bias 35
'blind' subjects 186
budget 145–6, 159–61, 168

case studies 183–4, 384–6
case-based sample 206
causal relationships 295–6
chi-square test 282–4
classroom report 472
clinical significance 297–8, 300, 489
cluster sample 205
code book of variables 254
coding data 255–8, 416
colleagues, managing 252
collection of data 154–6
   computers for 249–50, 416–17
   covert 107–8
   hints for 412–17

   preparing for 409–11
   qualitative research 373–400, 407–19
   quantitative research 207–32, 242–62
comparative descriptive research design 177–8
computers
   backing up 20
   for data analysis 266, 417, 426, 431–4, 438–40, 444, 445
   for data collection 249–50, 416–17
   for data management 416–17
   for data processing 254–8
   disks 417
   etiquette of using 21
   Internet and anonymity 109–10
   legal aspects of use 21
   for literature search 53–6
   structure of 18–19
   types of 19–20
concept 78
conceptual framework 87–8
conference paper 472
confidentiality 111–12
confirmability 380–1, 399
congruency 375–6, 455–6, 457
conservation principles 80–1
content analysis 217
context of data 376–7, 408
contingency table 284
control group 179, 186–7, 247–8
convenience sample 206
correlation 279–82, 295
correlation coefficient 279, 280
correlational research design 178
counterbalanced research design 193–4
credibility 380
critical ethnography 359–61, 368, 455
critical methodologies 16, 342, 367
   action research 151–2, 347–51, 368, 454, 455
   compared with poststructuralism 343–4
   critical ethnography 359–61, 368, 455
   differences from interpretative 310–11, 333, 455
   feminisms 352–9, 368, 455
   terms 345–6
critiquing
   analysis of data 70–1
   ethical requirements 70
   interpretation of data 70–1
   literature review 63–71
   methodology 66–7, 69–70
   qualitative research 68–71
   quantitative research 64–8
   research reports 63–71, 120

541

results of research   67–8
variables   66
crossover research design   193–4

data
  changing   258
  coding   255–8, 416
  context of   376–7, 408
  discussion of   61, 68, 71, 488–90, 500
  permission to collect   244–5
  skewed   276
  storage of   254, 415
  subjectivity of   408–9
  see also analysis of data; collection of data; interpretation of data; management of data; methods of obtaining data
deception of participants   107–8
deconstruction   362, 459
Delphi survey technique   228–9
Denyes's Self-Care Agency   81
dependent variables   39, 41, 179
descriptive research design   176–8
descriptive statistics   268–77
  interpreting   293–4
descriptive-level model   78
design of research
  case studies   183–4, 384–6
  comparative descriptive   177–8
  correlational   178
  counterbalanced   193–4
  crossover   193–4
  descriptive   176–8
  experimental   178–9, 183–94
  factorial   190
  longitudinal   192–3
  pre-experimental   179, 183–6
  pre-test post-test   184–5
  quasi-experimental   190–2
  simple descriptive   177
  statement of   137
directional hypothesis   40, 41
discourse analysis   362–6, 436–8, 445
discriminant analysis   288
discussion of data   61, 68, 71, 488–90, 500
disseminating findings   144–5, 158–9, 471–509
dissertation   472
double blind study   186

element of population   201
emancipation   345–6, 367
embryos/foetal tissue, ethics of research   112–13
empirico-analytical research see qualitative research
emplotment   435–6
empowerment   345
epistemology   306–7, 309–10, 332
equipment   242–3, 413
error in measurement   210–11
ethics   35, 143–4, 156–8, 169, 495–6
  codes and guidelines   98–9
  critiquing   70

definition of   96
  HRECs   98, 99, 100, 110, 114, 115–18
  NHMRC guidelines   98–9, 102, 104, 106, 107, 108, 110, 111, 112, 113, 114, 115
  principles of   98–112
  scientific misconduct   118–20
  in special cases   112–15
  unethical research examples   96–9
  whistleblowers   120
ethnography   324–8, 333
ethnonursing   324
evidence-based practice   187–8, 520–1
experience as data source   377
experimental mortality   180
experimental research design   178–9, 183–94
experimenter effect   182–3
extrapersonal stressors   83

factor analysis   286
factorial research design   190
feasibility   34–5
feminisms   352–9, 368, 455
fieldwork   386, 399
financial harm from research   101
findings   61
  critiquing   67–8
  disseminating   144–5, 158–9, 471–509
fittingness   380
focus groups   387–8
Foucauldian discourse analysis   436–7
fourteen-needs model   78
frequency count   274
frequency distributions   269
frequency polygon   275
functional health patterns   78
funding   166

grand theories   80–4, 311, 333, 368
graphs   269–70, 486
grounded theory   313–19, 333, 453
group processes and data   386–8

Hawthorne effect   182
hegemony   346, 368
Henderson's 14-needs model   78
histograms   269, 270, 486
historical research   328–31, 333
Human Research Ethics Committees (HRECs)   98, 99, 100, 110, 114, 115–18
hypotheses   39
  directional   40, 41
  null   40, 41, 278, 296
  and variables   66, 137–8

illustrations in report   485–8
image analysis   443
in vitro/in vivo research   112–13, 209–10
independent t-test   284–5
independent variables   39–40, 41, 179, 188
indexes as resource   52–3

indigenous participants   113–15
indirect measurement   209
inferential statistics   277–89
information as data source   216–32
informed consent   103–7
instrumentation   140–1, 182, 211–13, 234–5
integrity of data   415
Internet, research on   109–10
interpersonal stressors   82–3
interpretation of data
   critiquing   70–1
   different from analysis   450–2
   postmodern definition of   458–9
   qualitative   305–33, 450–66
   quantitative   293–4
   relevance of   463–4
   significance of findings   296–300
   synthesising interpretive and critical results   457–64
   truthfulness of   452–3
interpretive methodologies   15–16
   different from critical   310–11, 333, 455
   ethnography   324–8, 333
   grounded theory   313–19, 333, 453
   historical research   328–31, 333
   phenomenology   319–23, 333, 453, 454
intertextuality   362
interval scale   267, 268
interviews   230–2, 235, 388–90, 400
intrapersonal stressors   82

journal articles
   as resource   51–2
   writing   472, 473, 474, 506–7
journal keeping   390–1

legitimacy of research   35
Levine's Conservation Principles   80, 81–2
Likert scale   222, 267
literature as source of problems   31–2
literature review   31–3, 45–63, 72, 134–6, 148–52, 168, 478–80, 489, 493
   critiquing   63–71
literature search   53–6
logbook   253, 254
log-linear analysis   287–8
longitudinal research design   192–3

management of data
   coding   255–8, 416
   logging   254
   manipulating   258
   methods in proposal   142
   preparation for   248–9
   processing   255–8
   storing   254, 415
   using computer   416–17
manual analysis   428–30
Mateo Shira Model   514–15
maturation of subjects   181
mean score   273

measurement to obtain data   207–11
   differences and validity   182
   measurement-related error   210–11
median score   273
member checks   395
meta-analysis   217
metaparadigm of nursing   10, 22
methodology
   critiquing   66–7, 69–70
   detailed in proposal   137–43, 152–4, 168
   ethnographical research   324–5
   grounded theory research   313–16
   historical research   328–30
   meaning of   307
   phenomenological research   319–21
   qualitative research   274–97, 310–11, 340–66, 375–400
   quantitative research   176–95, 200–35
   in report   480–4, 493–4, 496–7
   see also research design
methods of obtaining data   207–32
   information (existing/new)   216–32
   instrumentation   140–1, 182, 211–13, 234–5
   measurement   207–11
   observation   181, 213–16, 393–6
   triangulation   232–4, 379–80
middle-range theories and models   80, 84–7
mode score   274
models   78
monograph   507
multiple regression   287
multi-stage sample   205–6

narrative   362
narrative analysis   435–6, 444
Neuman Systems Model   78, 80, 82–3
NHMRC guidelines   98–9, 102, 104, 106, 107, 108, 110, 111, 112, 113, 114, 115
nominal scale   267, 268
non-probability sampling   206–7
non-significant findings   296–7
normal curve   274–6
null hypothesis   40, 41, 278, 296
nursing knowledge   7–12, 22
nursing profession
   academic nursing   4–6, 22
   defining   8
   and ethics of research   118
   metaparadigm of   10, 22
   as source of problems   32, 33
nursing research
   aim of   37–8
   current scene   6–7
   examples of   316–61
   focus of   12
   history of   3–6, 22
   hypothesis   39
   levels of participation   2–3, 21
   as means of generating knowledge   305–6
   and nursing   2–3, 1–21, 77

postmodern influences on   16, 18
potential questions   38–9, 318–19, 323, 328, 331, 351, 358–9, 361
principles of   99–112
process   38–9
questions, formulating   38–9
relationship to theory   77–89
resources for   36
types of   12–21
use of theories and models   79–87
validity in   179–83
variables, identifying   39–40
NURSRES   21, 49

observation   181, 393–6
   types of   213–16
one-shot case study   183–4
ontology   306–7, 309–10, 332
oral presentations   472, 501–5
ordinal scale   267
Orem's Self-Care Deficit Nursing Theory   78, 79, 80–1

paired *t*-test   282
paradigms   12–13, 17–18
participants   139, 153–4, 167, 412
   allocating to groups   187–8, 247–8
   indigenous   113–15
   managing   251–2
   member checks   395
   mortality   294
   protecting rights   99–112
   recruiting   246–7
   special groups   106–7
Pearson Correlation Coefficient   279, 280
percentages   269
permission to collect data   244–5
phenomenology   319–23, 333, 453, 454
phenomenon   78
photography as data source   396
pie charts   270
pilot study   143, 216, 258–60, 262
place for data collection *see* setting for study
placebo   101, 102, 108, 181, 186, 193–4
placebo effect   181
plan of research   152, 168
population, defining   201–2
poster presentation   472–3, 504–5
postmodernism   16, 18, 22, 309–10, 332, 409, 454
   alternatives for qualitative methodologies   311–12
   compared with poststructuralism   344–5
   and interpretation   458–9
   key terms   362
   in nursing research discourse   362–6
poststructuralism
   compared with critical methodologies   343–4
   compared with postmodernism   344–5
praxis   346, 368
pre-experimental designs   179, 183–6

preliminaries   64–5, 69, 132, 146, 168, 474, 475–6, 493
pre-test post-test research design   184–5
primary sources   50
principles of research   99–112
privacy of information   110–11
probability   277–8
probability sampling   203–6
problem for research *see* question for research
proposal
   application forms   129
   approval   127, 128, 129, 130, 166–7, 168
   funding   166
   guidelines   129
   preliminaries   128–9, 168
   reasons for   127–8, 168
   submitting   129, 131, 165–6, 168
   unsuccessful   166
proposal (contents)
   abstract   132, 147
   aim   147
   altering   128
   analysis of data   142–3, 158
   appendixes   162
   background statement   133, 148
   body of proposal   132–46, 168
   budget   145–6, 159–61, 168
   collection of data   154–6
   design statement   137
   ethical implications   143–4, 156–8, 168
   hypothesis statement   137–8
   instruments and materials   140–1
   introduction   132–3, 168
   literature review   134–6, 148–52, 168
   management of data   142
   methodology   137–43, 152–4, 168
   objectives   132–3, 168
   participants   139, 153–4, 167
   pilot study   143
   plan   152, 168
   preliminaries   132, 146, 168
   procedures section   141–2
   for qualitative research   146–62, 168
   for quantitative research   131–46, 161–2
   questions   147–8
   references   161
   researchers, details of   146
   resources   145–6
   results, dissemination of   144–5, 158–9, 168
   sample procedure   139–40
   statement of significance   134, 147
   summary   132, 147, 168
   supporting material   161, 168
   time frame   145, 159
   title   146
   title page   476
   variables, definition of   138
proposal (writing)
   drafts   164–5
   headings   163–4

presentation 165
style 162–4, 168

Q-sort methodology 229
qualitative research 13–14
  analysis 417–18, 424–45
  collection and management 373–400, 407–19
  critiquing 68–71
  difference from quantitative 308–9, 332
  forms of data 407–8
  importance of people to 377
  interpreting findings 305–33, 450–66
  literature review 47–8
  methods 274–97, 310–11, 340–66, 375–400
  postmodern alternatives to 311–12
  process 14–15, 17
  in proposal 146–62, 168
  research design 176–7
  usefulness of data 408–11
  validity of 307
  words, importance of 407–8
  written report 474–5, 492–500
  see also critical methodologies; interpretive methodologies
quantitative research 13–15
  analysis 266–89
  collection and management 207–32, 242–62
  critiquing 64–8
  difference from qualitative 308–9, 332
  interpreting findings 293–301
  literature review 47
  methodologies 176–95, 200–35
  in proposal 131–46, 161–2
  research design 176–95
  written report 474–5, 476–92
quasi-experimental research design 190–2
questionnaires 218–28, 231–2, 235, 250–1, 255–6, 294
questions for research
  potential 318–19, 323, 328, 331, 351, 358–9, 361
  selection criteria 33–7
  sources of 29–33, 41
  stating 37–8, 147–8
quota sample 207

random assignment of subjects 187–8, 247–8
random sample 180, 204–5, 234, 244
range of scores 274
rating scales 222
ratio scale 267, 268
recommendations 500
references 68, 161, 490–1
regression line 279
relationship findings 294–6
reliability 16, 307, 378
replicating studies 32
report 471, 508–9
  critiquing 63–71, 120
  oral presentations 472, 501–5

  for publication 472, 473, 474, 506–7
  types of 472–3
report (contents) 472, 508–9
  abstract 476–7
  aims and objectives 493
  analysis and interpretation 497–500
  appendices 491–2
  body of 474, 475, 477–85, 493–7
  discussion 488–90, 500
  ethical requirements 495–6
  guidelines 474
  illustrations 485–8
  introduction 478
  literature review 478–80, 489, 493
  methodology 480–4, 493–4, 496–7
  preliminaries 474, 475–6, 493
  presentation 492
  qualitative 474–5, 492–500
  quantitative 474–5, 476–92
  recommendations 500
  references 490–1
  results 484–8
  structure 474–6
  supporting materials 474, 475
  target audience 473–4
  title 476, 493
  title page 476
research *see* nursing research; qualitative research; quantitative research; results of research; using research in practice
research contexts 376–7
research design *see* design of research
research proposal *see* proposal
researchers' details 146
resources for project 35–7, 145–6
results of research 61
  critiquing 67–8
  dissemination of 144–5, 158–9, 471–509
reviewing the literature *see* literature review
rights of participants 99–112
rigour in research 377–82, 399
Rogers's Unitary Human Beings Theory 79, 83–4
Roy's Adaptation Theory 80, 82

sampling 139–40, 202–7, 234
scales 222–3, 235, 267–8, 286
scattergram 279
science and research 13–14
scientific method 308–9
scientific misconduct 118–20
secondary sources 50
selection effects 181
self-report as data source 217–32
semantic differential scale 222
seminar paper 472
serendipitous findings 298
setting for study 139, 200–1
  access to 244–5, 251, 412–13
  preparation of 246
significant findings 297

Index 545

simple descriptive research design   177
skewed data   276
snowball sample   207
Solomon four-groups research design   189–90
standard deviation   276–7
statement of significance   134, 147, 489–90
static group comparison   185–6
statistical significance   278, 297–8, 489
statistics
  descriptive   268–77
  graphics of   269–73
  inferential   277–89
  means in one group   279–84
  means of more than two groups   285–6
  means of two groups   284–5
  measures of central tendency   273–4
  measures of variability   274–7
  more than one dependent or independent variable   286–8
  non-parametric   276
  parametric   276
  probability   277–8
  relationships in one group   279–84
  and scales   268
  uses   266
storage of data   254, 415
storytelling as data source   396–7
stratified sample   205
stressors   82–3
subjectivity of data   408–9
subjects of study *see* participants
submitting proposal   129, 131, 165–6, 168
sum (total)   268–9
supporting material   161, 474, 475
synthesising qualitative interpretive and critical results   457–64
systematic error   210–11
systematic sample   205

tables of data   271–3, 486
target audience   473–4
target population   201–2
testing effect   181
thematic analysis   426–8, 432, 433–4, 444

theories
  conceptual framework, using   87–8
  definition of   77–8
  developing from research   88
  grand   80–4, 311, 333, 368
  historical use of frameworks   79
  middle range   80, 84–7
thesis   51, 472
time frame   145, 159
time series research design   192–3
title of research   61, 146, 476, 493
title page   476
triangulation   232–4, 379–80
type I error   278
type II error   278

unethical research, examples of   96–9
unsuccessful proposals   166
using research in practice   514–15
  barriers to   516–19
  and clinical practice guidelines   522–3
  educating nurses in   523–4
  encouraging   519–20
  and evidence-based practice   520–1

validity   14, 179–83, 278, 307, 352–3
variables
  code book of   254
  critiquing   66
  defined in proposal   138
  dependent   39, 41, 179
  extraneous   183
  and hypothesis   66, 137–8
  identifying   39–40
  independent   39–40, 41, 179, 188
  and validity   180–3
videoconferencing   231
videotaping as data source   398
visual aids for oral presentation   501
visual analogue scale   223

words, importance in qualitative research   407–8
writing proposal *see* proposal (contents); proposal (writing)
writing report *see* report; report (contents)